Notice

This book has been withdrawn from health library stock for one or more of the following reasons:

- There is a more recent edition of the title
- The book is more than 10 years old and more current material on the topic is available

You are therefore strongly advised to check any information contained within this book before using it to inform patient care

VOLUME 1

Encyclopedia of Radiographic Positioning

STEVEN B. DOWD, Ed.D., R.T.(R.)
Program Director and Assistant Professor
Radiologic Sciences
University of Alabama—Birmingham
Birmingham, Alabama

BETTYE G. WILSON, M.A.Ed., R.T.(R.), R.D.M.S.
Assistant Professor
Radiologic Sciences
University of Alabama—Birmingham
Birmingham, Alabama

W.B. SAUNDERS COMPANY
A Division of Harcourt Brace & Company
Philadelphia London Toronto Montreal Sydney Tokyo

W.B. Saunders Company
A Division of
Harcourt Brace & Company

The Curtis Center
Independence Square West
Philadelphia, Pennsylvania 19106

Library of Congress Cataloging-in-Publication Data

Encyclopedia of radiographic positioning / [edited by] Steven B. Dowd, Bettye G. Wilson.

p. cm.

Includes index.
ISBN 0–7216–4202–0

1. Radiography, Medical—Positioning—Encyclopedias. I. Dowd, Steven B. II. Wilson, Bettye G.

RC78.4.E531 1995 616.07'572—dc20

DNLM/DLC 94–13891

Encyclopedia of Radiographic Positioning ISBN 0–7216–4202–0

Printed in the United States of America.

Last digit is the print number: 9 8 7 6 5 4 3 2 1

We dedicate this book, with love and appreciation,
to our parents:
Gerald and Maria Dowd
George and Velma Greene

Contributors

ERNA AGNARSDOTTIR, B.S.R.T.
Program Director, Diortic Instructor, The Icelandic College of Engineering and Technology; Radiologic Technologist, City Hospital, Reykjavik, Iceland

CHARLES B. BURNS, M.S.P.H.
Associate Professor, Division of Radiologic Science, University of North Carolina, School of Medicine, Chapel Hill, North Carolina

DONNA F. BURR, M.A.Ed., R.T.(R.)
Laboratory Instructor, Radiologic Sciences, Radiographer Program, Division of Medical Imaging and Therapy, University of Alabama at Birmingham, Birmingham, Alabama

JOLENE CARSON, M.A., R.T.(R.), F.A.S.R.T.
Speaker, Advanced Health Education Center, Houston, Texas; Formerly, Assistant Professor, Radiologic Technology Program, Northeast Louisiana University, Monroe, Louisiana

JOHN H. CLOUSE, R.T.(R.), B.S.R.S.
Radiography Faculty, Owensboro Community College, Owensboro, Kentucky

STEVEN B. DOWD, Ed.D., R.T.(R.)
Program Director and Assistant Professor, Radiologic Sciences, University of Alabama at Birmingham, Birmingham, Alabama

PATRICIA W. ENOS, A.A., A.A.S., B.A.
Clinical Coordinator, SUNY Health Science Center, College of Health-Related Professions, Syracuse, New York

KATHY L. FLOWERS, A.S., R.T.(R.)
Quality Film Control Specialist, Keesler Medical Center, Keesler Air Force Base, Mississippi

GUDRUN FRIDRIKSDOTTIR, R.T.
Clinical Instructor, The Icelandic College of Engineering and Technology; Chief Radiologic Technologist, Medical Imaging, Domus Medica, Reykjavik, Iceland

JANICE D. HALL, M.A.Ed., R.T.(R.)
Associate Professor and Director, Advanced Imaging Program, Division of Medical Imaging and Therapy, University of Alabama at Birmingham, Birmingham, Alabama

SHU IIZUKA
Department of Diagnostic Radiology, Cancer Institute Hospital, Toshima-Ku, Tokyo, Japan

WENDY B. LAVINE, M.B.T.(R.), B.Sc.
Lecturer and Clinical Coordinator, Radiography Program, The Michener Institute for Applied Health Sciences; Director, Diagnostic Imaging, Baycrest Centre for Geriatric Care, Toronto, Ontario, Canada

KAZUO MATSUTANI
Department of Diagnostic Radiology, Cancer Institute Hospital, Toshima-Ku, Tokyo, Japan

SAMMY L. MOORE, Jr., A.A.S.
Occupational Instructor, Community College of the Air Force, Maxwell Air Force Base, Alabama; Assistant Course Supervisor, Radiology Phase II, Keesler Medical Center, Keesler Air Force Base, Mississippi

REX PROFIT, M.A., B.S.
Sales Representative, Fuji Medical Systems U.S.A., Inc., Stamford, Connecticut

LUCINDA K. PRUE, R.T.(R.) (M.)
Instructor, Medical Technology Management Institute, Milwaukee; Chief Mammography Technologist, Department of Radiology, University of Wisconsin—Madison, Madison, Wisconsin

NOBUO SATO, R.T.
Department of Diagnostic Radiology, Cancer Institute Hospital, Toshima-Ku, Tokyo, Japan

BERNARD J. SHAPIRO, B.Sc., M.D., C.M., F.A.C.R., F.R.C.P.(C.)
Professor Emeritus, Faculty of Medicine, Department of Diagnostic Imaging, University of Toronto; Consultant, Mount Sinai Hospital; Baycrest Hospital; Toronto Hospital, Toronto, Ontario, Canada

CHARLENE E. SIRMAN, B.S., R.T.(R.), A.R.R.T.
Adjunct Clinical Instructor of Radiologic Technology, McNeese State University; Director of Radiological Services, Children's Clinic of Southwest Louisiana, Lake Charles, Louisiana

ROGER SMITH, D.C.R.(U.K.), R.T.(Canada)
Faculty (Retired) at British Columbia Institute of Technology, Vancouver, British Columbia, Canada

MASAYUKI WATANABE
Department of Diagnostic Radiology, Cancer Institute Hospital, Toshima-Ku, Tokyo, Japan

BETTYE G. WILSON, M.A.Ed., R.T.(R.), R.D.M.S.
Assistant Professor, Radiologic Sciences, University of Alabama at Birmingham, Birmingham, Alabama

Preface

This text is designed to be a current reference for positioning and procedures performed in radiography and to provide radiographers and students with the information they need to perform procedures in the modern practice of radiography. Radiography, as it is performed today, is certainly nothing like it was when we (the authors) graduated from school only a few decades ago; it is certain to change just as much in the near future.

The first part, "Introduction to Radiography," covers topics that a radiographer needs to know before beginning procedures—basic terminology, patient care, image production, equipment, radiation protection, and film evaluation. Although not designed as a textbook per se, we believe that this material will make the book useful in an introductory radiologic technology course as well as in courses in procedures and positioning.

The second part covers basic positioning of the upper and lower extremities, chest and bony thorax, abdomen, spine, and skull. Most of these topics, with the exception of the skull, are taught in introductory positioning courses (e.g., Procedures I and II); thus, this section would find use in such courses. In the third part, a variety of procedures loosely defined as "special procedures" are covered—primarily contrast studies, but also areas such as mammography, pediatric radiography, and for the first time in any text, geriatric radiography. Along with skull radiography, these typically form an advanced course in positioning/procedures (e.g., Procedures III). We have also included an extremely useful chapter on computed digital radiography by Charles Burns that originally appeared in another Saunders publication, *Seminars in Radiologic Technology*. More than just theory, it will help the practitioner use computed radiography effectively in conjunction with positioning and procedures.

Many of the chapters are written or cowritten by individuals who are expert in a certain area. This text also benefited from international authorship, which shows how radiography is basically the same throughout the world, although a country or area may perform some procedures differently. Such information is valuable to us in the United States to help us improve the performance of radiologic procedures. International connections will continue to increase, and these connections can help radiography grow as a profession.

As the editors of this text, we invested many years and thousands of hours in its production. We believe that radiography stands ready to—at last—show that it is, as a profession, more than "film-shooting." This text has attempted to, for example, provide additional information about pathology and diagnostic information not covered in other books. In a chapter such as "Genitourinary Tract," for example, we spend some additional time discussing the use of the plain (scout) film, and what that film should show. Our goal is not to intrude on the diagnostic realm of the radiologist but, instead, to work toward functioning as a physician's assistant in the production of a diagnostic film. The more a radiographer knows about diagnosis, the more he or she will be able to provide, simply put, good patient care.

We also believe that health care reform will provide many avenues for expanded practice of the radiographer. Authorities such as Dr. James Thrall predicted these trends about 2 years ago (see, e.g., his article, "Cut Costs by Increasing Technologists' Responsibilities," in Volume 15, Number 2 of *Diagnostic Imaging*) and we believe these trends will continue. In Great Britain, experiments continue with using radiographers to perform some basic screening. We would like to see radiography become a profession that includes expanded roles in patient care and some basic screening of films in addition to current responsibilities. We believe that radiographers are able to meet the challenges of health care for the year 2000 and beyond.

As an encyclopedia, this text must be authoritative. However, we have also attempted to describe, in only the briefest terms, procedures we feel to be outdated. Some information seemed best left to the archives rather than included in a modern text. We certainly welcome input from users of the text in order to revise subsequent editions; as a first effort, we cannot hope to be perfect.

There are a number of individuals and institutions to be thanked in the production of this text: Betty Canan, Ann Steves, Janice Hall, Maria Tyson, Lucille Boyd, Donna Burr, Audrey Harris, University of Alabama at Birmingham Hospital, The Children's Hospital of Alabama, Birmingham Veterans Administration Medical Center, St. Vincent's Hospital, Lakeshore and Spain rehabilitation centers, and radiography program students (Class of 1995) were some of those in Birmingham who provided support, input, or actual material for the text. In our families, we need to thank our spouses and children for their understanding of our responsibilities while we were working on this book. Once one chapter was completed, another demanded attention. A chapter such as "Skull Radiography" seemed as long as an entire book!

We also need to thank our authors for providing us with their expertise in subjects with which we have only a passing acquaintance. We hope that a chapter such as "Geriatric Radiography," written by a radiographer with many years of practical experience in working with older patients, will become required reading in schools and programs throughout the country. Not even a decade ago, geriatric radiography was not seen as an important topic; now we increasingly see it included in curricula in radiography programs.

Lisa Biello, an acquisitions editor who is perhaps best described as a combination talent scout, editor, and counselor, served as a guide in the development of this book. Her assistant, Peg Waltner, was, as always, extremely efficient in sorting out administrative details. Last, but certainly not least, Scott Weaver, a developmental editor at W.B. Saunders, patiently helped us put this text together. Without him, this book would never have been published. He is certain to have a bright future in the publication business.

I (S.D.) have dedicated this book to my parents, primarily for all the opportunities they have given and continue to give me. My success is due in no small amount to their efforts. As mentioned earlier, my wife, Lisa's, and son, Josh's, understanding must also be acknowledged; they have now suffered through many chapters and books with very little complaining. As most authors know, the majority of a book is not written at the office, but late at night at home. I appreciate their love and encouragement very much.

I (B.W.) have dedicated this book to my parents also. Although they are both deceased, it was my father who made me promise to grow up to put something after my name other than a period; and my mother taught me to look to my faith for direction and joy in all things. I must acknowledge as well that my husband, Willie, daughter, Kassaundra, and son, Byronn, were the ones who provided the encouragement and love necessary to keep me dedicated and self-confident. Special thanks to my son, Byronn, who used his artistic talent to provide some of the preliminary drawings for the text. May both of my children have brilliant careers in their chosen fields.

STEVEN B. DOWD
BETTYE G. WILSON

Contents

VOLUME 2

PART ONE

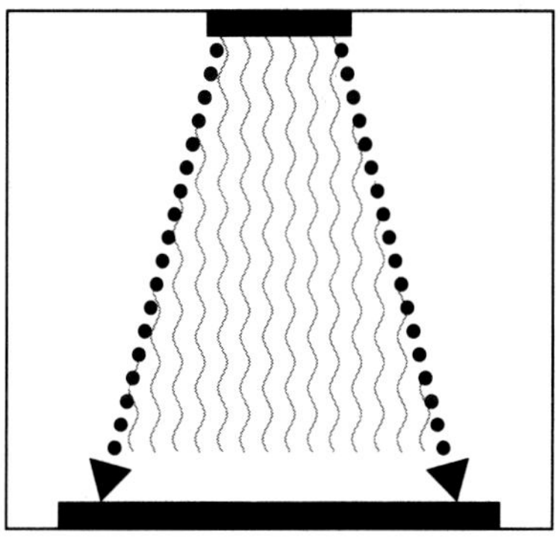

Introduction to Radiography

CHAPTER 1

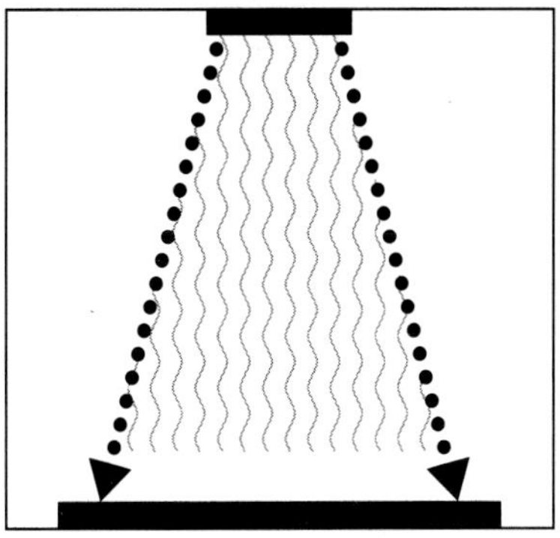

Steven B. Dowd, Ed.D., R.T.(R.)

Introduction to Positioning Terminology

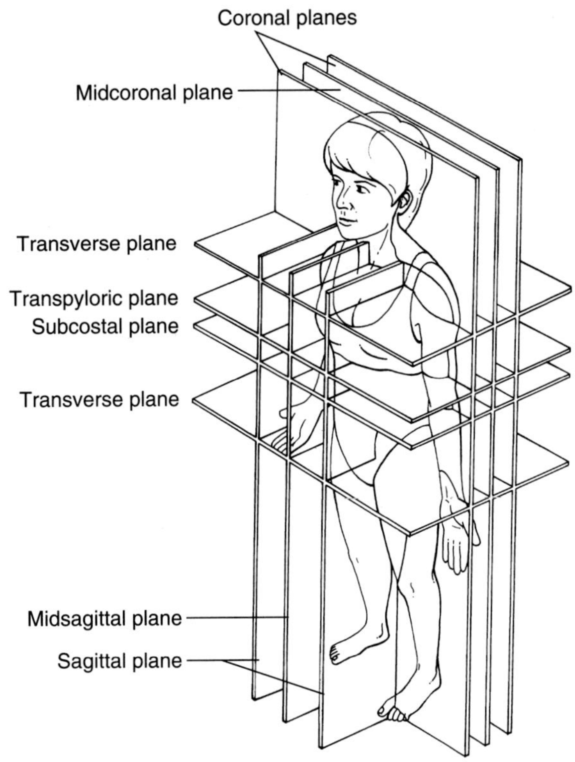

Figure 1.1. Anatomic planes.

This chapter reviews terminology needed for understanding positioning and the performance of radiographic procedures. It is designed to serve as a reference or review for graduate radiographers or as an introduction to radiographic terminology for student radiographers.

ANATOMIC PLANES

Anatomic planes are used as reference points in referring to the location of a structure or the position of the patient (Fig. 1.1).

Transverse plane—Any horizontal plane of the body that divides the body into upper and lower portions; a plane at right angles to the longitudinal axis of a structure.

Midsagittal or median plane—A plane that passes longitudinally through the middle of the body from front to back and divides it into right and left halves.

Sagittal plane—Any vertical plane that passes through the body parallel to the median plane or sagittal suture and divides the body into right and left portions.

Coronal or frontal plane—Any plane that passes longitudinally through the body from side to side, at right angles to the median plane, and divides the body into front and back parts.

Transpyloric plane—A horizontal plane halfway between the superior margins of the manubrium sterni and the symphysis pubis; does not usually correspond to the level of the pylorus.

Subcostal plane—A horizontal plane transecting the trunk at the level of the lower margins of the 10th costal cartilages.

Midcoronal or midaxillary plane—The coronal or frontal plane that divides the body into equal front and back halves.

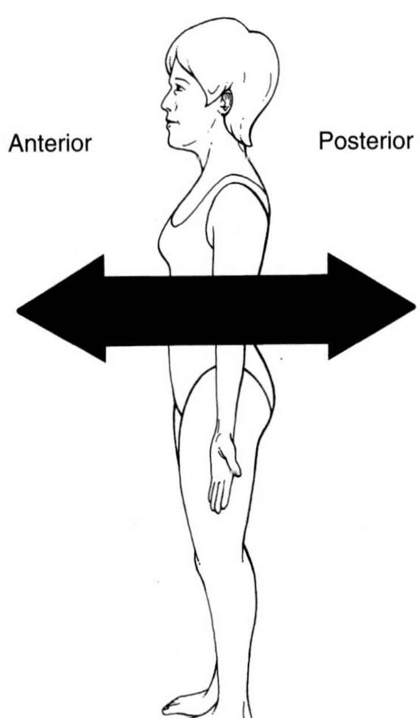

Figure 1.2A. Anterior and posterior.

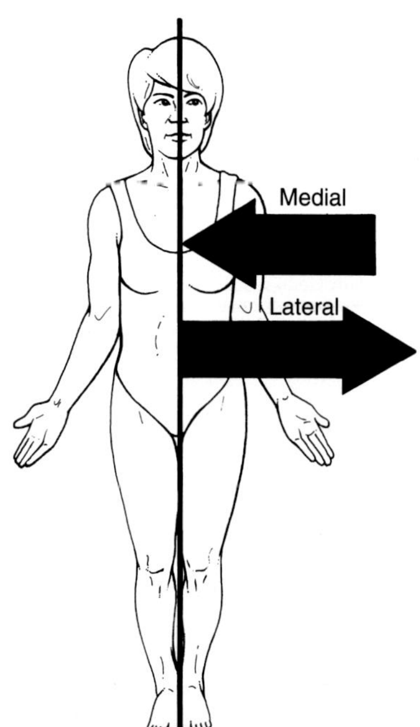

Figure 1.2B. Medial and lateral.

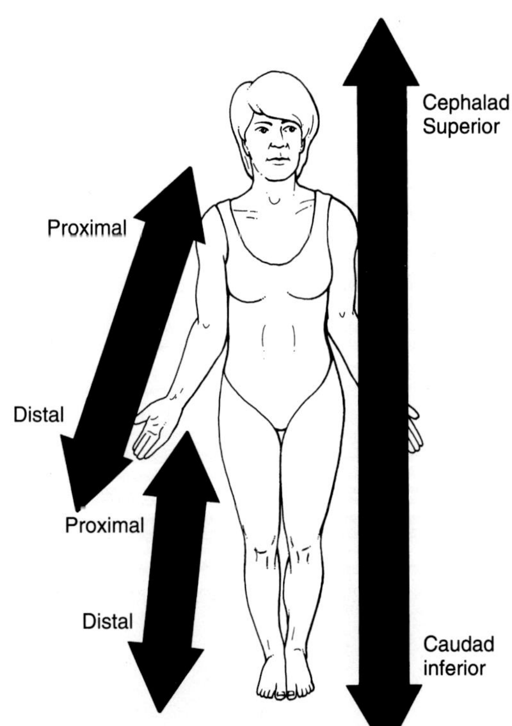

Figure 1.3. Proximal and distal; cephalad and caudad.

DIRECTIONAL TERMINOLOGY

Anterior—Situated in front of or in the forward part of an organ; used in reference to the ventral or belly side of the body (Fig. 1.2A).

Posterior—Situated in back of, or in the back part of, or affecting the back part of, a structure; used in reference to the back or dorsal surface of the body.

Medial—Pertaining to the middle; closer to the median plane or the midline of a body or structure (Fig. 1.2B).

Lateral—Denoting a position farther from the median plane or midline of a body or a structure.

Proximal—Nearest; closer to any point of reference; opposed to distal (Fig. 1.3). The point of reference for extremities is the point of attachment to the trunk.

Distal—Remote; farther from any point of reference; opposed to proximal.

Cephalad (cephalic; superior)—Toward the head; opposite to caudad.

Caudad (caudal; inferior)—Directed toward the tail; opposite to cephalad.

BODY CAVITIES

The body comprises two major cavities (Fig. 1.4): the dorsal cavity, located near the posterior aspect of the body, and the ventral cavity, located near the anterior aspect. The dorsal cavity is further subdivided into the cranial and the spinal cavities. The cranial cavity contains the brain, and the spinal cavity contains the spinal cord and the beginnings of the spinal nerves.

The large organs in the ventral cavity are called viscera. The ventral cavity is further subdivided into the thoracic (chest) cavity and the abdominopelvic cavity by the diaphragm. Some texts refer to the abdominopelvic cavity as two separate cavities (abdominal and pelvic), even though the abdomen and the pelvis are not divided by a wall.

ABDOMINAL DIVISIONS

The abdomen is divided into nine regions (Fig. 1.5) by four imaginary lines projected onto the anterior wall—two pass horizontally around the body (the upper at the level of the cartilages of the 9th ribs, the lower at the tops of the crests of the ilia) and two extend vertically on each side of the body from the cartilage of the 8th rib to the center of the inguinal ligament. This method of division is most commonly used by anatomists. The regions are:

Three upper: Right hypochondriac, epigastric, left hypochondriac.

Three middle: Right lumbar, umbilical, left lumbar. The lumbar regions are also called lateral regions.

Three lower: Right iliac, hypogastric, left iliac. (The iliac regions are also called inguinal regions. The hypogastric region is also called the pubic region.)

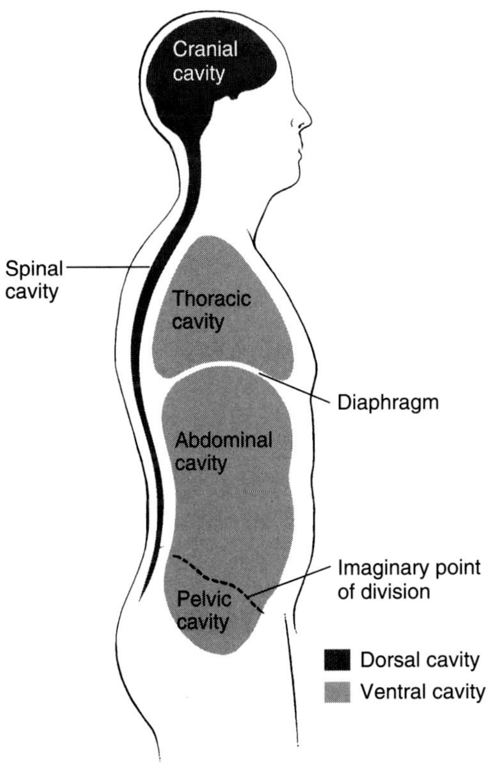

Figure 1.4. Body cavities.

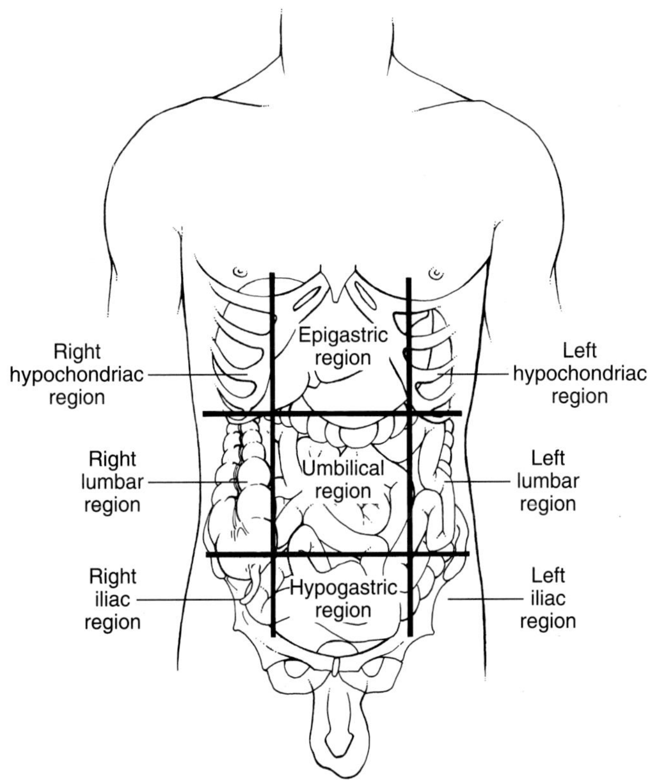

Figure 1.5. Nine regions of abdomen.

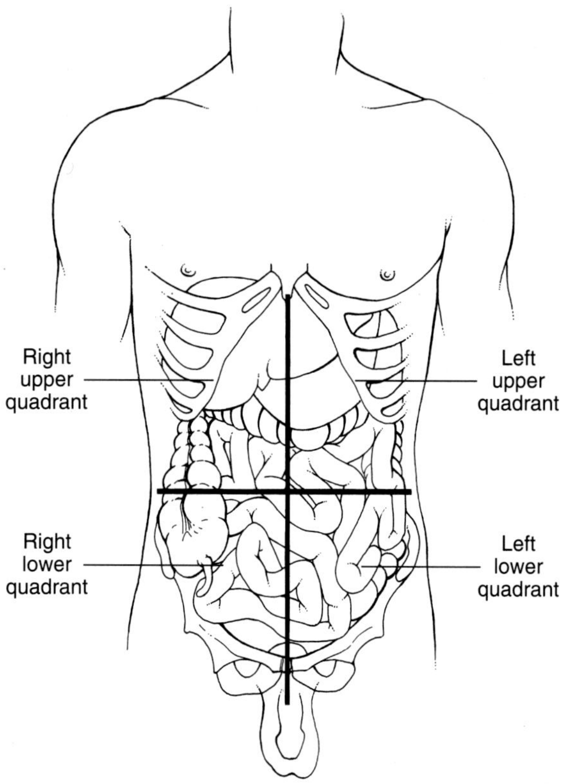

Figure 1.6. Four quadrants of abdomen.

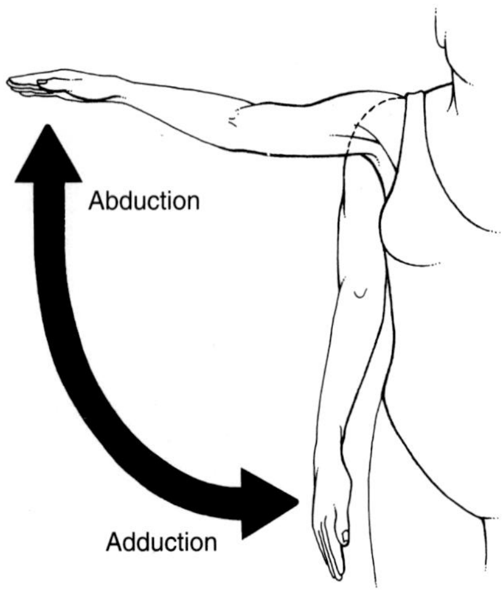

Figure 1.7. Abduction and adduction.

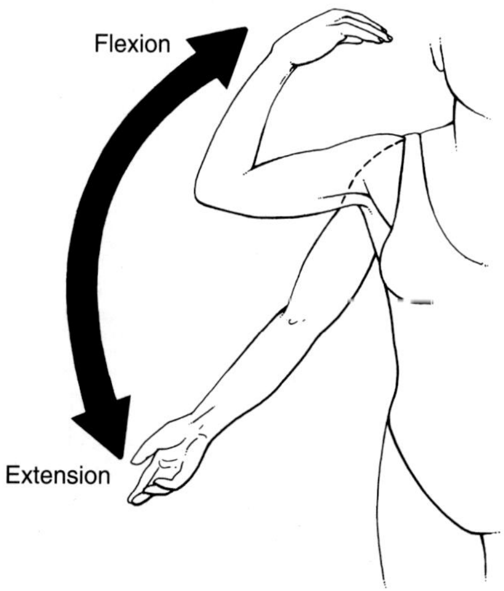

Figure 1.8. Extension and flexion.

The term hypochondriac means below the ribs. The popular use of the term hypochondriac as a person obsessed with illness and bodily functions stems from the fact that the ancient Greeks thought that this condition was due to a disturbed function of the upper abdominal organs.

The abdomen can also be divided into four quadrants (Fig. 1.6)—a right upper quadrant (RUQ), a left upper quadrant (LUQ), a right lower quadrant (RLQ), and a left lower quadrant (LLQ). The quadrant system is the one most commonly used in clinical practice of radiographers and other health professionals.

MOVEMENT

Abduction—A drawing away from the medial plane, or, in the digits, from the axial line of a limb (Fig. 1.7).

Adduction—A drawing toward the median plane, or, in the digits, toward the axial line of a limb. A useful tool in remembering the difference between abduction and adduction is the prefix ad-; when something is drawn toward the median plane, it is added to it.

Extension—The movement by which the two elements of any jointed part are drawn away from each other (Fig. 1.8).

Flexion—The act of bending or condition of being bent; bending movement of a joint in which the two elements of any jointed part are drawn toward each other.

Eversion—A turning inside out; a turning outward, as of the foot (Fig. 1.9).

Inversion—A turning inward.

Pronation—The act of assuming the prone position, or the state of being prone.

Prone—Lying with the face downward. This term also refers to turning the hand so that the palm is facing downward (Fig. 1.10).

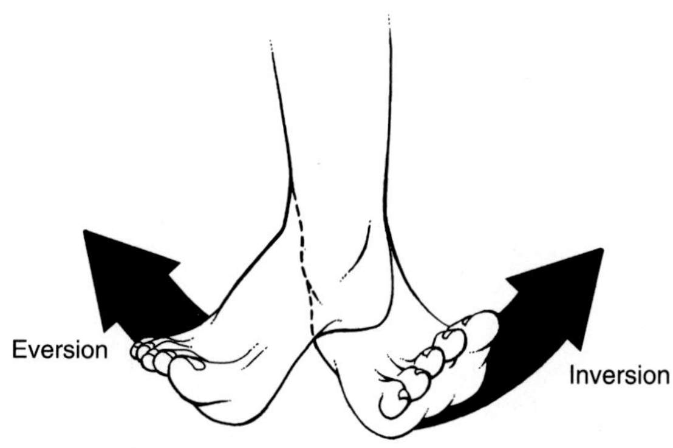

Figure 1.9. Eversion and inversion.

Supination—The act of assuming the supine position, or the state of being supine.

Supine—Lying with the face upward. This term also refers to turning the hand so that the palm is facing upward.

POSITIONING TERMS

In radiography, the term position refers to the position of the body or of the part being radiographed.

Anatomic position—The position of the human body, standing erect, with the palms of the hands turned forward; the position of reference in description of site or direction of various structures or parts as used in anatomic nomenclature. Radiographs are usually placed on a viewbox as if the patient were facing the viewer in anatomic position.

Supine—Lying with the face upward (Fig. 1.11).

Prone—Lying with the face downward (Fig. 1.12).

Lateral—Pertaining to the side; in positioning terminology, a position in which the side of the patient is next to the film (Fig. 1.13).

Oblique—Patient is rotated between supine and prone (Fig. 1.14).

Right anterior oblique (RAO)—Patient is semiprone or standing, with the right side closest to the film (Fig. 1.15).

Left anterior oblique (LAO)—Patient is semiprone or standing, with the left side closest to the film (Fig. 1.16).

Right posterior oblique (RPO)—Patient is semisupine or standing, with the right side closest to the film (Fig. 1.17).

Left posterior oblique (LPO)—Patient is semisupine or standing, with the left side closest to the film (Fig. 1.18).

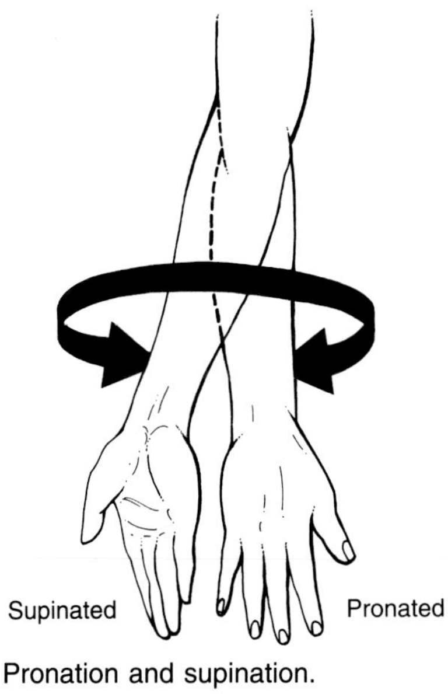

Figure 1.10. Pronation and supination.

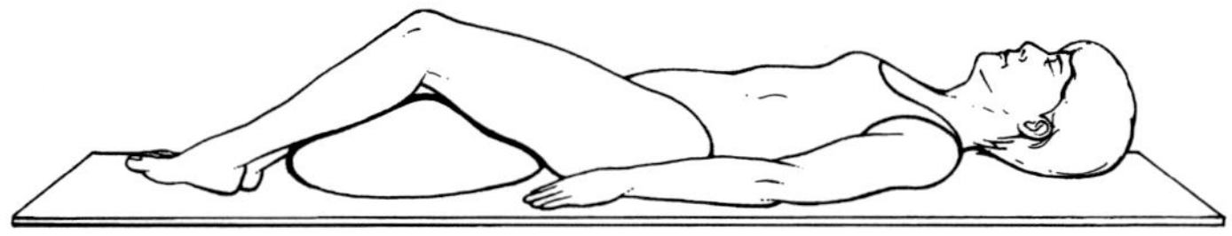

Figure 1.11. Supine.

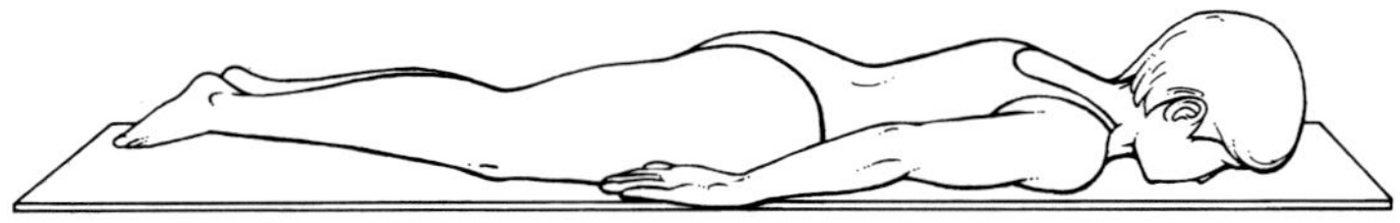

Figure 1.12. Prone.

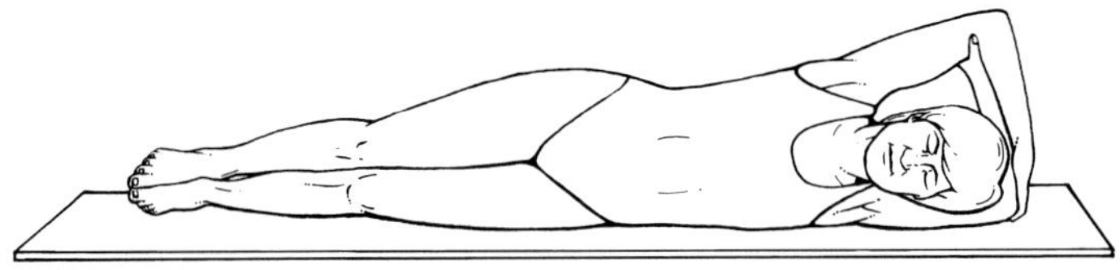

Figure 1.13. Lateral.

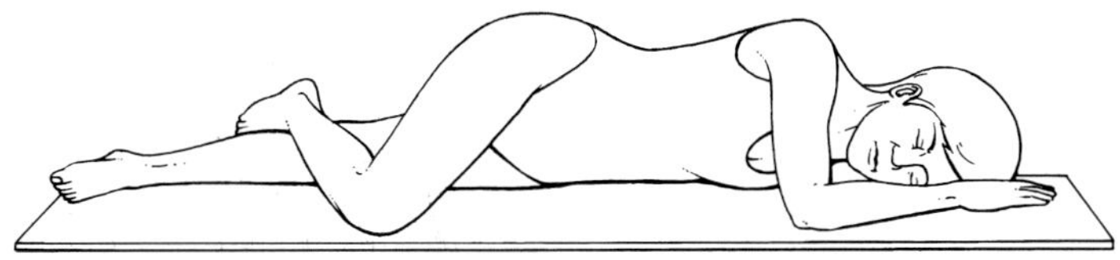

Figure 1.14. Oblique.

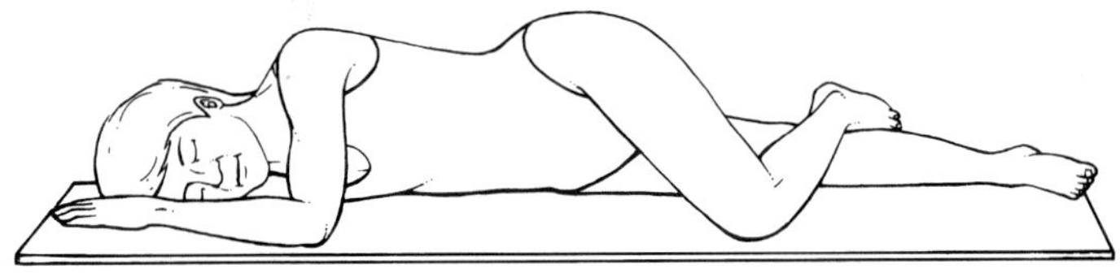

Figure 1.15. Right anterior oblique.

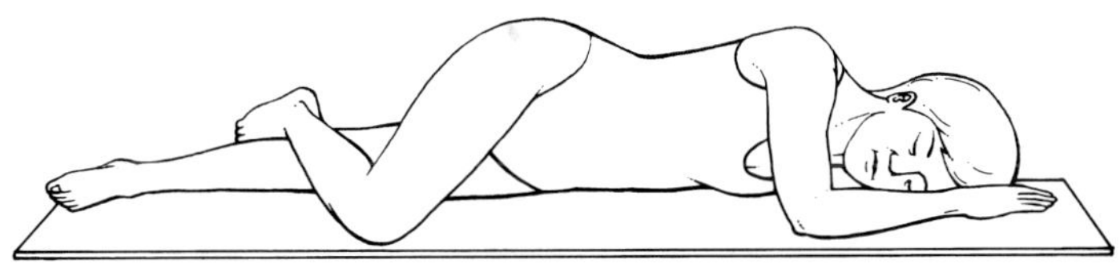

Figure 1.16. Left anterior oblique.

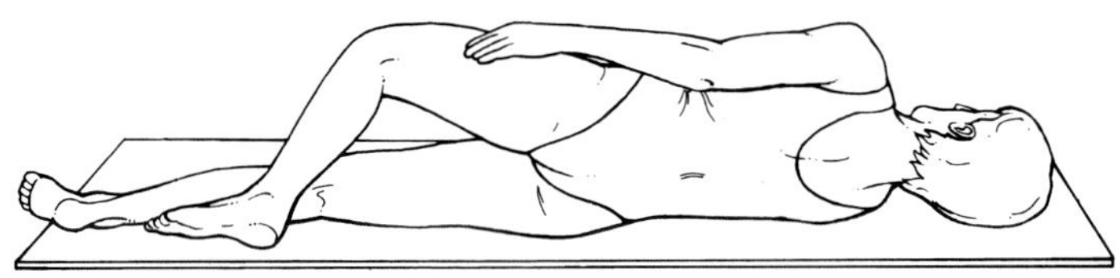

Figure 1.17. Right posterior oblique.

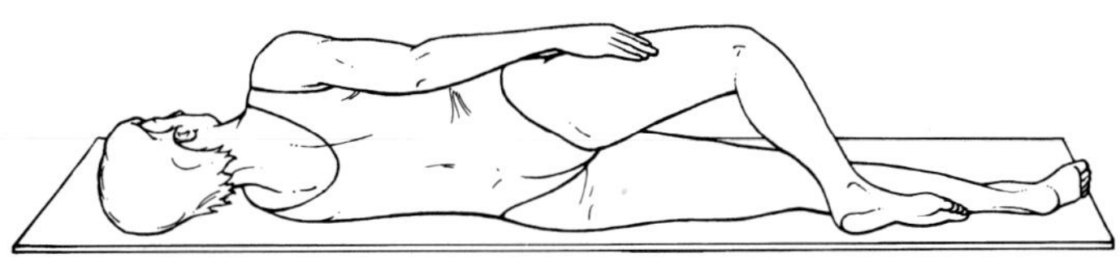

Figure 1.18. Left posterior oblique.

Decubitus—Patient is lying down; in positioning terminology, may also refer to the fact that the central ray is horizontal.

Dorsal decubitus—Patient is supine; the beam enters on one side of the patient (left or right) and exits from another (Fig. 1.19).

Ventral decubitus—Patient is prone; the beam enters on one side of the patient (left or right) and exits from another (Fig. 1.20).

Lateral decubitus—Patient is lying on either side (right or left). When the patient is lying on left side (right side is up), this is called a left lateral decubitus position. When the patient is lying on right side (left side is up), this is called a right lateral decubitus position. The beam enters on either the front or the back of the patient and exits from the other side (Fig. 1.21).

PROJECTIONS

The term projection refers to the path of the x-ray beam.

Anteroposterior (AP)—Beam enters the front (anterior) surface and exits through the back (posterior) surface. Patient is supine or standing, with the back against an upright filmholder/grid device (later called simply device; Fig. 1.22).

Posteroanterior (PA)—Beam enters the back (posterior) surface and exits through the front (anterior) surface. Patient is prone or standing, with the front surface against an upright device (Fig. 1.23).

Lateral—Patient is lying or standing, with one side against a table or upright device; named for the side that is against the table or upright device (Fig. 1.24).

Oblique—Projection named opposite from the position; thus, an RPO projection, with the right posterior side closest to the film, is a right AP oblique projection. An LPO is a left AP oblique; an RAO, a right PA oblique; and an LAO is a left PA oblique.

Axial—A projection with a longitudinal angulation of the central ray in relationship to the long axis of the body part (Fig. 1.25).

Tangential—A projection in which the central ray "skims" (passes between or by) body parts; projects anatomic structures in profile and free of superimposition (Fig. 1.26).

Because conventional radiography can only provide a two-dimensional view of a three-dimensional object, at least two projections as near as 90 degrees from each other as possible are usually required. Although radiologists are very adept at "looking through" superimposed anatomy, a variety of pathological conditions are well visualized on only one specific projection or by comparing two projections. When joints and articulations are of interest, three projections (AP or PA, oblique, and lateral) are often necessary.

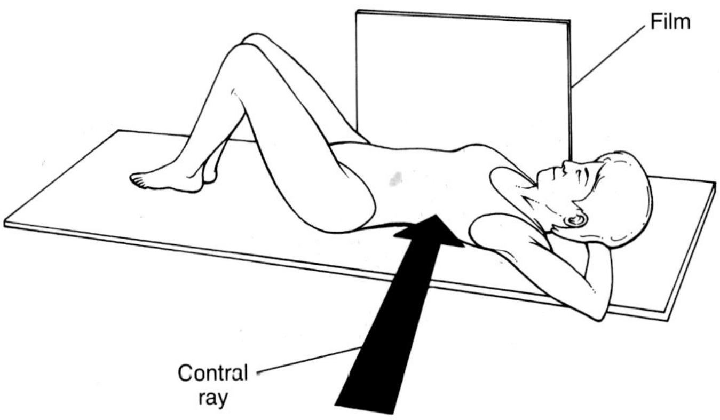

Figure 1.19. Dorsal decubitus.

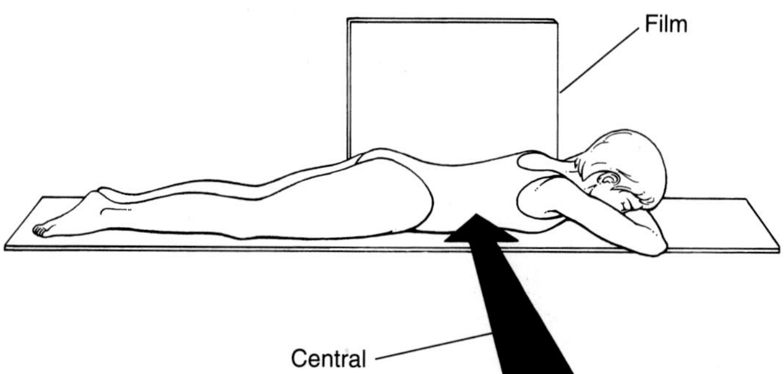

Figure 1.20. Ventral decubitus.

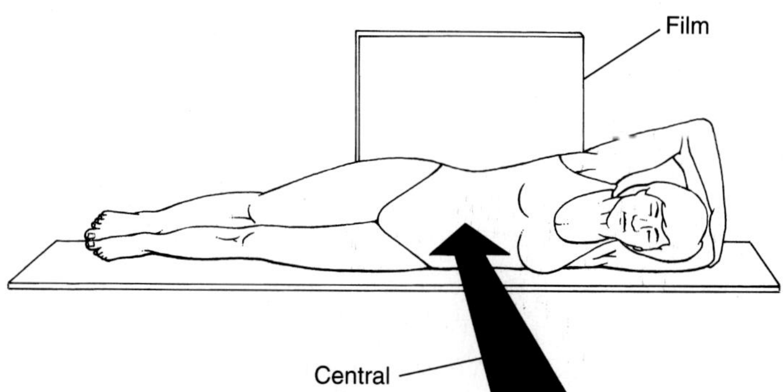

Figure 1.21. Lateral decubitus.

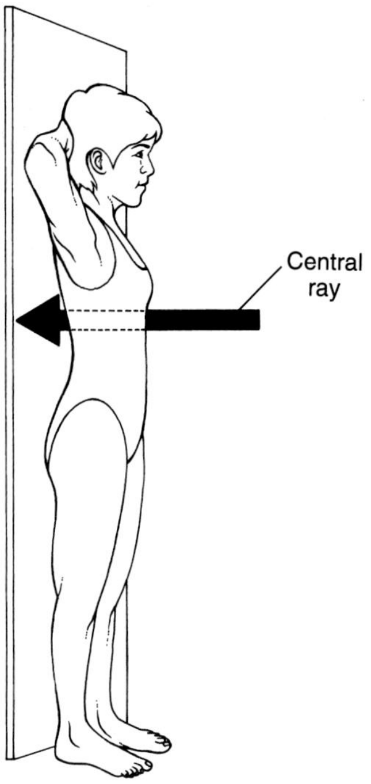

Figure 1.22. Anteroposterior.

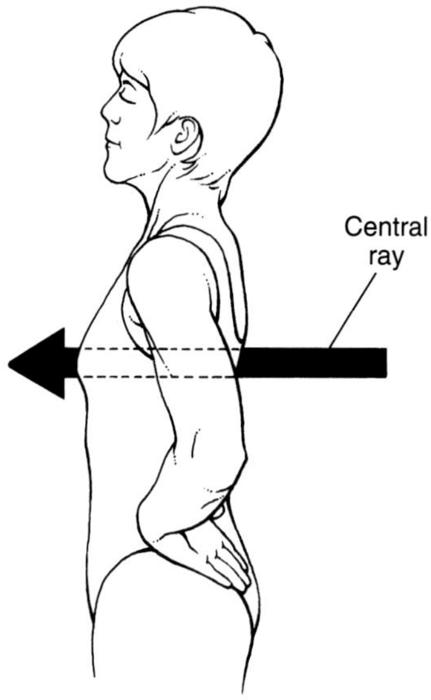

Figure 1.23. Posteroanterior.

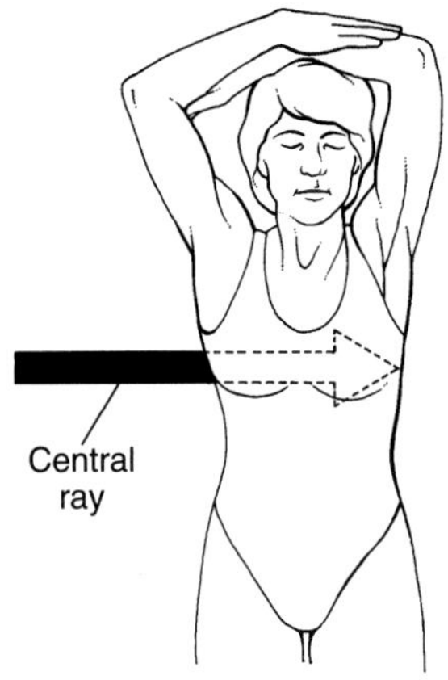

Figure 1.24. Lateral.

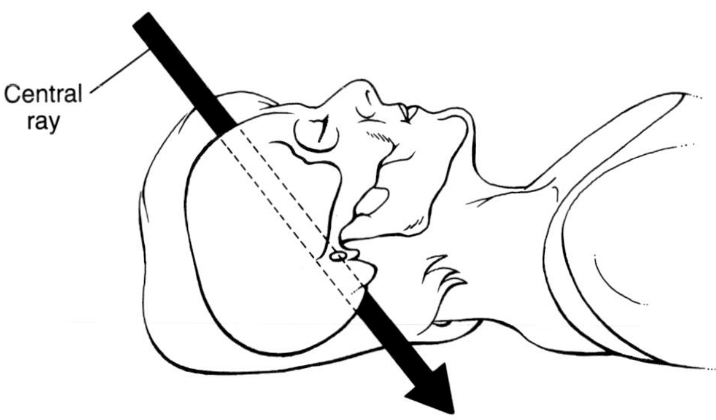

Figure 1.25. Axial.

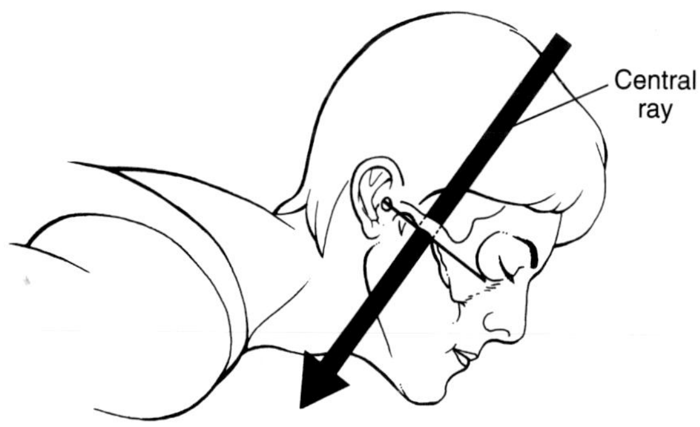

Figure 1.26. Tangential.

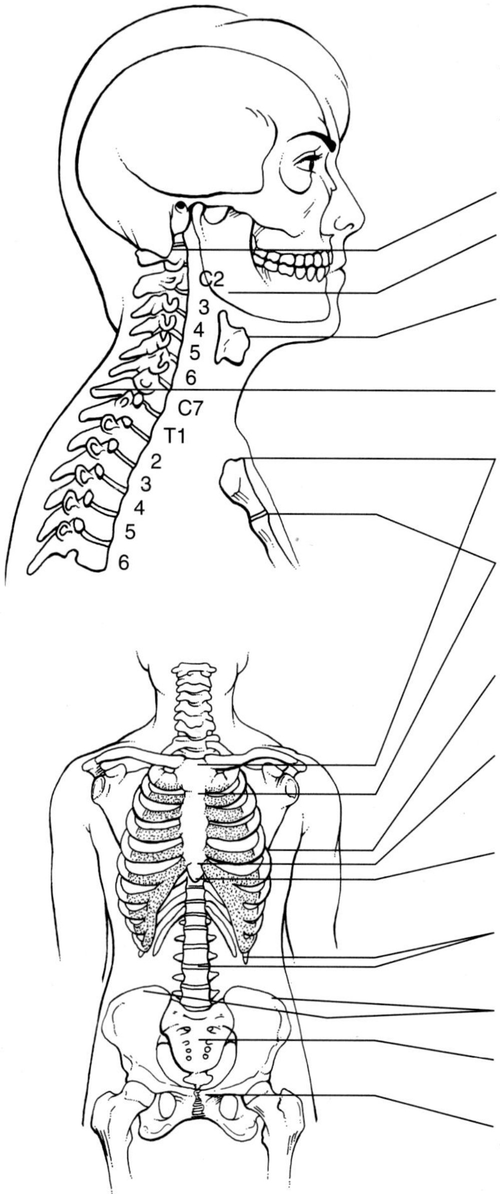

Palpable/Visible Landmark	Internal Structure
Mastoid tips	Body of C1
Angle of mandible (gonion)	Intervertebral disk space of C2–C3
Thyroid cartilage (Adam's apple)	Body of C4
Vertebral prominence	Body of C7
Sternal notch (angle of Louis)	T2–T3 intervertebral disk space
Sternal angle	T4–T5 intervertebral disk space
Inferior angle (tip of scapula)	Body of T7
Xiphisternal junction (junction of sternal body and xiphoid)	T9–T10 intervertebral disk space
Xiphoid tip	Lower portion of body of T10
Lower lateral costal margins	Body of L3
Iliac crests	L4–L5 intervertebral disk space
Anterior superior iliac spine (ASIS)	Second sacral segment
Symphysis pubis/greater trochanters	Coccyx

Figure 1.27. Landmarks: head, neck, and torso.

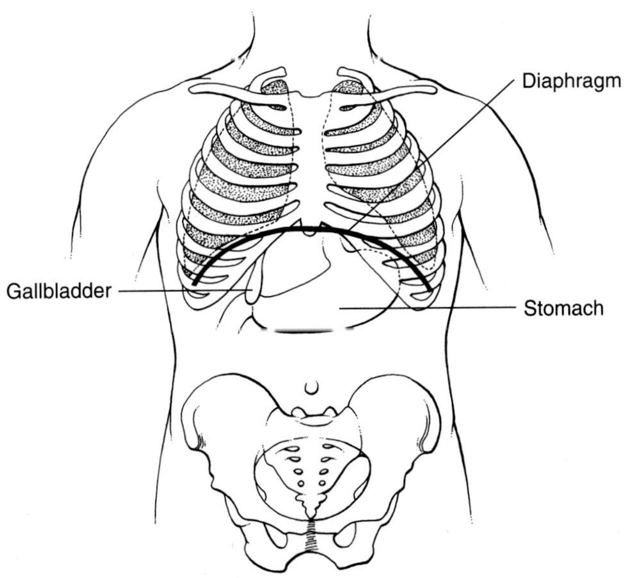

Figure 1.28. Hypersthenic.

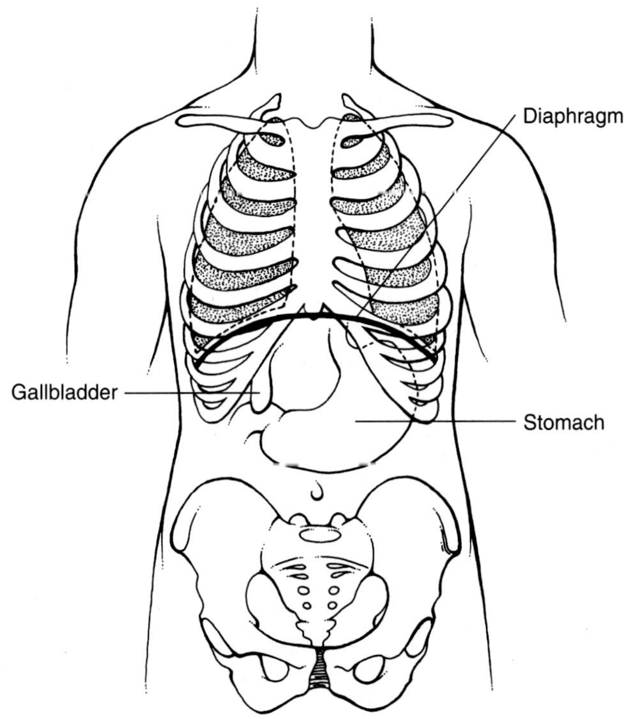

Figure 1.29. Sthenic.

VIEW

The term view is no longer part of accepted practice, except in certain circumstances. It referred to how the x-ray film "saw" the body; thus, an AP projection yielded a PA view. This term sometimes caused miscommunications between the physician and the radiographer, for example, when the physician would ask for a PA (without specifying view) and the radiographer would perform a PA projection, which actually gave an AP view.

METHOD

The term method has been used in reference to the originator of a position or projection. There has been a gradual movement in professional practice away from the use of named methods. In most cases, this text uses both the name of the position or projection and the name of the method.

RADIOGRAPHIC LANDMARKS

Radiographers use a variety of palpable (this refers to the use of touch) or visible landmarks to determine proper positioning and the location of internal structures (Fig. 1.27). Radiographers should remember that, to some patients, touch involves a violation of privacy. Patient permission to touch should be secured first. To sick patients, a "too-heavy" touch may be disturbing. Patient touching should be a positive form of communication.

BODY HABITUS

A knowledge of body habitus (physique; body build and constitution) helps the radiographer determine the location of internal structures, as well as their approximate shape and size. The most common categorization of body habitus used in radiography is listed here. These terms are used primarily for classification of abdominal viscera for positioning during upper gastrointestinal studies, as well as in some other studies such as radiography of the sternum.

Hypersthenic (Fig. 1.28)—About 5 percent of the population. Broad and deep thorax, ribs almost horizontal, shallow thoracic cavity. Short lungs, narrowed above and broad at bases. High diaphragm. Long abdomen, upper part broad, lower part small; stomach and gallbladder high, almost horizontal, and away from midline.

Sthenic (Fig. 1.29)—Accepted as the average body habitus; about 50 percent of population. Organs are in "normal" position.

Hyposthenic (Fig. 1.30)—About 35 percent of the population. Modification of asthenic type.

Asthenic (Fig. 1.31)—About 10 percent of the population. Narrow and shallow thorax, lower ribs slope downward sharply from the sternum, long thoracic cavity. Long lungs that extend well above clavicles, broader above than at bases. Long and narrow heart, with longitudinal axis almost vertical. Low diaphragm. Short abdomen, upper part narrow, lower part broad; stomach and gallbladder low, vertical, and toward midline.

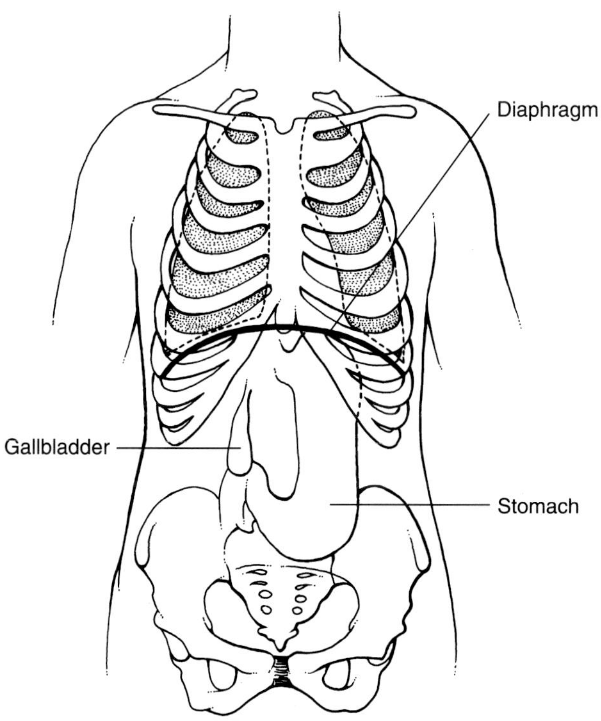

Figure 1.30. Hyposthenic.

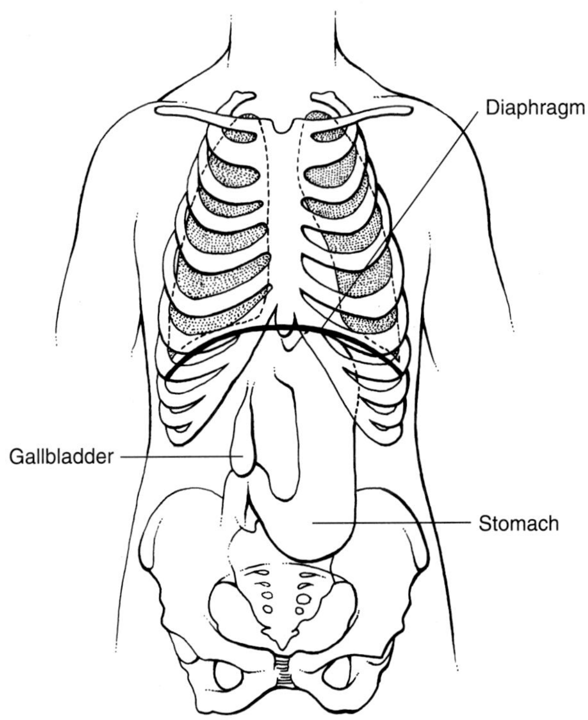

Figure 1.31. Asthenic.

Other Modifications to Body Habitus

The classifications of body habitus have been in use for many years, having been developed by Mills in 1917. Another means of body habitus determination is the body mass index (BMI; also called body build index), which is calculated by dividing the body weight by the square of the stature (height). This method of determining body habitus is often used to determine obesity. It is commonly used by exercise physiologists and other medical professionals.

Another determination of body habitus uses three categories based on tissue derivation from the germ layers of the embryo. The first type is the endomorph, in which tissues derived from the endoderm predominate. There is a relative preponderance of soft roundness throughout the body, with large digestive viscera and accumulations of fat, large trunk and thighs, and tapering extremities.

The second type is the ectomorph, in which tissues derived from the ectoderm predominate. This individual has a propensity to linearity and fragility. There is a large surface area, thin muscles and subcutaneous tissue, and slightly developed digestive viscera.

The third type is the mesomorph, in which tissues derived from the mesoderm predominate. This individual has a relative preponderance of muscle, bone, and connective tissue. There is usually a hard, heavy physique of rectangular outline.

In summary, there are various ways to express body habitus. Whether the traditional means used in radiography for years are the best or the only usable methods for radiography is not known. Perhaps some combination would be best. In any case, this would certainly be an interesting research study, especially for a practicing technologist or group of technologists. For example, Martensen (1992) analyzed the slope of the leg in relation to body size in order to determine the angulation needed for the AP knee radiograph. She used an anterior superior iliac spine (ASIS)–to–table top measurement to determine whether the central ray should be directed caudally 5 degrees, perpendicularly, or cephalically 5 degrees.

Bibliography

Dorland's Illustrated Medical Dictionary. 28th ed. Philadelphia, WB Saunders, 1994.

Leonard PC: Quick and Easy Medical Terminology. Philadelphia, WB Saunders, 1990.

Martensen KM: Alternate AP knee method assures open joint space. Radiol Technol 1992; 64:19–25.

Mills WR: The relation of body habitus to visceral form, position, tonus, and motility. AJR 1917; 4:155–169.

CHAPTER 2

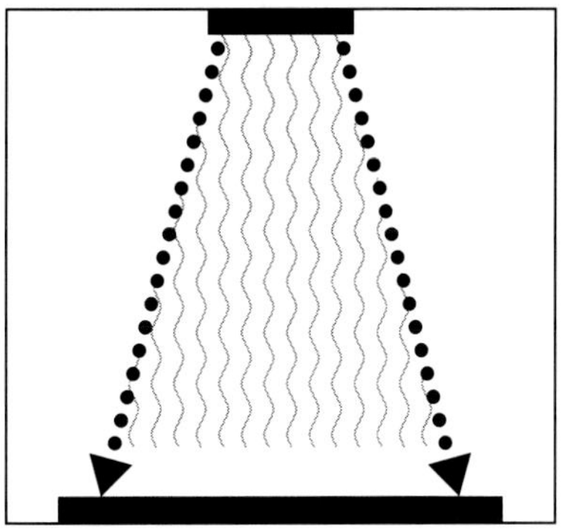

Patient Care

Steven B. Dowd, Ed.D., R.T.(R.)

Rex Profit, R.T.(R.)

The purpose of this chapter is to provide a basic introduction to patient care, including ethics, law, communications, patient safety and comfort, contrast media, and the handling of basic medical emergencies. Infection control is covered in a separate chapter. This chapter can provide only the basics of patient care; readers interested in a more detailed description should consult a text such as Adler and Carlton's *Introduction to Radiography and Patient Care* (1994).

One of the most import aspects of the radiographer's role in health care is patient care; it is as important as positioning, technique, and radiation protection. In some departments, a registered nurse (called the radiology nurse) assumes many patient care duties; however, these duties could be performed as well by a radiographer.

MEDICAL LAW AND ETHICS

Ethics

Ethics is the study of standards of conduct and moral behavior. This study translates into codes of ethics such as the one developed by the American Society of Radiologic Technologists (ASRT), which forms the basis for ethical practice among radiologic technologists (Fig. 2.1). This further translates into the Code of Ethics of the American Registry of Radiologic Technologists (ARRT), which governs the practice of all technologists registered by the ARRT. An understanding of the codes will assist the radiographer in professional practice. Ethics in health care are no longer seen as simple do or do not rules of behavior. Ethics exist to help the practitioner make hard decisions about professional practice. Craig (1994) makes the following observation about the former role of ethics in health care and its new application:

For many years the health care profession was governed by rigid, no-nonsense rules that discouraged any emotional or personal involvement with patients, and it demanded unquestioning obedience to authority figures. Formerly rigid professional role behaviors have become more sensible and flexible.

Medical codes of ethics are based on the principle of beneficence. The health professional should, first, "do no harm" to the patient and should promote the maximum benefit possible. This is the most important aspect of any medical code of ethics. Principle 7 of the ASRT Code, for example, holds the radiologic technologist responsible for protecting the patient from unnecessary radiation.

The flux between the concepts of autonomy (the patient's right to self-determination) and paternalism (the health care worker's desire to bring about a good patient outcome) is also reflected in the ASRT Code of Ethics. What we see as the best outcome for a patient is not necessarily the *true* best outcome. The patient is also covered under a bill of rights developed by the American Hospital Association (Fig. 2.2).

Records

Radiographs are legally considered to be medical records. Under most laws, they are retained at least 7 years, or in the case of minors, 7 years after the minor reaches legal age. Falsifying medical records is grounds for criminal indictment as well as for civil liability for damages suffered. Along with altering films, altering patient histories would constitute falsification. The key feature in diagnosing some conditions (e.g., trauma due to child abuse) is the relationship between the medical findings (on the films) and the history taken by the radiographer.

ASRT CODE OF ETHICS*

1. The Radiologic Technologist conducts himself/herself in a professional manner, responds to patient needs, and supports colleagues and associates in providing quality patient care.
2. The Radiologic Technologist acts to advance the principal objective of the profession to provide services to humanity with full respect for the dignity of mankind.
3. The Radiologic Technologist delivers patient care and service unrestricted by concerns of personal attributes or the nature of the disease or illness, and without discrimination, regardless of sex, race, creed, religion, or socioeconomic status.
4. The Radiologic Technologist practices technology founded upon theoretical knowledge and concepts, utilizes equipment and accessories consistent with the purpose for which they have been designed, and employs procedures and techniques appropriately.
5. The Radiologic Technologist assesses situations, exercises care, discretion and judgement, assumes responsibility for professional decisions, and acts in the best interest of the patient.
6. The Radiologic Technologist acts as an agent through observation and communication to obtain pertinent information for the physician to aid in the diagnosis and treatment management of the patient, and recognizes that interpretation and diagnosis are outside the scope of practice for the profession.
7. The Radiologic Technologist utilizes equipment and accessories, employs techniques and procedures, performs services in accordance with an accepted standard of practice, and demonstrates expertise in limiting the radiation exposure to the patient, self, and other members of the health care team.
8. The Radiologic Technologist practices ethical conduct appropriate to the profession, and protects the patient's right to quality radiologic technology care.
9. The Radiologic Technologist respects confidences entrusted in the course of professional practice, protects the patient's right to privacy, and reveals confidential information only as required by law or to protect the welfare of the individual or the community.
10. The Radiologic Technologist continually strives to improve knowledge and skills by participating in educational and professional activities, sharing knowledge with colleagues, and investigating new and innovative aspects of professional practice. One means available to improve knowledge and skills is through professional continuing education.

Courtesy of the American Society of Radiologic Technologists, Albuquerque, NM; ©1989.

*Adopted by The American Society of Radiologic Technologists and The American Registry of Radiologic Technologists.

Figure 2.1. ASRT Code of Ethics.

Usually the facility that performs the procedure owns the radiographs. Patients and physicians are entitled to the report generated and may pay for copies of the films. Facilities or physicians may refuse to release radiographs in their own best interests unless the radiographs are subpoenaed by a court.

Some facilities also release radiographs only to a physician, as they feel that a patient may attempt to read films on his or her own and come to a false diagnosis. The American College of Radiology has indicated that a patient has a right to his or her films on a loan basis, unless a medicolegal situation exists. It is easy to lose films that are loaned to patients or physicians, and it is for this reason, rather than a desire to withhold the films, that some facilities prefer not to loan out films.

Radiographs can be introduced as evidence in court. Radiographers may be asked to identify films in court. Although a radiographer would never diagnose from a film, if a radiographer failed to mark a film or marked a film incorrectly and then attached a removable sticker to indicate the side of interest, the credibility of the radiographer in taking a diagnostic film and the validity of the films could be questioned. The name of the patient, x-ray number, date, and place must be imprinted on the radiograph and right or left markers must be permanently developed onto the film.

Consent

To perform any procedure, a radiographer must secure patient consent. Consent is permission to perform a procedure granted by a person in his or her right mind. Informed consent is a procedure whereby patients may consent or refuse medical intervention based on information provided by a health care professional regarding the nature and possible consequences of the intervention. In radiology, informed consent is often used to refer only to written consent secured for invasive examinations.

Simple consent refers to a patient's agreement that an examination can be performed. Simple consent may be considered a baseline, with informed consent a "broader form" of consent coming from the patient's autonomy and the fiduciary duty of the physician. All consent must be voluntary, competent, and informed. Thus, before any examination is performed (with certain exceptions), consent must be secured. Always ask competent adult patients whether they agree to have a procedure performed. Patients may revoke consent at any time.

Other Medicolegal Definitions

Torts

Torts are acts that are covered by laws that govern the rights of individuals, or personal injury law. These laws cover noncriminal acts, including:

- Assault—A threat or the act of intentional injury. This involves injurious touch.
- Battery—This is touching another without permission. One purpose of licensure laws is to allow health professionals the right to touch patients.
- False imprisonment—Confinement without authorization.

■ Radiography Example

Restraining a patient without securing permission from the patient or other responsible party.

- Libel and slander—Written (libel) or oral (slander) defamation of character.

■ Radiography Example

Hanging an unfavorable report on the department bulletin board about a fellow radiographer (libel); talking with an acquaintance about a teenage patient who was admitted to the hospital for suspected pregnancy (slander). In the latter example, the radiographer might also be sued for invasion of privacy.

Negligence

Whereas torts are intentional injury, negligence refers to unintentional injury. Negligence is a breach of or a failure to fulfill the expected standards of care. If a health care professional is to be held liable for damages based on a finding of negligence, the following must be established:

1. The standard of care expected of the professional (duty).
2. A breach of duty by the professional.
3. The cause of injury is due to the negligence of the professional.
4. An injury must actually have occurred.

■ Radiography Example of Malpractice

Duty—Always lock stretcher wheels.
Breach of Duty—Radiographer does not lock stretcher wheels.
Injury—Patient falls during transfer owing to rolling stretcher.

Can the injury be attributed to the neglect of the radiographer? ***YES.***

Respondeat Superior

This doctrine is Latin for "let the master answer"; it holds the hospital or physician responsible for wrongful action committed by a person who is carrying out orders or serving the interests of the institution or person.

Personal Responsibility

Radiographers have their own legal responsibilities in health care. That is, simply if the physician, for example, is held to be "negligent" in a malpractice case, this does not excuse you from personal responsibility for any wrongful conduct of your own. The opposite is also true. Although this may be obvious, it means that a radiographer can be held separately responsible for wrongful actions committed on a patient. Some radiographers assume that their responsibilities end under respondeat superior; this is not correct. Craig (1994) notes that any failure to meet medicolegal standards of conduct "leaves the physician and *his or her agents* open to civil actions."

Borrowed Servant

In conjunction with respondeat superior, hospital employees are "borrowed" for a purpose. Thus, the physician rather than the hospital might be held responsible for orders given if a radiographer commits a wrongful action under the direction of the physician.

Res Ipsa Loquitur

Res ipsa loquitur means "the act (or thing) speaks for itself." Thus, it is obvious that sponges are not to be left inside a patient

A PATIENT'S BILL OF RIGHTS*

Introduction

Effective health care requires collaboration between patients and physicians and other health care professionals. Open and honest communication, respect for personal and professional values, and sensitivity to differences are integral to optimal patient care. As the setting for the provision of health services, hospitals must provide a foundation for understanding and respecting the rights and responsiblities of patients, their families, physicians, and other caregivers. Hospitals must ensure a health care ethic that respects the role of patients in decision-making about treatment choices and other aspects of their care. Hospitals must be sensitive to cultural, racial, linguistic, religious, age, gender, and other differences as well as to the needs of persons with disabilities.

The American Hospital Association presents *A Patient's Bill of Rights* with the expectation that it will contribute to more effective patient care and be supported by the hospital on behalf of the institution, its medical staff, employees, and patients. The American Hospital Association encourages health care institutions to tailor this bill of rights to their patient community by translating and/or simplifying the language of this bill of rights as may be necessary to ensure that patients and their families understand their rights and responsibilities.

Bill of Rights†

1. The patient has the right to considerate and respectful care.
2. The patient has the right to and is encouraged to obtain from physicians and other direct caregivers relevant, current, and understandable information concerning diagnosis, treatment, and prognosis.

   Except in emergencies when the patient lacks decision-making capacity and the need for treatment is urgent, the patient is entitled to the opportunity to discuss and request information related to the specific procedures and/or treatments, the risks involved, the possible length of recuperation, and the medically reasonable alternatives and their accompanying risks and benefits.

   Patients have the right to know the identity of physicians, nurses, and others involved in their care, as well as when those involved are students, residents, or other trainees. The patient also has the right to know the immediate and long-term financial implications of treatment choices, insofar as they are known.
3. The patient has the right to make decisions about the plan of care prior to and during the course of treatment and to refuse a recommended treatment or plan of care to the extent permitted by law and hospital policy and to be informed of the medical consequences of this action. In case of such refusal, the patient is entitled to other appropriate care and services that the hospital provides or transfer to another hospital. The hospital should notify patients of any policy that might affect patient choice within the institution.
4. The patient has the right to have an advance directive (such as a living will, health care proxy, or durable power of attorney for health care) concerning treament or designating a surrogate decision maker with the expectation that the hospital will honor the intent of that directive to the extent permitted by law and hospital policy.

   Health care institutions must advise patients of their rights under state law and hospital policy to make informed medical choices, ask if the patient has an advance directive, and include that information in patient records. The patient has the right to timely information about hospital policy that may limit its ability to implement fully a legally valid advance directive.
5. The patient has the right to every consideration of privacy. Case discussion, consultation, examination, and treatment should be conducted so as to protect each patient's privacy.
6. The patient has the right to expect that all communications and records pertaining to his/her care will be treated as confidential by the hospital, except in cases such as suspected abuse and public health hazards when reporting is permitted or required by law. The patient has the right to expect that the hospital will emphasize the confidentiality of this information when it releases it to any other parties entitled to review information in these records.
7. The patient has the right to review the records pertaining to his/her medical care and to have the information explained or interpreted as necessary, except when restricted by law.
8. The patient has the right to expect that, within its capacity and policies, a hospital will make reasonable response to the request of a patient for appropriate and medically indicated care and services. The hospital must provide evaluation, service, and/or referral as indicated by the urgency of the case. When medically appropriate and legally permissible, or when a patient has so requested, a patient may be transferred to another facility. The institution to which the patient is to be transferred must first have accepted the patient for transfer. The patient must also have the benefit of complete information and explanation concerning the need for, risks, benefits, and alternatives to such a transfer.
9. The patient has the right to ask and be informed of the existence of business relationships among the hospital, educational institutions, other health care providers, or payers that may influence the patient's treatment and care.
10. The patient has the right to consent to or decline to participate in proposed research studies or human experimentation affecting care and treatment or requiring direct patient involvement, and to have those studies fully explained prior to consent. A patient who declines to participate in research or experimentation is entitled to the most effective care that the hospital can otherwise provide.
11. The patient has the right to expect reasonable continuity of care when appropriate and to be informed by physicians and other caregivers of available and realistic patient care options when hospital care is no longer appropriate.
12. The patient has the right to be informed of hospital policies and practices that relate to patient care, treatment, and responsibilities. The patient has the right to be informed of available resources for resolving disputes, grievances, and conflicts, such as ethics committees, patient representatives, or other mechanisms available in the institution. The patient has the right to be informed of the hospital's charges for services and available payment methods.

The collaborative nature of health care requires that patients, or their families/surrogates, participate in their care. The effectiveness of care and patient satisfaction with the course of treatment depend, in part, on the patient fulfilling certain responsibilities. Patients are responsible for providing information about past illnesses, hospitalizations, medications, and other matters related to health status. To participate effectively in decision-making, patients must be encouraged to take responsibility for requesting additional information or clarification about their health status or treatment when they do not fully understand information and instructions. Patients are also responsible for ensuring that the health care institution has a copy of their written advance directive if they have one. Patients are responsible for informing their physicians and other caregivers if they anticipate problems in following prescribed treatment.

Patients should also be aware of the hospital's obligation to be reasonably efficient and equitable in providing care to other patients and the community. The hospital's rules and regulations are designed to help the hospital meet this obligation. Patients and their families are responsible for making reasonable accommodations to the needs of the hospital, other patients, medical staff, and hospital employees. Patients are responsible for providing necessary information for insurance claims and for working with the hospital to make payment arrangements, when necessary.

A person's health depends on much more than health care services. Patients are responsible for recognizing the impact of their lifestyle on their personal health.

Figure 2.2. The American Hospital Association's Patient's Bill of Rights.

A PATIENT'S BILL OF RIGHTS (Continued)

Conclusion

Hospitals have many functions to perform, including the enhancement of health status, health promotion, and the prevention and treatment of injury and disease; the immediate and ongoing care and rehabilitation of patients; the education of health professionals, patients, and the community; and research. All these activities must be conducted with an overriding concern for the values and dignity of patients.

**A Patient's Bill of Rights* was first adopted by the American Hospital Association in 1973. This revision was approved by the AHA Board of Trustees on October 21, 1992.

†These rights can be exercised on the patient's behalf by a designated surrogate or proxy decision maker if the patient lacks decision-making capacity, is legally incompetent, or is a minor.

Figure 2.2. *(continued)*

following surgery and no expert testimony is needed to prove a wrongful act.

■ Radiography Example

A radiographer leaves the room for 5 minutes to take a phone call. She has left a young infant in the room, who then falls and suffers a skull fracture. It is obvious that an infant should never be left alone in an x-ray room.

The accurate exchange of information, communication, from radiographer to radiographer is a very crucial role for all radiographers. This communication, from one individual to another, is a constant flow, by either verbal words, gestures, sounds, actions, visual images, or most important, appearance. A simple smile and clean appearance communicate as much as does the most articulate speech.

For communication to occur, there must be a sender, a receiver, and constant avenues for feedback from the messages. It is the radiographer's responsibility to establish this open communication immediately and to maintain it in such a fashion to always include the patient and his or her family. It is a challenge to provide accurate, genuine communication to all patients; however, children, geriatric patients, and non–English-speaking patients may pose an additional challenge. Everyone has the ability to communicate with another individual. It is the radiographer's responsibility to determine the most appropriate method of carrying out this exchange of information.

Radiographers have a limited amount of time to spend with patients; therefore, they must put forth a strong effort in the accurate exhange of information. This requires diligent concentration by the radiographer in order to secure information from the patient while assuring that the patient feels welcome and comfortable in the radiology department. This is a very difficult task and must be taken seriously. This communication, between the radiographer and the patient, is as important as the actual performance of the radiographic examination.

When establishing good communication, you must establish a friendly rapport with your patient immediately, within the first *three minutes*. This is accomplished with a warm smile and a friendly, sincere greeting. You must introduce yourself and tell the patient who you are: "Good morning. I'm John, the radiographer who will be working with you to complete your examination." Equally important, the radiographer must determine the correct pronunciation of the patient's name and how he or she prefers to be addressed: for example, Mr. Smith, Mrs./Ms. Jones. The initial introductions are crucial to establishing that friendly rapport necessary to complete the examination.

When communicating with patients, you must always put yourself at the same level as the patient. Do not tower over patients sitting in chairs, in wheelchairs, on carts, or on x-ray tables. Throughout this communication you must maintain eye contact and touch. Eye contact and gentle touch, a light hand on the shoulder, assure patients that their needs are your primary concern. However, you must be careful that you do not overdo the eye contact or touch. Too much can be as much a blockage to communication as not enough.

Thoroughly explain all the examinations to the patient in a language and in layperson's terms that can be easily understood. Be careful also not to "talk down" to the patient. This includes the proper dressing procedure. Patients are in a foreign environment and their fears may obstruct their listening and comprehension skills. So it may take a little extra patience to ensure they understand everything that has been explained to them.

During performance of the procedure, it is important that someone always be with, or very near, the patient to answer questions and provide assurance. Your constant presence and sincerity will communicate to patients that their care and comfort are your number one priority. Any breakdown in this will put up roadblocks to all future communication with the patient.

Other roadblocks or blockages to communication may be:

- Calling a patient by the incorrect name.
- Avoiding eye contact.
- Avoiding a patient's questions.
- Giving false assurances; for example, "Don't worry," "You'll be fine."
- Telling untruths; for example, "this won't hurt."
- Treating the patient as an object and not as a human being.
- Using a voice lacking sincerity.
- Showing a lack of concern for a patient's privacy and comfort.
- Not involving the patient in the examination.

There are many other blockages to communication. They all involve the radiographer and the inability to realize the importance of the patient. Every radiographer tends to become too involved in the completion of procedures and to forget about the needs of each individual patient. When this happens, all the patients suffer and do not receive proper care. It is every radiographer's responsibility to be aware of the comfort of all patients in the department.

A good sequence to follow in establishing a communication line and a comfortable rapport between radiographer and patient is:

1. Introduce yourself.
2. Tell patient who you are.
3. Determine patient's correct and preferred name.
4. Assist patient to dressing room.
5. Explain proper dressing procedure.
6. Assist patient to radiographic room.
7. Explain examination thoroughly (in a private area).
8. Obtain patient's history (in a private area).
9. Answer all questions and concerns.
10. Perform patient's examinations with continuous communication.
11. Maintain constant contact with patient.
12. Explain proper dismissal and follow-up procedures.
13. Assist patient to waiting room for discharge.

PATIENT SAFETY AND COMFORT

Body Mechanics

General rules of body mechanics are:

1. Preparation for lifting includes always maintaining good posture, evaluating the situation before lifting, and, most important, communicating with the patient before attempting to lift him or her.
2. When a patient or object is lifted, held, carried, or moved, stand as close as possible to the person or object. The more one leans away from the person or object to be moved, the harder muscles must work.
3. Keep the arms as close as possible to the body's vertical axis.
4. Stand with a fairly broad base, having the feet about 12 inches apart. One leg should be ahead of the other and the knees bent to aid in balance.
5. Pull when possible rather than pushing. Moving should be rhythmic rather than jerky.
6. Maintain the back straight and bend from the hips and knees, not from the shoulders or waist.
7. Stoop rather than bending at the waist when reaching down to the floor. Keep the back straight.

Patient Transfer

Patients in the hospital arrive in one of three ways: ambulatory (under their own power), by wheelchair, or by stretcher (gurney). Some general rules of transferring patients are:

1. Always explain the procedure to the patient and allow the patient to help as much as possible.
2. Always have enough people there to help.
3. Always lock wheels. The number one legal problem encountered by radiographers is patient falls resulting from not locking wheels on stretchers and wheelchairs.
4. Be cautious of footrests.
5. Follow general rules of body mechanics for yourself and for the patient.

Patient Restraint

Patient restraint is necessary at times in the radiology department. It may be due to the fact that the patient cannot cooperate (e.g., a very young patient or a confused patient) or cannot prevent voluntary motion of a part. Potential legal problems can result when restraints are used on adult patients against their will. Similar legal problems can result when the parents of young patients do not understand the use of restraint. Be sure that consent has been secured for restraint.

The Patient With Tubes

Intravenous Tubes

Intravenous (IV) tubes are used to infuse fluids into the patient's body. Many radiographers are learning venipuncture as a part of their education in order to participate fully in patient care. A radiographer should know to watch for the patients with IV tubes:

1. If the needle has been inserted into the hand or the arm, make sure that the arm stays straight.
2. The bag or bottle to which the tubing is connected should never be lowered below the level of the needle.
3. The following situations must be reported:
   - Complaints of pain or tenderness at the needle site.
   - Complaints of nausea, vomiting, rapid breathing, or an increase in pulse rate.
   - Unexpected removal of the needle.
   - Blood at the needle end of the tubing.
   - No flow of solution or if bottle or bag has run out of solution.
   - A rate that seems "too fast"—in patients with chronic obstructive pulmonary disease (COPD) or congestive heart failure, a too-fast flow rate can lead to pulmonary edema.

Nasogastric Tubes

Nasogastric tubes are passed via the nose into the gastrointestinal tract for a variety of reasons (Fig. 2.3), including reliev-

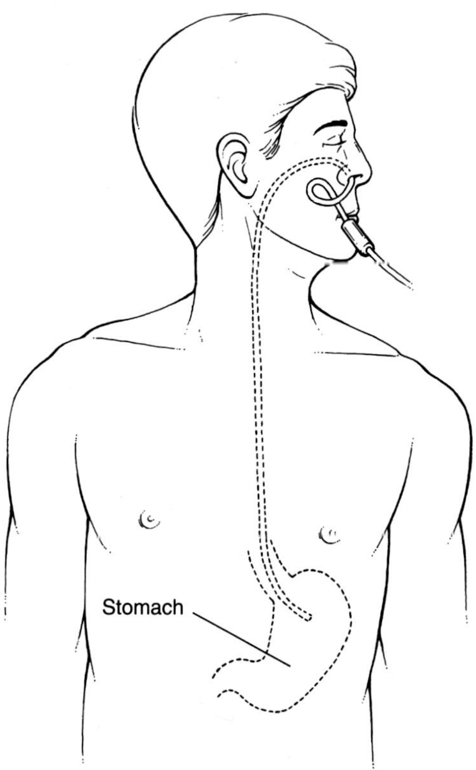

Figure 2.3. Nasogastric tube insertion.

ing gastric distention by removing gas, secretions, or food; instilling medication, fluids, or foods; and obtaining specimens for laboratory analysis. Fluoroscopy is sometimes used to confirm proper tube placement, and radiographers may assist in the placement of nasogastric tubes.

When patients come to the department with nasogastric tubes, it is important to maintain integrity of the tube. The tube is usually taped or pinned to the patient's clothing. Reinsertion of a nasogastric tube can be extremely painful.

Oxygen

Patients may need oxygen to alleviate respiratory difficulty. Oxygen should be considered a drug to be prescribed by the physician. Oxygen can be piped into the patient's room. When a patient needing oxygen is transferred to the department, a cylinder or tank is used.

The radiographer should note the rate of flow on the oxygen supply system; it is usually 3 to 5 L/minute for most patients and less than 3 L/minute for patients with COPD and emphysema. If the rate of flow seems incorrect, contact the patient's nurse, physician, or radiologist.

General rules for oxygen administration are:

- Know and observe all fire rules of the facility.
- Check the flowmeter and ensure that the water chamber is bubbling.
- Check the tubing to ensure that flow is constant.
- Secure the tubing.

Rules to follow with cylinders or tanks are:

- A cylinder must always be in a cart and secured.
- Cylinders should never be placed near heat.

Chest Tubes

Chest tubes are used to remove fluid, blood, or air from the pleural cavity so that the lung can reexpand. Pneumothorax is the primary indication for chest tubes. The exit end of the drainage system must be kept low and the integrity of the tubes maintained.

Tracheostomy Tubes

A tracheostomy tube is left in place following the tracheotomy (a surgical opening in the trachea creating an artificial airway) to provide a temporary or permanent opening. When radiographing a patient with a tracheostomy, never untie the tapes holding the tube in place. In many cases, the tube will need constant suctioning of secretions; this is often performed by a nurse or respiratory therapist, but it can be performed by a radiographer trained in proper suctioning technique.

Urinary Catheters

Urinary catheters are inserted through the patient's urethra and into the bladder (Fig. 2.4). The insertion of a urinary catheter is a sterile procedure performed only by trained personnel. Although radiographers rarely perform urinary catheterization, they more often remove urinary catheters following procedures such as various types of cystography.

Retention catheters are used to temporarily or permanently drain urine. Catheters should be taped to the patient. Some rules to follow with patients with urinary catheters are:

- Be sure that the drainage bag attached to the catheter is always kept lower than the patient.
- Check for kinking of the tubing; ensure that the patient does not lie on the tube.

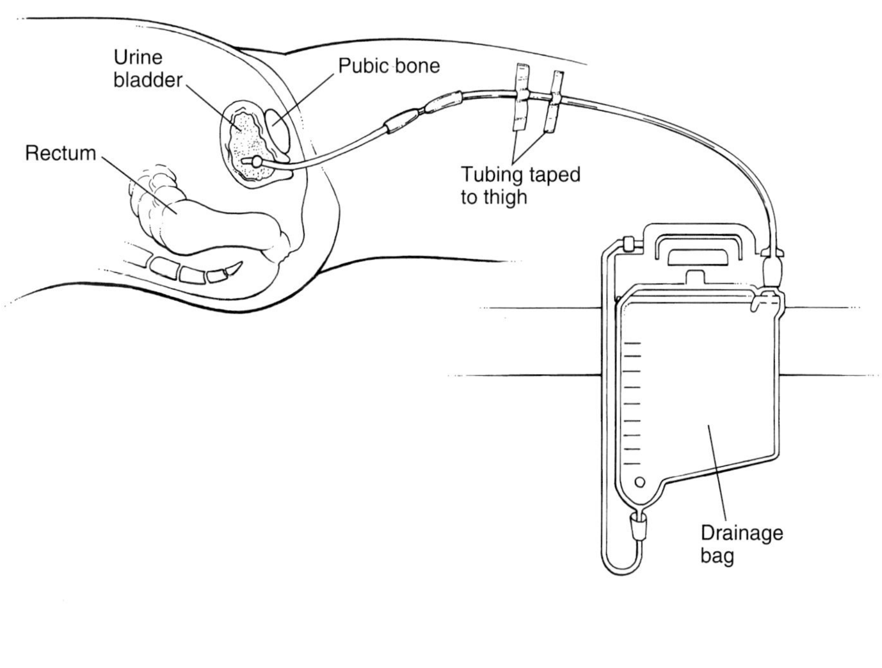

Figure 2.4. Urinary catheterization in a female patient.

MONITORING VITAL SIGNS

The term vital signs refers to temperature, pulse, respirations, and blood pressure. Additional information that should be secured in monitoring vital signs includes color, skin temperature, and patient comments.

Temperature

Body temperature is the result of a balance between heat production and heat loss. When the body temperature is below normal, this is called hypothermia; when temperature is above normal, it is called fever or pyrexia. The temperature under the tongue (oral temperature) is usually 98.6 degrees F (37 degrees C), although this can vary. A temperature 1 degree F above or 2 degrees F below this value can still be considered normal. An axial temperature (under the armpits) is about 0.5 degree F (0.28 degree C) lower than the oral temperature. Rectal temperatures are 0.5 to 1.0 degree F (0.28 to 0.5 degree C) higher than oral temperatures.

Pulse Rate and Rhythm

The pulse is the advancing pressure wave in an artery caused by the expulsion of blood when the left ventricle of the heart contracts. This wave occurs with each contraction of the ventricle and is an easy way to measure heart rate. The normal pulse rate in adult men is 70 to 74 beats/minute; and in adult women, 78 to 84 beats/minute. This depends on sex, age, exertion, body position, and health status. Along with rate, volume and quality should be observed.

The most frequent site for palpation of the pulse is the radial artery at the base of either thumb. Three fingers (not including the thumb) should be placed over the artery (Fig. 2.5). The pulse may also be counted at the carotid artery, the femoral artery, and the apex or tip of the heart (which requires a stethoscope).

Respirations

The process by which the lungs exchange carbon dioxide and oxygen is called respiration. The normal adult breathes at a rate of 16 to 20 breaths/minute. A radiographer must be able to note on a patient:

- Rate—Number of respirations per minute.
- Rhythm—A regular rate of breathing and a symmetric movement of the chest.
- Depth—The amount of air taken in with each respiration. Terms used are normal, shallow, and deep.
- Character—The quality of respirations (e.g., wheezing or coughing).
- Dyspnea—Difficulty in breathing, including difficulty in breathing in certain positions.

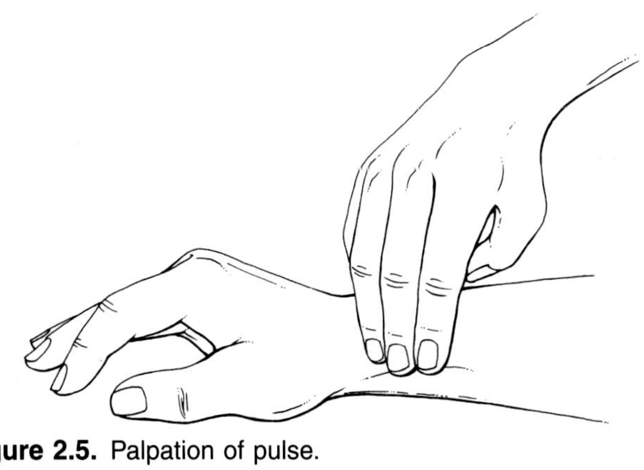

Figure 2.5. Palpation of pulse.

Blood Pressure

The pressure of circulating blood against arterial walls produced by the pumping action of the heart is blood pressure. The highest pressure is observed when the heart contracts (systolic pressure). The lowest pressure is observed at rest (between beats; diastolic pressure). The normal adult blood pressure is 120/80.

Shock

Shock is a condition in which the circulating blood volume and peripheral blood flow are inadequate and do not return enough blood to the heart. This lack of circulating blood does not allow adequate oxygenation of body tissue and organs.

There are a variety of means of classifying shock. The most common types are:

- Hypovolemic shock—Results from a loss of fluid or large amounts of blood, as following a car accident.
- Normovolemic shock—Amount of fluid is unchanged; the body's ability to pump fluid is impaired.
- Vasogenic shock—Similar to normovolemic; the vessels expand in a need for more blood; however, this need is not met.

Another type that may occur following contrast media administration is anaphylactic shock. This is due to an allergic reaction. The only effective treatment for anaphylactic shock is an injection to combat the agent causing the reaction.

The diagnosis of shock is established primarily through the evaluation of vital signs. Indications of shock include weak, thready pulse, tachycardia (heart rate greater than 100 beats/minute in adults), tachypnea (rapid breathing), decreased blood pressure, and decreased temperature.

CONTRAST MEDIA

Radiographers perform a variety of examinations that use contrast media to better delineate structures in the body. Various chapters in this text outline the performance of such examinations. Radiographers must also know the risks involved in these procedures, and be able to instruct patients in preparation for these examinations and give postprocedural instructions.

Types of Contrast Media

Contrast media are divided into two basic types:

1. Negative contrast media—Gases such as air in the patient's intestinal tract or room air introduced into a joint during arthrography.
2. Positive contrast media—Elements of high atomic number. Three types are:
   - Barium sulfate.
   - Oil-based contrast.
   - Water-soluble contrast.

Barium Enema

Barium solution is usually available in a prepared, prepackaged form as a powder (which must be mixed with water) or a suspension. Barium suspensions and solutions should have these characteristics:

1. Allow for rapid flow.
2. Allow for good adhesion to the mucosa.
3. Provide adequate radiographic density in a thin layer.
4. Provide an even, plastic coating.
5. Exhibit a lack of foam or artifacts.

The barium enema is used to diagnose pathological conditions of the colon, or lower gastrointestinal tract. A much larger catheter is required than that used for cleansing enemas to allow the more viscous barium to be instilled into the lower bowel. The catheter may have a plain tip or an inflatable cuff attached. The cuff is inflated after the tip is inserted to hold the catheter in place and to prevent involuntary expulsion of barium. Damage to the rectal wall from improper use of balloon catheters is the most common complication of a barium enema. Balloons should never be overinflated (the amount recommended varies from 30 to 90 cc of air). Balloons are contraindicated in cases of rectal narrowing. Other complications include breaks in the gastrointestinal mucosa owing to trauma or disease, which permits barium to enter the peritoneal cavity or bloodstream. Disease conditions such as ulcers, cancer, and diverticulitis can create minute asymptomatic perforations that can blow out under pressure. Then peritonitis or venous emboli may cause serious complications leading to fibrosis or barium granuloma, or even death.

Most often, preparation for a barium enema consists of,

1. Dietary restrictions, usually in the form of a lower minimum residue diet. This severely restricts the patient's intake of milk, overcooked meat, or eggs and prohibits consumption of fruit and raw or cooked vegetables.
2. Purgation using a variety of laxatives, including castor oil, bisacodyl, magnesium citrate, and Picolax.
3. Overhydration (clear fluids). A clear liquid diet is often prescribed for the 24-hour period prior to a barium examination. This includes carbonated beverages, clear gelatin, clear broth, and coffee or tea with sugar. Whole-grain cereals, bread, vegetables, fried foods, and milk are excluded.
4. Cleansing water enema.

Patient instructions are of extreme importance following a barium enema because barium retention can cause fecal impaction or intestinal obstruction. Barium has hygroscopic qualities, which means that it will absorb fluid from the bowel. Extreme dehydration as a result of preparation for the test is another possible postprocedural complication. In geriatric patients, fluid imbalance may lead to altered mental status.

Stools will often be white or very light-colored until all the barium is expelled. Some physicians regularly prescribe a laxative medication or an enema following barium studies. In any case, the lack of a bowel movement within 24 hours would indicate that the personal physician should be contacted. The importance of eliminating the barium cannot be overly stressed to the patient. Tell the patient not once, but two or three times, that this is *extremely* important.

The patient should increase fluid intake and dietary fiber for several days unless medically contraindicated. The patient should be instructed to rest following the examination.

The Patient Should Immediately Contact His or Her Personal Physician If Any of the Following Occurs After a Barium Enema:
Weakness or fainting.
Abdominal pain, constipation, or rectal bleeding.
Not passing flatus.
Polyuria, nocturia, or abdominal distention.

Oil-based contrast agents are so named because they contain iodine within a poppy-seed oil. They are relatively safe; their main disadvantage is that they remain in the body for long periods of time.

A variety of water-soluble iodinated contrast agents exist, including:

1. Gastrografin—Used in place of barium sulfate in cases of suspected bowel perforation.
2. Biliary agents—Given in tablet form for imaging the gallbladder and liver.
3. Intravascular agents—Used to visualize the urogenital system or nervous system, and, in some cases, in computed tomography studies.

Reactions to Contrast

The four types of reactions to iodinated contrast are:

1. Mild—No treatment necessary. Observation is of greatest importance. The patient may exhibit:
   - "Metallic" taste in mouth.
   - Flushing of skin.
   - Nausea.
   - Numbness around face and mouth.
   - Vomiting.
   - Mild urticaria (hives).
2. Moderate—Require some treatment, such as antihistamines, but patients do not have to be hospitalized. The patient may also exhibit:
   - Urticaria of increased severity.
   - Mild drop in blood pressure.
3. Severe—Require hospitalization and are possibly life-threatening. The patient may exhibit:
   - Prolonged drop in blood pressure.
   - Collapse of circulatory system.
   - Angina (chest pain).
   - Cardiac arrhythmia.
   - Coma, convulsions, and paralysis.
4. Fatal—The rarest type, occur about one in every 20,000 examinations.

About 5 percent of patients have reactions (usually mild) to water-soluble contrast media. Reactions to the other types of contrast media are rarer. If the patient has a history of allergies, there is about a 4-fold increase in the risk of reaction to water-based contrast over that in patients with no history of allergies. A history of asthma increases the potential incidence of a reaction by 5 times. Once a patient has a history of reactions, his or her potential to have another reaction increases by 11 times. Infants, patients with heart disease or an abnormal resting electrocardiogram and individuals with diabetes, heart disease, and sickle cell anemia are also more susceptible.

SINGLE–RESCUER CARDIOPULMONARY RESUSCITATION

Cardiopulmonary resuscitation (CPR) is a combination of artificial respiration and artificial circulation (Fig. 2.6). Its function is to provide enough oxygen to the body's tissues to sustain life. All radiographers involved in the care of patients must be certified in CPR. A brief overview of single-rescuer CPR is:

- Assess the situation.
- Call for help to bring assistance.
- Open the airway by head-tilt/chin-lift method (Fig. 2.6A).
  - Place one hand on forehead.
  - Place fingers of other hand under bony part of jaw.
  - Tilt head and lift jaw.
- Assess for respirations—Look, listen, and feel 5 seconds (Fig. 2.6B).
  - Give two full breaths, each breath being 1 to 1.5 seconds long (Fig. 2.6C).
  - Check carotid pulse on the side nearer you for 5 seconds (Fig. 2.6D).
  - Begin compressions if no pulse—Rate of 15 compressions to every 2 full breaths.

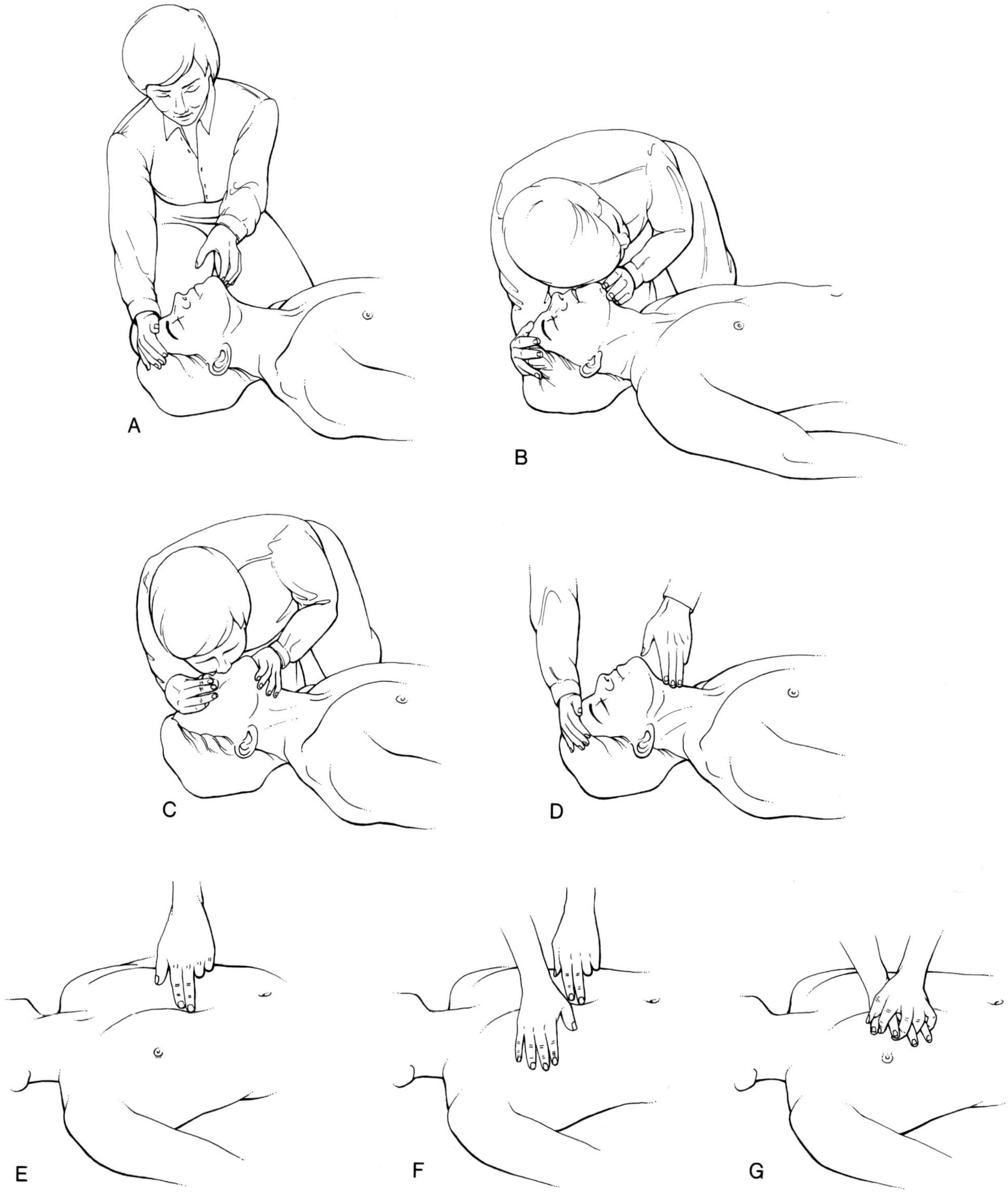

Figure 2.6. Cardiopulmonary resuscitation. *A*, Head-tilt/chin-lift. *B*, Look, listen, and feel for breathing. *C*, Mouth-to-mouth ventilation. *D*, Check carotid pulse. *E*, Place middle finger of hand closer to feet in sternal notch, index finger next to middle finger. *F*, Place heel of remaining hand on sternum next to index finger. *G*, Remove first hand and place over second with only heel on the sternum, fingers off the chest.

- Kneel facing victim's chest.
- Locate the sternal notch with hand closer to victim's legs.
- Place middle finger in notch, index finger next to middle finger (Fig. 2.6E).
- Place heel of remaining hand on sternum next to index finger (Fig. 2.6F).
- Remove first hand and place over second with only heel on the sternum, fingers off the chest (Fig. 2.6G).
- Compress with straight arms, locked elbows, straight down.
- Count out loud: "one and two and three" to fifteen.
- Continue for four cycles and recheck pulse.
- Continue CPR if no pulse. If pulse is present, discontinue CPR and check vital signs.
- CPR should be started within first 6 minutes to prevent irreversible brain damage.
- Compress to a depth of 1.5 to 2 inches (4 to 5 cm) for an adult at a rate of 80 to 100/minute. If you hear ribs cracking, reposition hands. Each time you leave the chest to give a breath, you must relocate correct hand position.

Compressions are of no value without oxygen.

TRAUMA

Radiographers often work with patients who have experienced a variety of injuries. Trauma is the fourth leading cause of death in the United States, and the leading cause of death among individuals aged 1 to 44 years. In the United States, 340,000 individuals are permanently maimed each year by trauma. Chapter 24 details trauma and mobile radiography. Some of the types of trauma seen by radiographers include fractures of bones, especially extremities; spinal injuries; motor vehicle accidents; abdominal trauma; and gunshot wounds.

According to Drafke, there are a variety of general problems associated with trauma radiography. These include obtaining AP and lateral projections in an immobilized and supine patient; placement of cassette and central ray; moving the patient or certain limbs; immobilization; radiation protection; body fluid isolation; and planning. Most problems in trauma radiography can be solved through appropriate planning.

Bibliography

Adler A, Carlton R (eds): Introduction to Radiology and Patient Care. Philadelphia: WB Saunders, 1994.
Chandler GM: Squash mammography "horror stories." RS Wavelength 1993; 4:12.
Craig M: Introduction to Ultrasonography and Patient Care. Philadelphia: WB Saunders, 1994.
Dowd SB: Nonaseptic techniques. *In* Adler A, Carlton R: Introduction to Radiography and Patient Care. Philadelphia: WB Saunders, 1994.
Drafke MW: Trauma and Mobile Radiography. Philadelphia: FA Davis, 1990.
Ehrlich RA, McCloskey ED: Patient Care in Radiography. 4th ed. St. Louis: CV Mosby, 1993.
Gibbons M: Trauma care centers in need of emergency financial care. ADVANCE for the Radiologic Science Professional 1993; 6:13, 17.
Rayman R: The Body in Brief: Essentials for Health Care. El Paso, TX: Skidmore-Roth, 1989.

CHAPTER 3

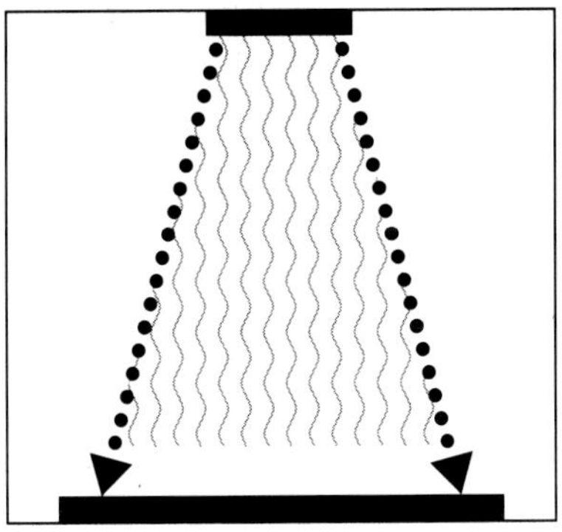

Steven B. Dowd, Ed.D., R.T.(R.)

Practicing Universal Precautions and Infection Control in the Radiology Department

It has become increasingly important for the radiographer to both understand and be able to practice infection control. A variety of diseases, including acquired immunodeficiency syndrome (AIDS), hepatitis B, and tuberculosis have necessitated an increased awareness of infection control. In the past, radiographers had to follow relatively simple guidelines to prevent the spread of infection. Today, radiographers must understand the cause of diseases and how diseases are transmitted and must know means to minimize their own risk of contracting a disease. As a professional health care practitioner, a radiographer must be able to separate the sense from the nonsense in areas such as human immunodeficiency virus (HIV) infection, for which misconceptions and rumors abound.

The first part of this chapter discusses the implementation of universal precautions in the radiology department. The two causative agents that led to the Centers for Disease Control and Prevention's (CDC) recommendations for universal precautions, HIV and hepatitis B virus (HBV), are described in terms of their nature, transmission, and risk factors. Universal precautions in general terms are discussed, and the role of regulatory agencies in enforcing or recommending standards for universal precautions is presented.

The next three sections of this first part describe the responsibilities of certain individuals—managers, radiographers, and educators—in the radiology department. Model universal precautions guidelines tailored specifically for a radiology department are presented. As attitudes have been shown to have a strong impact on the education and practice of universal precautions, this is also discussed. Finally, guidelines for development of an educational program are presented.

In the second part of the chapter, general guidelines for isolation procedures are presented. These are based on the CDC's guidelines.

UNIVERSAL PRECAUTIONS

Human Immunodeficiency Virus (HIV)/Acquired Immunodeficiency Syndrome (AIDS)

Nature

AIDS was first identified in 1981 at the University of California at Los Angeles (UCLA) School of Medicine. The disease, caused by a virus, is the manifestation of an immunosuppressive disease that allows life-threatening infections. The origin of the virus is thought to be Africa, perhaps as long as 90 years ago. The cases at UCLA involved 5 young gay men hospitalized with a very rare infection for healthy young people—*Pneumocystis carinii* pneumonia. Later, they also developed other opportunistic infections normally seen only in the severely immunodepressed. At the same time, researchers from New York University published a report that showed a sudden unexplained rise in the incidence of Kaposi's sarcoma in gay men. Kaposi's sarcoma is a form of cancer that rarely affected North American men under the age of 50 years before AIDS was identified.

Cases were further documented in Haitian immigrants in 1982, and the first European cases were reported in 1982. Heterosexuals were first diagnosed in 1983 when two female partners of intravenous (IV) drug use were reported to have AIDS.

The causative agent of AIDS is a retrovirus, HIV. Viruses are humankind's most primitive, yet most numerous, enemy. They can multiply only in a living cell and use the cell's metabolic machinery to reproduce themselves. All viruses have a preference as to location (e.g., cold viruses prefer the upper respiratory system) and have the same two basic components—nucleic acid (DNA or RNA) and a surrounding protein layer called the capsid.

As a retrovirus, HIV reverses the normal flow of genetic information. HIV carries RNA as genetic material along with an enzyme known as reverse transcriptase. HIV is closely related to a known cancer-causing virus. When the virus invades a cell, its RNA forms a template that will develop DNA genes with the transcriptase. DNA corresponding to the viral RNA is then assembled. This DNA is then integrated into the host cell's chromosomes. This may remain latent for years until activated, whereupon it will make new virus particles that will eventually kill the cell.

HIV prefers white blood cells, and the T4 lymphocyte, regulator of the immune response, is the most common host to HIV. This severely depresses and compromises the immune system. T lymphocytes are produced in bone marrow and are conditioned in the thymus. They are able to perform very specialized and complex duties known as cell-mediated immunity.

Transmission

In infected persons, the blood is a chronic carrier of HIV, although the virus has been isolated from other body fluids, such as semen, saliva, vaginal secretions, tears, breast milk, cerebrospinal fluid, and urine. Isolating HIV from tears and saliva has been extremely difficult, and transmission and infection through these routes have not been proved. One recent case has indicated that breast milk *may* occasionally be infectious, but this is still unconfirmed. Three basic means of transmission are:

1. Sexual—Transmission may occur between both homosexuals and heterosexuals. Risk factors include multiple partners and rectal intercourse.
2. Perinatal—Pregnant women may transmit the virus to the fetus.
3. Exchange of blood, body substances, or tissues—The most frequent form of transmission by this means is between drug users who share needles. This is also the means by which health care workers not otherwise at risk may contract the infection.

Infectious and noninfectious body substances are listed in Table 3.1. Note that *all* body substances should be considered potentially infectious under universal precautions for maximum safety.

HIV follows, as do all infectious diseases, the "eyeglass" model

Table 3.1 Infectious and Noninfectious Body Substances

Infectious	Noninfectious*
Blood	Breast milk†
Bloody fluids	Sweat
Pus/purulent fluids	Nasal secretions
Semen	Tears
Vaginal secretions	Saliva‡
Cerebrospinal fluid	Sputum
Synovial fluid	Urine
Pleural fluid	Stool
Peritoneal fluid	
Pericardial fluid	
Amniotic fluid	

*If stool is contaminated with blood (infectious material), for example, then it is also considered infectious.

†Considered to be "usually noninfectious." (Data from Update: Universal precautions for prevention of transmission of HIV, hepatitis B virus, and other blood-borne pathogens in health care settings.MMWR 36:377, 1987.)

‡May be considered infectious in the dental setting, where saliva is contaminated with blood (see first note).

of epidemiology shown in Figure 3.1. An organism is contained within a reservoir and there must be a portal of exit, as well as a portal of entry to the potential host, for transmission to occur. The most common means of spreading HIV is by direct contact, in which the victim actively and directly contacts the infection source. In all sexually transmitted diseases, such as AIDS, an exit site must contact the entry site—*no other* means of transmission has been proved.

Only very small numbers (one study listed 0.0016 percent) of reported AIDS cases have involved exposure in the health care workplace. Almost every single case has definitely involved a loss of anatomic integrity (i.e., nonintact skin or mucosa). The risk of infection after a single needlestick is considered to be 0.5 percent. This lends much credence to the implementation of universal precautions.

Risks

In a study of 770 health care workers actually exposed to the virus, only 3 developed HIV seropositivity (Dept. of Labor, OSHA, 1987). Only 1 of these 3 individuals actually seroconverted to develop full-blown AIDS. In 1990, the total number of health care workers showing AIDS antibodies, both seroconverted and nonseroconverted, was 69, according to the CDC.

Hepatitis B

Nature

There are at least four types of viral hepatitis, with hepatitis B being spread by exposure to body fluids containing the virus. Usually called an infectious disease, hepatitis B is actually a contagious disease. Thus, it is spread by direct contact with a person, infected blood, or possibly, infected body fluids.

An estimated 200,000 people in the United States develop hepatitis B infection every year. About 60 percent of cases are subclinical; that is, no symptoms are reported, or the affected person describes only a general feeling of malaise. Forty percent of cases are acute, which may lead to a 6-month acute period, with 6 additional months possibly needed for recovery. Hepatic failure is possible if the case leads to fulminant hepatitis B. Ninety percent of cases will resolve, however.

Transmission

The proven, laboratory-replicable mechanisms of HBV are:

1. Direct percutaneous inoculation—Accidental needlesticks with contaminated serum or plasma.
2. Contamination of mucosal surfaces—Most commonly, mouth pipetting or accidental eye splashes.
3. Contamination of minute cutaneous scratches or abrasions.

Airborne transmission has been postulated but not replicated in the laboratory setting. Most probably, suspected airborne transmission has involved droplet contamination.

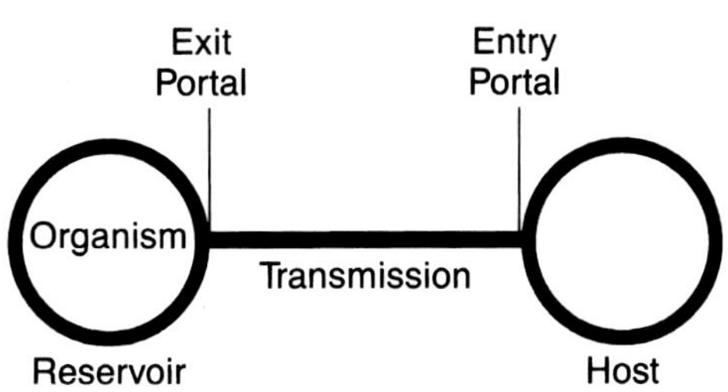

Figure 3.1. Eyeglass model of infectious disease.

Two items are related to the efficiency of transmission. First, there is what has been termed an extraordinary viral load. That is, the amount of HBV needed for infection is low, with most infected individuals having 100 million times the amount needed in the blood. Second, HBV is an extremely stable virus in the environment. It has been shown to retain infectivity after drying for 7 days at 25° C and 42 percent relative humidity. HBV is considered to be relatively sensitive to disinfection.

Risks

As a group, health care workers are from 5 to 15 times more likely to contract HBV infection than the general public. There is a greater risk of mortality among health care workers exposed to HBV compared with HIV. Approximately 12,000 health care workers are infected each year with HBV, with 220 to 265 of these individuals dying from acute and chronic effects of the infection. This translates into a mortality rate of about 1.85 to 2.2 percent. The risk of infection after accidental exposure to HIV is less than half that, about 0.75 to 0.5 percent. In further contrast, the risk of infection from HBV is 12 to 17 percent for unvaccinated individuals.

Implementing Universal Precautions

In 1987, the CDC recommended the use of barrier precautions with all patients when contact with blood or body substances is expected. This means that *all patients should be considered infectious for HIV and other blood-borne pathogens.* The American Hospital Association (AHA) has since endorsed these procedures, now commonly called universal precautions.

A synopsis of the CDC guidelines and the recommendations of the AHA is:

1. Education of personnel regarding epidemiology, modes of transmission, and prevention of HIV infection is paramount.
2. Barrier precautions (gloves, gowns, and protective eyewear) are appropriate for all personnel who perform or assist in procedures involving contact with blood, mucous membranes, or nonintact skin of patients.
3. When sharp objects, such as needles and scalpels, are to be used, extra care is needed to prevent injuries. Two-handed capping of needles should *never* be performed. If instruments to perform one-handed capping are unavailable, the "scoop" method should be performed—place the cap on a flat surface, "scoop" it up with the needle, elevate the capped needle to a 90-degree position, and then snap the cap with the free hand.
4. Exudative skin lesions on health care workers or weeping dermatitis of their hands are reasons for their exclusion from procedures in which contact with blood or body fluids may occur.
5. Mouth-to-mouth resuscitation should be avoided, with ventilation devices available.
6. Sterilization and disinfection procedures currently used are adequate to sterilize and disinfect instruments and devices contaminated with blood and body fluids of patients infected with HIV. Most commonly, a solution of 5.25% sodium hypochlorite diluted 1:10 with water is used.
7. Workers should be tested if there is a parenteral or mucous membrane exposure or if extensive exposure of intact skin to blood or body fluids occurs with a patient who has tested positive for HIV.

Table 3.2 lists radiographic examinations that have a potential for exposure to body fluids.

Table 3.2 Radiologic Examinations With Potential Exposure to Body Substances

Infectious Material	Examination
Tissue	Biopsy; x-ray examination of trauma victim.
Bile	Percutaneous transhepatic cholangiography; stone extraction
Vaginal secretions	Vesicoureterography; hysterosalpingography; vaginography
Tears	Lacrimography
Saliva	Bronchography; laryngography; esophagography; upper gastrointestinal studies; sialography; endoscopic retrograde cholangiopancreatography; gastrointestinal tube placement
Peritoneal or amniotic fluid	Herniography; amniocentesis
Urine	Fistulography; cystography; vesicoureterography; nephrostomy; stone extraction
Pus or serum	Enema studies; fistulography; lacrimography; lymphography; nephrostomy; foreign body removal; gastrointestinal tube placement; abscess drainage; stone extraction
Feces	Enema studies; fistulography
Joint fluid	Arthrography
Cerebrospinal fluid	Lumbar puncture
Blood	All of the above *except* laryngography; esophagography; upper gastrointestinal studies; sialography; cystography

Regulatory Agencies and Universal Precautions

OSHA (the Department of Labor's Occupational Safety and Health Administration) is now also involved in monitoring employee exposure to HIV and HBV. In 1986, various unions petitioned OSHA, owing to the risk of contracting HBV and HIV, to implement emergency standards to protect workers from occupational exposure to blood-borne diseases. Radiologic technologists are considered by OSHA to fall in the category of high-risk health care workers.

Institutions or departments may now be inspected and are expected to have protection standards that conform to what are considered "existing guidelines":

1. CDC recommendations for prevention of HIV transmission in health care settings.
2. The joint advisory notice of the Departments of Labor and of Health and Human Services.
3. OSHA's own compliance document—C.P.L. 2–2.44c (1987).

The focus of current inspections is on health care workers with potential for body substance contacts, body substances recognized by the CDC to transmit HIV and HBV, and infection control programs. Inspections may be unprogrammed (which can occur following employee complaints, fatalities, reports of imminent danger, or hospitalization of five or more employees) or programmed. Programmed inspections occur at random, with 10 to 15 facilities in an OSHA region visited per year.

Radiology Department Managers' Responsibilities

Radiology department managers' responsibilities for infection control include:

1. Identify both workers and tasks that have potential for exposure.
2. Following such identification, develop procedures for these tasks.
3. Provide both orientation and continuing education to those with a potential for exposure.
4. Provide protective equipment—facilities for hand washing, sharps disposal, resuscitation devices, disinfectant, and bleach for blood spills.
5. Develop methods for exposure reporting and follow-up.
6. Monitor compliance, through incident reports, observation, and surveys of employees.

The first step to be undertaken is the last mentioned. Employees must be surveyed to determine their current practices. Along with identifying compliance, surveys provide the basis for educational programs. Sample questions that are asked of employees in an OSHA inspection are provided in the box on this page. A sample survey questionnaire is given in Figure 3.2.

Second, supplying personal protective equipment is not enough. OSHA mandates that the employer enforce the use of these materials. Also, it is the responsibility of the employer to evaluate the safe design and construction of personal protective equipment.

Radiographers' Responsibilities

Radiographers must be willing to undergo the educational programs offered by their institutions, and willing to implement universal precautions in their practice. Universal precautions will be implemented in slightly different ways in different practice settings.

With the wide range of practice settings for radiographers (e.g., hospitals, clinics, physicians' offices, or the various specialties such as angiography), it is imperative that each practitioner understand and be able to implement universal precautions as they relate to specific professional settings. Mueller and colleagues (1989) describe their use of the universal precautions tray in interventional radiology. The potential of mammographic equipment to transmit HIV and HBV has been the subject of American Society of Radi-

SAMPLE QUESTIONS ASKED OF EMPLOYEES DURING AN OSHA INSPECTION

- Does your job require you to come in contact with blood or body fluids?
- Do you know what the phrase "universal precautions" means?
- Has management provided you with training for the use of personal protective equipment such as gloves, masks, eyewear, or other clothing?
- Have you ever had to clean up a blood spill?
- What did you wear and use to clean up the spill?
- Do you always wear gloves during procedures in which body fluids will be handled?
- Have you had appropriate size and quantity of disposable gloves in the last 6 months?
- Do you wear eye protection, masks, aprons, or gloves in situations involving blood splashes or splatters?
- Are containers for waste disposal constructed so they do not leak?
- Have you been informed by management of appropriate guidelines for handwashing, sharps disposal and handling, the disposal of contaminated materials, and cleaning reusable equipment?
- Do you know the procedure to follow after needlesticks or blood exposure?
- Have you received the hepatitis B vaccine while an employee here?

ologic Technologists publications, most notably the August/September 1991 *Wavelength*. Although the need for their use has not been confirmed, Uniflex (Hicksville, NY) has developed Protex-ray cassette covers for protection against "HIV, HTLV [human T-cell lymphoma virus], and other hazardous situations." Hansen and coworkers (1994) found that the practice of universal precautions in interventional radiology was quite variable.

The integrity of gloves has also been a subject of recent debate in professional journals. Some authors (e.g., Laudicina [1991]) have called for the use of radioactive material to test gloves; this is probably poor strategy. Those interested in more traditional means of testing gloves should consult the article by Kornewicz and associates (1989).

Please answer the questions below to the best of your ability. This survey is confidential, so do *not* sign your name.

	Always	Usually	Never	N/A
1. I wear gloves for direct contact with blood and other body fluids as well as for contact with mucous membranes and nonintact skin.				
2. I wear masks and protective eyewear or face shields when contact with droplets of blood is anticipated.				
3. I wear gowns or aprons when blood may splash or splatter. Also, I clean up all spills with bleach.				
4. I place all patient specimens in sturdy leakproof containers with a secure lid.				
5. I use mouthpieces, resuscitiation devices, or other ventilation devices when resuscitation is needed.				
6. I will (or have) refrain from direct patient care if I have exudative lesions or weeping dermatitis.				
7. I understand and use our incident reporting system when exposed to blood or body fluids.				
8. I understand and use proper sharps disposal methods.				
9. The following are available in this department:				
a. Gloves.				
b. Masks and protective eyewear.				
c. Protective apparel such as gowns and aprons.				
10. When involved in any invasive procedure, I routinely use universal precautions.				

Comments:

11. I feel that I have a good knowledge of universal precautions. **YES** **NO**

12. I did not understand, and/or have a question regarding, item # ________ of the first ten items.

13. I would like to have more information regarding the topic(s) listed below.

____

____

14. I have the following general comments:

____

____

____

____

____

Figure 3.2. Sample survey questionnaire. (From Dowd SB: AIDS, the technologist, and universal precautions. Radiol Technol 1991; 62:281.)

Educators' Responsibilities

Educators must assure themselves that students have received education sufficient to practice universal precautions before the students assume responsibilities for patient care in the clinical setting. This education will of course vary, as does the practice of universal precautions, with the educational setting. In most cases, however, it is to be expected that this education must be equivalent to that received by radiologic technologists in the clinical setting.

A Model for Universal Precautions in Radiology

A guide for radiology departments in applying universal precautions is:

1. Survey employees at 1-year intervals regarding knowledge and application of universal precautions. Use the results to modify educational and training programs, as well as to evaluate personal protective equipment.
2. Provide a training in-service program at initial employment of all technologists, as well as any other workers exposed to body fluids. "Ward clerks" are excluded from the categories of high-risk or at-risk employees; however, if they perform tasks related to body fluids, they should be included. OSHA strongly recommends *task evaluation* in the implementation of universal precautions. An example applied to home health care can be found in Rice (1993) and can serve as a beginning guideline.
3. Provide educational opportunities for workers relevant to transmission of HBV and HIV and universal precautions.
4. Evaluate all tasks relevant to those guidelines in Table 3.2 or, as further information becomes available, other guideline(s).
5. Provide personal protective equipment. Use could be monitored through periodic inspection of employees, as well as the self-reported use of surveys.
6. Assure yourself that your incident reporting system is adequate in a universal precautions environment.
7. Most importantly, maintain documentation relevant to all of these.

The Attitudinal Side of Universal Precautions

Patient Care as Task and Attitude

Some articles have noted that radiographers are sometimes seen as "uncaring" members of the health care team. This statement is of course patently false, but it may relate to radiographers' typical approach to patient care. McKenna-Adler (1990) has noted, for example, that a focus on high technology may limit our ability to provide "high-touch" care. Equipment has become, she notes, our barrier to care.

A profession such as nursing is often described, using Talcott Parsons' role delineation (1955), as primarily an *expressive* profession—that is, concerned with acts designed to help the patient reduce and tolerate the psychological discomfort of illness or treating the patient as a person rather than a case. At the same time, nurses recognize the *instrumental* side of helping—acts that give the patient technical assistance to solve a particular health problem or get well. Although the literature has not delineated a primary role for radiographers based on Parsons' concept, it is probable that we are most often concerned with the pragmatics of cases and instrumental in our approach to patients.

A need exists to view patient care as both task *and* attitude, especially in today's customer service environment in health care.

Universal Precautions as a Barrier to Patient Care

Universal precautions can serve as a barrier to patient care. Starr (1988) has noted that an increased reliance on infection control isolation, with its use of gowns, gloves, and masks, limits our ability to communicate. Frequently, he stated, patients in isolation are the ones who need the most support. We need to "devise ways of overcoming these necessary handicaps to communication."

The Effect of Phobias and Prejudice on Patient Care

The folklore of AIDS was the subject of an interesting article by Helwig in the *Canadian Medical Association Journal* (1989). The author contends that whenever "knowledge is scant or conflicting, folklore takes over." Many jokes and apocryphal stories are associated with AIDS—signifying poor knowledge of, and phobic attitudes toward, AIDS and AIDS patients. "Photocopier lore"—that is, stories passed from office to office by photocopies—has produced a virtual explosion of AIDS-related texts, according to the author. For example, one tongue-in-cheek memo stated: "All internal mail may only be licked by registered blood donors who have not changed sexual partners in the last 4 years." Such folklore influences health professionals and future health professionals and will have a strong impact on entry-level and continuing education.

Leisner (1989) notes that there are many "voices" of AIDS—medical, legal, financial, ethical, and spiritual. Although we may have a primary interest in hearing the strictly medical voices of AIDS, lack of knowledge in other areas makes us view the process impersonally. The tendency of radiographers to sometimes "depersonalize" their involvement with patients has been described. All radiographers are familiar with at least one fellow practitioner who refers to patients as examinations (e.g., "the foot") or by physical appearance (e.g., "the moose").

In our own profession, a case study documented by Pauley and Sedillos (1989) has shown the negative effect such ignorance can have on patient care:

> *When the technologist arrived to escort me to the radiology clinic, she was fully suited in mask, gloves, and gown; the only thing missing was eye goggles. I realize that not much was known then [1985] about the disease, but no one else had used such extreme precautions. This technologist was only going to transport me to the x-ray clinic; she was not going to perform an invasive procedure on me!*

Knowledge of and Attitudes Toward AIDS and Universal Precautions

In general, studies have found negative attitudes toward AIDS patients and the implementation of universal precautions. Results are equivocal regarding knowledge of AIDS and universal precautions—for example, one study found good general knowledge of AIDS and universal precautions, but a poor knowledge of how to apply universal precautions to the specific clinic area where these individuals worked. Also, most health care workers severely overestimate their personal risk of contracting AIDS while severely underestimating their risk of contracting hepatitis B.

One study specifically focused on radiographers and radiography students, finding generally negative attitudes toward and poor knowledge of AIDS and universal precautions (Dowd, 1991). One graduate radiographer in this study thought that the virus could be transmitted through intact skin.

Changing Knowledge and Attitudes

AIDS and universal precautions education is a challenge owing to the preconceptions each individual has along with her or his knowledge base. We must (1) address the fear and anxieties of individuals; (2) reduce that fear; and (3) increase the genuine concern individuals must have to effectively care for AIDS patients. In radiologic technology, a useful outline for teaching about AIDS and universal precautions has been developed by Clements (1989). It begins with 1 hour on history/epidemiology; continues with 1 hour on biology and transmission and 1 hour on AIDS/HIV infection in radiology; and shifts gears at the end for 1 hour on caring for the AIDS patient. An interesting preassignment for the final lecture is a 1- to 2-page values clarification essay on how students feel about having to treat AIDS patients and the responsibilities of health care workers. A study testing this curriculum found it to be effective in enhancing knowledge and changing attitudes, except in the area of homophobia.

Developing an Education Program

OSHA, the CDC, and the AHA have specific goals and objectives regarding appropriate educational programs. There must be an initial orientation prior to beginning duties, with periodic education and training based on policy. The dates and content of all educational and training programs (there is a difference between the two, training focusing on tasks and education on knowledge), the presenters, and all attending the program must be documented. The content must include:

1. General infection prevention and control practices, to include handwashing.
2. Modes of transmission of HBV and HIV.
3. Need for universal precautions as recommended by the CDC for all patients.
4. Location, indications, and proper use of personal protective clothing and equipment.
5. Methods for removal, handling, and decontamination or disposal of contaminated equipment or personal protective clothing.
6. Practices in the workplace related to the specific duties of employees, such as cleaning of blood spills, handling of contaminated sharps, and disposal of infective or contaminated waste.
7. Procedures that relate to exposures to blood or body substances, emergency corrective action, reporting procedures, and medical follow-up.
8. The availability of and recommendations for hepatitis B vaccine. (*Author's note*: OSHA defines "exposure potential" as exposure to blood and/or body fluids once or more a month.)

Additional AHA recommendations include the development of special teams able to answer questions relative to AIDS/HIV and appropriate work practices and to provide support to personnel and patients. Also, information may be provided to families of employees, and the hospital may wish to serve as a resource for community education.

There is a known resistance on the part of established health care workers to the implementation of universal precautions. Along with the attitudinal concerns discussed in previous sections, programs should focus on the lessons AIDS has taught epidemiologists. First of all, as mentioned earlier, HIV has been known to exist for many years, not just a decade. The virus was previously isolated to Africa. Simply put, the question must now be asked—how many other viruses like this are there? Knowledge often brings more questions than it answers, and AIDS has been no exception.

Summary

This part of the chapter has presented the concept and practice of universal precautions holistically for practitioners and students. AIDS and hepatitis B are problems of clinical practice that will remain, and perhaps increase in the future. There are no simple solutions to these problems, and to date, the practice of universal precautions is the best possible solution for the protection of the patient *and* the health care worker.

ISOLATION PROCEDURES

Radiographers work with patients both in the isolation unit (often a private room in the hospital) and in the department. The term isolation refers to the fact that the patient has been separated from those unaffected for the period during which a disease is communicable to others. Although isolation techniques and types of isolation vary slightly between hospitals, it is important that radiographers understand isolation and become skilled in isolation techniques. This is to protect themselves as well as the patient. Professional radiographers do not shy away from working with potentially infectious patients, but must learn means to protect themselves and their patients.

Proper disinfection techniques and conscientious handwashing are the most important factors in preventing the spread of infection. The hands are used for many tasks in patient care and can be a source of infection if not washed before and after each patient contact or after contact with contaminated articles.

An additional consideration for radiographers is whether to undergo certain immunizations to prevent the possibility of infection. Although this is a personal decision, recommendations are listed in Table 3.3.

All hospitals must practice universal precautions against blood and body fluids. Most hospitals also supplement these precautions with one or more isolation systems that deal with diseases not covered under universal precautions. Although general guidelines are presented here, it is the responsibility of each individual to learn the specific guidelines of their facility.

In 1983, the CDC developed guidelines for two types of isolation systems. One type is based on revised categories of isolation. These are described here.

Table 3.3 Immunizations Recommended for Health Care Workers

All Workers	Workers With Chronic Diseases or Other Personal Risk Factors
Hepatitis B	Influenza
Measles	Pneumococcal disease
Mumps	
Rubella	
Poliomyelitis	
Tetanus	
Diphtheria	

The second type is based on disease-specific isolation precautions. This type uses a single instruction card on which specific precautions are written or checked as appropriate. Since the development of these recommendations, the CDC has also published recommendations for universal blood and body fluid precautions. These are discussed, as well as the category of reverse or protective isolation, no longer described in federal guidelines.

Hospitals may choose to use either system as proposed, to modify one of the systems, or to develop a system of their own. This section reviews the seven guidelines and universal precautions and concludes with general guidelines for radiographing isolated patients.

Strict Isolation

Strict isolation is designed to prevent the transmission of highly contagious or virulent infections that can be spread by air and contact.

Masks, gowns, and gloves are indicated. Hands must be washed after touching the patient or potentially contaminated articles and before taking care of another patient. Infective material must be discarded or bagged and labeled before being sent for decontamination and reprocessing. A private room is indicated unless patients share the same organism. The door should remain closed.

Care must be taken to avoid needlestick injuries. Used needles must not be recapped or bent but placed in a prominently labeled, puncture-resistant container designated specifically for such disposal.

■ Examples of Diseases Requiring Strict Isolation

Pharyngeal diphtheria
Lassa fever and other viral hemorrhagic fevers, such as Marburg virus disease
Methicillin-resistant *Staphylococcus aureus* infection
Pneumonic plague
Smallpox
Varicella (chickenpox)
Disseminated zoster

Contact Isolation

When an infection is highly transmissible, but strict isolation is not warranted, contact isolation is used.

Masks are indicated for those coming close to the patient, with gowns required if soiling is likely and gloves recommended for touching infected material. Handwashing is required, and articles must be discarded or labeled and bagged as previously described.

■ Examples of Diseases or Conditions Requiring Contact Isolation

Acute respiratory infections in infants and young children
Gonococcal conjunctivitis in newborns
Cutaneous diphtheria
Endometritis due to group A streptococci
Furunculosis due to staphylococci in newborns
Herpes simplex, disseminated or neonatal
Impetigo
Influenza in infants or young children
Multiply-resistant bacterial infection
Pediculosis
Pneumonia, viral, in infants or young children
Rabies
Rubella
Scabies
Ritter's disease
Skin, wound, or burn infection
Vaccinia

Respiratory Isolation

Respiratory isolation is used to prevent transmission of disease through direct contact or over short distances through droplet transmission in air. Direct contact could occur through soiled linen or tissues. Airborne droplet transmission could occur when droplets are coughed, sneezed, or exhaled.

Gowns and gloves are *not* indicated; masks are. Handwashing is required, and articles must be disposed or labeled and bagged as described. A private room is indicated. Patients with the same organism may share a room.

■ Examples of Diseases Requiring Respiratory Isolation

Epiglottitis due to *Haemophilus influenzae*
Erythema infectiosum
Measles
Meningitis
Meningococcal pneumonia
Meningococcemia
Mumps
Pertussis
Pneumonia due to *H. influenzae* in child of any age

Acid-Fast Bacilli Isolation

This isolation category is for patients with current pulmonary tuberculosis (TB) who have a positive sputum smear or chest x-ray that strongly suggests current (active) TB. Laryngeal TB is also included in this category. Acid-fast bacilli (AFB) precautions are used instead of TB isolation to protect patient privacy. In some cases, there is still a stigma attached to having TB. Some people associate TB with poor hygiene.

In actuality, TB is a chronic pulmonary and extrapulmonary infectious disease. It is acquired by inhaling a dried-droplet nucleus containing a tubercle bacillus into the alveoli. The disease is characterized by stages of early infection that are frequently asymptomatic, latency, and a potential for recurrent postprimary disease. Outbreaks of TB are increasing worldwide, especially among the homeless, migrants, persons with AIDS, and prisoners in correctional facilities. In addition to immunosuppression (e.g., AIDS), frequent exposure to active TB can increase one's risk of contracting TB. At least 10% of new TB cases are now multidrug-resistant. CDC guidelines now require the wearing of masks by employees exposed to TB. The ideal mask is a High-Efficiency Particulate Air Respirator (HEPA). Patients with contagious TB should be transported with valveless particle respirators.

Masks are indicated; gowns and gloves are not, barring special circumstances. Handwashing is required, and articles must be discarded, cleaned, or sent for decontamination and reprocessing. A private room with special ventilation is indicated unless patients share the same organism.

Enteric Precautions

Enteric precautions prevent infections transmitted by direct or indirect contact with feces.

Masks are *not* indicated; gowns are if soiling is likely. Gloves are if infective material is touched. Articles contaminated with infective material must be discarded or bagged and labeled. A patient with poor hygiene should have a private room.

■ Examples of Diseases Requiring Enteric Precautions

Amebic dysentery
Cholera
Coxsackievirus disease
Diarrhea, acute, with suspected infectious etiology
Encephalitis
Enteroviral infection
Various forms of gastroenteritis
Hand, foot, and mouth disease
Viral type A hepatitis
Poliomyelitis
Typhoid fever

Drainage and Secretion Precautions

Draining and secretion precautions prevent infections transmitted by direct or indirect contact with purulent material or drainage from an infected source. Some diseases that involve contact with these types of material are covered under one of the previous categories with stricter requirements.

A private room is not needed. Masks are not needed. Gowns are needed if soiling is likely. Gloves are needed for touching infective material. Contaminated articles must be discarded or bagged and labeled before being sent for decontamination and reprocessing.

■ Examples of Diseases and Conditions Requiring Drainage and Secretion Precautions

Minor limited abscess
Minor limited burn infection
Conjunctivitis
Infected minor or limited decubitus ulcer
Minor or limited skin infection
Minor or limited wound infection

Blood and Body Substance Precautions

This was discussed in the first part of this chapter. Examples of diseases that require blood and body fluid precautions are listed.

■ Examples of Diseases and Conditions Requiring Blood and Body Substance Precautions

AIDS and AIDS-related complex (ARC)
Arthropod-borne viral fevers
Babesiosis
Creutzfeldt-Jakob disease
Hepatitis B; hepatitis C
HIV-positive serology test
Leptospirosis
Malaria
Rat-bite fever
Relapsing fever
Syphilis

Reverse Isolation

This involves an individual with limited immune status, such as a burn patient or organ transplant recipient. As a category, protective or reverse isolation was eliminated from federal guidelines in 1983.

Isolation is still required for such compromised patients. Thorough handwashing is required *before* touching anything in the room. A modification of surgical technique is required, with masks, caps, gowns, and gloves. Specific precautions should be posted or described in the patient's chart.

General Guidelines for Isolation

For the radiographer working with the patient in isolation, the first step is to determine the type of isolation. It is advisable to have two people perform isolation procedures. Then one radiographer can remain clean and the other dirty. In this context, the term clean means that the object handled is free of organisms causing the patient's illness. After the examination, *everything* must be decontaminated for safety.

Procedures for transporting the isolation patient to the department will vary. For respiratory isolation, the patient will wear a mask. Often, the room in which the examination will be performed will be prepared *before* the patient is brought to the department.

These general guidlines are recommended as a step-by-step procedure in radiographing the isolation patient:

1. *WASH HANDS*—This is the most important, *never* overstated, principle of infection control.
2. One worker will come in contact with the patient and another will touch only the machine and contaminated objects.
3. Put on cap (covering all hair), then gown, then gloves.
4. The worker coming into contact with the patient will hold open a protective cover (a pillowcase is most common) and the other worker will "drop" the cassette gently into the covering.
5. The worker coming into contact with the patient will explain and perform the procedure.
6. Hand the cassette to the other worker by pulling back the cover.
7. After removing and discarding the gown, *WASH HANDS* again.
8. The *entire* machine must be cleaned before returning to the department, if the equipment is portable. If the examination is done in a radiographic room, the machine and surrounding area must be cleaned.

Bibliography

About Viral Hepatitis. South Deerfield, MA: Channing L. Bete, 1986.

American Hospital Association (AHA) Special Committee on AIDS: AIDS/HIV Infection: Recommendations for Health Care Practices and Public Policy. Chicago: American Hospital Association, 1988.

Becker MH, Janz KN, Band J, et al: Noncompliance with universal precautions policy: Why do physicians and nurses recap needles? Am J Infect Control 1990; 18:232–239.

Cleary PD, et al: Compulsory premarital screening for the human immunodeficiency virus. JAMA 1987; 258:1757–1762.

Clements M: Teaching outline for presenting an AIDS module in a radiologic technology course. *In* Hopp JW, Rogers EA (eds): Instructor's Guide for AIDS and the Allied Health Professions. Philadelphia: FA Davis, 1989.

Cuteri R: Another way to do testing. ADVANCE for Radiologic Science Professionals, July 8, 1991, p 4.

Department of Labor/Department of Health and Human Services: Joint Advisory Notice: Protection against occupational exposure to hepatitis B virus (HBV) and human immunodeficiency virus (HIV). Fed Reg 1987; 52(210):41818–41823.

Department of Labor, Occupational Safety and Health Administration: Compliance Document C.P.L. 2–2.44c, 1987.

Department of Labor, Occupational Safety and Health Administration: Occupational exposure to hepatitis B and human immunodeficiency virus. Fed Reg 1987; 52:45438–45441.

Dowd SB: AIDS knowledge and attitudes of health professionals: An annotated bibliography. ERIC document # ED 324535. Abstract in Res Educ, March 1991.

Dowd SB: Developing and evaluating a departmental universal precautions policy. Radiol Management 1991; 13:28–32.

Dowd SB: Do we care? RT Image 1990; 3(33):16–17.

Dowd SB: An evaluation of the effectiveness of a educational program in improving attitudes and knowledge of acquired immunodeficiency syndrome in radiography students. A practicum submitted in partial fulfillment of the requirements for the degree of doctor of education. Ft. Lauderdale, FL: Nova University, 1991.

Dowd SB: The knowledge and attitudes of radiologic technologists and allied health students regarding AIDS and AIDS patients. Can J Med Radiat Technol 1991; 22:19–22.

Dowd SB: Teaching about AIDS poses real challenge. ADVANCE for Radiologic Technologists, October 15, 1990, p 13.

Elder HA: Transmission of HIV and prevention of AIDS. *In* Hopp JW, Rogers EA (eds): AIDS and the Allied Health Professions. Philadelphia: FA Davis, 1989, p 63.

Favero MS: Preventing transmission of hepatitis B infection in health care facilities. Am J Infect Control 1989; 17:168–171.

Friedland GH, Klein RS: Transmission of the human immunodeficiency virus. N Engl J Med 1987; 317:1125–1135.

Goodlad J: Understanding hepatitis B. Nursing Times 1989; 85(24):69–71.

Gordon KF: OSHA enforcement for occupational exposure to HBV and HIV. ASCP Teleconference, May 1990.

Grimes D: Infectious Diseases. St. Louis: CV Mosby, 1991.

Hammond JS, Eckes JM, Gomez GA, et al: HIV, trauma, and infection control: Universal precautions are universally ignored. J Trauma 1990; 30:555–561.

Hansen ME, McIntire DD, Miller GL, et al: Use of universal precautions in interventional radiology: Results of a national survey. Am J Infect Control 1994; 22:1–5.

Heller RM, Horev G, Kirchner SG, et al: AIDS awareness in the conduct of radiologic procedures: Guidelines to safe practice. Radiology 1988; 166:563–564.

Helwig D: AIDS tales: When knowledge is scant or conflicting, folklore takes over. Can Med Assoc J 1989; 140:1084–1085.

Hepatitis: Everything from A to D. Abbot Park, IL: Abbot Laboratories, no date.

Korniewicz DM, Laughon BE, Butz A, et al: Integrity of vinyl and latex procedure gloves. Nurs Res 1989; 38:144–146.

Laudicina PF: Nuclear medicine agent pinpoints defects in disposable gloves. ADVANCE for Radiologic Science Professionals, May 30, 1991.

Leisner K: Educational strategies for dealing with AIDS. Emerg Med Services 1989; 17:48–51.

Lewis JE: History of the acquired immunodeficiency syndrome (AIDS) epidemic. *In* Hopp JW, Rogers EA (eds): AIDS and the Allied Health Professions. Philadelphia: FA Davis, 1989, p 2–18.

Loudin A: HIV transmission: Should the healthcare worker worry? RT Image 1990; 3(18):45.

McKenna-Adler A: High technology: Miracle or malady for patient care? Radiol Technol 1990; 61:478–481.

Moskop JC: AIDS and hospitals: The policy options. Hosp Health Services Admin 1990; 35(2):166.

Mueller PR, Silverman SG, Tung G, et al: New universal precaution aspiration tray. Radiology 1989; 173:278–279.

Pauley D, Sedillos RT: AIDS and health care workers: Case studies. *In* Hopp JW, Rogers EA (eds): AIDS and the Allied Health Professions. Philadelphia: FA Davis, 1989, p 267.

Parsons T: Family Socialization and Interaction Processes. Glencoe, IL: Free Press, 1955.

Poteet M: New disease precautions lead to equipment maintenance concerns. RS Wavelength 1991; 2(6):1, 9.

Prince NA, Beard BJ, Ivey SL, et al: Perinatal nurses' knowledge and attitudes about AIDS. JOGNN 1989; 5:363–369.

Recommendations for prevention of HIV transmission in health care settings. MMWR 1988; 37:35.

Rice R: Principles of universal precautions/body substance isolation. Home Healthcare Nurse 1993; 11(4):55–59.

Starr MD: Touch as a communication in ministry. Care Giver 1988; 5:69–77.

Update: Universal precautions for prevention of transmission of HIV, hepatitis B virus, and other blood-borne pathogens in health care settings. MMWR 1987; 36:377.

Watts N: Foreword to Purtilo R: Health Profession/Patient Interaction. 3rd ed. Philadelphia: WB Saunders, 1984.

CHAPTER 4

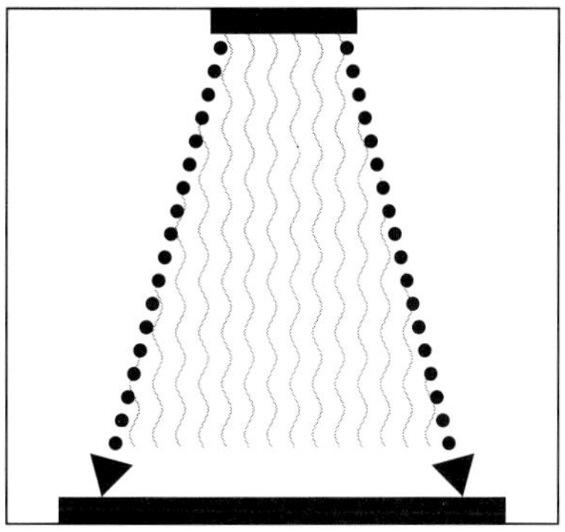

Radiation Protection

Steven B. Dowd, Ed.D., R.T.(R.)

THE BASIS FOR RADIATION PROTECTION

As with all human activities, the use of ionizing radiation to diagnose disease carries both risks and benefits. We freely decide to engage in activities such as airline travel because we perceive the benefit of such an activity to outweigh the potential risk. Similarly, the amount of information provided by a diagnostic radiograph ordered by a physician who has reason to suspect a disease process far outweighs the potential risk.

Radiation protection is an art based on sound scientific principles. The goal of radiation protection is to limit the exposure of patients to a level that is as low as reasonably achievable that still provides a maximum amount of diagnostic information. The professional on the health care team who is primarily responsible for radiation protection of the patient, in conjunction with physicians and radiologic physicists, is the radiographer.

X–RAY PRODUCTION

X-rays are a form of radiation (see later in this chapter) produced in an x-ray tube by accelerating electrons toward a target. When the electrons are stopped by the tube, they give off energy in the form of x-rays. The electrons are produced at the filament or anode of the tube by the application of a low-voltage current (milliampere-seconds, or mAs) and are accelerated by a high-voltage current (kilovolts peak or kVp).

X-rays penetrate matter in relation to the density and atomic number of that matter. The human body is made up of a variety of substances, some of which, such as bone, almost totally attenuate (absorb) x-ray. Other substances, such as air, allow much of the radiation to pass through. These different densities, or shadows, are recorded on film.

The radiographer can control a variety of factors, including the x-ray beam, to produce a diagnostic image. These factors must also be manipulated to provide radiation protection to the patient. Thirteen of these factors are discussed later in the section on Protecting the Patient.

IONIZING RADIATION

Radiation is a general term used to describe the process of emitting radiant energy in the form of waves or particles. Ionizing radiation produces positively and negatively charged particles. Sources of ionizing radiation can be manufactured (e.g., x-ray, nuclear power, and nuclear waste) or natural background (e.g., cosmic rays from the sun or the radioactive material in the earth's crust).

Radiation Units

Four units are used to express the intensity of radiation (Table 4.1.) The roentgen (R; traditional unit) or coulomb per kilogram (C/kg; SI unit) is a measure of the ionization of air produced by x-radiation and gamma radiation. In the United States, it is still customary to use the traditional units; in most other countries, SI (Système International d' Unites) units are used.

The rad (an acronym for *r*adiation *a*bsorbed *d*ose; traditional) or the gray (Gy; SI) is used to express the absorbed dose. The rem (*r*adiation *e*quivalent *m*an; traditional) or the sievert (Sv; SI unit) expresses dose equivalence, or the absorbed dose times a quality factor (in essence, a measure of the biologic effect) for personnel radiation monitoring. The last unit, the curie (Ci; traditional) or becquerel (Bq, SI), is not strictly a measure of radiation intensity but instead measures radioactive decay of a material. Only the first three are of interest to the diagnostic radiographer working with x-radiation.

Table 4.1 Radiation Units

Quantity	Traditional Unit	SI Unit
Exposure (measured in air)	Roentgen (R)	C/kg
Absorbed dose	Rad	Gray (Gy)
Dose equivalent (occupational)	Rem	Sievert (Sv)
Radioactivity	Curie (Ci)	Becquerel (Bq)

Radiation Detection Instruments

Two general classes of instruments are used to detect ionizing radiation: Field survey instruments, such as ionization chambers and Geiger counters, record the amount of ionizing radiation in air. Personnel monitors measure personal exposure to radiation on a regular basis. Three basic types of personnel monitors are: film badges, thermoluminescent dosimeters, and pocket ionization chambers. The desirable characteristics of personnel monitoring devices are: (1) portability; (2) ruggedness; (3) sensitivity; (4) reliability; and (5) low cost.

Film badges have been in use since the 1940s. A small piece of film is placed inside a badge containing a variety of metal filters that allow estimation of the radiation dosage and energy. Film badges should be changed every month, as they can fog easily owing to temperature and humidity changes. They are sensitive to about 10 mrem (0.1 mSv).

Thermoluminescent dosimeters (TLDs) use lithium fluoride, which stores radiant energy that is released when the TLD is heated. TLDs can be worn for up to 3 months and are more sensitive than film badges (to about 5 mrem or 0.05 mSv). Their main disadvantage is cost.

Pocket ionization chambers have the advantage of providing immediate readings, but they are not in wide use because they must be recalibrated daily and if the exposure exceeds the range of the dosimeter, the additional amount of exposure cannot be determined. Also, they are easily affected by trauma. Ionization chambers are generally used in short-term situations, for example, when a nurse or other health care worker visits the department.

INTERACTIONS WITH MATTER

As x-ray beams pass through matter, they undergo a process called attenuation. Some x-rays pass through matter and do not interact with the atom, some interact with the entire atom, some with the nucleus, and some with an orbital electron. Thus, there is a reduction in the original number of x-rays. This reduction is based on the energy of the x-rays and the density and atomic number of the absorbing material.

In bone, for example, a process known as the photoelectric effect is common. Here the x-ray photon interacts with an inner shell of the atom. The x-ray photon is totally absorbed and the electron is ejected from the shell. As the shells seek to reach equilibrium by filling the shells with electrons from outer orbits, x-ray photons are given off. Most of these photons are absorbed in tissue, so they contribute little or nothing to the image, but they can cause biologic changes.

Compton scattering occurs when the x-ray photon interacts with a loosely bound outer-shell electron. The electron is ejected, and the photon is scattered in another direction. This scatter radiation is a primary cause of image degradation and occupational exposure to the radiographer.

BIOLOGIC EFFECTS

Radiation effects are classified as either early (short-term) or late (long-term) to humans in addition to the known effects to the fetus. This outline is an adaptation of Bushong's (1993), listing the known biologic effects of radiation:

A. Early effects
   1. Acute radiation syndromes (doses above 200 rad or 2 Gy whole body)
      a. Hematologic syndromes
      b. Gastrointestinal syndromes
      c. Central nervous system syndromes
   2. Local tissue damage
      a. Skin
      b. Gonads
      c. Extremities
   3. Hematologic depression
   4. Cytogenetic depression
B. Late effects
   1. Leukemia
   2. Other malignant disease
      a. Bone cancer
      b. Lung cancer
      c. Thyroid cancer
      d. Breast cancer
   3. Local tissue damage
      a. Skin
      b. Gonads
      c. Eyes
   4. Life span shortening
   5. Genetic damage
      a. Cytogenetic damage
      b. Doubling dose
      c. Genetically significant dose
C. Fetal irradiation
   1. Prenatal death
   2. Neonatal death
   3. Congenital malformation
   4. Childhood malignancy
   5. Diminished growth and development

A variety of problems exists in quantifying the biologic effects of low doses of ionizing radiation, such as are received by most patients and radiation workers. First, there is usually a long latent period of 5 to 20 years between the exposure and the manifestation of any potential long-term effect. Second, effects are not radiounique—that is, anything that can be caused by radiation can be caused by a variety of other factors. Third, there is a lack of available data at low doses. To study the effect of 1 rem (10 mSv) on the body—what the typical radiation worker receives in 1 or 2 years—would require a population sample of one million individuals followed for over 20 years. To adequately study the genetic effects of such a small dose would require at least three generations worth of data. Thus, most of our knowledge of the effects of low-level radiation is drawn from population samples having received high doses of radiation and studies of laboratory animals.

RISK VERSUS BENEFIT

Maximum Permissible Doses/ Dose Equivalent Limits

Maximum permissible doses (MPDs) were established to quantify what are considered to be "safe" doses. For the occupational worker, the MPD was considered to be that dose of radiation, if received over a 50-year working lifetime, that would not result in radiation injury.

Although many individuals continue to use the term MPD, it should not be employed because it indicates that there is an acceptable (maximum permissible) dose. The term dose equivalent limits is now preferred.

The linear, nonthreshold dose response relationship was the basis for the MPD and remains a common model for quantifying the risks from ionizing radiation. It assumes that any dose of radiation, no matter how small, will have some effect. It is an extremely conservative model, and probably overestimates the risk from low doses of radiation. This is in accordance with prudent practice.

The concept of the lack of a threshold has led to risk versus benefit considerations for both patients and operators of radiologic equipment. Frankel (1975) noted that, if a threshold is not assumed, then *every* use of radiation involves a small risk but "use of radiation in the healing arts results in such numerous benefits that if judiciously used the benefits of radiation greatly exceed the very small risk to the individual." Without ionizing radiation, the health of the population would decline because we would lack the ability to diagnose disease and pinpoint trauma. Payne and Loken (1975) thus proposed a bell-shaped curve in which the health of the population was seen as low with a nonuse of ionizing radiation, high when radiation was well-used, and declined when radiation was overused.

A similar concept applied to the individual is the risk-benefit continuum (Fig. 4.1). Obviously, there is no need for an examination if it carries only a risk, and the patient should refuse the

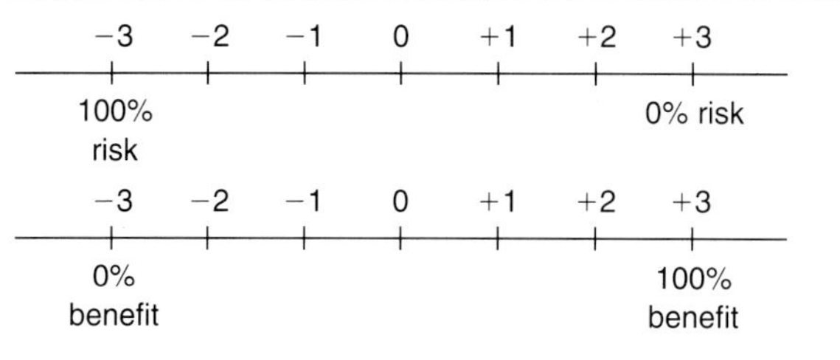

Total
- −6 Patient should not undergo examination
- −3 Patient and physician may decide that patient should not undergo examination because of high risk-benefit ratio
- 0 Difficult decision for patient and physician; risk and benefit equal
- +3 Good risk-benefit ratio; patient probably should undergo examination
- +6 Patient should undergo examination

Figure 4.1. Risk-benefit continuum. (From Dowd S: A continuum for evaluating risks and benefits of ionizing radiation. Appl Radiol 1984; 13:81.)

examination. But when the risk is small, and the potential benefit great, the patient should have the examination. Most radiologic examinations carry a very small risk in relation to the potential benefit. It is important that patients know that their physicians have made such an analysis in the decision to order the examination and that the patient has the right to refuse an examination based on a personal risk-benefit analysis. The risk-benefit continuum is a useful tool for personal and classroom learning of risk versus benefit. For example, what personal, numerical value would the radiographer assign to a career in radiation work? At 500 mrem (5 mSv) per year from age 20 years, the stated risk is 7 days of life expectancy lost. What values are to be attached to being a radiographer and what numerical value can be assigned to the benefits? From this, the need to make personal choices from risks and benefits is illustrated.

Agencies and advisory groups that have contributed to the formation of the MPD and dose equivalent limits include the International Commission on Radiologic Protection (ICRP), the National Council on Radiation Protection and Measurements (NCRP; a United States agency), the National Academy of Sciences Advisory Committee on the Biological Effects of Ionizing Radiation (BEIR), and the United Nations Scientific Committee on the Effects of Atomic Radiation (UNSCEAR).

The development of an MPD was crippled in the early years of radiography by the lack of units to express radiation intensity. At first, the *erythema* dose (the amount of radiation needed to redden the skin) or a dose based on the fogging of radiographic plates was used. Not until the roentgen was first used in the 1920s were radiation exposures adequately quantified. In 1931, the MPD was an equivalent of 200 mrem (2 mSv) per day; in 1936, it was lowered to 100 mrem (1 mSv); and it reached today's level of approximately 20 mrem (0.2 mSv) per day in 1959.

Most countries have adopted a 5-rem (50 mSv) per year *maximum* dose limit for occupationally exposed individuals. In Germany, a total lifetime cumulative occupational dose limit of 40 rem (400 mSv) is allowed. In the United States, recommended values are contained in *NCRP Report No. 91: Recommendations on Limits for Exposure to Ionizing Radiation* (Table 4.2). The lifetime dose in the United States is the worker's age in rem, or 10 times the age for the dose in mSv.

In the United States, facilities are also expected to conform to the principle of ALARA—*as* low *as* *r*easonably *a*chievable in terms of radiation dose. This basic philosophic principle emphasizes the need to minimize exposure to patients and all other individuals involved in radiologic procedures. Thus, workers and facilities have a responsibility to keep exposure low; this responsibility is contained in the professional Code of Ethics of radiographers.

Table 4.2 Recommendations on Limits for Exposure to Ionizing Radiation

Type of Exposure	Dose
Annual occupational	5 rem (50 mSv)
Cumulative lifetime	Age in years (rems) 10 × age in years (mSv)
Fetal Exposures	
Gestational period	0.5 rem (5 mSv)
Monthly dose equivalents	0.05 rem (0.5 mSv)*

Data from National Council on Radiation Protection and Measurements: Recommendations on Limits for Exposure to Ionizing Radiation. Report No. 91. Washington, DC: US Government Printing Office, 1987.

*NCRP Report No. 116 (1993) recommends an 0.5 mSv monthly limit only.

Radiation Exposure and Pregnancy

Risk-benefit considerations are also used in the special situation of radiation exposure and pregnancy. To prevent radiation exposure to the fetus in the earliest days of pregnancy, some facilities use the "10-day rule," also known as "elective booking." Elective x-ray examinations of the abdominopelvic area should be postponed until 10 days after the onset of menstruation to minimize the possibility of pregnancy. These include lumbar spine, pelvis, abdomen, barium enema, hysterosalpingography, pelvimetry, uro/pyelo/cystography, and hip and femur examinations.

Many facilities post signs indicating to patients that they need to tell the radiographer whether they may be pregnant. According to Holmes (1991), in the United Kingdom it is the responsibility of the individual exposing the patient, whether radiographer or physician, to ascertain the pregnancy status of a patient. The United Kingdom Ionising Radiation Regulations specifically legislate dose limits for women of reproductive capability and the abdomen of a pregnant woman at work.

PROTECTING THE RADIOGRAPHER

Although the patient should be the only individual exposed to the primary beam, personnel may be exposed to scatter/secondary radiation or leakage radiation from the tube. Examinations with a possibility of exposure to the worker include interventional procedures, fluoroscopy, and mobile radiography.

Radiographers should not routinely hold patients who are unable to cooperate during a procedure. If immobilization devices are unavailable or cannot be used, assistance should be secured from nonradiation workers, preferably a family member or friend. No hospital worker should ever routinely hold patients. The individual holding the patient should remain at right angles to the primary beam. This individual should also wear a lead apron, and, if possible, lead gloves.

The three cardinal or most important principles of radiation protection are time, distance, and shielding. These are discussed in greater detail.

Time

The radiographer must reduce the amount of time spent in the area of the radiation source. Time and radiation exposure are directly proportional. If the amount of time spent in the area of the source doubles, radiation intensity doubles.

Most fluoroscopic equipment is equipped with 5-minute reset timers to remind the operator that a certain recommended time limit has elapsed for beam on-time. Also, fluoroscopic foot switches are designed to terminate the exposure once the foot is released from the swtich; they should be operated in an on-off pattern rather than continually on.

Distance

Distance is the most effective means of reducing radiation exposure. At a distance of 1 meter from the scattering object (the patient), the intensity of radiation in fluoroscopy decreases to 0.1 percent of the original value. Ruegsegger (1982) found that the intensity of radiation 1 meter from the patient in a neonatal intensive care unit was so small that a nurse or radiation worker standing at this distance would have to be exposed to 2000 films a month to reach the dosage allowed the general public. This low level would not excuse a lack of protection measures; it merely indicates safe operating practice.

The inverse square law, which states that radiation intensity varies to the inverse of the square of the distance, holds true for the primary beam, which is considered a point source of radiation, and after about 1 meter for scatter/secondary radiation. Thus, an intensity of 100 mrad (1 mGy) at 20 inches diminishes to 25 mrad (0.25 mGy) at 40 inches. This does not hold true for scatter/secondary radiation because the patient is an extended source of radiation. However, the basic concept is the same—*Remain as far from the source (patient) as possible.*

Shielding

Shielding consists of either fixed structural barriers (made of lead or concrete, or both) or devices such as mobile shields. Shielding is measured in terms of half-value layers (HVLs; the amount of material needed to reduce radiation exposure in half) and tenth-value layers (TVLs). Most lead aprons consist of 1 or 2 HVLs. For lead aprons to be effective, the lead must not be cracked; thus, aprons should not be handled carelessly or folded. Most protective curtains that drape the image intensifier used in fluoroscopy consist of 2 TVLs.

Fixed barriers are classified as either primary or secondary. A primary barrier can be struck by the primary beam. Secondary barriers can only be struck by scatter/secondary radiation. This means that the beam cannot be directed at the barrier. The control booth is usually considered a secondary barrier; the ceiling always is.

The Pregnant Radiographer

Recent legal decisions have indicated that pregnant radiographers cannot be transferred out of radiation areas, fired, or laid off owing to pregnancy. The pregnant radiographer *can be* required to sign forms indicating a knowledge of the risks involved and may ask for a transfer to areas of less exposure. Regulations use the term *declared pregnant woman*, indicating that a worker must advise her employer *voluntarily* and *in writing* of (1) her pregnancy and (2) her estimated date of delivery. Formal, voluntary, and prompt notification are the only means by which the employer can assure that fetal dose can be limited during pregnancy.

PROTECTING THE PATIENT

The foundations of the profession of radiography are production of a diagnostic image and radiation protection of the patient. Thirteen basic principles (Table 4.3), many of which are under the control of the radiographer, can be used to minimize patient exposure while retaining a diagnostic image.

Technique Selection

Tube current (milliampere; mA), time (s), and kVp should be selected in unison to produce an image that is diagnostically acceptable to the physician while maintaining good radiation protection practices. High kVp is preferred, yet it should not be so high as to degrade image quality through the production of excess scatter/secondary radiation and excessively long-scale contrast. Most examinations have an optimum kVp setting beyond which contrast scale is degraded. Increased kVp *increases* internal organ dose through the production of additional scatter/secondary radiation, but this is compensated for by the reduction in skin dose.

When techniques are selected manually, the time of exposure should be minimized to keep the degrading effects of motion as low as possible. Tube current (mA) can be increased to compensate in direct proportion. A technique of 100 mA and 0.1 second (10 mAs) is equivalent to 200 mA and 0.05 second. Doubling mAs would double the amount of radiation produced.

When techniques are phototimed (automatic exposure control devices are used), it is important to use a balance between mA and time that could not potentially overexpose the patient. In general, 1.5 to 2 times the required manual technique should be set for phototimed exposures. When problems occur with phototimed exposures, the radiographer should always switch to manual methods.

Table 4.3 Summary of Factors That Influence Patient Dose and the Potential Effect of That Factor on Image Quality

Factor	Effect of Factor on Patient Exposure	Potential Effect on Image Quality
Technique selection	Increased kVp with decreased mAs decreases exposure	Longer-scale contrast*
Filtration	Increased filtration decreases exposure	None
Projection	Proper use of projections decreases exposure	Increase or decrease†
Image receptor	Faster speeds with decreased mAs to compensate decreases exposure	Longer-scale contrast
Beam limitation	Decreases exposure	Improves image quality through shorter-scale contrast
Shielding	Decreases exposure	Properly applied, has no effect
Grids	Not a radiation protection device; proper use limits exposure	Improves image quality through shorter-scale contrast
Immobilization	Fewer repeats decreases exposure	Lack of motion increases image quality
Patient instructions	Increased cooperation decreases repeats	Improves overall image quality
Repeat exposures	Fewer repeats decreases exposure	Increases overall image quality
Patient doses	None directly; shows concern for patient	None
Equipment	Proper use and quality control decrease exposure	Increases image quality in short-term *and* long-term
Certification/ education	Certified and educated operators provide less exposure to patients	Increases image quality

Key: kVp, kilovolts peak; mAs, milliampere-seconds.

*In many cases, long-scale contrast is seen as detrimental; in others, such as chest radiography, long-scale contrast is beneficial.

†Although a projection may be beneficial from a radiation protection standpoint, image quality can be affected by placing the area of interest farther from the film (magnification).

Filtration

A filter is a device placed at the x-ray port to absorb low-energy radiation that would not contribute to the diagnostic value of the image as the rays would be absorbed within the patient. Removing these low-energy photons decreases overall patient dose.

Compensating Filtration

Compensating filters are used to adjust for variations in patient density. For example, wedge filters are used in foot radiography with the thick portion of the wedge over the toes and the thin portion toward the heel to provide for even density on the film. Woodruff (1991) noted that chest radiography of obese, large-breasted women could require two films because the bottom of the first film will be too light. Instead, a compensating filter can be used. Use of such a filter in this instance will (owing to the large amount of technique that must be used for the second film) cut the patient's dose by one third.

Other means of employing compensating filtration include the use of special cassettes made up of two types of intensifying screens or the addition of a piece of paper to a screen to limit the amount of light produced in one section.

Grids

Grids are placed between the patient and the image receptor to absorb scatter/secondary radiation. They are usually used when the thickness of a part exceeds 10 to 13 cm. This usually depends on the preferences of the radiologist. Using a grid requires an increase in technique factors; it is not a device to minimize radiation exposure. It does improve image quality by removing unwanted scatter/secondary radiation. It is the responsibility of the radiographer, if various grid ratios are available, to choose the lowest possible ratio that will reduce scatter, yet not require overly high technical factors.

Projection

Certain projections are superior in terms of radiation protection. In some cases, these are standard; in others, the radiographer should adapt positioning as needed for specific patients.

■ Examples of Preferred Projections

PA projections for chest and sternal radiography—Reduce radiation exposure to the sternum (active bone marrow).

PA skull—Reduces radiation exposure to the lens of the eye (minimizing the possibility of cataracts) by 95 percent over the AP projection.

Intravenous pyelogram (IVP) or a cystogram—Contrast-filled bladder serves as a gonadal shield for female patients in the AP projection.

Image Receptors

As the speed of an image receptor increases, the amount of radiation needed to expose the film decreases. In x-ray, intensifying screens are used to expose film with light and x-ray rather than just x-ray. On a negative note, as the speed of the film/screen system increases, diagnostic quality decreases. The highest possible film/screen combination still able to achieve the needed diagnostic quality should be selected in balance to minimize risk (radiation exposure) and maximize benefit (the quality of the examination).

Beam Limitation (Collimation)

Most modern equipment is fitted with positive beam limitation (PBL), which automatically collimates or limits the beam to the size of the film when using the Bucky grid. Most such equipment allows the radiographer to further minimize the beam size. Proper collimation reduces patient exposure *and* improves image quality. Other means of collimation include cones and cylinders, which are attached to the tube housing to further limit beam size; aperture diaphragms, which are used for machines lacking collimators; and lead blockers, which are placed in the beam to absorb scatter/secondary radiation.

Shielding

One of the most important means of minimizing the potential effects of radiation exposure on future generations is shielding of the ovaries and testes (gonads). This is important for all individuals of reproductive age (which is not as narrow as was once assumed) and younger.

Some facilities routinely use gonadal shielding, unless it will interfere with the diagnostic quality of the beam, to minimize patient anxiety associated with radiation exposure. As a rule, gonadal shielding should be used when the gonads are within 5 cm (2 inches) of the primary beam unless this would compromise diagnostic quality.

Three basic types of gonadal shields are: Flat contact shields, usually made of lead-impregnated vinyl, are placed directly over the patient's gonads. Shaped contact shields are used for male gonadal shielding. These are cup-shaped to provide for maximum protection in a variety of settings. Shadow shields cast a "shadow" in the beam and are mounted on the tube.

Male gonadal shielding should be used in examinations of the pelvis, hip (except obliques), and upper femur, unless it will interfere with the examination. Male gonadal shielding is not usually used on retrograde urethrograms, voiding cystourethrograms, and visualization of the rectum.

Other types of shielding include contact lens shields for the lens of the eye and breast shields for juvenile scoliosis examinations. Shielding can be used in conjunction with other methods to further minimize exposure. In addition to the real value of shielding, the public relations value of shielding patients should not be underestimated.

Immobilization

Patients unable to cooperate must be immobilized. A patient's ability to cooperate must be ascertained by the radiographer, who will then decide on appropriate means of immobilization. An adult may be unable to hold the forearm still and may need sandbags applied to each end of the arm to prevent image-degrading motion. Obviously a 6-month-old infant will be unable to cooperate and may need immobilization.

Patient Instructions

It is extremely important that the patient who is able to cooperate be allowed to do so. Experienced radiographers know the value of securing patient cooperation and the extent to which this minimizes repeat examinations. Taking a few extra seconds to secure patient cooperation and consent and instill a sense of trust in the radiographer can easily save the radiographer 15 minutes on repeat films.

Repeat Exposures

An "average" repeat rate for radiographs ranges from about 5 to 15 percent, although authors appear to give a variety of rates. Bushong (1993), for example, feels that 4 percent is the average rate for a busy department, whereas others list the higher number as accurate. Eight to 10 percent is probably an acceptable and fairly average repeat rate. A variety of factors influence repeat rate, including the experience level of the radiographer and the radiologist's view of image quality.

A very low repeat rate might indicate that poor-quality films are being passed. Repeat exposures owing to improper film processing, poor positioning, improper exposure factors, and poor patient instruction are under the control of the radiographer. In line with risk-benefit, considerations, radiographs should only be repeated when the quality of the film is unacceptable.

Patient Exposures

The radiographer should be familiar with estimated exposures of representative examinations. Because the radiographer is able to control factors that lead to this exposure, and the patient may be interested in the exposure, this information is valuable to the professional.

Patients may be informed about the exposures they receive in several ways. In some departments, this information is released only by the radiologist or physicist. In any case, the radiographer should know what type of information is to be provided to patients about dose and who is to provide it, as well as knowing representative exposure values for professional use. Some of these values, with a historical perspective on how they have changed since the 1950s, are listed in Table 4.4. Owing to improved equipment, better methods of quality control, and increased education of radiographers, patient exposures have decreased up to 97 percent.

Equipment

The radiographer should report all equipment problems as soon as possible. The radiographer may also be involved in quality assurance checks of equipment. For some procedures, a diagnostic radiation physicist should assess the radiation safety characteristics of the machine. Chapter 8 of this volume describes the basics of quality assurance and quality control. These procedures increase the overall quality of images and protect the patient from excess radiation.

Table 4.4 Representative Patient Exposures

Examination	Sante (1954): Incident Exposure	Statkiewicz-Sherer (1993): Permissible Entrance Skin Exposure
PA chest	50 mR	12–26 mR
Lateral skull	1300 mR	105–240 mR
AP abdomen	1300 mR	375–698 mR
Extremity	250–1000 mR	8–327 mR

Certification/Education

As professionals, radiographers should only perform procedures for which they are qualified. Various reports have shown the value of training in radiation protection to the patient; for example, Tilson found that radiographers who engaged in continuing education were more likely to provide radiation protection to patients.

Williamson and Le Heron (1989), in New Zealand, found that limited radiography in small practice settings, as performed primarily by nurses, led to a 55 percent rejection rate by radiologists. Although only 18 percent of these radiographs were "completely undiagnostic," patients should be provided only with films that are completely *diagnostic*.

In the United States, the organization responsible for certifying radiographers is the American Registry of Radiologic Technologists (ARRT). In addition to certifying radiographers, this organization also offers certification examinations in cardiovascular and interventional radiography (CVIT) and mammography, and plans examinations for computed tomography, magnetic resonance imaging, and quality assurance.

CONCLUSION

The majority of this text focuses on the role of positioning in producing quality radiographs. The focus of this chapter was to concentrate on another, related role of the radiographer—that of radiation protection of the patient and radiographer in accordance with risk versus benefit and *as low as reasonably achievable* (ALARA).

Bibliography

American Society of Radiologic Technologists (ASRT) Code of Ethics. Available from the ASRT, 15000 Central Avenue SE, Albuquerque, NM 87123.

Barnett M, Eccleston R.: Radiation Protection During Medical X-Ray Examinations. Rockville, MD: US Department of Health, Education, and Welfare, 1976.

Bushong SC: Policies for managing the pregnant employee. Radiol Management 1984; 6(3):2–7.

Bushong SC: Radiation protection. *In* Ballinger PW (ed): Merrill's Atlas of Radiographic Positions and Radiologic Procedures. 5th ed. St. Louis: CV Mosby, 1982.

Bushong SC: Radiologic Science for Technologists. 5th ed. St. Louis: CV Mosby, 1993.

Butler PF, Thomas AW, Thompson WE, et al: Simple methods to reduce patient exposure during scoliosis radiography. Radiol Technol 1986; 57:411–417.

Carroll QB: Fuchs's Principles of Radiographic Exposure, Processing, and Quality Control. 3rd ed. Springfield, IL: Charles C Thomas, 1985.

Code of Ethics. Can J Med Radiol Technol 1991; 22(1):6.

Cusworth RJ: Quality Assurance in Diagnostic Radiology: An Eight-Step Methodology. Denver: Multi-Media Publishing, 1983.

DeVos D: Basic Principles of Radiographic Exposure. Philadelphia: Lea & Febiger, 1990.

Donohue DP: An Analysis of Radiographic Quality. Baltimore: University Park Press, 1980.

Dowd SB: A continuum for evaluating risks and benefits of ionizing radiation. Appl Radiol 1984; 13(2):81–82.

Frank E, Stears J, Gray J, et al: Use of the PA projection: A method of reducing x-ray exposure to specific radiosensitive organs. Radiol Technol 1983; 54:343–347.

Frankel R: Radiation Protection for Radiologic Technologists. New York: McGraw-Hill, 1975.

Holmes P: Off beam. Nurs Times 1991; 87(4):20.

The Ionising Radiation Regulations 1985. HMSO ISBN 0–11–057333–1.

Land CE: Estimating cancer risks from low doses of ionizing radiation. Science 1981; 209:1197–1203.

Martigoni K, Nitschke J: A new radiation protection dose limit for occupationally exposed personnel in the Federal Republic of Germany. Radiologe 1991; 31(5):235–239.

McLemore J: Quality Assurance in Diagnostic Radiology. Chicago: Year Book Medical, 1981.

Mole RH: The ten-day rule: A misnomer. Radiography 1984; 50:229–230.

National Council on Radiation Protection and Measurements: Recommendations on Limits for Exposure to Ionizing Radiation. Report No. 91. Washington, DC: US Government Printing Office, 1987.

Payne JT, Loken MK: A survey of the risks and benefits of ionizing radiation. CRC Crit Rev Clin Radiol Nucl Med 1975. Cleveland: CRC Press.

Proposed rules, specific area gonad shielding, guidelines for use on patients during medical diagnostic x-ray procedures. Fed Reg 1975; 40(180):42749.

Rossi RP: Radiation protection. *In* Carlton RR, Adler A: Principles of Radiographic Imaging: An Art and a Science. Albany, NY: Delmar, 1992.

Ruegsegger DR Jr: Radiation exposure levels in an intensive care nursery. Pediatr Nurs 1982; 8:244–247.

Sante LR: Manual of Roentgenological Technique. Ann Arbor, MI: Edwards Brothers, 1954.

Statkiewicz-Sherer MA, Visconti PJ, Ritenour ER: Radiation Protection in Medical Radiography. 2nd ed. Denver: Multi-Media Publishing, 1993.

Tilson ER: Educational and experiential effects on radiographer's radiation safety behavior. Radiol Technol 1982; 53:321–325.

Williamson BDP, Le Heron JC: Radiographic quality and radiation protection in general medical practice and small hospitals. N Z Med J 1989; 102(863): 104–107.

Woodruff K. Here's a way to make filters. ADVANCE for Radiologic Science Professionals 1991; 4(36):23.

CHAPTER 5

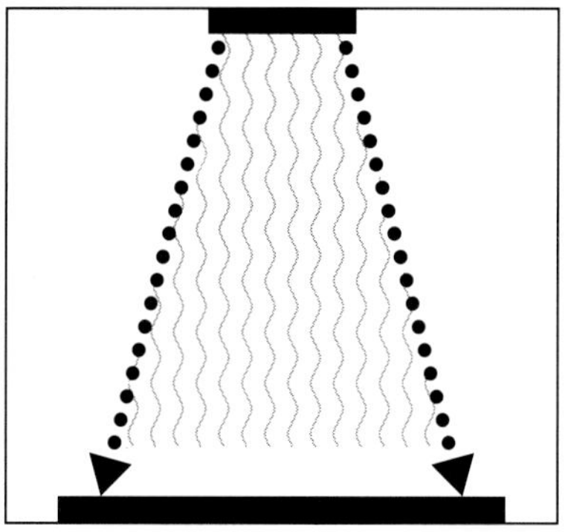

Equipment

Steven B. Dowd, Ed.D., R.T.(R.)

Roger Smith, R.T.(R.)

The purpose of this chapter is to overview equipment commonly used in radiology departments. Along with imaging equipment and accessories used, the production of a radiograph as well as the properties of x-ray is reviewed.

STEPS IN THE PRODUCTION OF A RADIOGRAPH

It is appropriate to review the steps in the production of the diagnostic film called a radiograph produced by a radiographer.

1. Review the requisition and other patient records. Set up the radiographic room according to the needs of the patient and examination. This would include having available a clean table, markers, contrast media if needed, and appropriate film cassettes.
2. Greet the patient and verify patient's identification (ID) by wrist ID and verbal verification. Put the patient at ease (ensuring later patient cooperation) by explaining the examination. Check for contraindications such as pregnancy.
3. Based on communication with the patient, as well as on requisition and records and visual clues, ascertain any special needs: Are there multiple injuries that will preclude certain positions? Will the patient require special instructions? Will restraint be necessary? Will pathology require a change in technical factors?
4. Select the technical factors required based on the parameters of the examination: Bucky or tabletop, film-screen speed, anatomic part, automatic exposure control or manual factors, pathology.
5. Place the patient in the proper position. Continue to communicate with the patient throughout this process. Check factors such as centering of tube to table, correct film size, correct use of left and right markers, and bucky tray pushed in as far as possible.
6. Reassess factors such as body habitus while moving back to the control panel. Change technical factors if necessary. Continue to communicate with the patient. Give instructions, such as respiration, and expose the film.
7. Continue to communicate with the patient. Indicate the end of the examination or begin the process of exposing another film.

CONTROL PANEL

The radiographer manipulates a variety of items on the control panel (Fig. 5.1), including milliamperage (mA), time of exposure (s), kVp (peak kilovoltage), and in the case of units with automatic exposure controls, density controls that will control the density of the film. When using the automatic exposure control, a backup time must be selected. This is the maximum time that the exposure can run, and it should be set as low as possible. In general, the backup timer should be set so that it will terminate when 1.5 times the expected manual technique is reached.

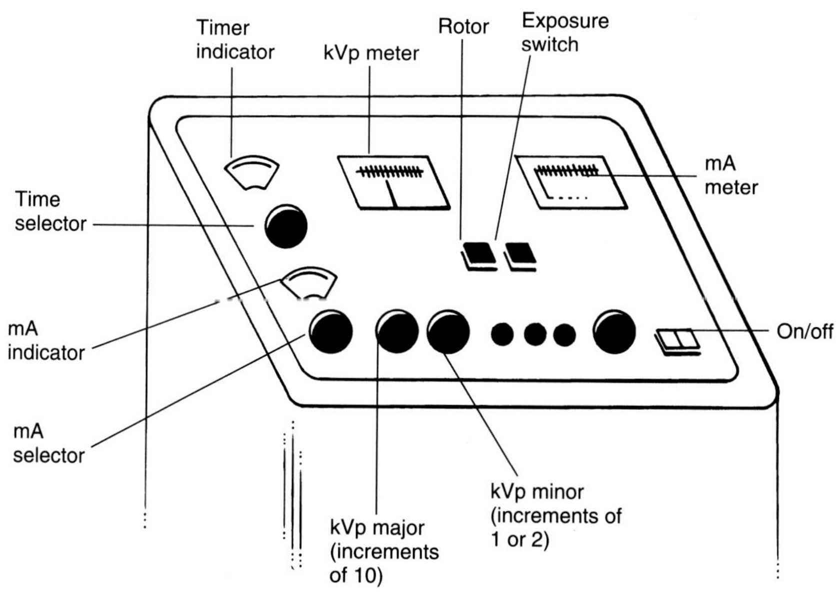

Figure 5.1. Basic control panel showing controls routinely manipulated by radiographer. Rotor and exposure switch may be on panel or on a hand-held device.

RADIOGRAPHIC TUBE

Overhead Tube (Radiographic)

The device used to produce x-rays of diagnostic energy is the x-ray tube (Fig. 5.2). Since it hangs above the x-ray table, it is sometimes called the overhead tube (as opposed to the fluoroscopic tube, usually housed in the x-ray table), and films taken using this tube are sometimes called overhead films, especially those taken after fluoroscopy.

Three basic components to an x-ray tube are (1) the cathode, or source of electrons; (2) the anode, or target; and (3) an evacuated glass envelope to allow for the free flow of electrons. The electron cloud is generated by applying a low-voltage current to the cathode (milliampere-seconds; mAs) and is accelerated through application of a high-voltage current (peak kilovoltage; kVp).

The x-ray beam that exits the tube housing is called the primary beam. On entering the patient, the primary beam may be absorbed, produce other types of radiation (secondary and scatter), or pass through to expose the film. The portion of the primary beam that passes through the patient and exposes the film is called the remnant beam.

Collimator

The collimator is a device used to limit the size of the x-ray beam. Most modern x-ray equipment is also equipped with positive beam limitation (PBL; also called automatic collimation) that limits the beam to a size no larger than the cassette inserted into the bucky tray.

Filtration

All x-ray tubes have filtration designed to absorb low-energy x-rays that would only interact in the patient (increasing patient dose) and would not contribute to the image. On some tubes, the filtration can be selected according to the needs of the examination.

Fluoroscopy

Fluoroscopy is dynamic radiography, or radiography of motion. Examinations that use fluoroscopy include upper gastrointestinal examinations, barium enemas, and angiography. Fluoroscopy uses a fluorescent screen that emits light when struck by x-rays to produce the image. The fluorescent screen and the x-ray tube are kept in alignment by a device called a **C**-arm (Fig. 5.3).

A device called an image intensifer amplifies the image and converts the x-ray photons into visible light. This device improves the quality of the image. The images may be viewed on a television monitor as they are made. Permanent images are recorded using the spot film device, which stores a cassette in the fluoroscope, or another method, such as camera film or videotape.

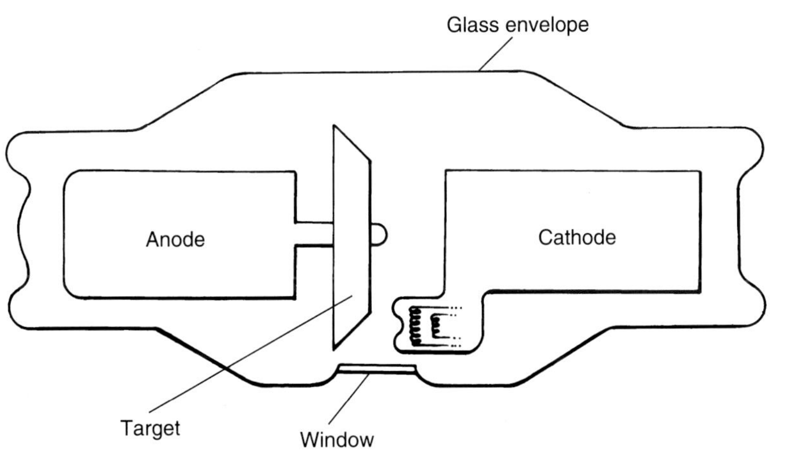

Figure 5.2. Basic design for x-ray tube.

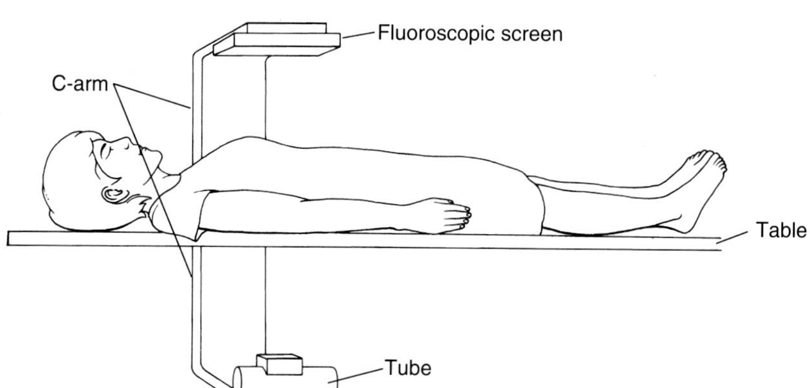

Figure 5.3. Basic C-arm setup for fluoroscopy.

PROPERTIES OF X-RAYS

Although they have no mass or charge, x-rays have the capacity to "behave" as both waves and particles. The physical properties of x-rays are:

1. Extremely penetrating electromagnetic waves. X-rays are a part of the electromagnetic spectrum, similar to light, but of shorter wavelength. The ability of x-rays to pass through matter is one of the bases of medical imaging.
2. Heterogeneous (many different wavelengths) and polyenergetic (many different energies). Since x-rays consist of many different energies, they are not equally absorbed in a material. This factor, along with patient habitus, determines the differential absorption of the beam.
3. Cannot be focused by a lens. This necessitates the use of other means to focus the beam, including collimation and filtration.
4. Will cause some crystals to give off light (fluoresce). This is the basis of operation for intensifying and fluoroscopic screens.
5. Will affect photographic film. Another basis for medical imaging, it also allows for the use of film badges as a radiation-monitoring device.
6. Will ionize gases. This is the basis of operation for one type of automatic exposure control. It measures the amount of air ionized and terminates the exposure at a preset level.
7. Will cause biologic changes. This necessitates the use of radiation protection practices. Since these changes cannot be exactly predicted, radiation exposures must be kept as low as reasonably achievable (ALARA).
8. Will produce secondary and scattered radiation when interacting with matter. This will decrease the quality of the image, and constitutes most of the radiographer's exposure to radiation.
9. Electrically neutral. A fact that separates x-ray from some other forms of ionizing radiation, such as alpha and beta radiation.
10. Will travel in all directions, in a diverging straight line, at the speed of light. This necessitates shielding of the tube to prevent exposure from leakage radiation.

PATIENT

Calipers and Angligners

Calipers are measuring devices used to determine the size of an anatomic part (Fig. 5.4). They should always be used when setting manual techniques in conjunction with the generator's technique chart. Angligners are devices used to measure the angulation of the head for skull positioning (Fig. 5.5).

Immobilization Devices

When patients cannot cooperate, the part must be immobilized. Figure 5.6 shows a variety of devices that can be used to immobilize a variety of anatomic parts.

RADIOGRAPHIC FILM AND SCREENS

Film

The basic components of x-ray film are a support base and emulsion layers (Fig. 5.7). Present-day film bases are made of polyester to which a blue tint has been added to aid the eye in visualizing film contrast. The emulsion is coated on both sides of the base. It is composed of a gelatin binder and a recording medium of silver halide crystals. An antiabrasion coat on the emulsion helps to protect the film from scratches and other damage.

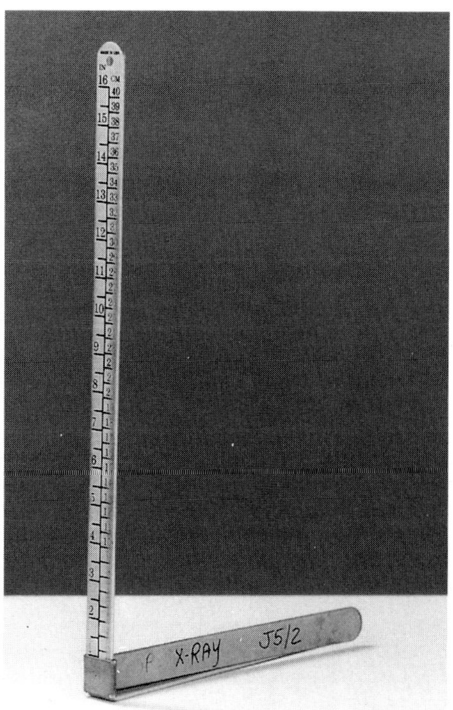

Figure 5.4. Calipers.

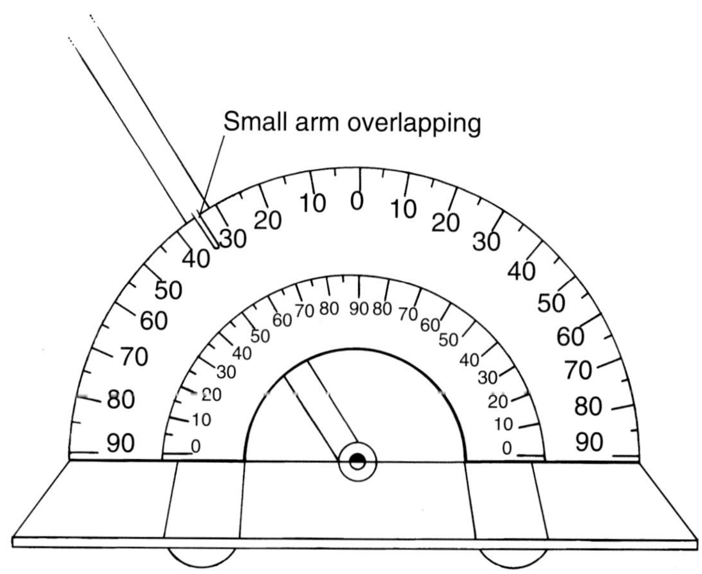

Figure 5.5. Angligner. *Note:* The measurements on the outer side begin at 90° and decrease in 5° increments to the center (0°); the measurements on the inner side begin at 0° and increase in 5° increments to the center (90°).

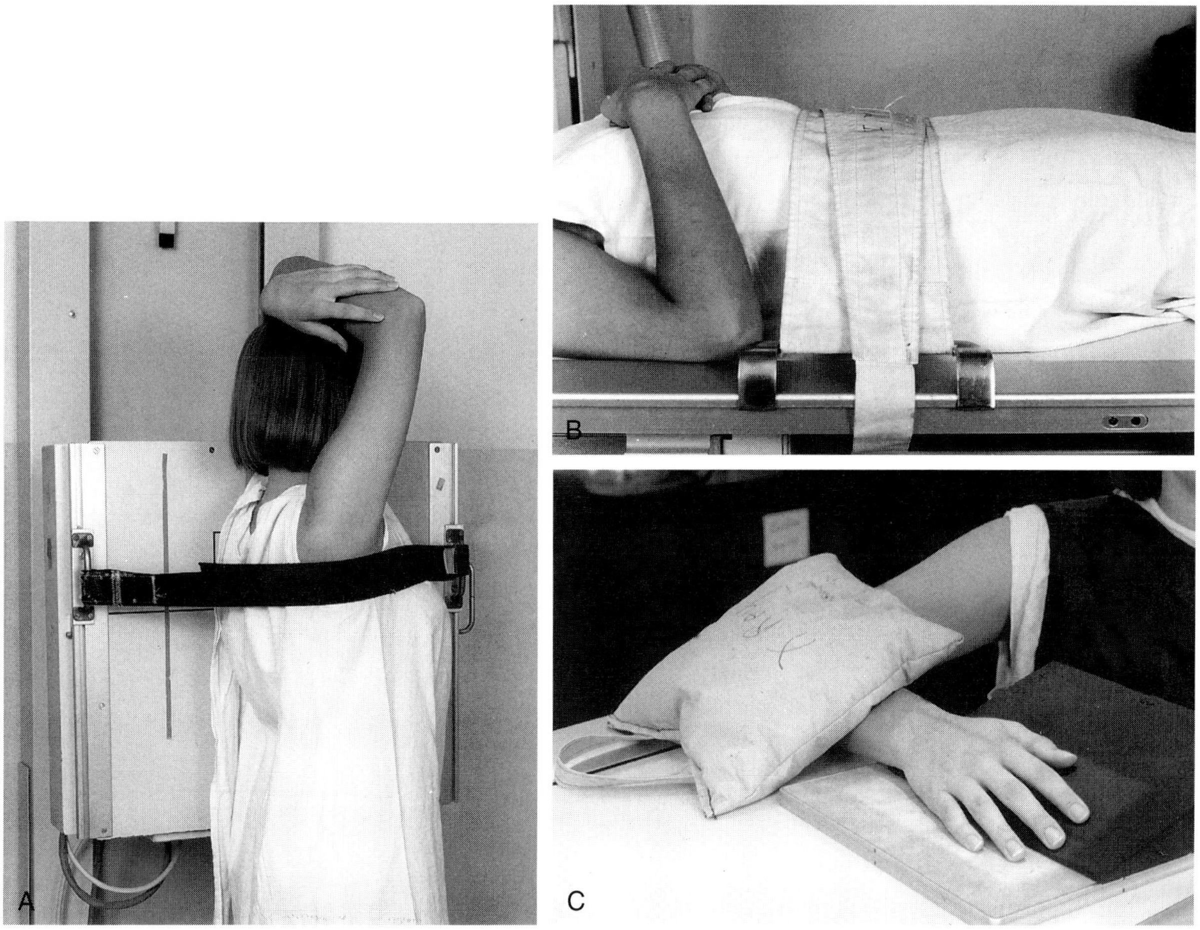

Figure 5.6. Immobilization devices. *A*, Straps used for lateral chest radiograph. *B*, Velcro straps used on patient lying supine on table. *C*, Sandbag to hold arm steady. (*A–C*, From Adler A, Carlton R: Introduction to Radiography and Patient Care. Philadelphia: WB Saunders, 1994, pp 166, 167.)

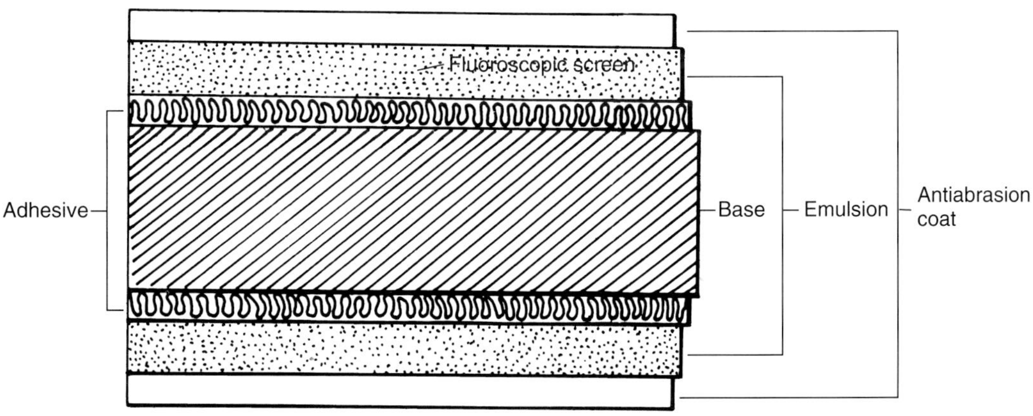

Figure 5.7. Basic cross-section of double-emulsion film. The two basic components are the base and the two emulsions. An adhesive binds the emulsion to the base and an antiabrasion coat on top of each emulsion layer protects the emulsion.

Cassettes

X-ray cassettes (Fig. 5.8) contain intensifying screens, sheets of plastic embedded with phosphorescent crystals. The film is sandwiched between the screens. The light given off by the screens exposes the film.

The common sizes for x-ray cassettes in the United States are 14 × 17 inches, 7 × 17 inches, 14 × 14 inches, 11 × 14 inches, 10 × 12 inches, 9.5 × 9.5 inches, 8 × 10 inches, and 5 × 7 inches. In other countries, x-ray cassettes are available in similar, but not always identical, metric sizes.

RADIOGRAPHIC TABLE

Basic Construction

A standard table used in a combination radiographic/fluoroscopic room (also called an R and F room; Fig. 5.9) consists of:

1. A width of about 30 inches (76 cm), about 75 to 90 inches (190 to 229 cm) long, and about 34 inches (86 cm) in height.
2. A heavy base that can support a great deal of weight.
3. A radiolucent (easily penetrated by x-ray) top made of materials such as bakelite (a type of plastic), foam, or carbon fiber.
4. A drive mechanism that allows the table to be tilted and "floated" to allow for a variety of patient positions.
5. A spot film changer or other recording device for making permanent fluoroscopic images.
6. A bucky tray beneath the tabletop.
7. A detachable footrest to assist the patient in standing when the table is tilted.

Radiographic tables are not known for their comfort, and the radiographer must be sure to make every effort to ensure the comfort of the patient. This is especially acute with older or emaciated patients.

Grids and Bucky Tray

Grids are devices designed to remove scatter radiation from the film. The grid is composed of alternating strips of lead with a radiolucent substance. Remnant radiation can pass through, whereas unfocused scatter will be absorbed by the lead strips. Stationary grids (in which the grid does not move during the exposure) are used in situations for which a movable grid, such as the Potter-Bucky diaphragm (called the Bucky for short), is not practicable.

The movement of the grid is designed to blur out the grid lines noticeable on a radiograph when a stationary grid is used.

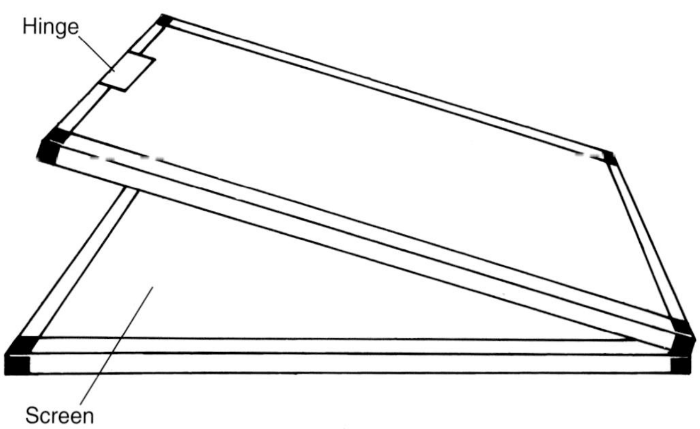

Figure 5.8. X-ray cassette showing bottom screen.

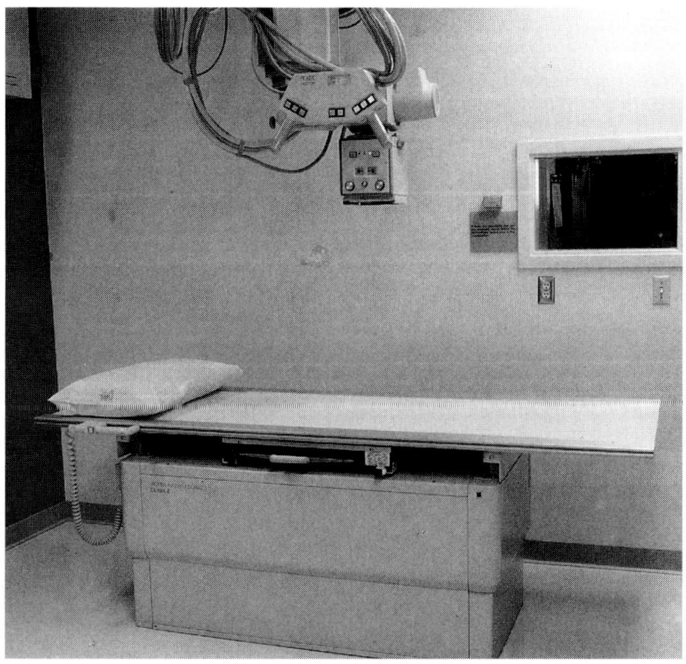
Figure 5.9. X-ray table.

DARKROOMS

Although many departments are switching to so-called daylight processors—in which cassettes are inserted into a device that removes the film from the cassette, stamps an identification on the film, routes the film into the processor, and then reloads the cassette with film—some departments still have radiographic darkrooms (Fig. 5.10).

McKinney (1988) notes that a radiographic darkroom must be a "scientific laboratory," since so many factors can alter radiographic film, including heat, light, humidity, static electricity, pressure, chemical fumes, and radiation. A darkroom must be kept free of these contaminants.

Processors

A processor (Fig. 5.11) is a device that develops, fixes (makes the image permanent), washes, and dries the x-ray film. The rate of film development is controlled by time and temperature. Chemicals used in the processor must be replenished as needed. To maintain film quality, processors must be evaluated daily.

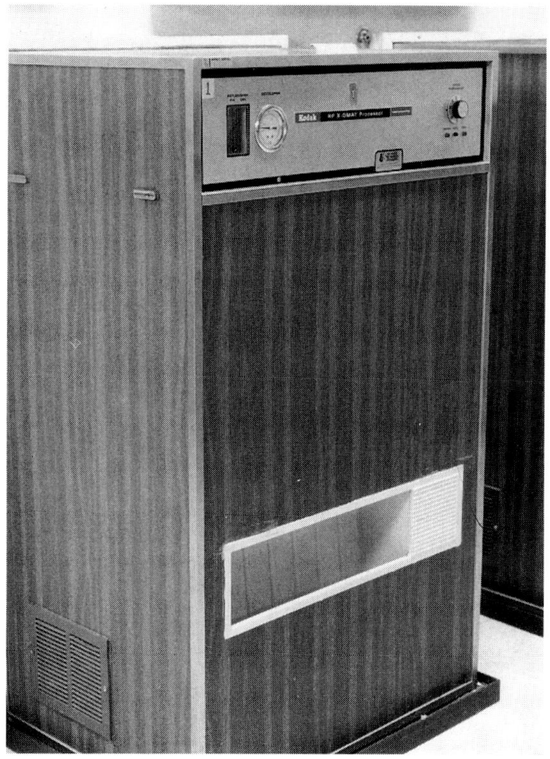

Figure 5.11. Processor.

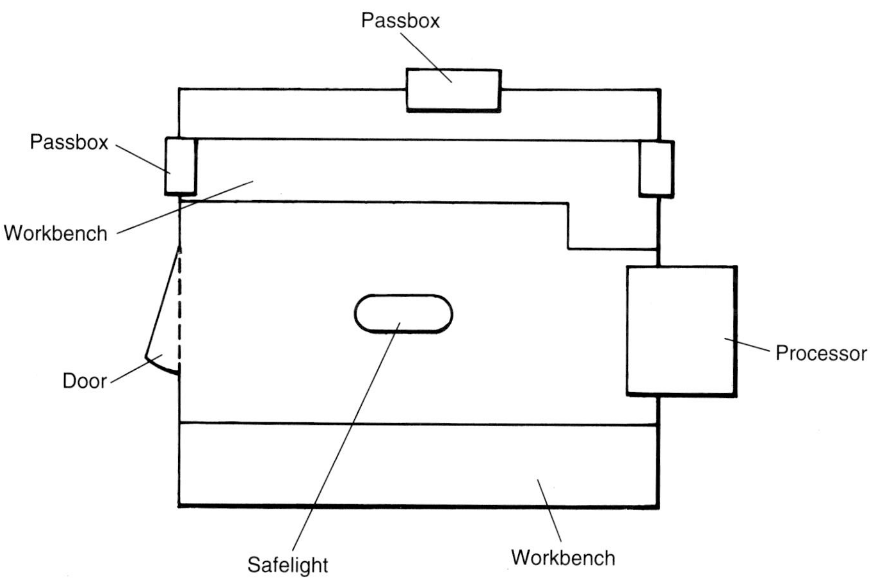

Figure 5.10. Basic design for a radiographic darkroom. The door must be light-tight. Passboxes allow films to be passed to darkroom without opening the door. The processor will usually open into a viewing area. Safelight allows enough light to work without exposing the films.

VIEWBOXES

Radiographic films are generally viewed on viewboxes (Fig. 5.12). The light source generated by a viewbox or set of viewboxes in a department must be consistent, else the films may be seen as substandard.

SPECIALIZED IMAGING EQUIPMENT AND MODALITIES

Although this text covers primarily routine ("plain-film") radiography and fluoroscopy, there are a variety of other imaging modalities that should be familar to the radiographer.

Computed Tomography

In computed tomography (CT), the emergent x-ray beam is measured by a detector array. The electrical signals produced by the detector array are converted to digital form and then processed by a computer. The computer reconstructs an image from the data, and displays the image on a cathode-ray tube. CT is non-invasive and has high contrast resolution, replacing some radiographic studies that required the use of contrast media. Another advantage of CT, and other forms of imaging using computers, is the ability to manipulate the image *after* exposing the patient.

Magnetic Resonance Imaging

Magnetic resonance imaging (MRI) allows visualization of body tissues by applying an external magnetic field. This makes it possible to distinguish between hydrogen atoms in different environments. Since the MRI image gives information about the chemical makeup of tissues, it is possible to distinguish between normal, cancerous, atherosclerotic, and traumatized tissue masses.

Digital Imaging

Mallott and Fodor (1993) describe digital radiography (also called computed radiography) as a "relatively recent introduction that allows the direct acquisition of images in a digital format." The information provided by an x-ray beam after it passes through the patient is analog (continuous) in nature; to present images digitally requires a method that can reduce those continuous data into discrete units. One such method is the photostimulable phosphor plate, an image receptor that stores the image until they are processed by a computer. Digital imaging is discussed in greater detail in Chapter 28.

Nuclear Medicine

Nuclear medicine is a branch concerned with the use of radionuclides in the diagnosis and treatment of disease. Nuclear medicine is particularly useful in demonstrating function; for example, a technique known as positron emission tomography (PET) can show the metabolic activity of the brain and heart.

Sonography

Sonography allows for the visualization of structures within the body by recording the reflections or echoes of pulses of ultrasonic waves directed into the body. Diagnostic ultrasound uses frequencies of 1 to 10 MHz (megahertz).

Ultrasound is particularly useful in obstetric and gynecologic imaging, in which exposure to ionizing radiation is a concern. It

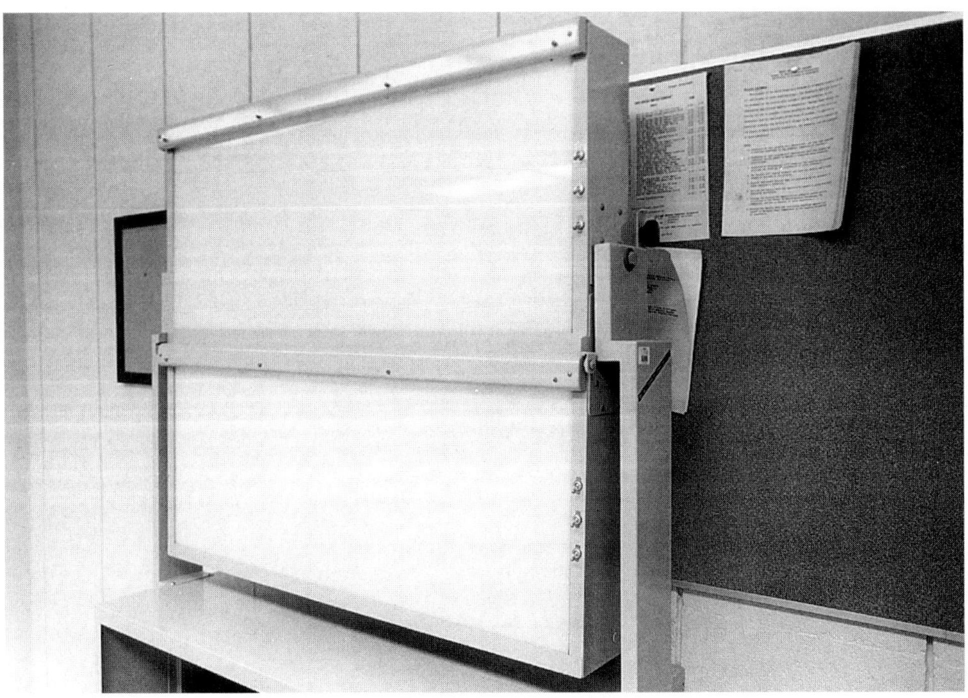

Figure 5.12. Viewbox.

can evaluate fetal size and maturity as well as the position of the fetus and the pelvis. Ultrasound also has uses in imaging of the heart and major blood vessels, size and structural changes in the abdominopelvic cavity, the evaluation of tumors, and the evaluation of foreign bodies in the eye.

COMPUTER TECHNOLOGY IN THE RADIOLOGY DEPARTMENT

Along with the previously discussed methods of imaging using digital techniques, radiology departments are becoming increasingly reliant on computer technology to run the department. Most radiology departments use a radiology information system (RIS) to run the department. Functions performed by an RIS include patient registration and tracking, film tracking, and analysis of employee productivity. Many RISs can interface with the hospital information system (HIS).

Another use of computer technology is the picture archiving and communications system (PACS), which allows all images to be stored in a digital format and allows images to be transmitted anywhere using a modem.

Bibliography

Burns EF: Radiographic Imaging: A Guide for Producing Quality Radiographs. Philadelphia: WB Saunders, 1992.
Chesney DN, Chesney MO: X-Ray Equipment for Student Radiographers. 3rd ed. London: Blackwell Scientific Publications, 1984.
Hagler M: The Pocket Rad Tech. Philadelphia: WB Saunders, 1993.
Malott JC, Fodor J III: The Art and Science of Medical Radiography. 7th ed. St. Louis: CV Mosby, 1993.
McKinney WEJ: Radiographic Processing and Quality Control. Philadelphia: JB Lippincott, 1988.
O'Toole M (ed): Miller-Keane Encyclopedia and Dictionary of Medicine, Nursing, and Allied Health. 5th ed. Philadelphia: WB Saunders, 1992.
Thompson MA, Hall J, Hattaway P, Dowd SB: Principles of Imaging Science and Protection. Philadelphia: WB Saunders, 1994.
Tortorici M: Concepts in Medical Radiographic Imaging. Philadelphia: WB Saunders, 1992.

CHAPTER 6

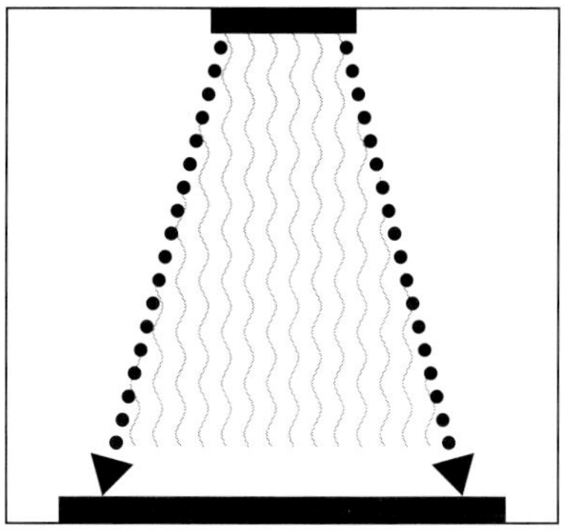

Steven B. Dowd, Ed.D., R.T.(R.)

Image Production and Technical Factor Selection

This chapter is an overview of image production and factors that influence the production of a diagnostic image. According to Burns (1992), the responsibilities of a radiographer in producing a diagnostic image are to ensure:

1. Exposure factors are adequate.
2. There has been adequate penetration of the part of interest.
3. Sufficient radiographic density and contrast are present.
4. Field size is appropriate.
5. Motion is eliminated during exposure.
6. The anatomic part is properly positioned.
7. Proper accessories have been selected.

The primary focus of this text is on aspect #6, proper positioning of the anatomic part. However, the practice of radiography requires a knowledge of all of the responsibilities listed. Each chapter contains information related to technical factor selection as well as to evaluation of the image for acceptability. The intent of this chapter is to provide background material on imaging for the chapters on positioning. Following a description of the image and properties of the image, the effects of technical factors on the image are presented. Important terms are indicated in **boldface type.** They are defined in the glossary. If their usage is still not clear, the reader is referred to a text covering imaging, such as Burns' *Radiographic Imaging: A Guide for Producing Quality Radiographs* (1992) for more information.

THE RADIOGRAPHIC IMAGE

The image produced on a film due to exposure to x-ray is called a **radiograph.** Radiographers manipulate a variety of technical factors—most notably **kilovoltage, milliamperage, time** of exposure in seconds or milliseconds, and **distance**—to produce a quality image. Figure 6.1 shows three examples of radiographs. There are two major properties of a radiograph—**photographic** and **geometric.**

Photographic Properties

The term photographic properties refers to radiographic **density** (the amount of blackness on the film) and radiographic **contrast** (differences between adjacent densities). Photographic properties make definition visible; they do not actually influence the geometry of image formation.

The primary factors affecting density are the combination of milliamperage and time (milliampere-seconds; known as **mAs**), kilovolts peak **(kVp)**, and distance. The primary factors affecting radiographic contrast are kilovoltage, **filtration, beam restriction, grids,** and **tissue thickness** and **composition,** which affect **subject contrast**; and **film, processing,** and **screens,** which affect **film contrast.**

Radiographic Density

Density refers to the amount of blackening on a film. It is the amount of **opacity** on a processed film. Opacity is an inability to be penetrated by light. In this regard, a radiograph is similar to an overhead transparency used in classroom instruction, in that dark areas do not allow light to pass through, whereas the clear areas do, forming a type of image. The amount of exposure reaching the film determines the amount of density on the processed radiograph. The controlling factor for density is mAs.

Theoretically, mAs *is* mAs. That is, the combinations of mA and time are unimportant so long as the mAs values are the same. Thus, 100 mA at 0.1 second is the same as 200 mA at 0.05 second as both are 10 mAs. However, with extremely long (6 seconds) and extremely short exposure times (less than 10 msec), the reciprocity law does not hold true with intensifying screens. This is called **reciprocity law failure.**

Measuring density on a film is termed **densitometry.** Density is measured through the formula:

$$\text{Optical density} = \text{Log}_{10} \frac{\text{Incident light intensity}}{\text{Transmitted light intensity}}$$

The **incident light** refers to the light that passes through the viewbox; **transmitted light** refers to the intensity of light from the film. On a clear film, 100 percent of light would be transmitted through a film and the density value would be 0.0. As density is based on $\log_{10}$, a density of 1.0 means that 10 percent of the light has been transmitted through the film, 2.0 = 1 percent, and 3.0 = 0.1 percent.

The diagnostic range varies depending on the text consulted. Most commonly, 0.25 to 2.0 is given. This means that the useful densities for a film range from 0.25 to 2.0.

Three factors can be used to manipulate the density on a radiograph. The primary factor is mAs. There is a linear, direct proportion of radiographic density and mAs. Thus, doubling mAs doubles density. kVp can also be used to control density, as a 15 percent change in kVp will halve or double density. It is not a preferred change in most cases because it also influences scale of contrast. Distance can also be used, but this is a rare choice because distance changes must be calculated according to the inverse square law and this also affects geometric properties of the image.

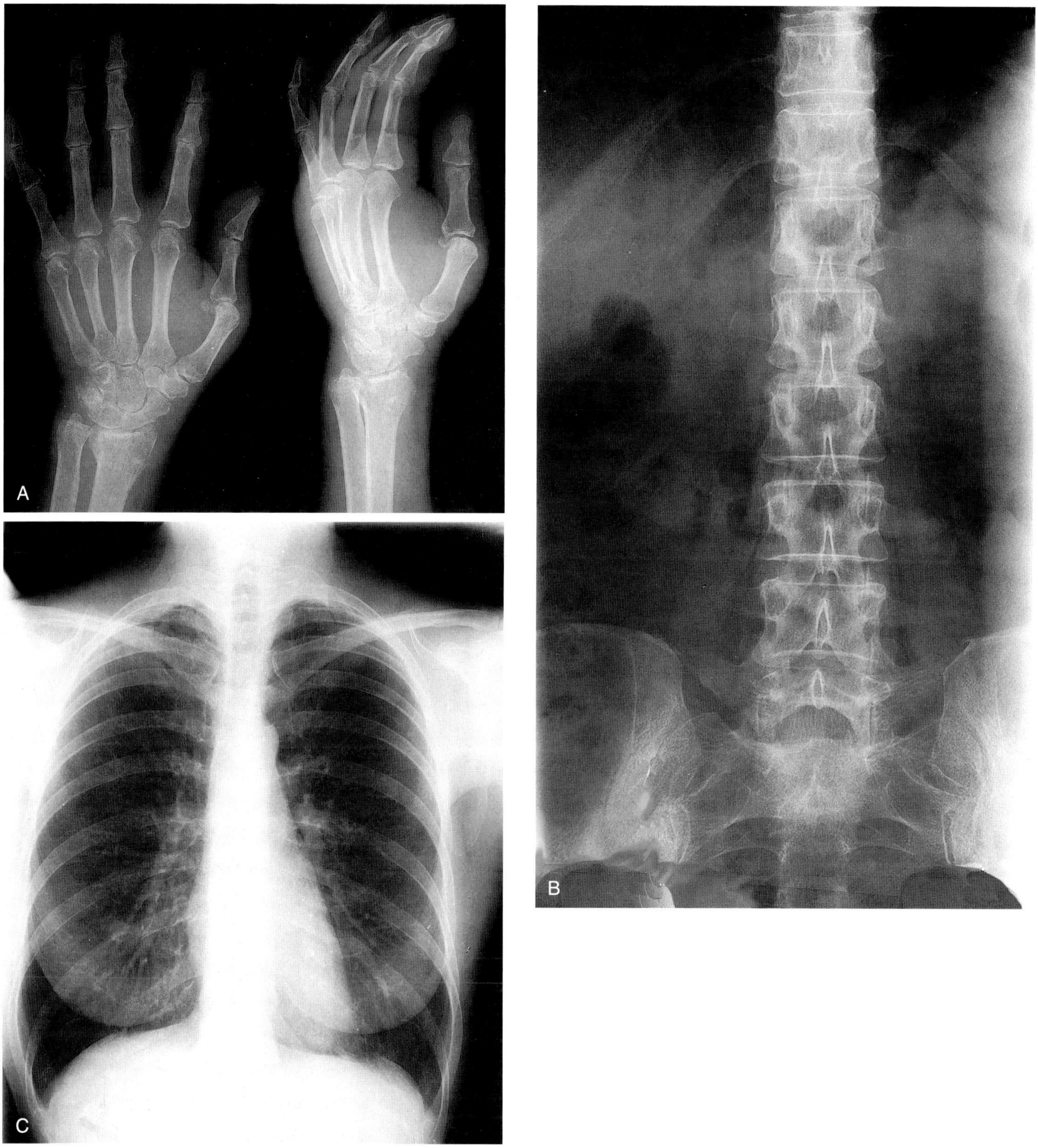

Figure 6.1 Three radiographs: A, hand; B, lumbar spine; C, chest.

Radiographic Contrast

Density alone will not produce an image; obviously there must be differences in density for an image (Fig. 6.2). The function of contrast is to make detail visible. The primary factor controlling contrast is the penetrating ability of the beam (kVp).

There are two basic types of contrast. **Film contrast** is the difference between adjacent radiographic densities based on the response of a given x-ray film emulsion type to exposure and processing. **Subject contrast** is the result of attenuation (absorption) of the x-ray beam by differences in tissue composition. The term radiolucent refers to objects that allow x-rays to easily penetrate. The term radiopaque refers to objects that attenuate or absorb much of the beam.

Exposure latitude is the range of exposures that may be used to obtain a radiograph demonstrating acceptable visibility of image detail. It is associated with subject contrast in that when high kVp is used, **low** or **long-scale contrast** results (many shades of gray), giving a wide exposure latitude. This gives the radiographer a greater margin of error in technique selection. The opposite is also true—low kVp is associated with **high-** or **short-scale contrast** (blacks and whites), giving a narrow exposure latitude (Fig. 6.3).

Geometric Properties

Geometric properties are factors related to the geometry of image formation that affect the actual **recorded detail** instead of visibility of detail. The term **definition** refers to the clarity and **sharpness** of the image. The opposite of definition and sharpness is the **unsharpness** of the image. Burns lists the characteristics of definition as recorded detail, **distortion,** and **visibility of detail.** These terms are sometimes vague, sometimes confusing, and often used interchangeably by practitioners and text authors.

Recorded Detail

Penumbra refers to the area of image unsharpness, whereas **umbra** refers to the sharpness of image details (Fig. 6.4). The principal factors affecting the geometric properties of image formation are: **focal spot size, focal-film distance,** and **object-film distance,** which affect **geometric unsharpness; film-screen contact** and **phosphor layer thickness,** which affect **screen unsharpness;** tube movement, object movement, and film movement, which affect **motion unsharpness;** object-film distance and focal film distance, which affect **size distortion;** and alignment of tube, object, and film, which affects **shape distortion.**

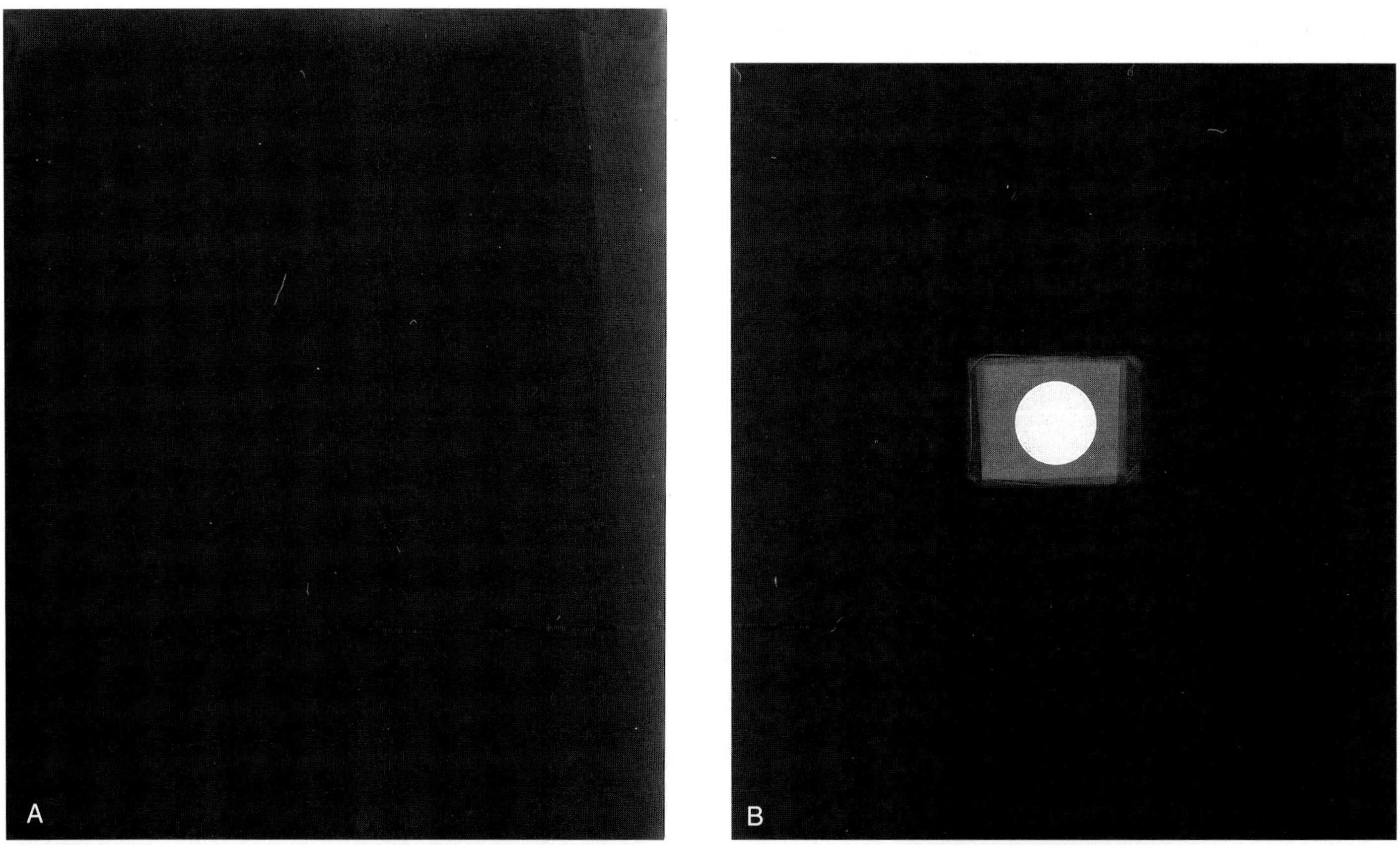

Figure 6.2 A, A radiograph with density (blackness) only. B, A radiograph of a coin embedded in a block of paraffin wax, showing low density at the paraffin and no density at the coin.

The three basic components of unsharpness are:

- Geometric unsharpness is defined as the unsharpness in a radiographic image due to the relative distance between the focal spot, object being radiographed, and film.
- Screen unsharpness is a result of phosphor thickness of intensifying screens or of poor screen-film contact. Faster-speed screens tend to have a thicker screen layer, except for rare earth screens.
- Motion unsharpness is the loss of recorded detail in a radiographic image as a result of movement of the x-ray tube, patient, or recording medium. It is controlled by immobilization techniques or short exposure times, or both. Involuntary motion of organs can only be controlled by short exposure times.

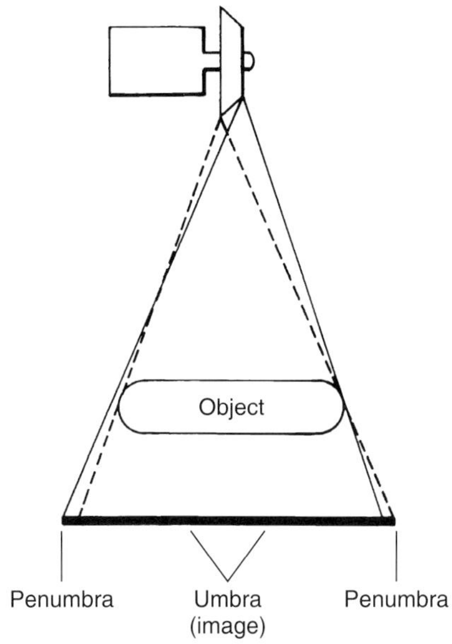

Figure 6.4 This shows the formation of umbra (the image) and penumbra (surrounding unsharpness).

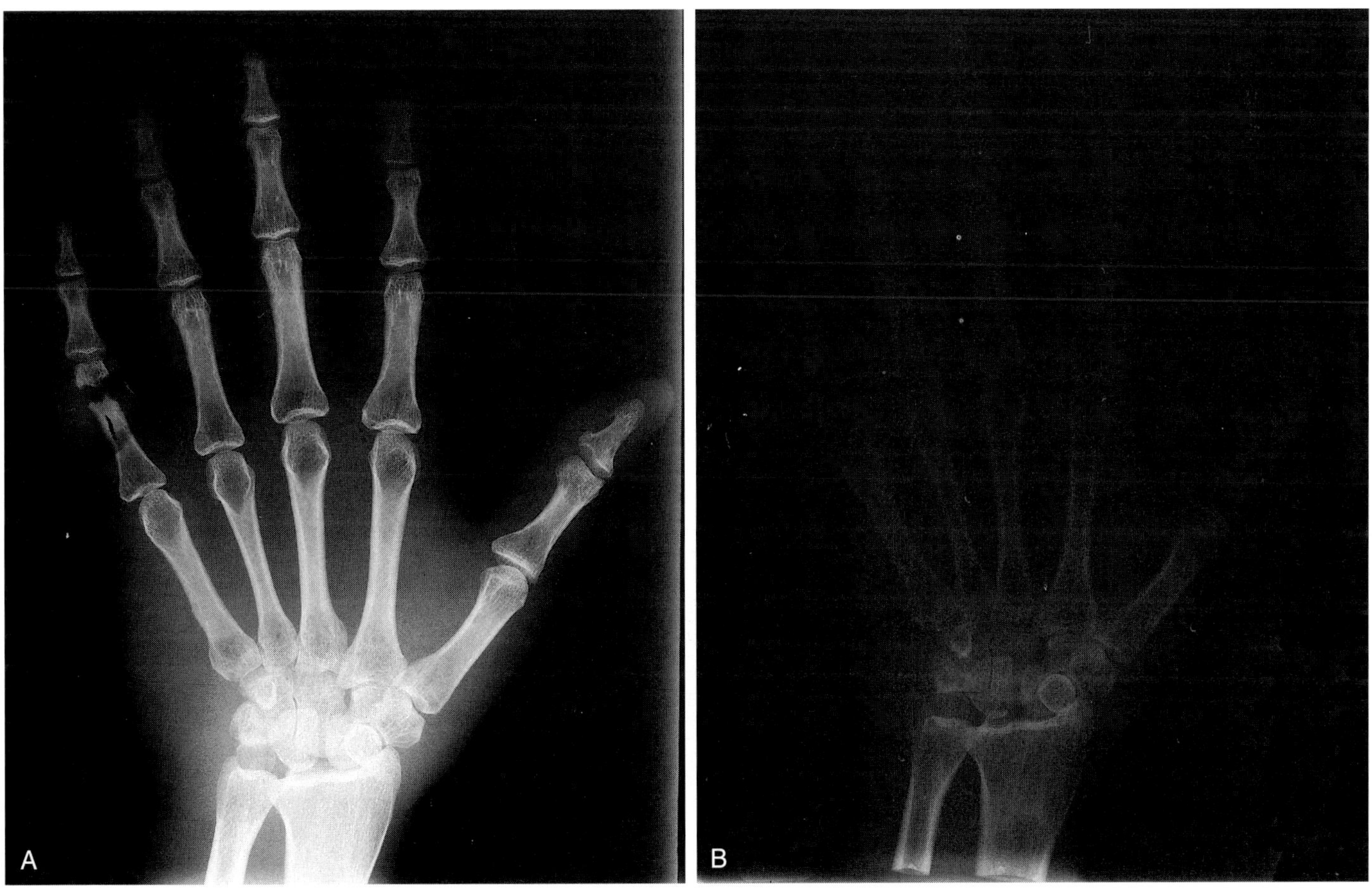

Figure 6.3 Two radiographs of a hand. A, At 40 kVP (kilovolts peak), shows mostly black and white; B, at 65 kVp, shows a greater range of densities for a longer scale of contrast.

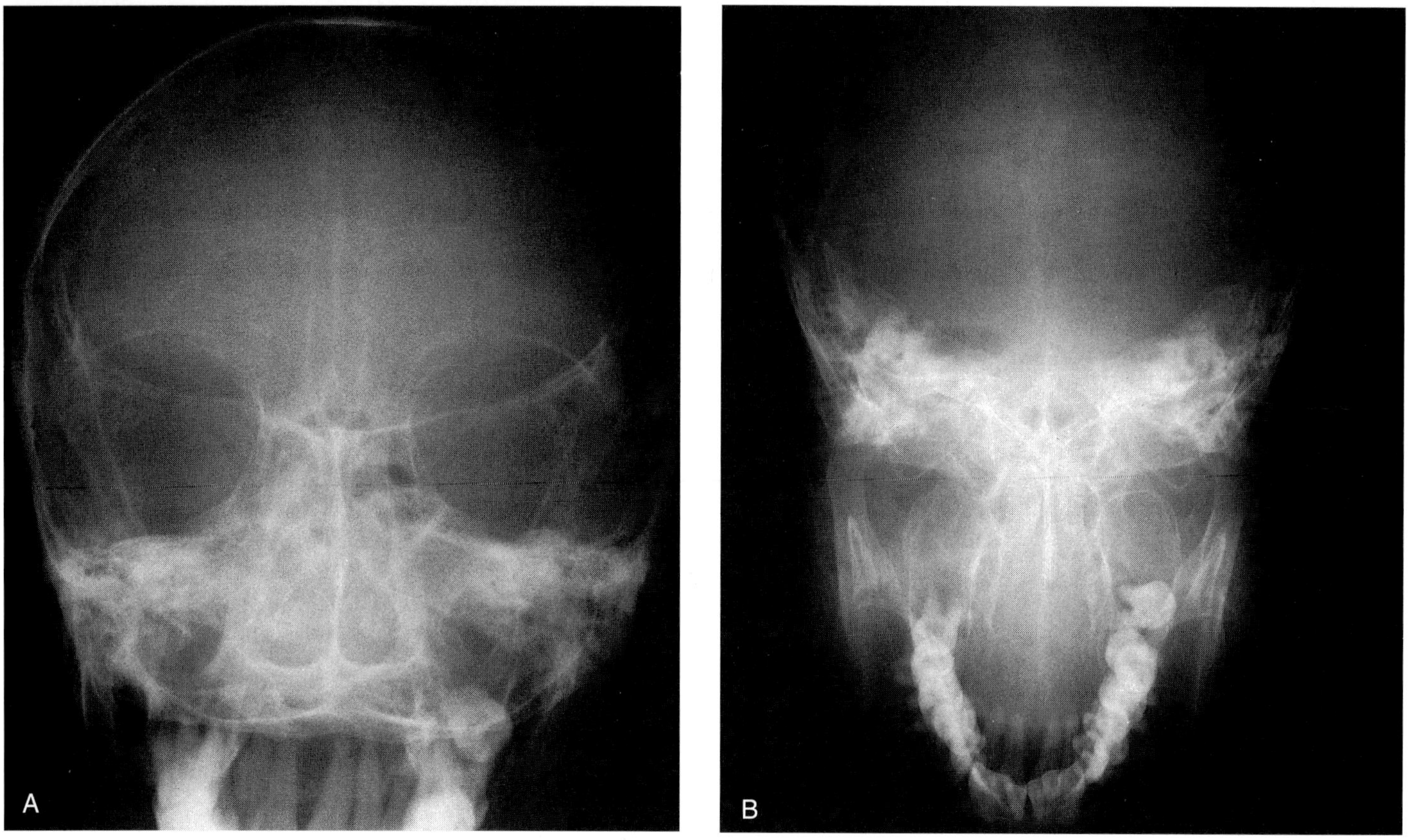

Figure 6.5 A, A regular anteroposterior (AP) radiograph of a skull. B, A posteroanterior (PA) axial radiograph of the same part using tube angulation to advantage.

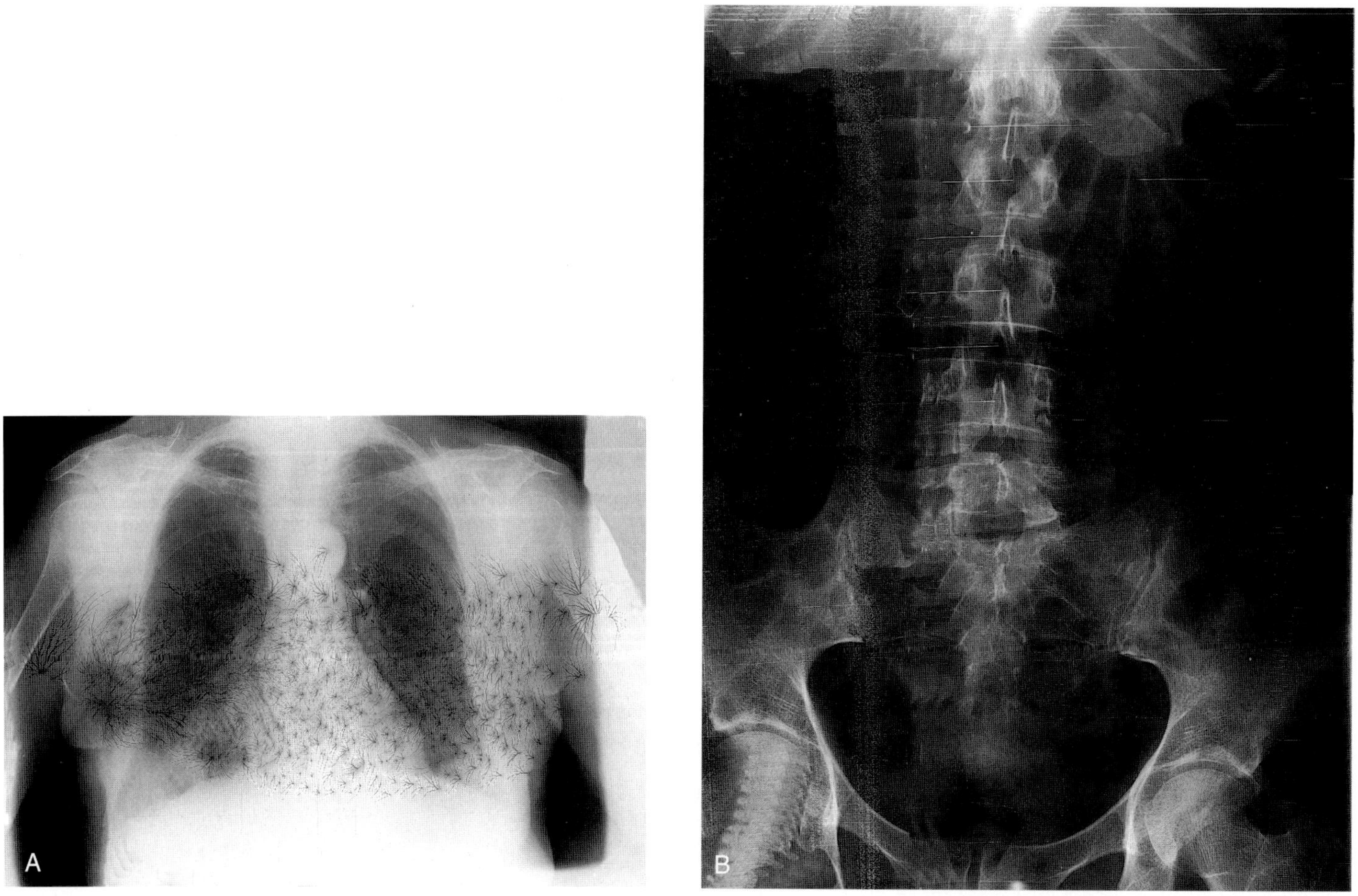

Figure 6.6 Film artifacts. A, Static (sensitized); B, scratches (non-sensitized).

Distortion of Image Details

Size distortion is the radiographic enlargement of the actual size of the structural details of the radiographic image due to increased object-film, decreased focus-to-object, or decreased focal-film distance. It decreases sharpness of the image by increasing the penumbral effect.

Shape distortion is the misrepresentation of the true image through foreshortening or elongation of the structural details of the radiographic image. Sometimes this is used to advantage, as in the PA semiaxial projection of the skull (Fig. 6.5).

PERCEPTUAL PROPERTIES OF IMAGE QUALITY

Radiographic Noise

An **artifact** is anything other than patient anatomy that was not intentionally meant to be imaged on the radiograph. Thus, patient pathology might be an "unwelcome surprise," but it is *not* an artifact. Artifacts are classified as sensitized, nonsensitized, or physical (Fig. 6.6).

Quantum mottle (Fig. 6.7) is a form of noise or unwanted information due to two factors. First, x-ray beams use multiple energies. Also, screens use light rather than x-ray, only to expose a film. Light produced across a screen is not always uniform. Using a fast imaging system with a high kVp and a low mAs can produce sufficient mottle to obscure recorded detail.

Figure 6.7 Quantum mottle on a computed radiograph.

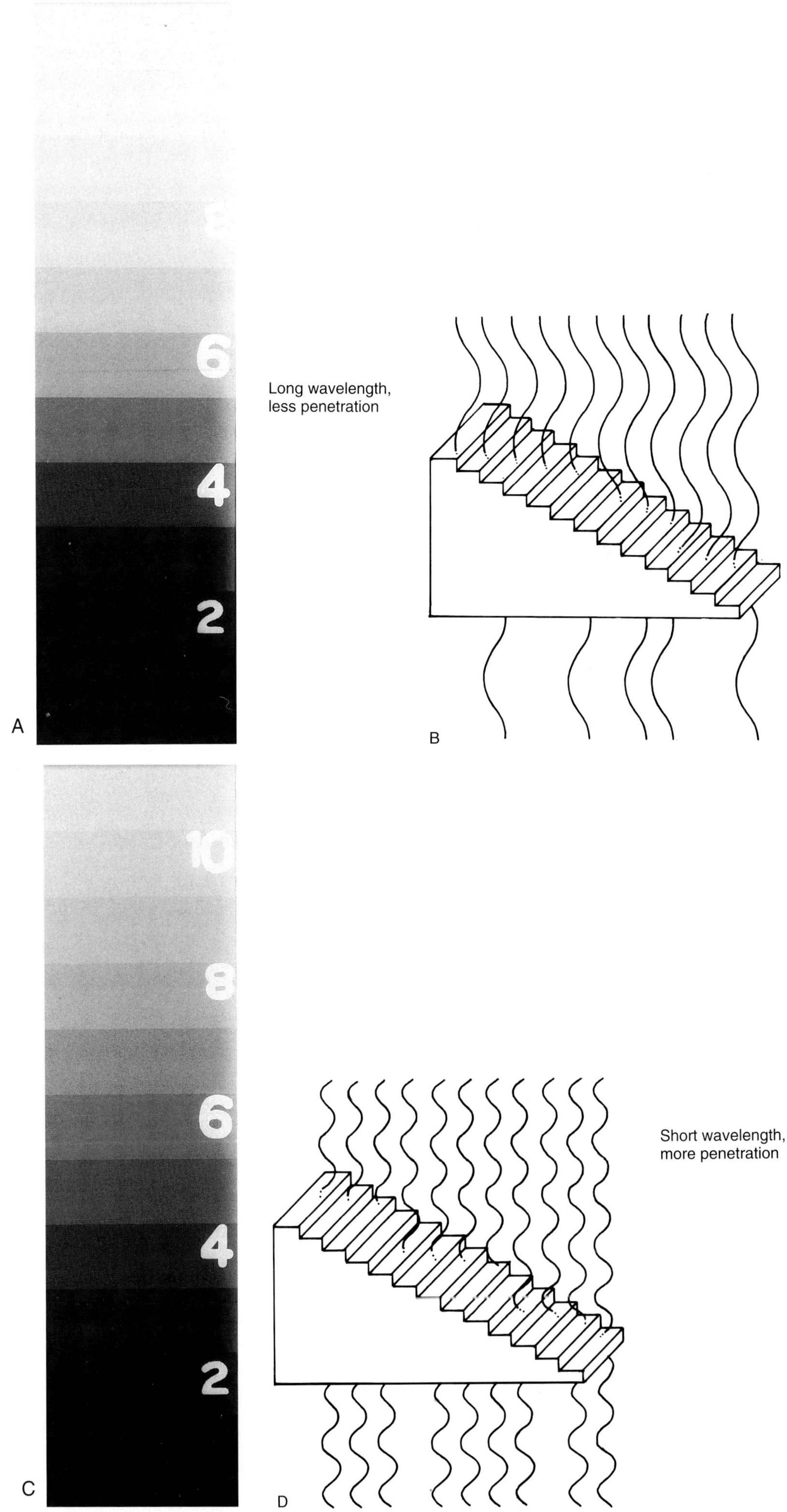

Figure 6.8 *A* and *B*, A lower-energy beam with longer wavelength and less penetration. *C* and *D*, A lower-energy beam with shorter wavelength and more penetration.

Viewing Conditions

Sight, environment, distance, and display format are important considerations for viewing conditions. A radiologist's viewbox may be brighter than the one in the departmental viewing room. Also, individuals have their own subjective view of image quality. There is no one perfect film—this is a value judgment.

Evaluating Radiographic Quality

Radiographic quality should be evaluated on three primary criteria: Radiographic, geometric, and perceptual. This subject is covered in greater detail in the next chapter.

Some reasons why a radiograph might be repeated are:

1. Patient motion or excessive size distortion.
2. Machine failure.
3. Tube-part-film misalignment.
4. Processor failure.
5. Excessive overexposure or underexposure.
6. Obscured anatomy owing to positioning errors.
7. When an artifact might be suspected pathology.

Reasons why radiographs should *not* be repeated are:

1. No evidence of gonadal shielding.
2. Wrong film size (too large) used.
3. Radiograph incorrectly marked.
4. Improper orientation of views.

These are all compromises of effective patient care, but repeating a radiograph under these conditions will only further compromise patient care through excess radiation exposure.

THE EFFECT OF KILOVOLTAGE ON THE RADIOGRAPH

kVp is the abbreviation for kilovolts peak. Increasing kVp will result in x-rays of shorter wavelength, higher frequency, and deeper penetration (Fig. 6.8). An increase in kVp will increase radiographic density. It is not the primary factor to be used in increasing density because it will also affect scale of contrast.

Contrast refers to differences in densities on the radiograph. Contrast scale will be heightened by decreasing kVp (a shorter scale of contrast, or more blacks and whites). A higher kVp will give a longer scale of contrast (more grays in the image).

Kilovoltage directly affects the exposure latitude. This means that at a higher kVp, there is a greater tolerance for mAs variations, or ability to make an error in selecting mAs. Thus, at a high kVp, exposure latitude is wide.

kVp does not affect recorded detail, size distortion, or shape distortion.

THE EFFECT OF MILLIAMPERE–SECONDS ON THE RADIOGRAPH

The combination of mA and time (mAs) affects the number of photons produced. Thus, if 20 mAs produces a number of photons (x), 40 mAs will produce twice as many photons (2x). Doubling the number of photons by doubling the mAs will also double the density on a film (Fig. 6.9). Thus, a film will appear twice as dense after doubling mAs, or will appear half as dense after halving the mAs. There is a direct relationship between mAs and image density; any change in mAs will have the corresponding effect on image density.

mAs does not affect recorded detail, size distortion, or shape distortion.

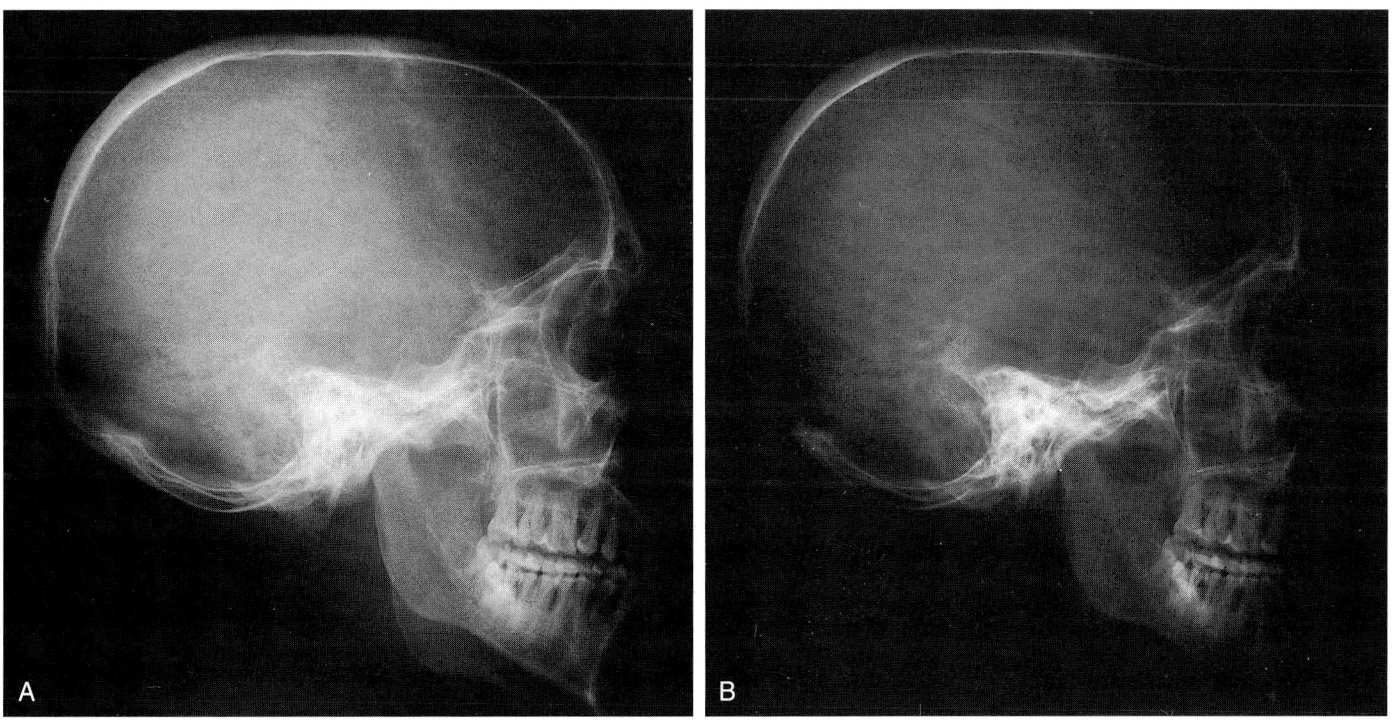

Figure 6.9 From A to B, the effect on a radiograph of doubling mAs (milliampere-seconds).

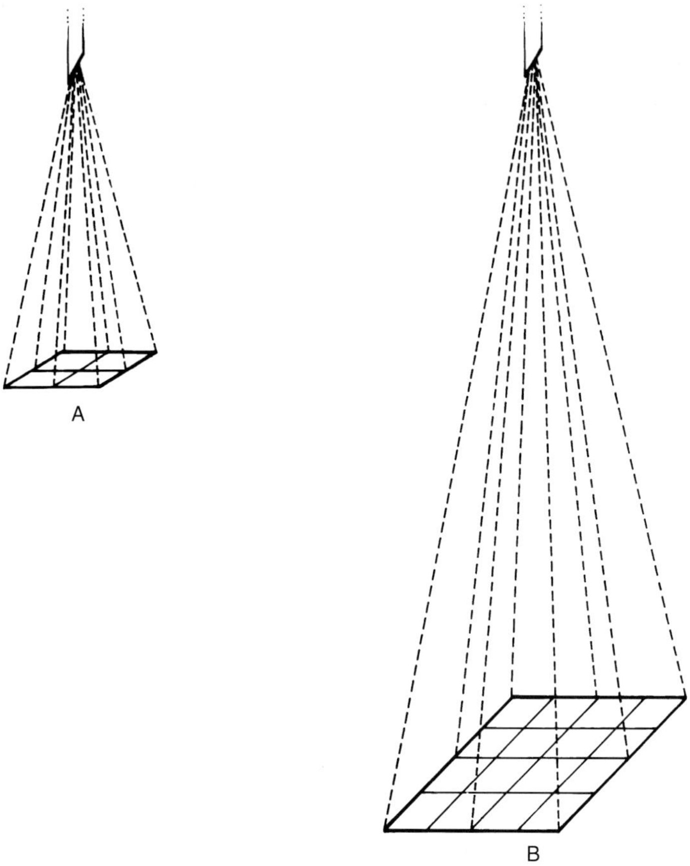

Figure 6.10 Illustration of inverse square law. Doubling the distance (e.g., from 20 to 40 inches) spreads radiation over four times as great an area. This reduces beam intensity to one-fourth the original value.

THE EFFECT OF DISTANCE ON THE RADIOGRAPH

There are two forms of distance. **Focal-film distance,** or **FFD** (also called **source-to–image receptor distance** or **SID**) refers to the distance from the focal spot (source) of the x-ray tube to the film. The distance from the object being imaged to the film is the **object-film distance** or **OFD** (also called **object-to–image receptor distance** or **OID**).

Inverse Square Law

If SID is doubled from a point source of radiation such as an x-ray tube, the intensity of radiation (as measured in roentgens) decreases by one fourth (Fig. 6.10). If distance is halved, intensity increases by a factor of 4. This is known as the **inverse square law:**

$$\frac{I_1}{I_2} = \left(\frac{D_2}{D_1}\right)^2$$

I_1 = first intensity D_1 = first distance
I_2 = second intensity D_2 = second distance

Thus, as distance is changed, the amount of radiation is changed *not* in exact proportion, but by the *inverse* of the square. The two most common distances used in radiography are 40 inches and 72 inches. Their relationship according to the inverse square law is 3.24. This means that:

1. If distance is changed from 40 to 72 inches, *increase* mAs (to compensate for the loss in intensity) by 3.24 (multiply by 3.24).
2. If distance is changed from 72 to 40 inches, *decrease* mAs by 3.24 (divide by 3.24).

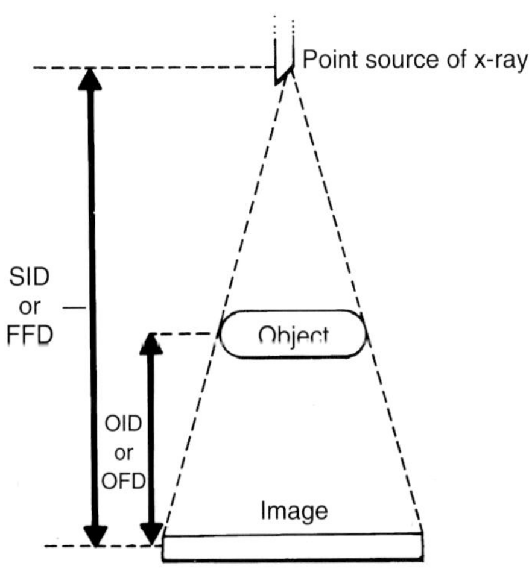

Figure 6.11 Diagram showing how projected object will increase in size because of source-to-image receptor distance (SID) and object-to-image receptor distance (OID).

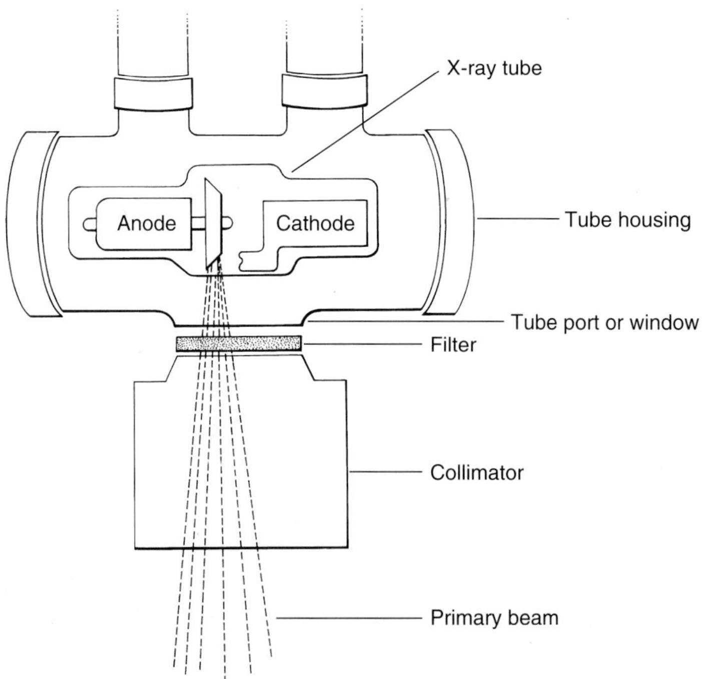

Figure 6.12 X-ray tube, tube housing, and collimator illustrating placement of filter designed to remove low-energy radiation.

Air Gap Technique

The **air gap** is an alternative to the use of a grid. It uses a 6- to 10-inch gap between the patient and the film. This takes advantage of the fact that scatter radiation will not travel in a straight line, whereas the primary beam will. Special techniques such as angiography and, in some cases, chest radiography make use of the air gap to improve image quality.

Magnification

All radiographs show an increase in the size of the image, known as **magnification.** As SID increases, magnification decreases. As OID increases, magnification increases (Fig. 6.11). Thus, the ideal situation for optimum radiographic quality is a long SID and a short OID. This is expressed as:

$$\text{Magnification} = \frac{\text{SID}}{\text{SID} - \text{OID}}$$

THE EFFECT OF FOCAL SPOT SIZE ON THE RADIOGRAPH

The focal spot is the area of the x-ray target actually hit by electrons. Most x-ray tubes have a large and a small focal spot. The smaller the focal spot size, the greater the image sharpness. Owing to the amount of heat produced by high mA's, high mA stations (usually 200 and above) require use of a large focal spot. Some assume that, since larger mA stations require the large focal spot, focal spot size influences density. In actuality, focal spot size will not affect density, contrast, size, or shape distortion.

THE EFFECT OF FILTRATION ON THE RADIOGRAPH

Collimator Filtration

Filtration refers to the use of metal filters placed in the path of the x-ray beam to eliminate low-energy photons (Fig. 6.12). Filters protect the patient from excessive radiation exposure, especially on the skin. Increasing the thickness of a filter requires an increase in exposure factors, especially kVp.

Compensating Filters

Compensating filters are placed between the tube and the part. Their function is to provide a more even distribution of the beam to parts, such as the foot, that do not have an even distribution of tissue. A **wedge filter** is a type of compensating filter in which the thick part of the filter is placed over the thinnest part of the anatomy (Fig. 6.13).

THE EFFECT OF BEAM RESTRICTION ON THE RADIOGRAPH

Beam restriction refers to limiting the size or area of the beam (Fig. 6.14 shows the use of **collimation** to limit the size of the beam). This is the most effective means of reducing **scatter** to the film. As the size of the field decreases, scatter radiation decreases, as does density, and a shorter scale of contrast is produced. Beam restriction improves the visibility of detail *and* reduces patient dose.

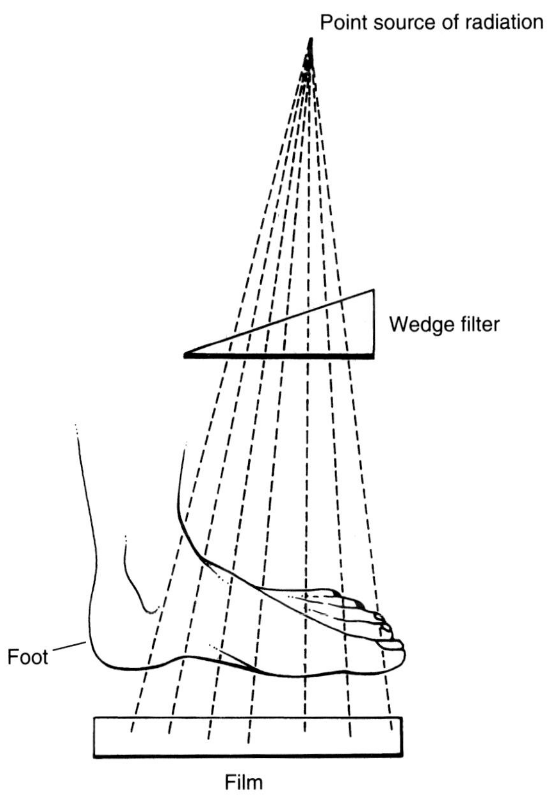

Figure 6.13 Compensating (wedge) filter used in foot radiography. The thin portion of the foot (toes) is placed under the thick end of the filter to compensate for the decreased tissue density.

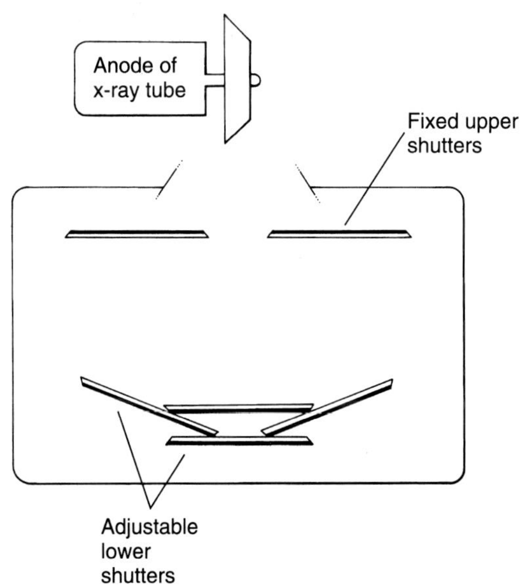

Figure 6.14 Use of collimation for beam limitation. The upper shutters are fixed; the lower shutters can be adjusted to increase or decrease beam size.

THE EFFECT OF ALIGNMENT OF TUBE, OBJECT, AND FILM ON THE RADIOGRAPH

Proper alignment of tube, object (part), and film minimizes distortion. Improper alignment can result in magnification, elongation, and foreshortening (Fig. 6.15).

THE EFFECT OF THE PATIENT ON THE RADIOGRAPH

The structure and composition of body tissue can affect density by changing the attenuation of the beam. This can be additive, meaning that technical factors must be increased, or destructive, meaning that technical factors must be decreased. Each chapter describes how pathology can alter positioning of the patient or technical factor selection. Also, body habitus differences such as obesity will produce radiographs with a longer scale of contrast. Tissue filled with gas or air will show greater contrast (shorter scale).

Grids

Grids are used to decrease the density on the film that is produced by scatter radiation (Fig. 6.16). This improves image quality. Using a grid will require an increase in exposure factors to maintain density owing to the added absorption of radiation. Grids are made by placing many lead strips vertically or slanted. They have a radiolucent interspacing. A Potter-Bucky diaphragm, also known simply as a Bucky, is a type of grid that moves. This eliminates the grid lines seen with a stationary grid.

Grids are selected by grid ratio (a measure of the height of the lead strip to the width of the interspace material) according to part thickness and exposure factors used. In general, grids are used for body parts in excess of 10 cm.

THE EFFECT OF FILM AND SCREENS ON THE RADIOGRAPH

As the speed of the film-screen system increases, the amount of radiation needed to expose the film decreases. As the speed of the screen increases, the greater the contrast (shorter scale). The greater the resolving power of the imaging system, the greater the recorded detail. Resolving power is greatest in slower-speed screens.

THE EFFECT OF MOTION ON THE RADIOGRAPH

Motion will result in image blur (Fig. 6.17). This is usually prevented through patient instruction or immobilization. It is also possible to have movement of the tube housing or the image receptor, although this is rare.

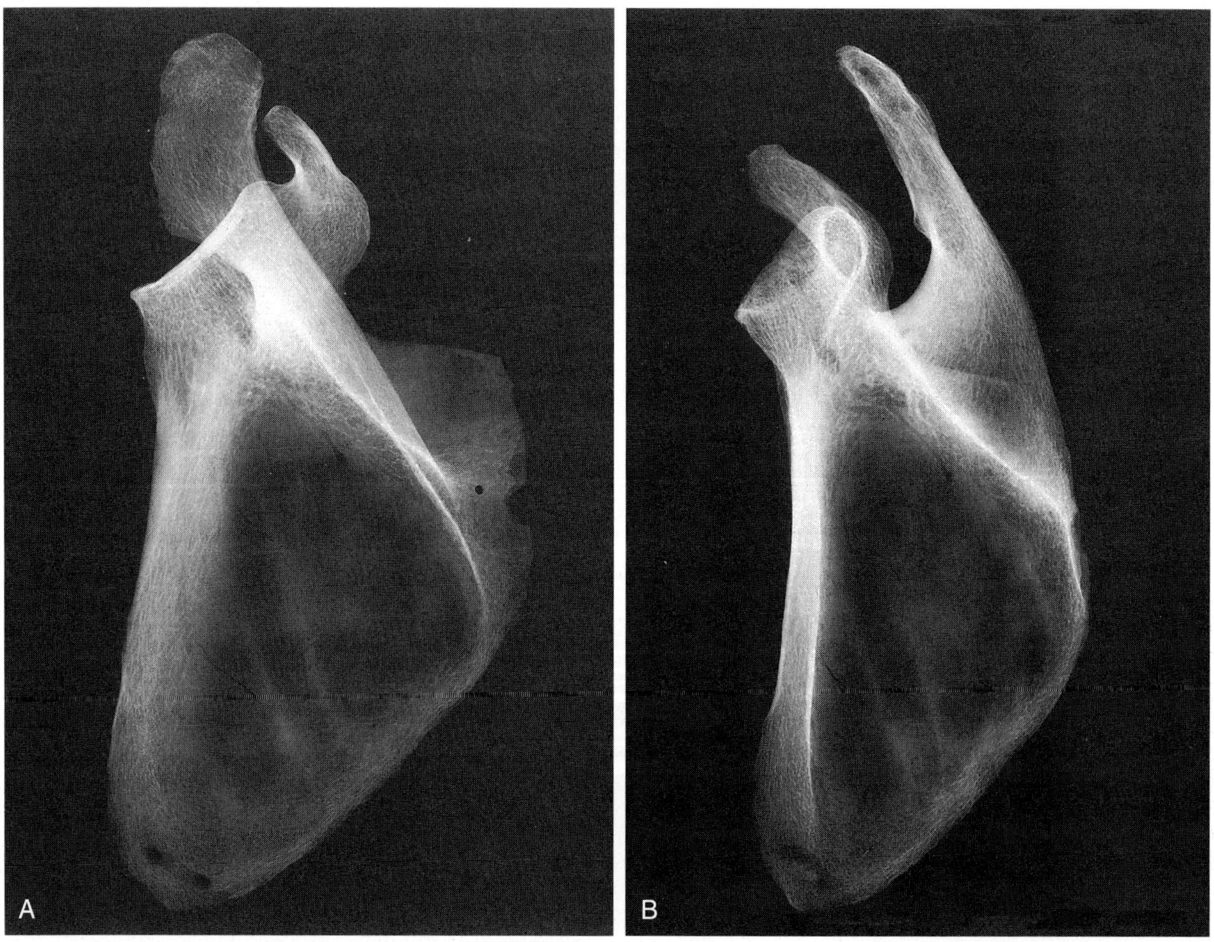

Figure 6.15 A and B, Foreshortening of a part owing to part angulation.

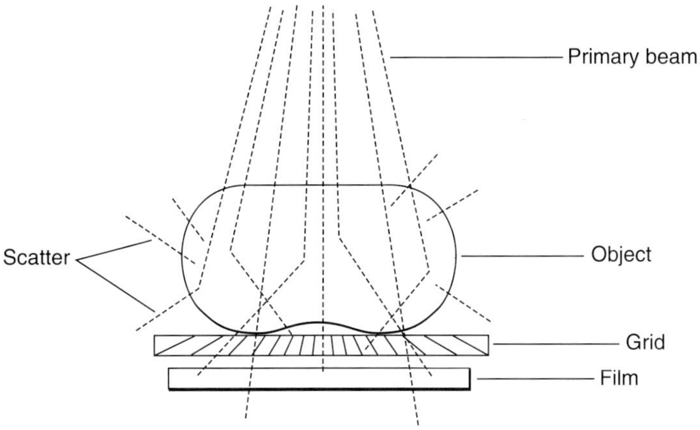

Figure 6.16 Elimination of scatter (unfocused radiation) with a grid. Note that this grid has angled the strips to compensate for the divergence of the primary beam.

THE EFFECT OF FILM PROCESSING ON RADIOGRAPHIC QUALITY

Processing an exposed x-ray film changes the **latent image** (which is not visible) to a **visible image**. Processing involves **development, fixation, washing,** and **drying**. Development is the process that actually makes the image visible. Fixation neutralizes the developer and hardens the emulsion of the film. The most important aspect of processing is maintaining control of time and temperature.

Increases in developer time or temperature increase radiographic density. The time-temperature relationship can also affect film contrast. If developer temperature is too high, fog results (Fig. 6.18). Underdevelopment owing to insufficient time or temperature can also prevent the film from building an adequate scale of contrast.

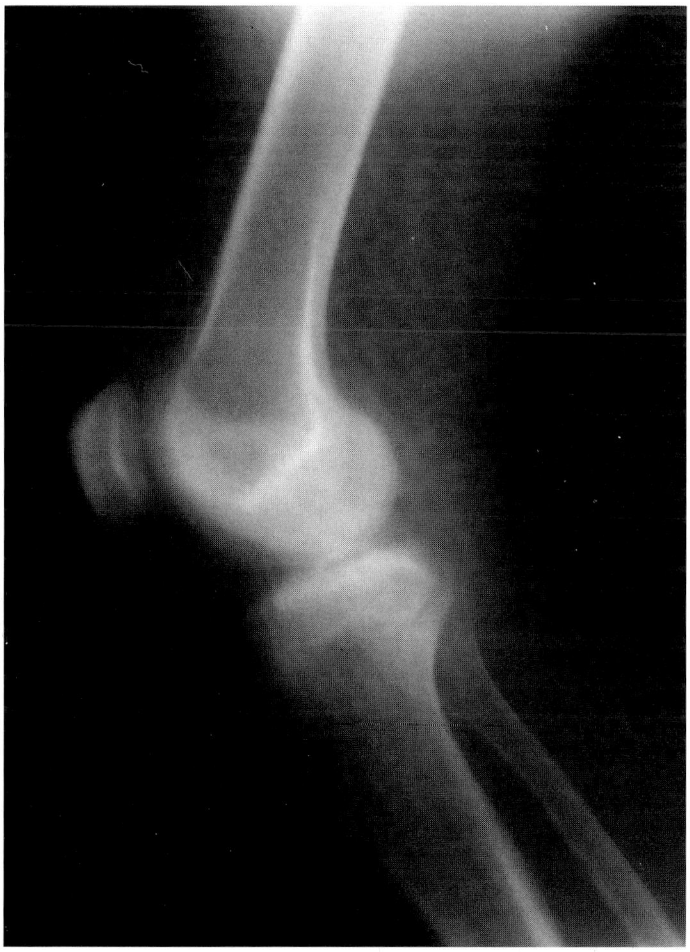

Figure 6.17 Motion unsharpness.

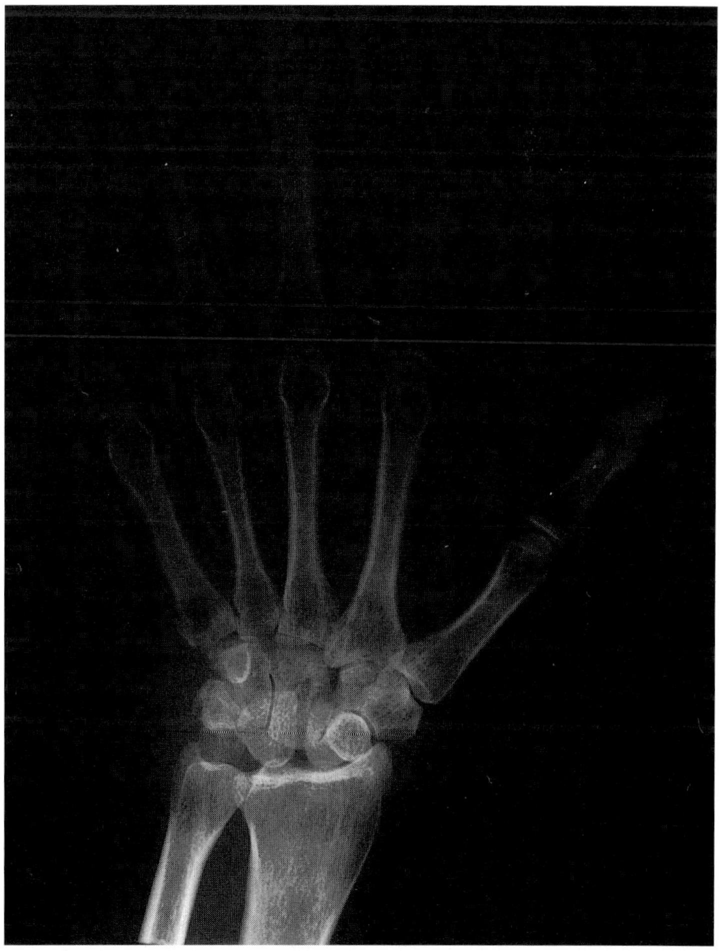

Figure 6.18 Fog due to increased developer temperature.

CONCLUSION

A variety of factors affect the image. Many of these are manipulated by the radiographer, who also is responsible for the evaluation of film quality. Although the focus of this text is on patient positioning, these concepts are important for a holistic understanding of the imaging process.

Bibliography

Burns EF: Radiographic Imaging: A Guide for Producing Quality Radiographs. Philadelphia: WB Saunders, 1992.

Bushong SC: Radiologic Science for Technologists. 5th ed. St. Louis: CV Mosby, 1993.

Carroll Q: Fuchs's Principles of Radiographic Exposure, Processing, and Quality Control. 3rd ed. Springfield, IL: Charles C Thomas, 1985.

Cullinan A: Producing Quality Radiographs. Philadelphia: JB Lippincott, 1987.

CHAPTER 7

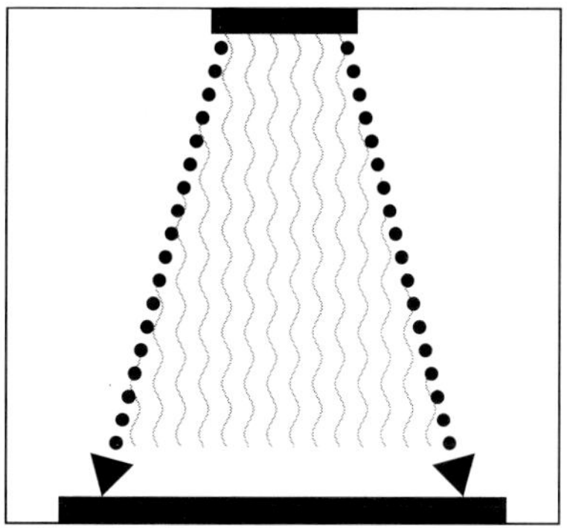

Radiographic Film Evaluation

Nobuo Sato

Masayuki Watanabe

Kazuo Matsutani

Shu Iizuka

Steven B. Dowd, Ed.D., R.T.(R.)

Bettye G. Wilson, M.A.Ed., R.T.(R.), R.D.M.S.

Radiographers are autonomous professionals, working for radiologists and as patient advocates rather than under the direct supervision of physicians. One aspect of this role is the independent production of a diagnostic image. Radiographers must understand the needs of radiologists in order to produce a film of diagnostic quality. This is a delicate balance, and requires a methodology for radiographic film critique (also called film evaluation) that:

1. Defines the relationship between radiology and radiography.
2. Defines film critique as a process.
3. Sets standards for acceptable radiographs.

THE RELATIONSHIP BETWEEN RADIOLOGY AND RADIOGRAPHY

Radiology is the detection and diagnosis of disease and injury from images of anatomic structures and physiologic and metabolic processes in the body. These images are visual patterns that reveal information about the underlying conditions of health, disease, and injury to the patient. For optimum conversion of patterns into information, images should be presented in a manner closely matched to the sensitivity characteristics of the human visual system.

New technology can of course improve the quality of images. One means by which technology development improved the imaging process in a measurable way was the development of image intensification for fluoroscopy. Prior to this, radiologists had to dark-adapt to view the dim fluoroscopic screen, which gave off no more light than that in a dimmed movie theater. Phototopic visual acuity (day vision) is so different from scotopic or night vision that it can be considered a separate visual system.

In general, the medical imaging process is highly inefficient. For example, Tuddenham found that the image conversion efficiency of fluoroscopy (number of photons generated in relationship to number of photons used by the brain to interpret images) was 0.00005 percent. Although techniques such as digital imaging hold obvious great potential in improving the diagnostic process, it is not known which images are of greatest value to the radiologist. In some cases, physicians have been known to not accept newer methods of imaging because they are so different from custom. The human abilities of the radiographer to provide a diagnostic image are currently of greater value than technology.

Radiology is a difficult discipline to learn. Along with knowledge requirements, the student must learn at a personal level how to arrive at radiologic diagnoses. This is currently done in an apprenticeship system (residency), an extremely inefficient process that cannot be replaced until we better understand the cognitive processes involved in doing radiology.

Radiography is a similarly difficult discipline to learn. Much of this profession is also still taught in an apprenticeship system (clinical experience) in which the student learns how to by actually doing radiography. Thus, many students learn the art of film critique by observing experienced radiographers practice this skill. It is often difficult for radiographers to explain this intuitive process to students.

In their text *Principles of Radiographic Imaging: An Art and a Science,* Carlton and Adler (1992) state:

> *Radiographers should strive toward developing an understanding of the perceptual problems that radiologists encounter when attempting to interpret radiographic images. Through this understanding the radiographer can work toward producing images that provide maximum assistance to the radiologist in the diagnostic process.*

Pattern recognition in terms of diagnosing pathology is the domain of the radiologist, who has the requisite medical knowledge to be competent in this area. The radiographer's skill in terms of pattern recognition lies in determining to what extent the image is of value to the radiologist. There are obviously gray areas here. For example, what knowledge of pathology must a radiographer possess in order to be able to effectively critique the image in terms of technical factors?

FILM CRITIQUE IN RADIOGRAPHY

The art of film critique is the application of science to image production and subsequent evaluation. This process seems at times, especially to students who have learned only "facts" relevant to radiography, to be unscientific. However, more often it is simply a matter of the radiographer, having internalized the theory, now applying it in a manner that works well in a practice setting. Similarly, the radiologist's skill in interpreting images seems at times to be almost magical. In reality it is an intuitive application of science matched with experience.

Film critiquing is defined by Carlton and Adler (1992) as "an analytical process that involves many of the steps involved in diagnostic decision making." Meschan and Ott (1984) describe nine basic roentgen signs that the radiologist observer uses to determine pathology:

1. Alterations in size of organ.
2. Alterations in number.
3. Changes in density.
4. Changes in shape from normal.
5. Changes in position from normal.
6. Changes in internal and external environment.
7. Alterations in organ functioning.
8. Changes with respect to time (sequential radiographs).
9. Changes due to treatment.

These are certainly all areas in which the radiographer must have some knowledge. If the radiographer is not able to ascertain when an organ differs in position from the normal, unnecessary repeat radiographs will result. Many portable technologists must regularly evaluate whether changes seen in the regular 6 AM chest radiograph are the result of technical problems, such as improper part-film-beam alignment, or new pathology.

The primary factors of an effective film critique as described by Carlton and Adler are: first the image is classified in terms of acceptability. Then the cause of the problem must be determined: whether it is (1) a technical factor problem in terms of a photographic problem with visibility of detail or a geometric problem with detail; (2) a procedural factor problem in terms of patient positioning (tube, part, or film alignment) or patient preparation; or (3) an equipment malfunction problem. Finally, corrective action is recommended.

Visual Perception in Terms of Image Diagnosis

Visual perception must be understood in order to have a complete grasp of film critique. Hendee proposes three models to describe the human visual system. First, there is the signal-to-noise ratio, which describes the observer's ability to extract simple signals from a uniform visual background. Then, there is the computational model, which proposes that visual stimuli are rapidly assembled into first a "primal sketch," which is then refined into a complete image. Finally, the most widely accepted model is the signal-channel model, in which the visual system is assumed to consist of a variety of channels tuned to receiving specific information. This is the model used here.

Relating the Signal-Channel Model to Film Critique

Based on Hendee's description of the signal-channel model of perception and Carlton and Adler's method of film critique, there appear to be four basic "signals" to which the radiographer must be attuned: (1) photographic properties, (2) geometric properties, (3) positioning, and (4) equipment malfunction.

This would produce a film critique process that, in a step-by-step manner, would be:

1. The radiographer always evaluates the entire image.
2. The image is evaluated in terms of photographic and geometric properties, positioning, and possible equipment problems.
3. The image is accepted or causes for the substandard image are theorized.
4. The theory is "tested."
5. From these "tests" of theory, the most plausible cause(s) is/are accepted.
6. The image is repeated with appropriate corrective factors.

CRITERIA FOR ACCEPTABLE RADIOGRAPHS

The remainder of this chapter describes criteria for acceptable radiographs in the areas of general radiography, tomography, mammography, and upper and lower gastrointestinal (GI) studies. Some of these were developed and published by the Japanese Society of Radiological Technology in 1992. Each institution may have specific criteria for accepting radiographs. The information here is presented as a guideline for professional practice. These guidelines will help the radiographer determine whether radiographs produced are acceptable. This information should be used in unison with the material presented in Chapter 6, on imaging, and in the next chapter, which discusses quality control and common equipment malfunctions.

What Is a Good Radiograph?

Radiographers want to produce the best possible radiograph with a minimum of radiation exposure and discomfort to the patient. Thus, in their education, radiographers learn about the following subjects in order to provide that radiograph.

- *Patient care.* This provides the radiographer with a knowledge of the patient, including proper communication. Ability to communicate with the patient and secure cooperation is imperative to the production of a quality radiograph.
- *Human structure and function.* A knowledge of anatomy is essential to the production of a quality radiograph. Radiographers must possess an ability to "see through" the patient in order to determine the effects of positioning.
- *Radiographic procedures.* Positioning and knowledge of procedures, including means of altering positioning to meet special needs, are areas given primary emphasis in the curriculum.
- *Radiation physics and imaging equipment.* Imaging equipment continues to increase in sophistication. A lack of understanding of how equipment works will limit the radiographer's ability to choose technical factors or determine whether a poor quality radiograph is due to human or technical factors.
- *Radiographic film processing.* One of the most important variables that must be kept under control in the radiology department is the development of radiographs. Failure to do so will lead to variable quality and increased radioation dose to the patient.
- *Radiation protection and biology.* A knowledge of the potential biologic effects of radiation and how to minimize radiation dose is a primary professional responsibility of the radiographer.
- *Radiographic pathology.* Without a knowledge of pathology, and the appearance of pathology on a radiograph, the radiographer will be unable to determine whether the cause of a substandard image is pathology.
- *Quality assurance.* Quality assurance is a systematic process designed to ensure quality in the radiology department—including the production of quality radiographs. Understanding common causes of repeats, for example, will help the radiographer minimize the number of repeats.

The production of a radiograph is not simply a psychomotor skill, or as has been popularly stated, "button-pushing." Bressler (1981; cited in Ireland, 1994) found that just three factors—kVp selection, mAs selection, and beam collimation—would lead to 82,000 technique option combinations. This does not take into accounty many other factors that may influence the production of the radiograph. This means that the intellectual rigor to produce a radiograph is high, and on a par with other intellectually demanding activities such as chess, where literally thousands of options have to be limited to come up with the best option. In chess, for example, a master player will have these thousands of options (moves) at his or her disposal, and will limit these to a best move or sequence of moves that lead to a preferred option such as checkmate or winning a piece. Similarly, the radiographer will limit the thousands of technical, positioning, and patient options to one set of factors designed to produce a diagnostic radiograph as the preferred option.

In this text, each positioning chapter details the specific qualities necessary for each position under the heading of Evaluation Criteria. These assist the radiographer in determining whether a radiograph meets standard professional criteria for acceptance. Figure 7.1 shows a specific criteria for certain examinations—*A* is a good stomach image showing the gastric area, *B* a good colon image showing what is called a "fine network pattern," and *C* is the dotlike pattern of reticular connective tissue as is seen in a good image of the outer margin of the breast.

In addition to those criteria, the following are general criteria for quality radiographs:

- Photographic properties of density and contrast are appropriate for examination.
  Density—For multiple examinations on one film or sequential examinations, for example, densities should be similar. Where both bone and soft tissue are to be shown, density should be appropriate for both tissues.
  Contrast—For example, for many examinations, short-scale contrast is preferred (e.g., extremities). For others, such as chest, a longer scale is often preferred.

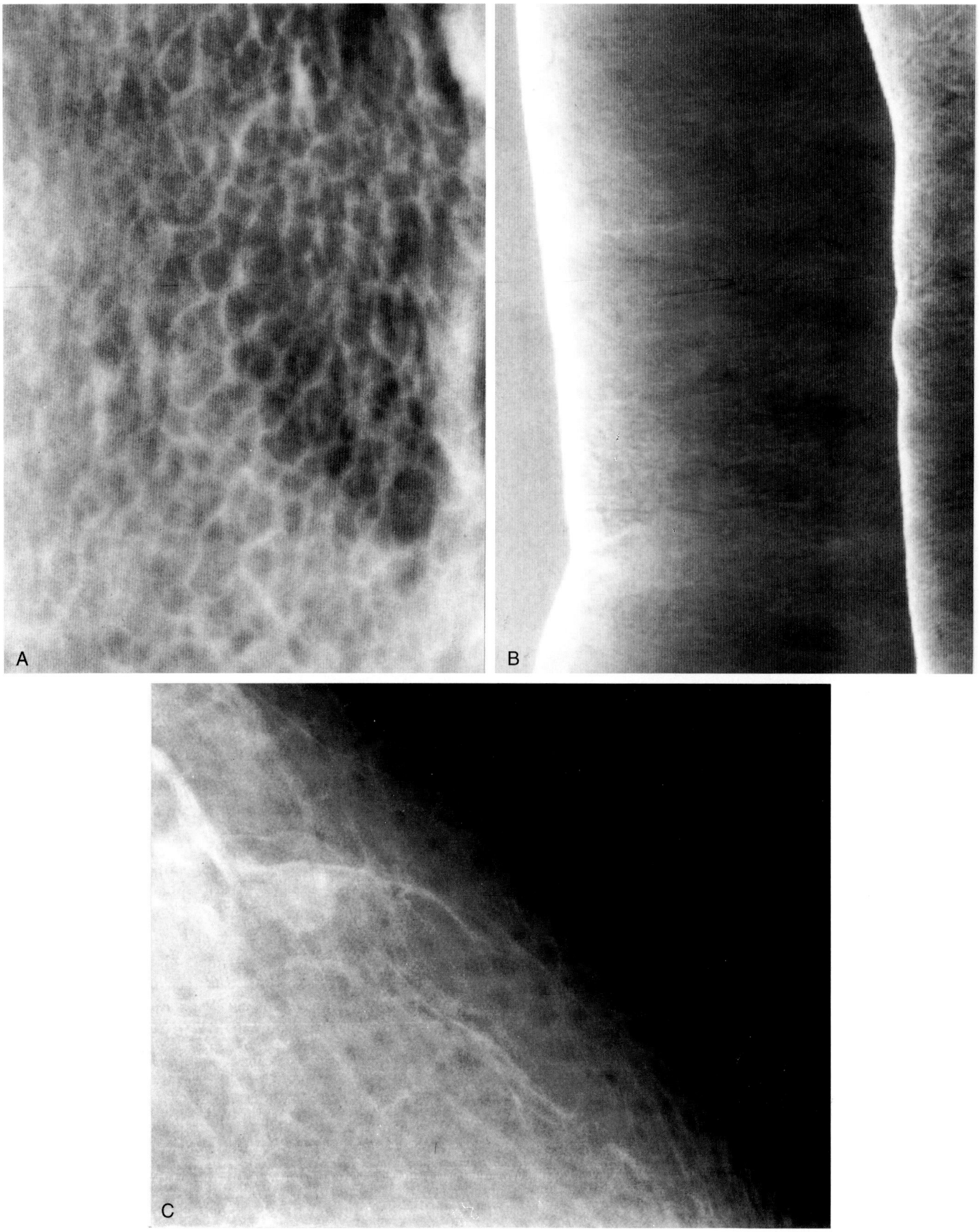

Figure 7.1. A, "Gastric area" visible in a good stomach image. B, "Fine network pattern" visible in a good colon image. C, Dot-like pattern of reticular connective tissue visible in a good image of the outer margin of the breast.

- Collimation (beam restriction) is appropriate for examination. Beam size should never exceed film size, for example, and in many cases, collimation should be much smaller than the film.
- Film markers are evident, and in proper place.
- Geometry is appropriate. Proper focal spot. Lack of blurring due to patient motion.
- Other technical factors. For example, lack of grid lines or artifacts.

What Is a Poor Radiograph?

Simplistically, a poor radiograph can be defined as one lacking one or more of the general or specific criteria listed. In some cases, however, one or more of the criteria can be missing, and the radiograph may still be judged "acceptable," although not of good quality. This is discussed further.

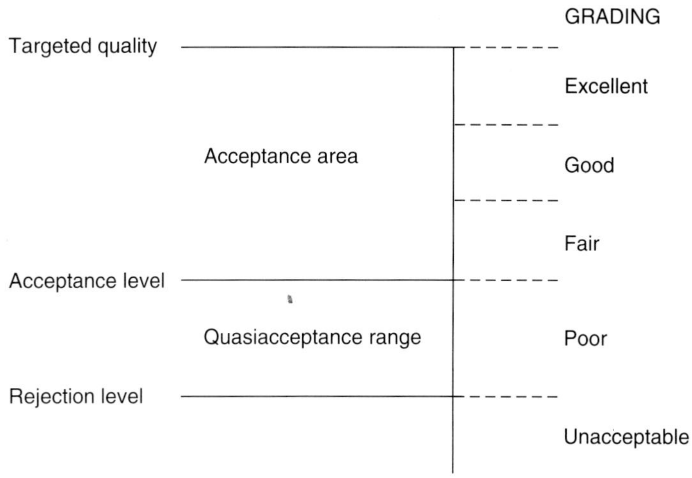

Figure 7.2. Quality levels.

What Is an Acceptable Radiograph?

Since standardization of patients is rare, and in some cases standardization of equipment and technical factors also cannot be achieved, radiographs not of quality may still be considered acceptable if they show the desired pathology or lack of pathology. Also, since radiographs are accepted by human beings, who show tolerance for ambiguity, quality standards do vary. This concept of acceptability is reflected in clinical competancy examinations for student radiographers, where some actions result in failure of the competency (e.g., anatomy clipped), whereas others may not (e.g., marker placement).

The determination of acceptability for radiographs is typically interdepartmental. Radiographers must determine the acceptability of radiographs as set forth by their department, but must also remember that, as professionals, they may be hel to the same standards of quality as other radiographers. In legal terms, this is oftern referred to as "standard of care."

An example of quality levels as determined by the Japanese Society of Radiological Technology is shown in Figure 7.2. This also illustrates what is called a "quasiacceptance range" in which some images that should ordinarily be rejected are accepted. An example of the use of quasiacceptance levels is in GI studies where patients may be allowed to leave before the study is completed—thus, taking repeats is not practical unless the study lacks diagnostic value.

Utilization of Specific Criteria

Figures 7.3 to 7.13 illustrate the use of specific evaluation criteria for radiologic examinations as developed by the Japanese Society of Radiological Technology for general radiography, tomography, and mammography. Note that these standards may vary slightly from United States criteria; however, in general, the criteria are similar.

Film Evaluation in Fluoroscopy

Recent experiments have begun using radiographers to perform some basic fluoroscopic screening. In Great Britain, radiographers pursuing master's degrees are currently being taught some basic screening. In Japan, radiographers may perform fluoroscopy (upper GIs) under the indirect supervision of radiologists who entrust them to follow a fixed sequence. In the United States, radiographers employed at University Hospital in Birmingham, Alabama, have been taught some basic screening techniques on an on-the-job basis, and one goal of the baccalaureate program in radiography at the University of Alabama at Birmingham is to educate radiographers in the basic theory of fluoroscopy and other types of screening so that they may assume such roles. Since fluoroscopy involves some diagnosis, an even higher standard of film evaluation is required.

Examples of general and specific criteria for upper GI studies (Figs. 7.14 to 7.18) are

General Criteria

I. Rejection criteria
  A. Wrong film size used
  B. Incorrect collimation used
II. Adequacy of exposure factors
  A. Density of region of interest (ROI) adequate for diagnosis
III. Adequacy of contrast techniques
  A. Appropriate amount of barium and air
  B. Sufficient coating of barium
  C. No remaining bubbles
IV. Positioning is adequate
  A. ROI is demonstrated
V. Overlapped images are present/not present
  A. No obstructive shadows overlapping ROI are present
VI. Image sharpness is adequate
  A. Motion blur due to peristalsis and patient movement is minimum
  B. Geometric blur due to incorrect placement of spot-film device against patient is minimal
VII. Artifacts
  A. No obstructive artifacts such as scratches, dust, or fog are present

(text continued on page 81)

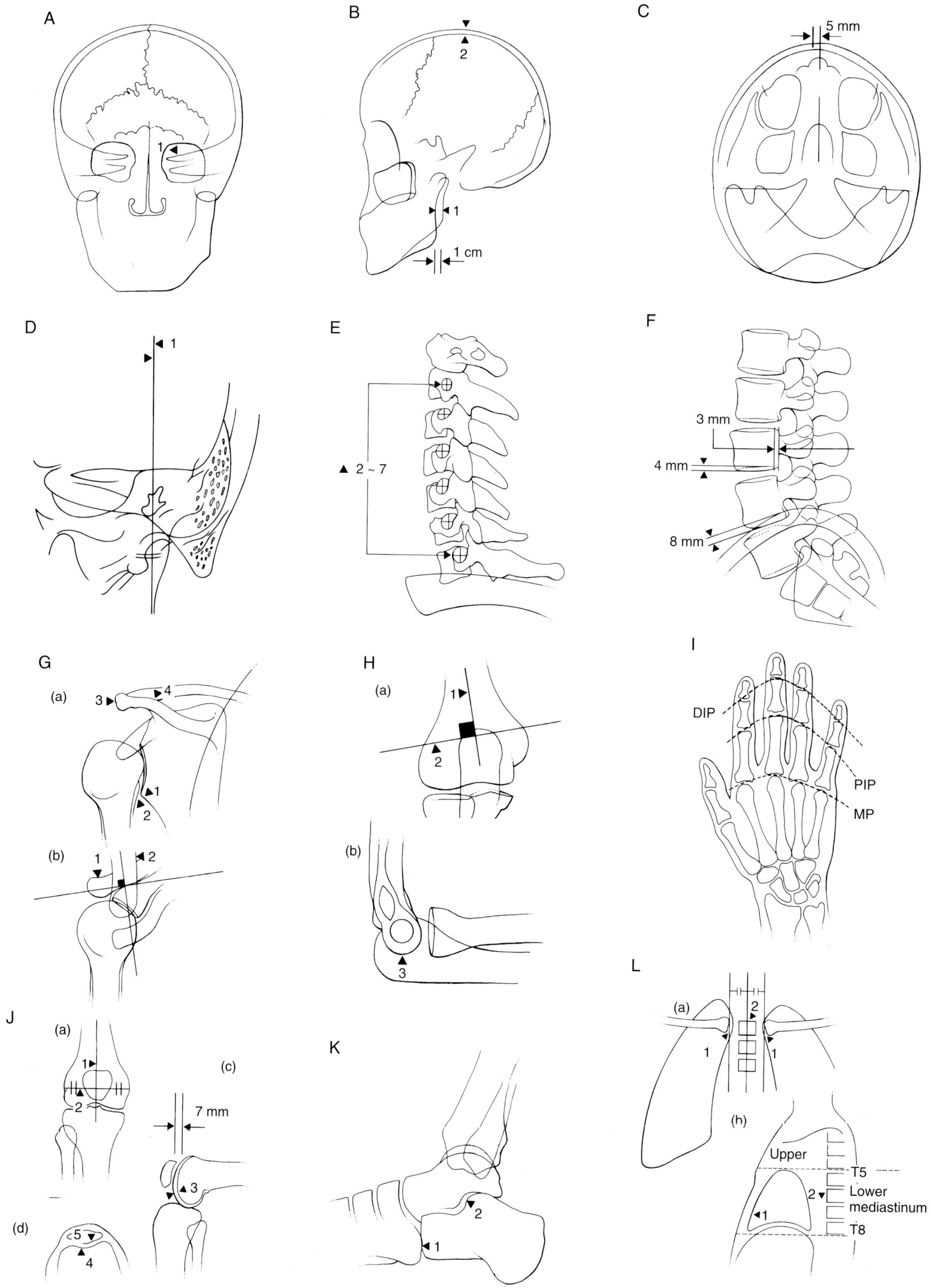
A
1
B
2
1
1 cm
C
5 mm
D
1
E
2 ~ 7
F
3 mm
4 mm
8 mm
G
(a)
3
4
1
2
(b)
1
2
H
(a)
1
2
(b)
3
I
DIP
PIP
MP
J
(a)
1
2
(c)
7 mm
3
(d)
5
4
K
2
1
L
(a)
2
1
1
(h)
Upper
T5
2
Lower
mediastinum
1
T8

Figure 7.3. A, AP or PA projection of the skull. (1) The distance from the lateral border of the skull to the lateral border of the orbit should be equal bilaterally. (2) Internal auditory meatus (▲1) should be positioned around orbital center. (3) Technical factors set so that petrous pyramids are visible.
B, Lateral projection of the skull. (1) Anterior and posterior clinoid processes of sella turcica are well aligned, and two sides of mandibular rami (▲1) are separated by no more than 1 cm. (2) Technical factors set so that inner and outer tables of skull (▲2) are visible.
C, Towne's projection. (1) Difference of the distance from center of foramen magnum to lateral border of temporal bone no more than 5 mm. (2) Dorsum sellae projected in foramen magnum. (3) Technical factors set so that internal structures of petrous pyramids are visible.
D, Auditory organs (Schuller's projection). (1) Entire mastoid process and mastoid cells included. (2) Technical factors set so structures inside mastoid cells are clearly visible.
E, Oblique cervical vertebrae. (1) Intervertebral foramina from C2 to C7 included (▲2–7). (2) Technical factors set so that bone trabeculae of cervical bodies are visible.
F, Lateral projection. (1) Vertebrae are lateral from C1 to the superior margin of C7. (2). Technical factors set so that bone trabeculae of cervical bodies are visible.
G *(a)*, AP projection of shoulder joint. (1) Glenoid fossa (▲1) and humeral head (▲2) should be separately visible. (2) Acromion (▲3) and clavicle (▲4) should overlap each other, with a wide subacromial space. (3) Technical factors set so that intertubercular sulcus between greater and lesser tubercles is visible.
G *(b)*, Axial projection of shoulder joint. (1) Relationship between humeral head and glenoid fossa should be clearly observable. (2) Horizontal portion of coracoid process (▲1) should cross clavicle (▲2) at right angle. (3) Parts of acromion and clavicle should overlap humeral head.
H *(a)*, Elbow—AP projection. (1) Technical factors set so tuberosities are visible. (2) Contour of olecranon overlapping distal end of humerus fully visible. (3) Long axis of humeral shaft (▲1) and line connecting medial and lateral condyles (▲2) should form right angle.
H *(b)*, Elbow—Lateral projection. (1) Technical factors set so that tuberosities are visible. (2) Trochlea (▲3) fully visible.
I, Fingers—AP/PA and lateral projections. (1) Distal interphalangeal joint, proximal interphalangeal joint, and metacarpophalangeal joint clearly visible. (2) AP/PA and lateral projections should be at right angles to each other.
J *(a)*, Knee—AP projection. (1) Patella observable on a line (▲1) that bisects the line between the medial and the lateral epicondyles of the femur.
J *(c)*, Knee—Lateral projection. (1) Separation between bilateral medial and lateral condyles (▲3) should be no more than 7 mm.
J *(d)*, Knee—Axial projection. (1) Wide articular space observable. (2) Patellar surface of femur (▲4) and patella (▲5) should be separately visible. (3) Technical factors set so that contour of patella is clearly visible.
K, Calcaneus—lateral projection. (1) Talocalcaneonavicular joint (▲1) and talocalcaneal joint (▲3) visible.
L *(a)*, Chest—PA projection. (1) Entire thorax including pulmonary apices and costophrenic angles well demonstrated. (2) Lung markings visible to distal ends; recognizable even with overlapping rib and clavicular shadows. (3) Edges of both sternoclavicular joints (▲1) should be equally distant from the shadow of spinous processes of thoracic vertebrae (▲2).
L *(b)*, Chest—lateral projection. (1) Technical factors set so that anterior (▲1) and posterior (▲2) mediastina are clearly visible. (2) Technical factors set so that trachea overlapping cardiac shadow is observable. (3) Body positioned so that median plane of trunk is parallel with film.

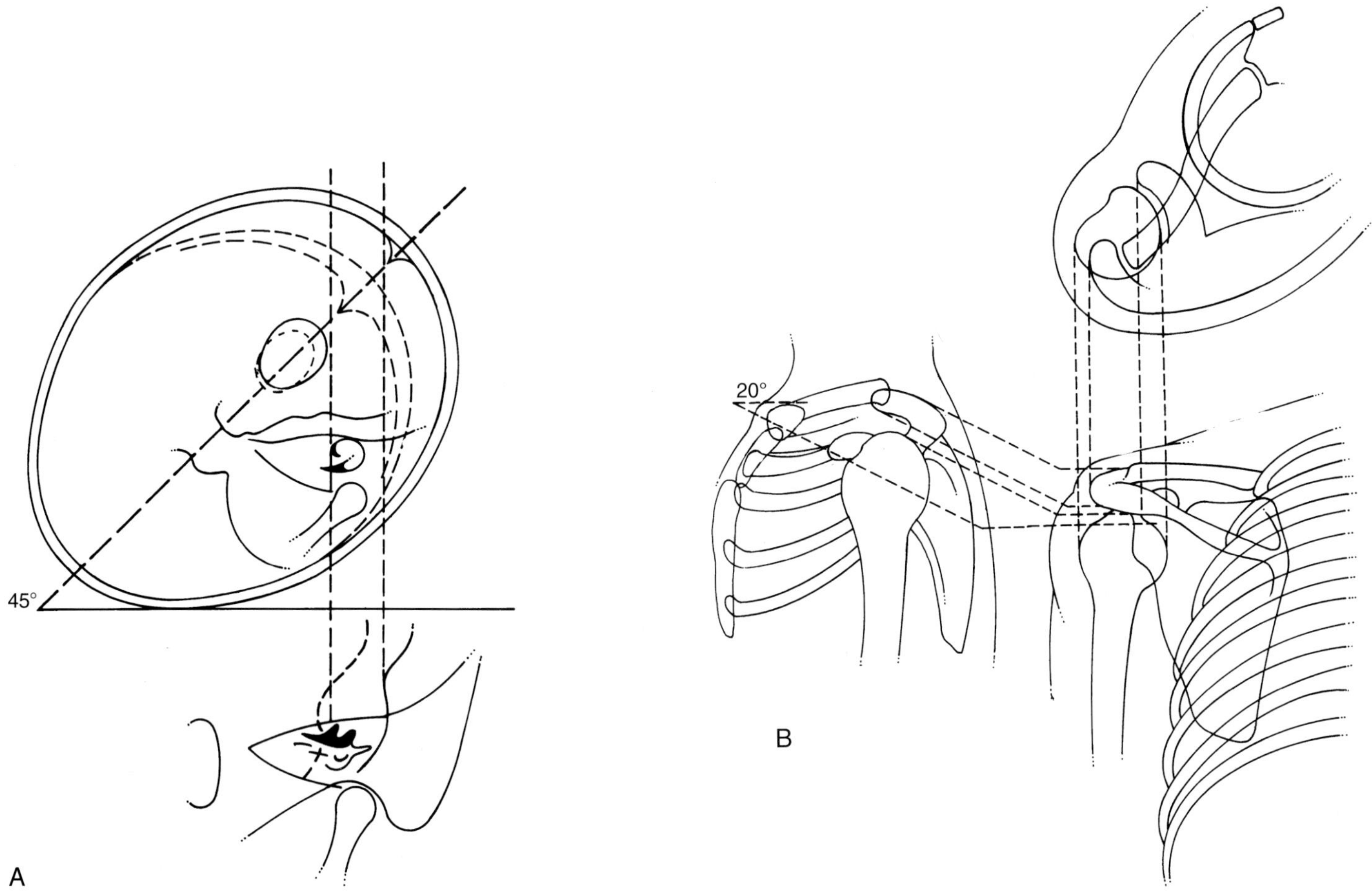

Figure 7.4. Variations are shown. A, Stenvers' projection. Brachycephalic skull and internal occipital crest are shown in *dashed lines* with the semicircular canals in *black*. B, Shoulder joint (frontal projection). The angle shown was selected to open the subacromial space and let the beam pass through the glenohumeral joint at a right angle.

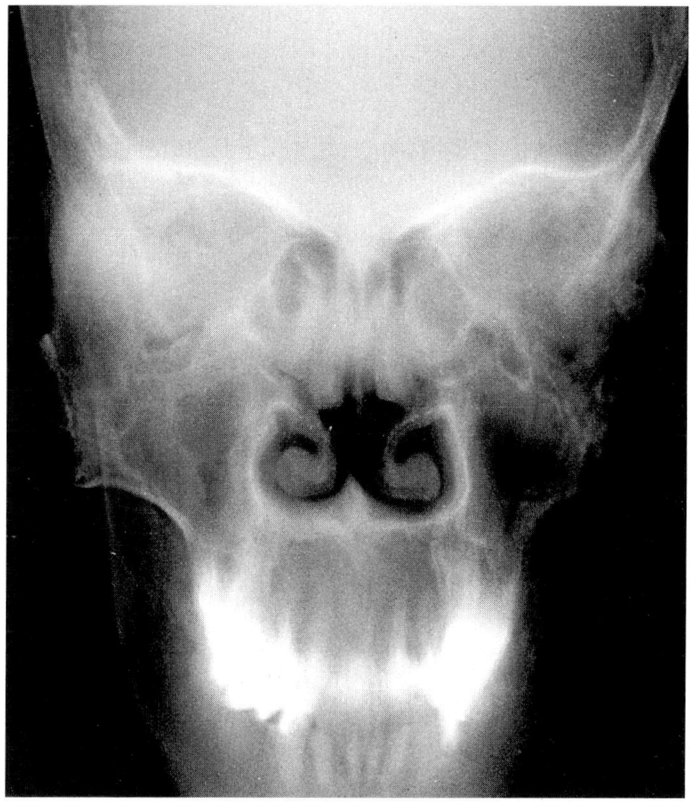

Figure 7.5. Paranasal sinuses—AP or PA projection (tomography). (1) Both maxillary sinuses demonstrated symmetrically. (2) Technical factors set so that mucoperiosteum is visible.

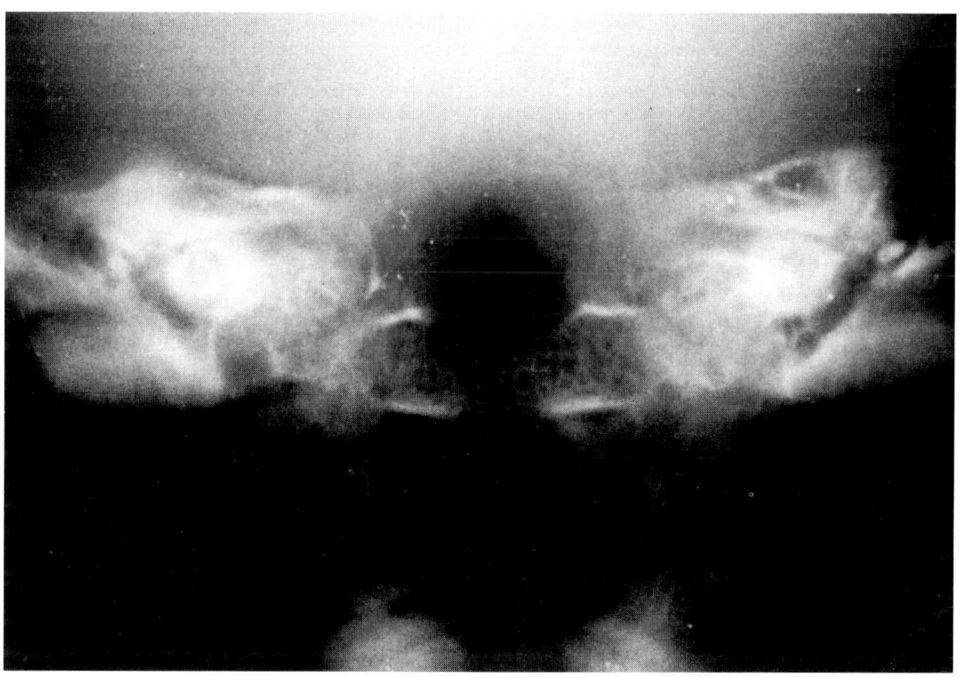

Figure 7.6. Internal auditory canal (tomography). Superior and lateral semicircular canals and cochlea visible symmetrically.

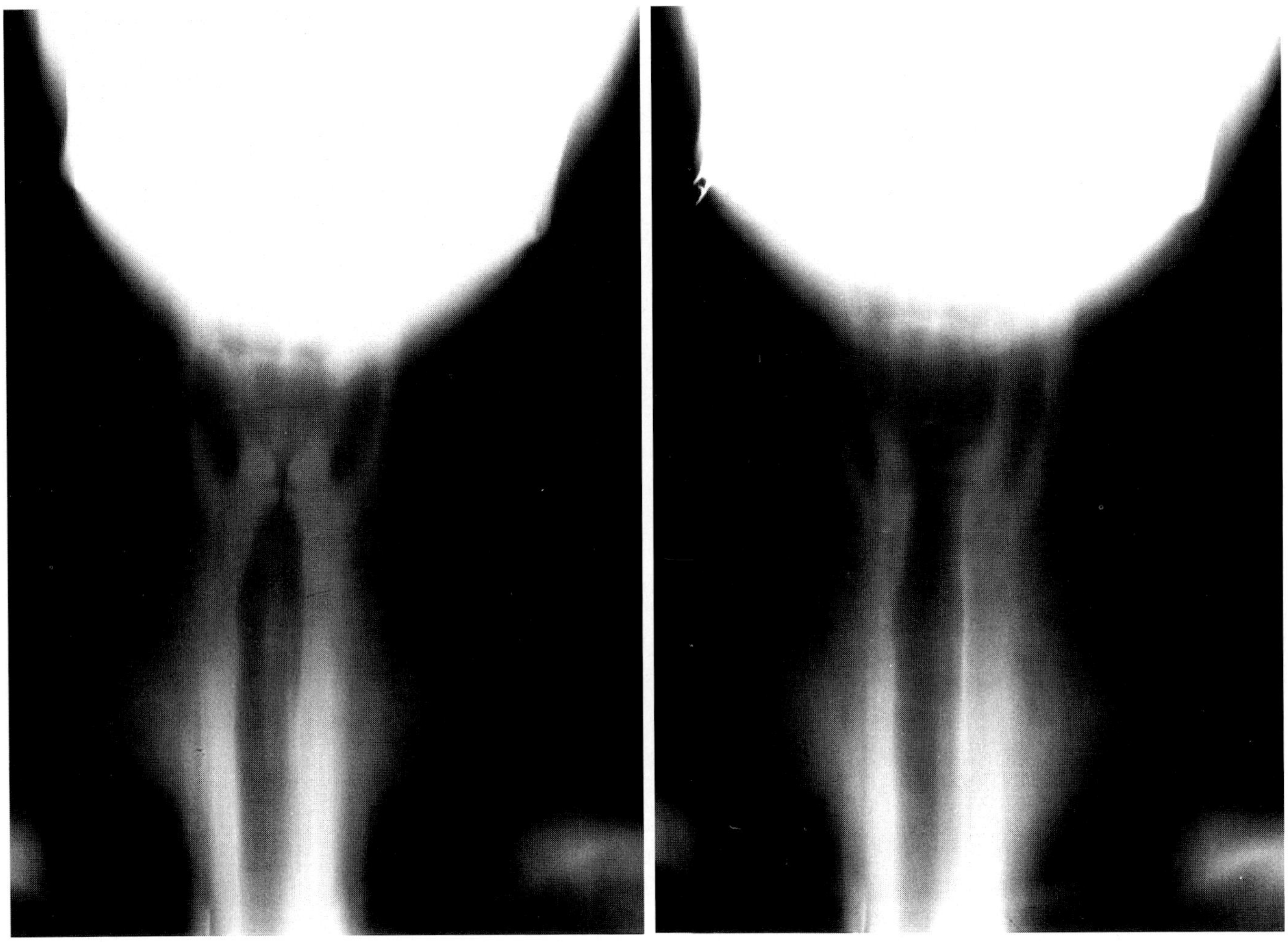

Figure 7.7. Larynx—AP or PA (tomography). Notches of laryngeal ventricle should be visible either breathing in or in phonation.

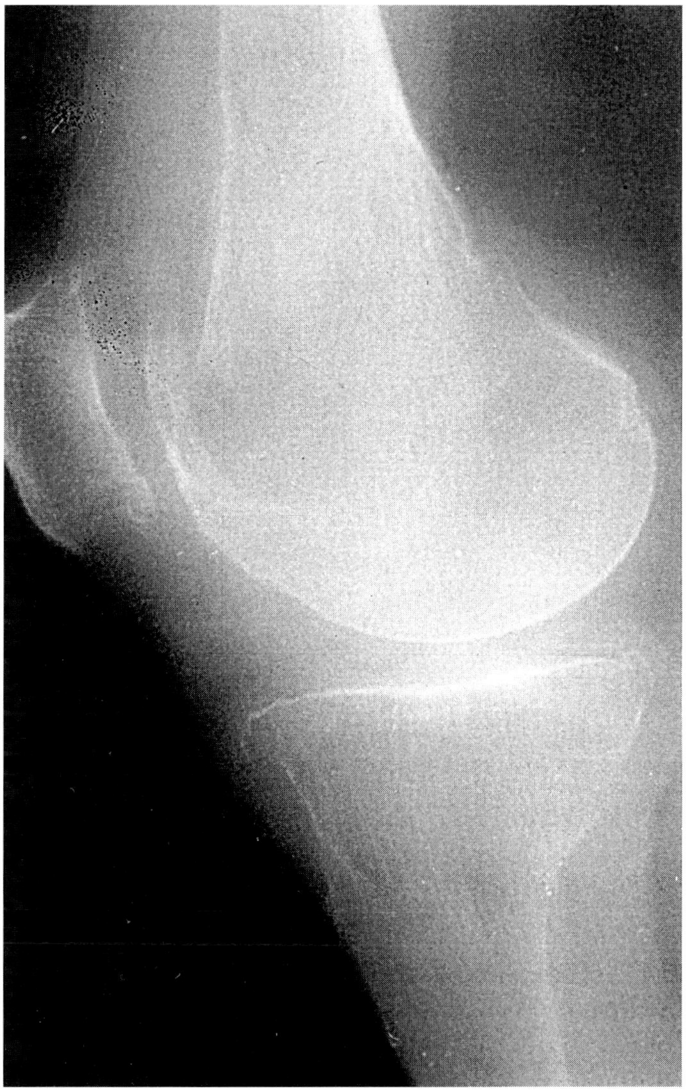

Figure 7.8. Upper and lower extremities—AP/PA projections. Margins and bone cortex of epiphysis should be clearly observable.

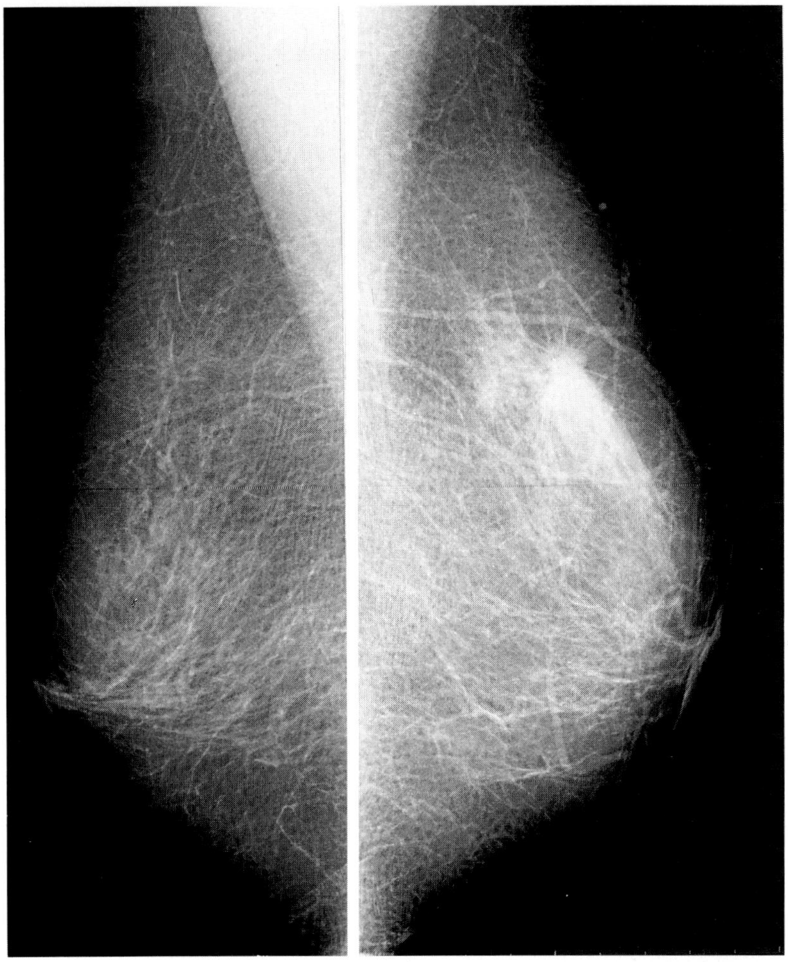

Figure 7.9. A part of the pectoral muscle (*top*) and soft tissue under the breast. In this figure and Figure 7.10, in the lateral projection, at the immediately lower part of the breast, part of the soft tissue should be included or, if not included, expected to be just out of view. This can be determined by the contour of the immediately lower part of the breast being concave, not convex.

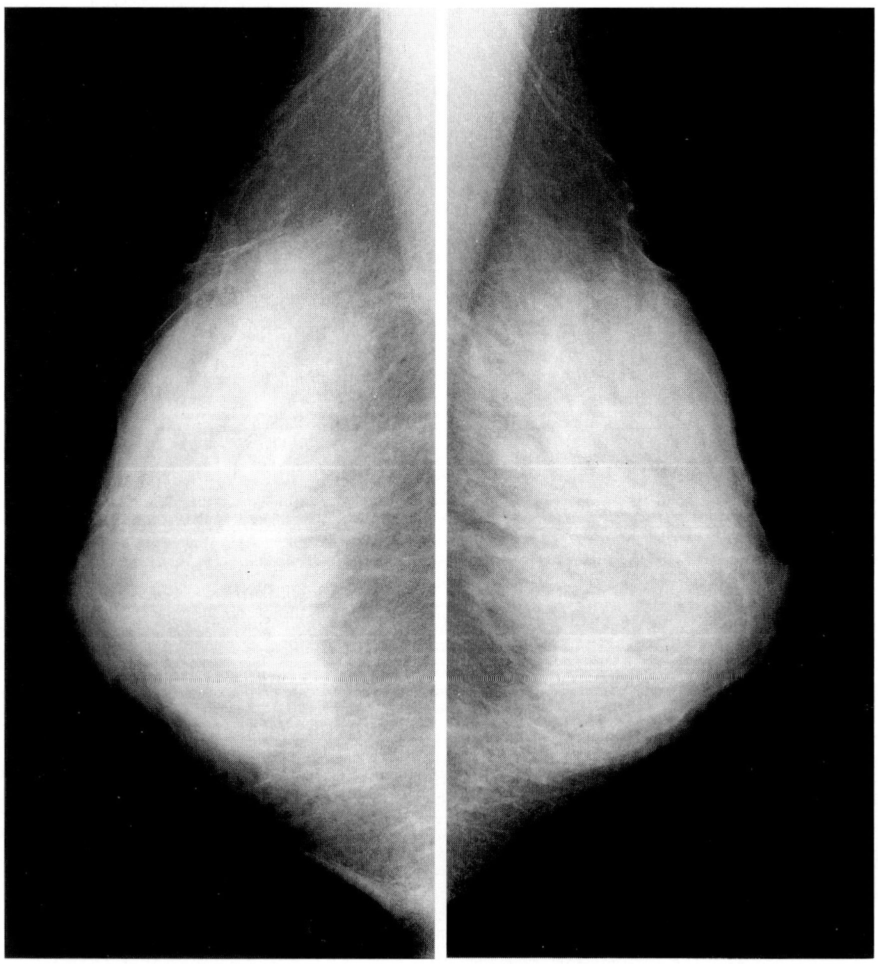

Figure 7.10. This figure does not show soft tissue under the breast, but in concave.

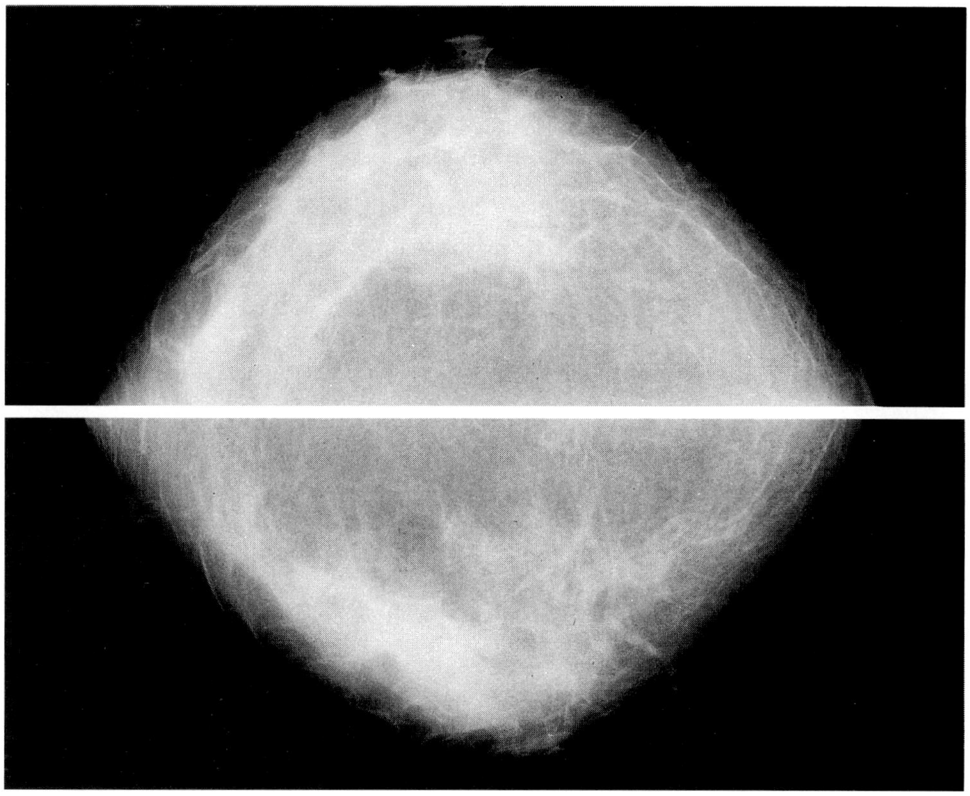

Figure 7.11. Craniocaudal projection of the breast in Figure 7.10. Width of the breast (chest wall to nipple) should not be less than 80% of its width in the lateral projection. For the post-menopausal and atrophic breast, as shown here, the reticular connective tissue showing the fine network should be seen at the outer margin.

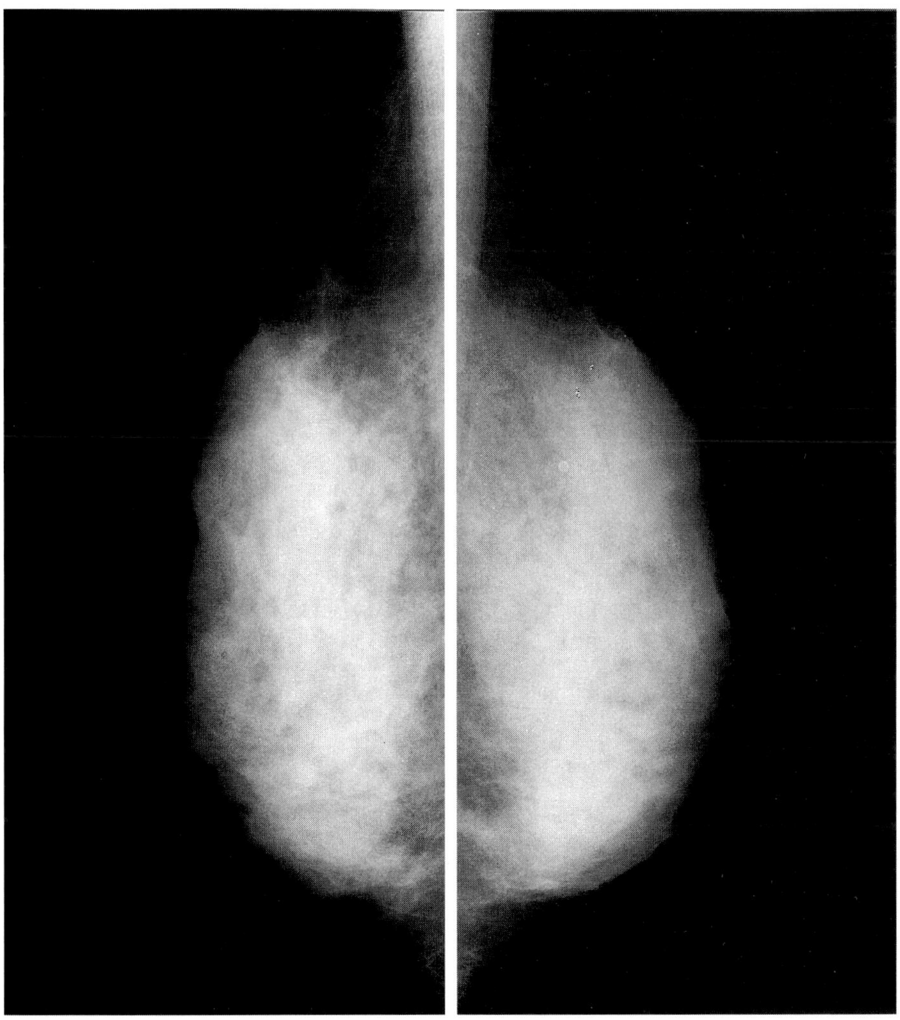

Figure 7.12. In a dense breast, even if the subcutaneous adipose tissue is blurred, at least its inner margins should be determined by the superficial fascia. The glandular tissue should be dissolved rather than forming a solid pattern, so as to provide part of the trabecula and blood vessel images through the patched dark areas.

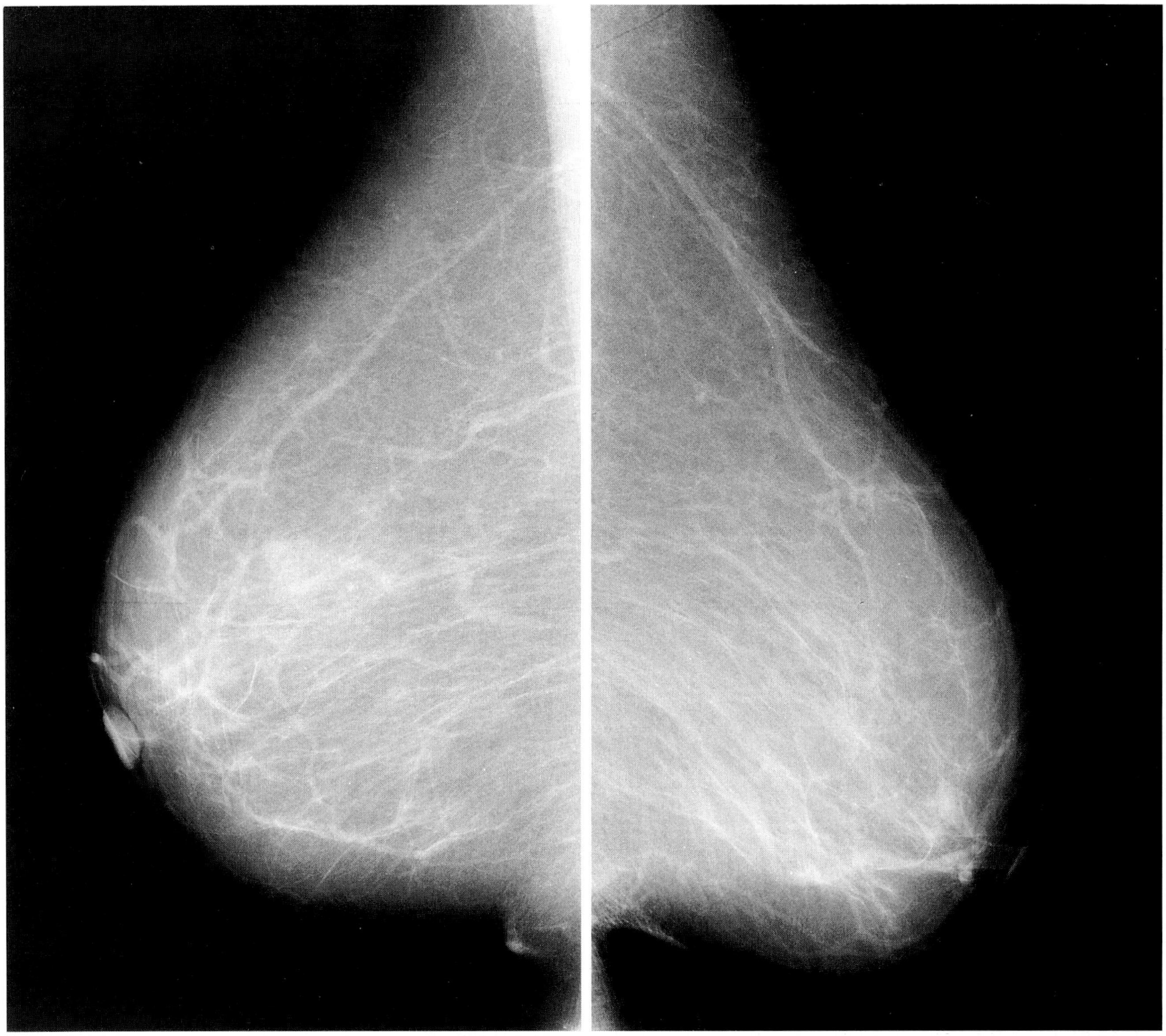

Figure 7.13. *Right,* A concave breast that has not had sufficient compression. *Left,* A more compressed breast that is still not convex.

Specific Criteria

I. Mucosa of anterior wall
   A. Mucosal relief method (Fig. 7.14*A*)
      1. Mucosal folds should be sufficiently expanded
      2. Mucosal surfaces from lower gastric body to pyloric antrum should be clearly recognizable
   B. Barium thin-layer method
      1. Mucosal surface from upper gastric body to pyloric antrum should be clearly recognizable
      2. Amount of air should be adequate

II. Double-contrast radiograph of esophagus (Fig. 7.14*B*)
   A. RAO position
      1. Esophagus should be expanded, providing a double-contrast image, especially at middle and lower intrathoracic esophagus
      2. No overlapping of thoracic vertebrae should be present

III. Barium-filling method
   A. Upright frontal position (Fig. 7.14*C*)
      1. Gastric angle should be depicted at widest possible point
      2. Margins of barium-filled image should be clearly recognizable
      3. Regions from lower gastric body to pylorus should be sufficiently filled with barium
   B. Prone position (Fig. 7.14*D*)
      1. Pylorus and duodenal bulb should be sufficiently filled with barium without overlapping each other

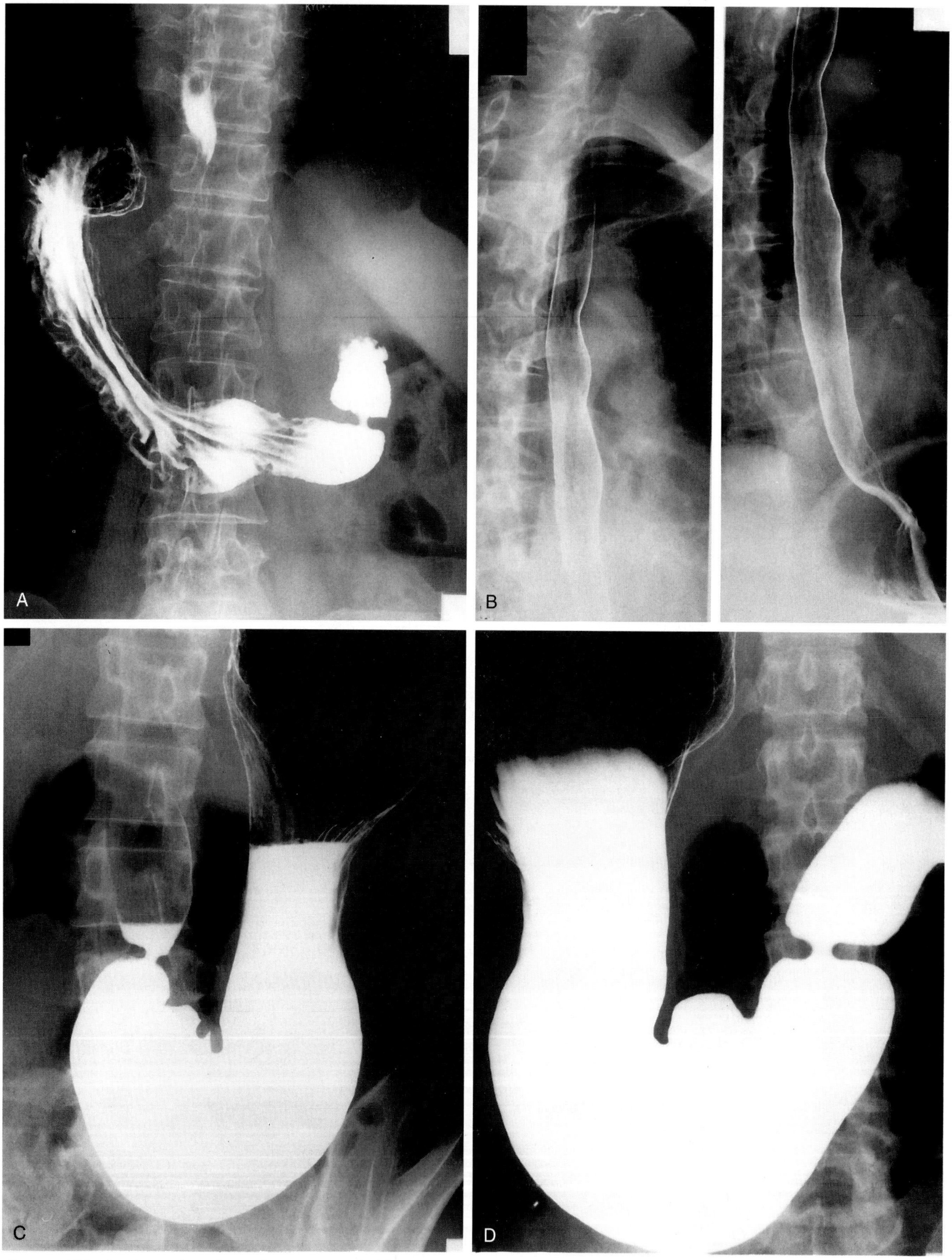

Figure 7.14. Radiographs taken prior to using double-contrast technique for stomach images. A, Mucosal relief method. B, Double-contrast image of esophagus. C, Barium-filling method, upright position. D, Barium-filling method, prone position.

IV. Double-contrast radiograph
   A. AP or PA supine position (Figs. 7.15*A* and 7.16*A*)
      1. Regions from middle gastric body to pyloric antrum should be well depicted
      2. Angular portion should be depicted at widest point
   B. Supine RAO position (Figs. 7.15*B* and 7.16*C*)
      1. Angular portion should be positioned free from vertebral shadow and, along with the pylorus, should be well depicted
   C. Supine LAO position (Figs. 7.15*C* and 7.16*B*)
      1. Gastric angle should be positioned free from vertebral shadow
      2. Regions from upper gastric body to middle gastric body should be well depicted
      3. When pyloric antrum is radiographed with table tilted down, regions from gastric angle to pylorus should be well depicted (show antra at the side of greater curvature)
   D. Semiupright LAO position (Figs. 7.15*D* and 7.17*C*)
      1. Cardiac orifice should be clearly identifiable

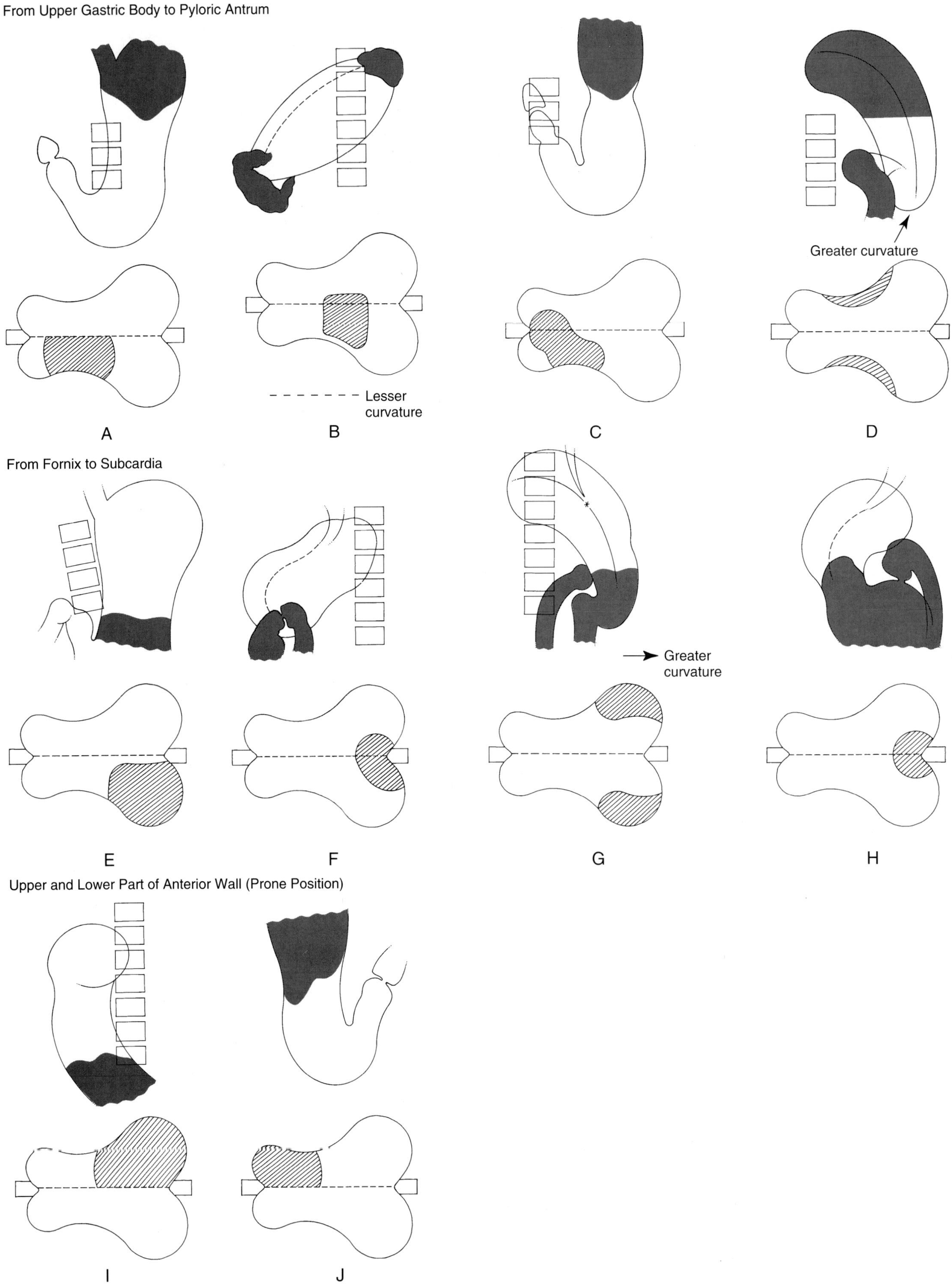

Figure 7.15. A–J, Diagnosable area (*shaded area*) using double-contrast technique. (See text for explanation.)

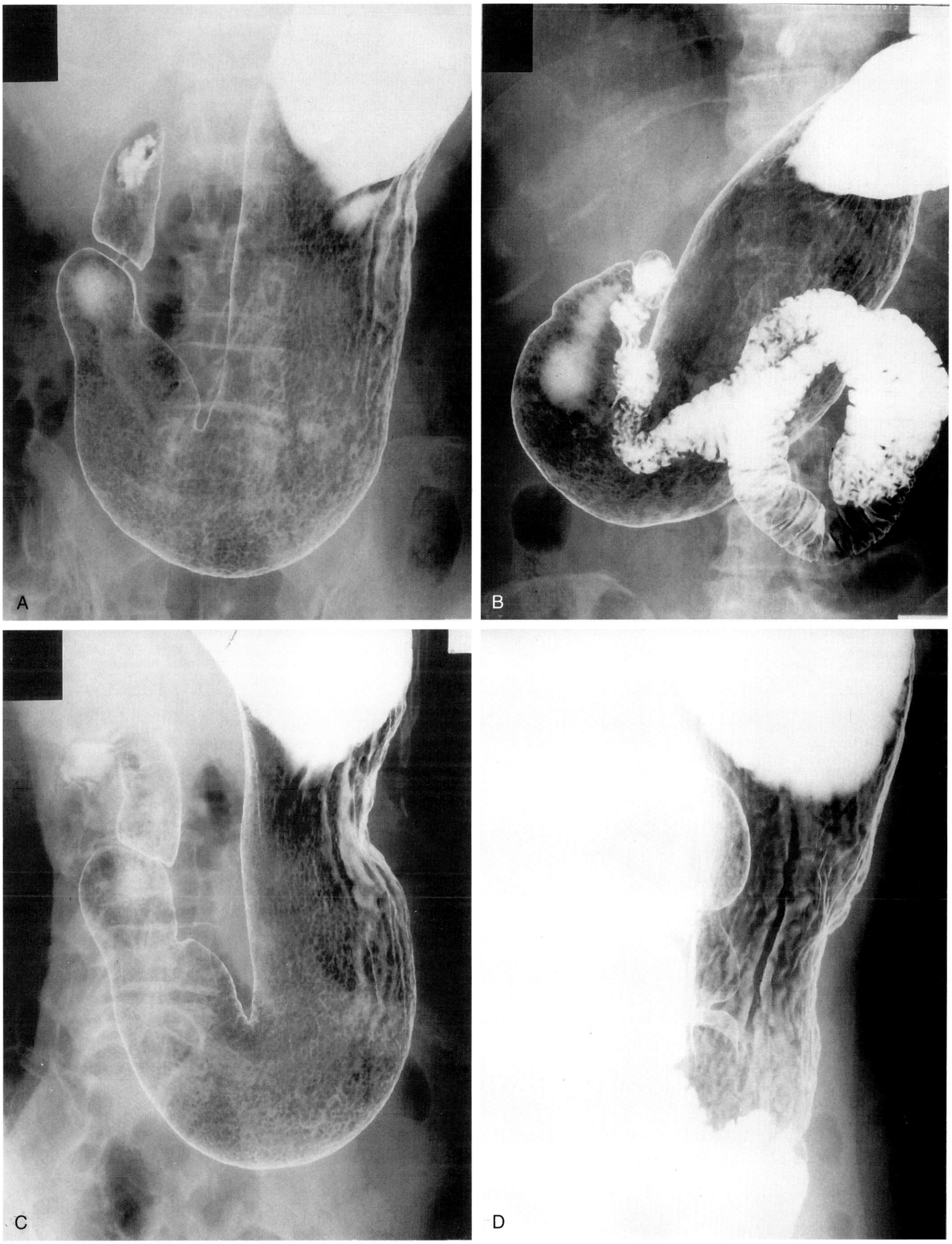

Figure 7.16. Double-contrast radiographs of middle to lower part of stomach. A, Frontal supine. B, Supine LAO. C, Supine RAO. D, Left recumbent.

V. Double-contrast radiograph of upper part of stomach
  A. AP or PA upright position (Figs. 7.15*E* and 7.17*A*)
    1. Fundus should be well coated with barium
    2. Air volume should not be decreased by belching or other means
  B. Upright RAO position (Figs. 7.15*F* and 7.17*B*)
    1. Same as A.1 and 2
  C. Upright LAO position (Fig. 7.15*G*)
    1. Same as A.1 and 2
    2. Take radiograph, after patient has drunk barium, to conincide with descent of barium

VI. Compression method
  A. Upright or semiupright position (Fig. 7.15*H*)
    1. Entire regions from middle gastric body to duodenal bulb should be compressed in sequence
    2. Strength of pressure should be adequate (applying both strong and weak pressures is required)

VII. Supplementary double-contrast radiograph
  A. Right recumbent position (Figs. 7.15*I* and 7.17*D*)
    1. Shows AP or PA projection of lesser curvature
  B. Left recumbent position (Figs. 7.15*J* and 7.16*D*)
    1. Greater curvatures from middle to inferior regions of gastric body should be shown en face
  C. Prone position (upper part) (Fig. 7.18*A*)
    1. Shows anterior wall in a tilt-up position
  D. Prone position (lower part) (Fig. 7.18*B*)
    1. Regions from lower to pyloric antrum should be depicted. Shows anterior wall in a tilt-down position.

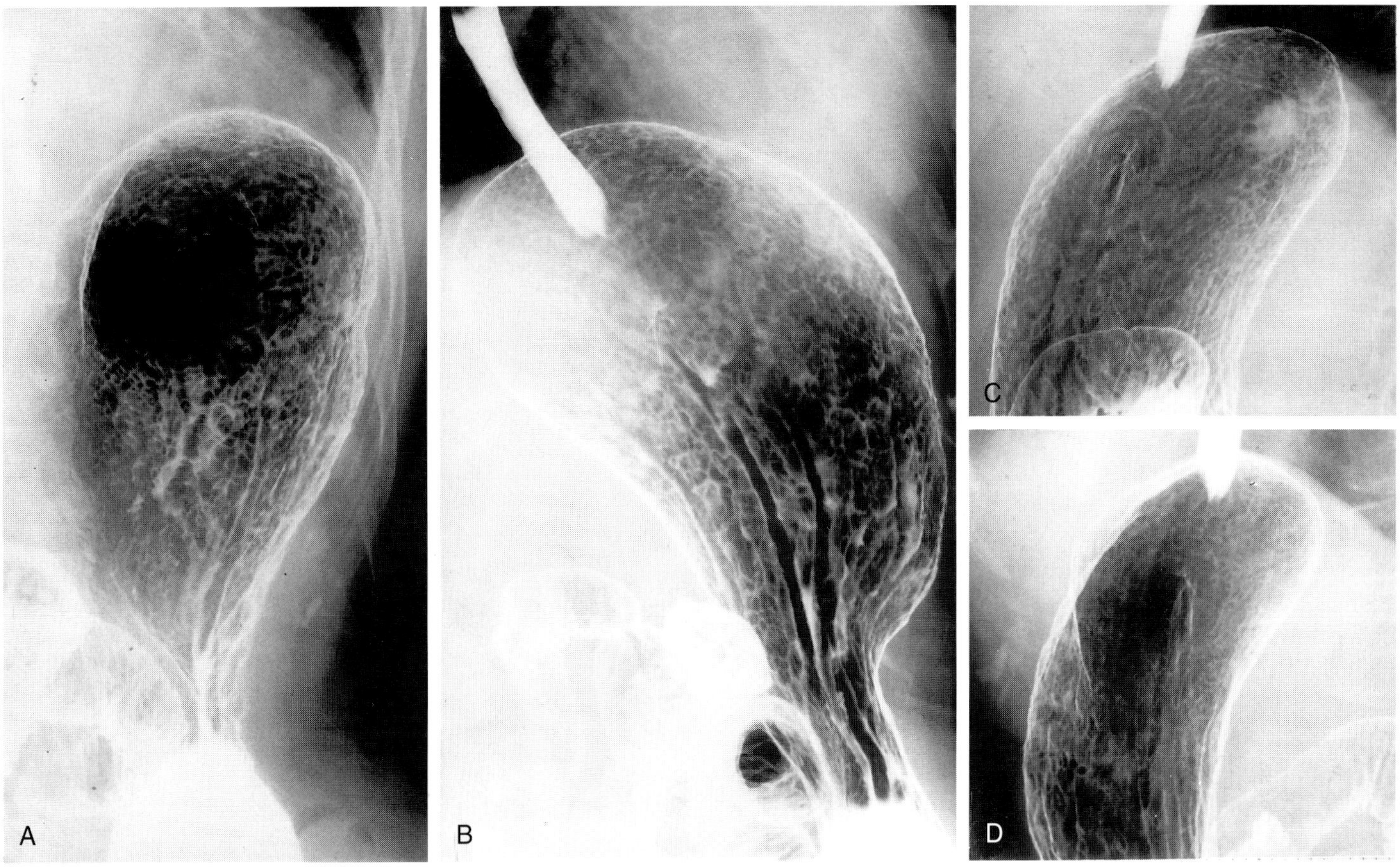

Figure 7.17. Double-contrast radiographs of upper part of stomach. A, Frontal upright. B, Upright RAO. C, Semiupright LAO. D, Right recumbent.

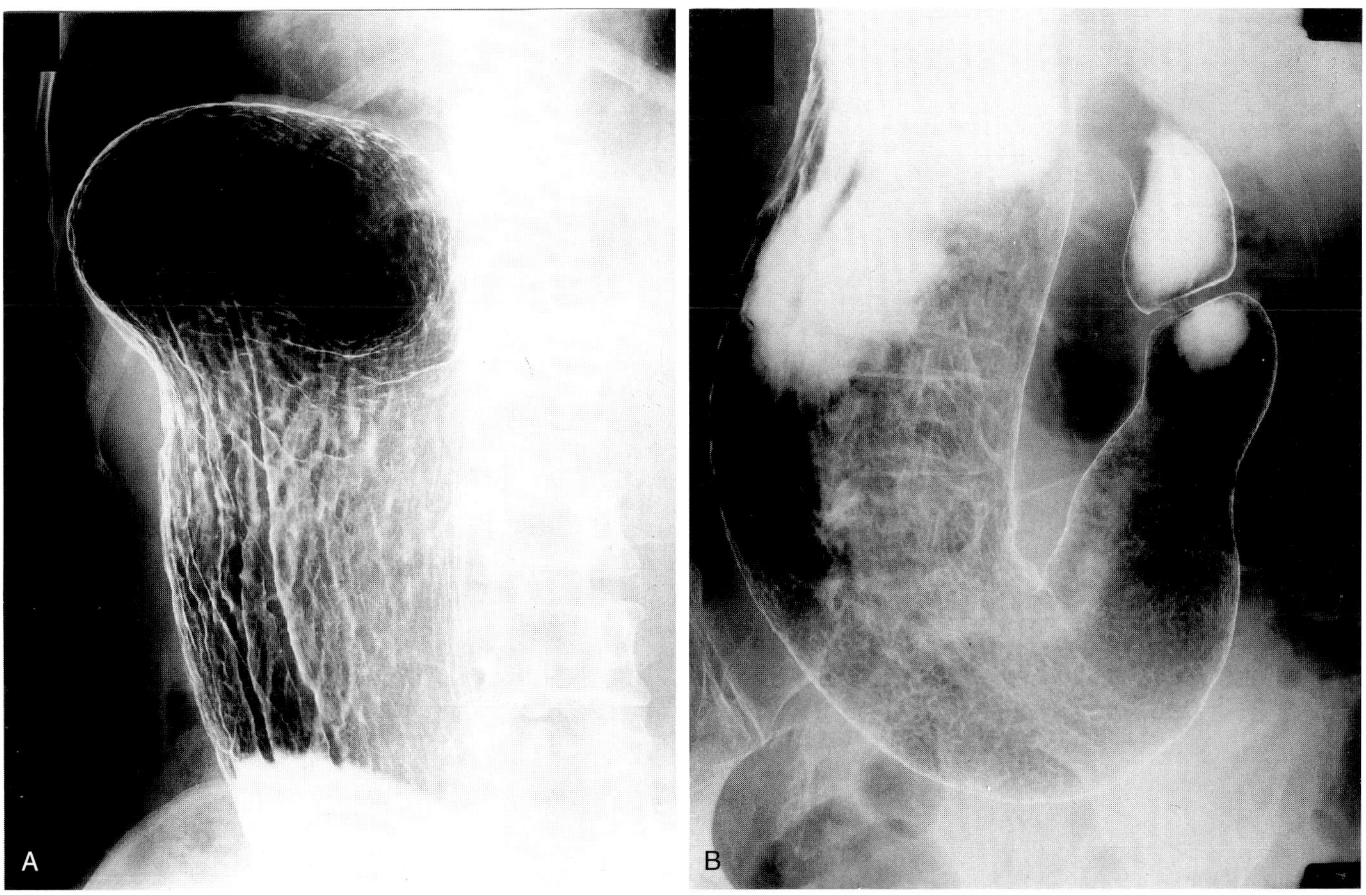

Figure 7.18. Double-contrast radiographs of anterior wall in prone position. A, Upper part. B, Lower part.

The recent trend is to eliminate the mucosal examination and replace it with the double-contrast technique in the prone position as described in VII.C and D. The key to double contrast is that the ROI has been washed by a bolus of barium, accomplished by rotating the patient several times in order to ensure both an adequate coating of the mucosa with barium and a minimum of gastric juice. This barium-coating procedure involves tilting the examination table at various angles in combination with patient movement (Fig. 7.19). This movement ensures complete coverage of the gastric wall, as was seen in Figure 7.14. The area to be examined is always the lower wall of the stomach or the area proximal to the table when the patient is in the recumbent position.

Even when a radiograph is taken of the upper part of the stomach in the upright position, either the anterior or the posterior wall has to be coated with barium before the table is tilted up. Figure 7.20 shows a diagram of the stomach incised along greater curvature, positioned with the distal end on the left and the proximal end on the right. Consequently, the anterior wall is the upper half and the posterior wall is the lower half, with the lesser curvature in the center. The stomach is positioned in the body in the three-dimensional setting that makes it difficult for one to determine the diagnosable area according the a patient's movement. An easy way to understand which area is to be examined is to make a loose grip with your right hand and hold it against your chest with your palm facing inward (Fig. 7.21). Twist or bend your body, keeping your hand against your chest. With your hand in this position, your fingers represent the fundus of the stomach and your thumb represents the antrum. The side of your index finger represents the lesser curvature, and the angle between your index finger and your thumb demonstrates the gastric angle. Consequently, the side of your little finger represents the greater curvature, with your palm as the posterior wall and the back of your hand as the anterior wall.

General and specific criteria for lower GI studies are shown in Figures 7.22 to 7.25.

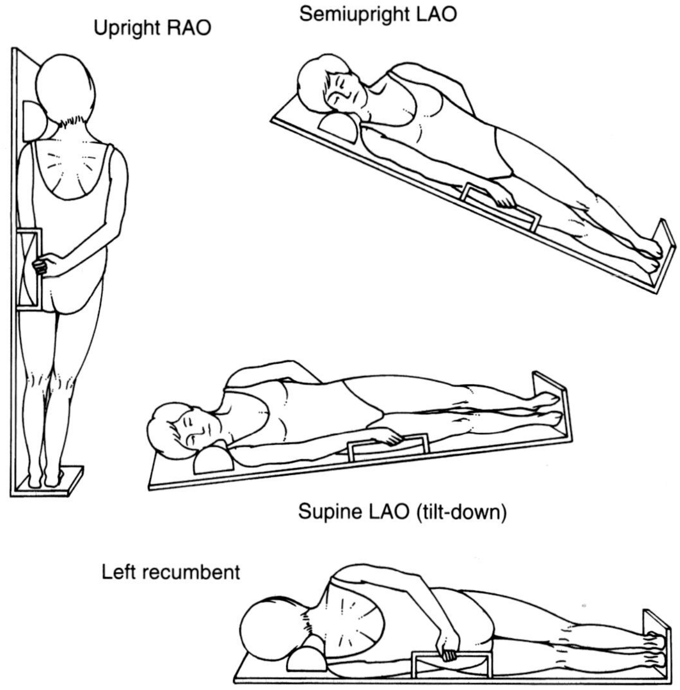

Figure 7.19. General body and table positioning for upper gastrointestinal examination during fluoroscopy for spot films.

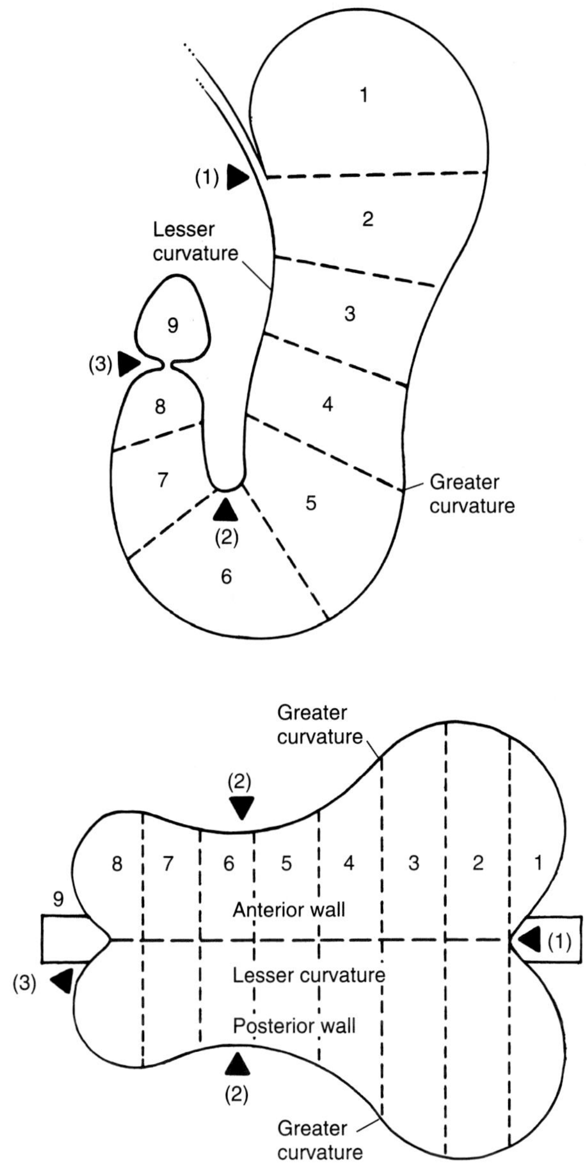

1. Fornix (fundus)
2. Subcardia
3. Upper gastric body
4. Middle gastric body
5. Lower gastric body
6. Angular portion
7. Antrum
8. Pyloric antrum
9. Duodenal bulb

▲ (1) Cardia
▲ (2) Gastric angle
▲ (3) Pylorus

Figure 7.20. Segmentation of stomach illustrated after the manner proposed by the National Cancer Center in Japan.

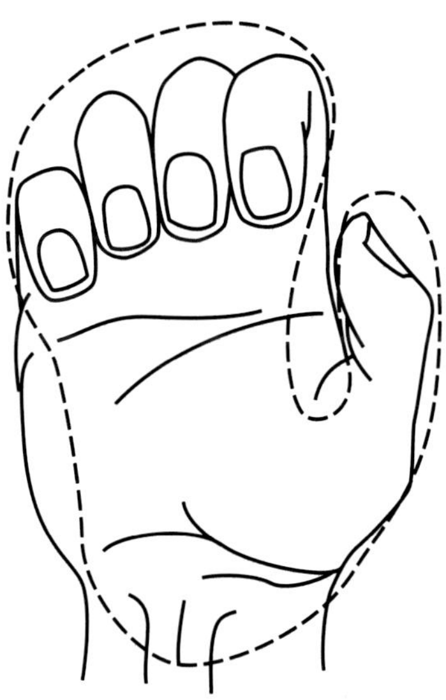

Figure 7.21. Right-hand configuration for simulating the shape of the stomach.

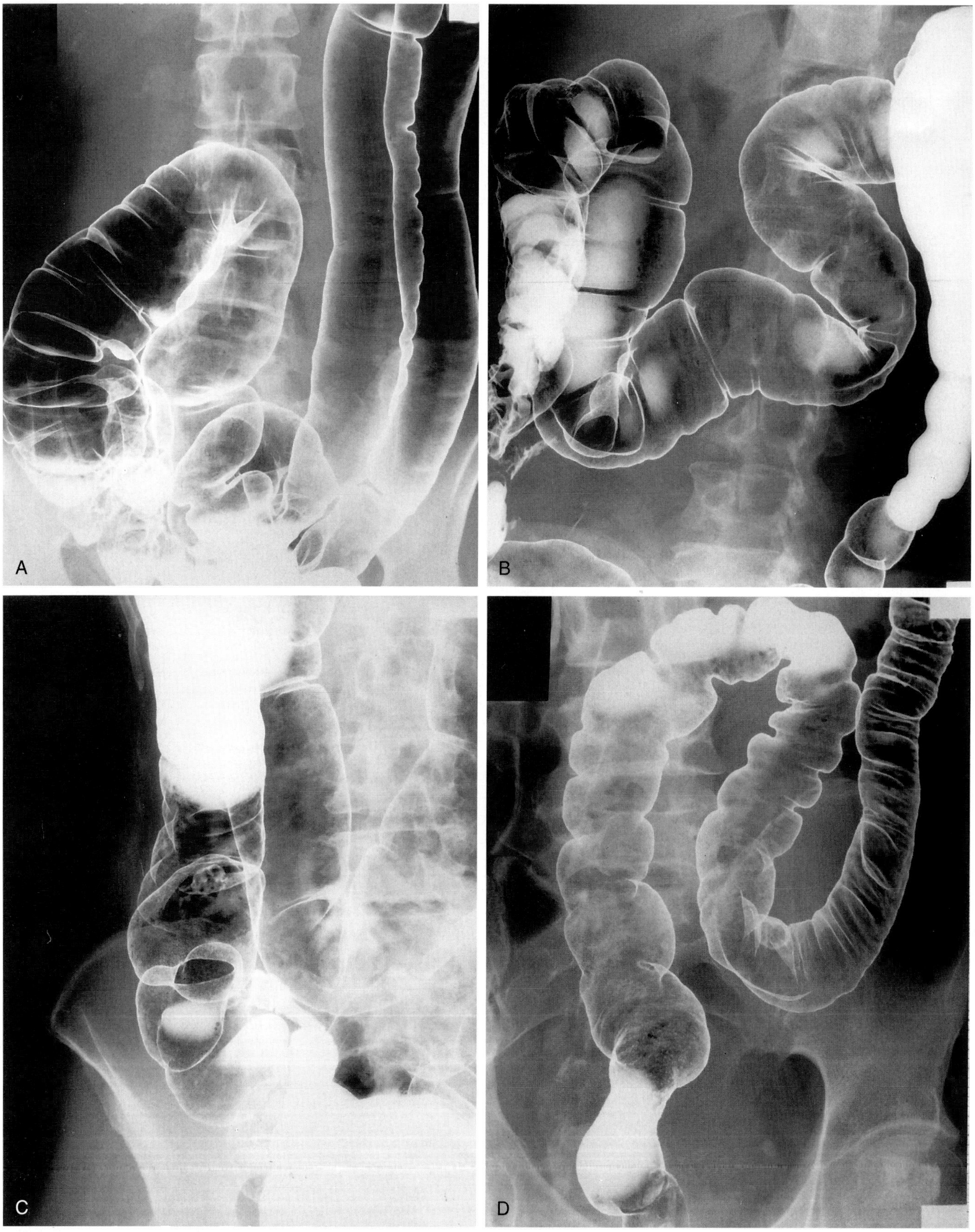

Figure 7.22. Double-contrast radiographs of large bowel. A, Transverse colon. B, Descending colon. C, Ascending colon. D, Sigmoid colon.

General Criteria

Same as those for upper GI studies, except:

I. Continuity of the tract
   A. One should aim for continuity of the tract, except for the sigmoid colon (Fig. 7.22)
   B. Overlapping of the sigmoid colon and the left and right flexures should be minimized.
   C. The same part of the tract should be radiographed from different angles.

II. Barium coating of the tract
   A. A "fine network pattern"* should be observable in at least one of the colon segments. (One should abide by the rule that air must push the mass of barium through the tract.) (See Fig. 7.1*B*.)
   B. The thin layer of contrast medium on the colonic mucosa should not crack owing to extended examination or to the highly concentrated barium medium.
   C. If two tracts are unavoidably overlapped, the frontal tract should be barium-coated thinly enough so that the tract behind can be observed.
   D. The cecum should be fully distended at the final stage to show sufficient air in all of the segments (see Fig. 7.22)
   E. The ileocecal region should be fully filled with barium without allowing any air to get in (see Fig. 7.22)

III. Other
   A. In the rectosigmoid area, the image should include the bottom of the anal tube, the sacrum, and the coccyx (Fig. 7.23)
   B. If there seems to be residual fecal matter on the colonic wall, it should be confirmed by taking another image showing its movement

*A double-contrast view of the innominate grooves and the minimum demonstrable radiological unit equivalent to "area gastricae" on the gastric mucosa.

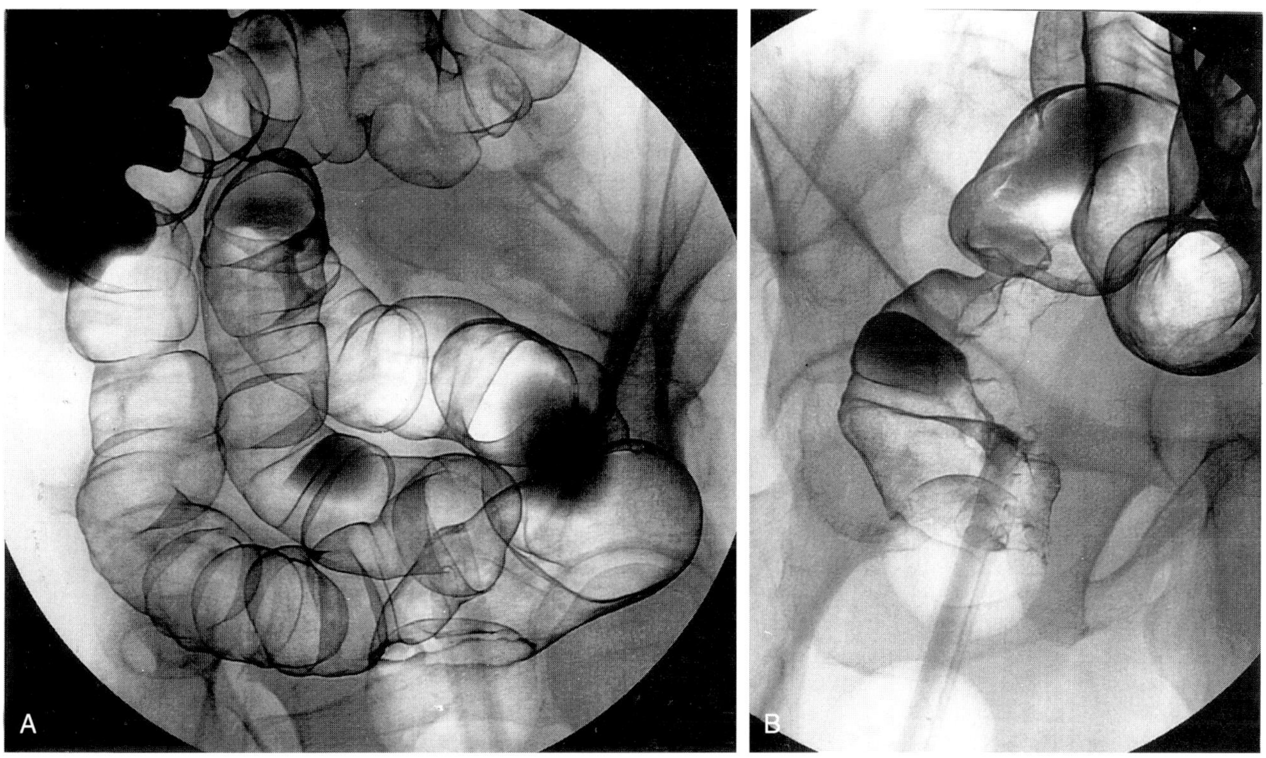

Figure 7.23. Complex sigmoid colon and rectum with distal end sealed using double balloons inflated with air. A, Sigmoid colon. B, Rectum.

As shown in the model, the transverse colon lies in front of the descending and ascending colons. When radiographs are taken of the splenic flexure, the left oblique projection is necessary so that as wide a gap as possible exists between the two adjacent colons. On the other hand, the right oblique position is necessary for getting a satisfactory radiograph of the hepatic flexure without overlap (Fig. 7.24). This is especially true in the case of the tract shown in this radiograph, which shows a model of the most difficult courses (clockwise loop for splenic flexure and counterclockwise loop for hepatic flexure) (Fig. 7.25).

As both flexures are superior in position, the table is tilted up so that unnecessary residual barium moves downward and air replaces it, thus allowing good double-contrast images. When the ascending colon is imaged with the patient in the supine position, some amount of unnecessary residual barium can be moved back to the transverse colon by rotating the patient left side down and tilting the table up. Repeat this procedure until satisfactory results are achieved.

The sigmoid colon is also positioned in front of the descending colon so that a left oblique position is usually necessary for preventing overlap. The sigmoid tract shown on the model represents a difficult N-shaped pattern at the junction of the descending and sigmoid colons.

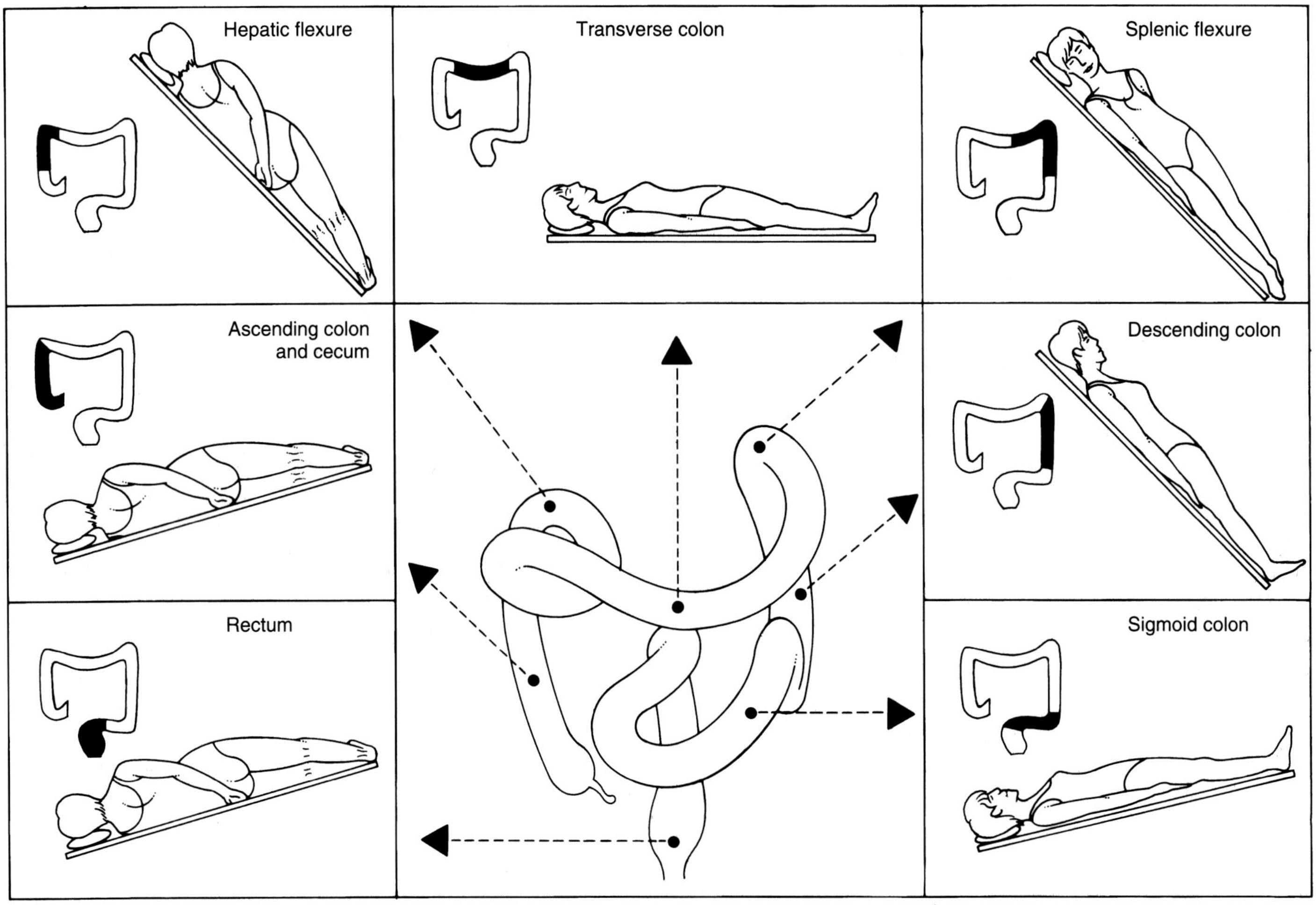

Figure 7.24. Various patient positions and their corresponding diagnosable parts of the colon. *Middle,* Three-dimensional colon is illustrated for better understanding of barium movement. (Courtesy of I. Ehara.)

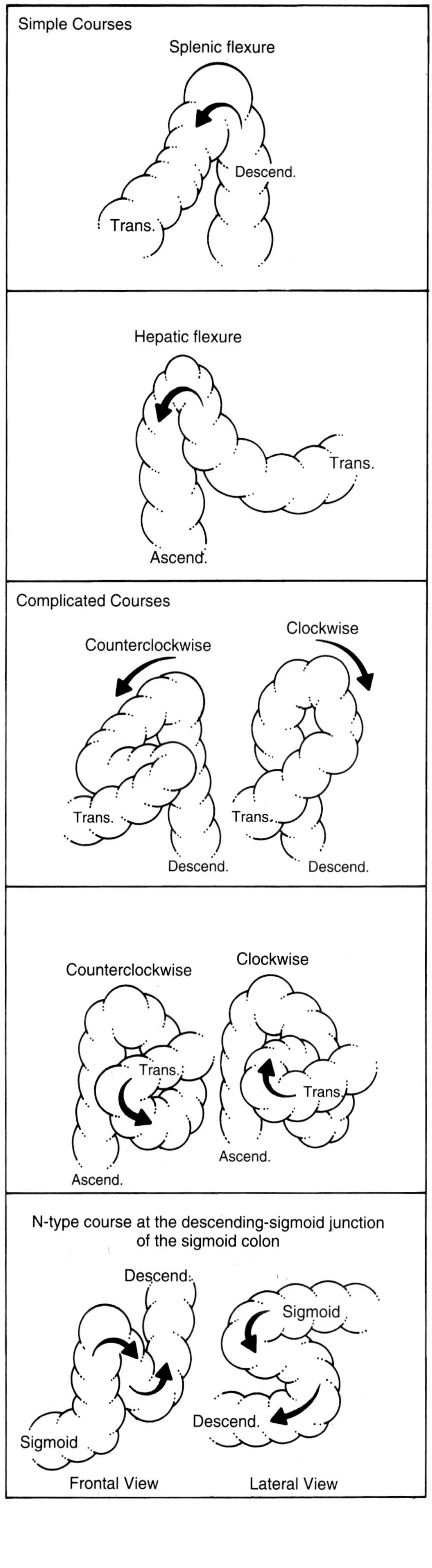

Figure 7.25. Various courses of the colon. Trans., Transverse colon; Descend, descending colon; Ascend, ascending colon. (Courtesy of I. Ehara.)

Bibliography

Bressler EC: Statutory Credentialing of Health Care Personnel. ASRT Fellow Thesis. Albuquerque, NM: American Society of Radiologic Technologists, 1981.

Carlton RR, Adler AM: Principles of Radiographic Imaging: An Art and a Science. Albany, NY: Delmar Publishers, 1992.

Curry TS, Dowdey JE, Murry RC: Christensen's Physics of Diagnostic Radiology. 4th ed. Philadelphia: Lea & Febiger, 1990.

Hendee WR: The human visual system and its application to perception of radiologic images. Invest Radiol 1988; 24:25.

Hendee WR, Manaster BJ, Harnsberger HR, et al: Oncologic imaging. *In* Holleb AI, Fink DJ, Murphy GP: American Cancer Society Textbook of Clinical Oncology. Atlanta: American Cancer Society, 1991.

Ireland SJ: Integrated Mathematics of Radiographic Exposure. St. Louis: CV Mosby, 1994.

Meschan I, Ott DJ: Introduction to Diagnostic Imaging. Philadelphia: WB Saunders, 1984.

Tuddenham WJ: The visual physiology of roentgen diagnosis. AJR 1957; 78:116–123.

CHAPTER 8

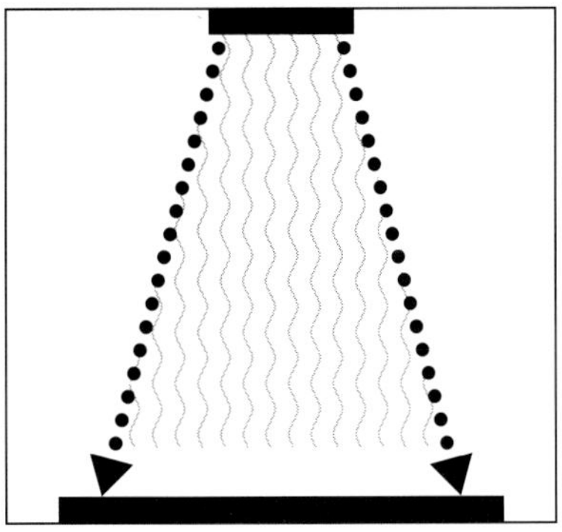

Quality Control

Steven B. Dowd, Ed.D., R.T.(R.)

Radiology departments must carry out a quality assurance program to ensure that services delivered are of high quality, with radiographs of diagnostic quality produced with a minimum of exposure to patient and personnel. This chapter discusses basic concepts of quality assurance and quality control (QC), describes QC tests, and concludes with a discussion of basic equipment malfunctions. This chapter, as an introduction, describes these procedures only in the most general terms and using a conceptual basis. Readers wanting more specific information are encouraged to consult the sources listed in the bibliography.

QUALITY ASSURANCE

Quality assurance is carried out by a team of individuals in the radiology department—radiologist, radiographers, administrators, and other employees. It is an important factor in receiving hospital wide accreditation by the Joint Commission on the Accreditation of Healthcare Organizations (JCAHO).

QUALITY CONTROL

QC is one aspect of total quality assurance. It refers to tests that ultimately should lead to improvement of image quality and consistency and a reduction of repeat rates, examination costs, and patient radiation exposure.

QC TEST PROCEDURES

There are three basic levels of QC testing. First-level tests are commonly carried out by technologists using inexpensive equipment. Second-level tests use more complicated types of equipment and are performed by a technologist specially trained in QC testing. Third-level tests are commonly performed by a physicist, and require some disassembly of equipment. They are not described here.

Basic QC Testing

A simple QC program can be carried out using a step-wedge (Fig. 8.1) and a metal thermometer, a dedicated QC cassette, eight pennies, and a variety of lead markers. Even the smallest of facilities can carry out basic QC testing.

Basic Penetrometer QC Check

A first step in basic testing involves the production of a step-wedge (Fig. 8.2) after the processor is cleaned and filled with fresh, properly mixed chemicals. Using 70 to 80 kV, the strip should show densities from almost clear at one end to black at the other. Technical factors used are recorded, and this strip is kept as a reference. Each morning a strip is exposed, and if the densities vary by more than one step, there is a problem in the imaging chain.

Potential Problem If Parameters Are Out of Alignment
A variety of causes for this problem are possible, including equipment and processor. More detailed testing is required to determine the root of the problem.

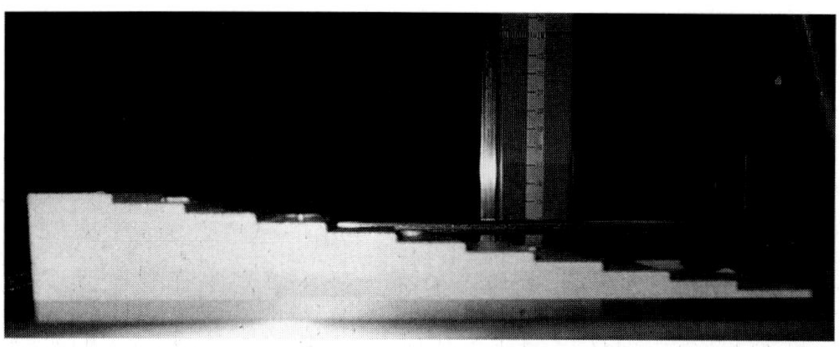

Figure 8.1. Step-wedge.

Figure 8.2. Radiograph of step-wedge.

Processor QC

Without a processor QC program, it is difficult to accurately determine the cause of substandard images. This variable must be controlled.

Chemical Activity

Chemical activity is typically assured by accurate mixing of solutions and routine checking of replenishment rates and activity. Also, films that are fed in the wrong direction may produce underreplenishment or overreplenishment of chemicals.

Potential Problems If Parameters Are Out of Alignment

1. Underreplenishment will result in loss of density or contrast.
2. Overreplenishment will waste chemicals and may cause significant changes in contrast.

Cleaning and Maintenance

A routine procedure must be followed for startup and shutdown of the processor. This is typically contained in the manual provided with the processor; a routine can be found in Burns and Dowd (1994b). This is the surest, and possibly the simplest, means of avoiding artifacts and reducing the chance of failure of the processor transport system.

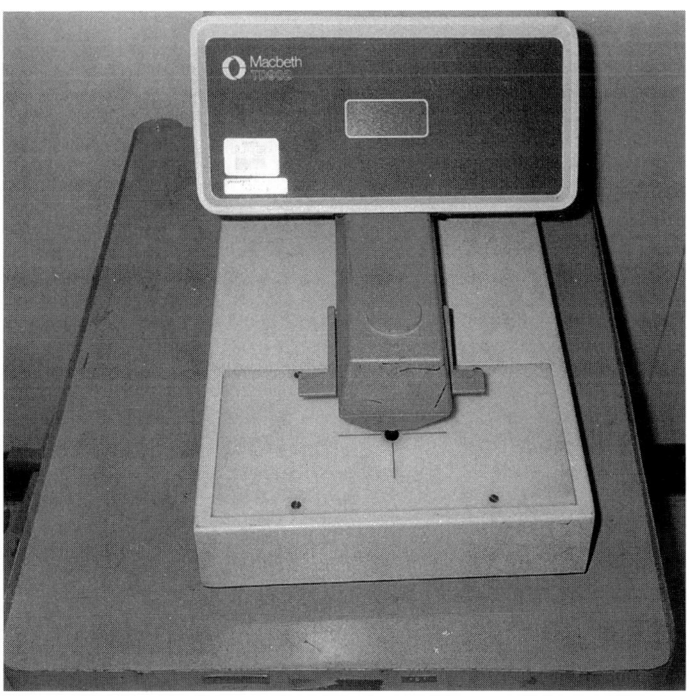

Figure 8.3. Densitometer.

Monitoring

Use of a sensitometer and densitometer (Fig. 8.3) is necessary for proper processor monitoring. The sensitometer is a reliable exposure source that can isolate problems observed to the processor; the densitometer is used to measure the film density. Four density values are measured:

1. Base plus fog is measured in the clear area adjacent to the strip.
2. The speed index (S), which should be 1.0 above base plus fog (about 1.2).
3. The high-density step (H), which should be 2.0 above base plus fog (about 2.2).
4. The low-density step (L), which should be 0.25 above base plus fog (about 0.45).

H minus L is the contrast index. Trend charts (Fig. 8.4) are used to monitor changes in the processor. Values must fall into these ranges: Base plus fog ± 0.05, speed index ± 0.10, and contrast index ± 0.10.

Once the functioning of the processor is known, other QC tests using film can be used to monitor the equipment.

Potential Problems If Parameters Are Out of Alignment

1. Low-contrast images due to increased base plus fog.
2. Changes in speed index may cause overexposure or underexposure of film and patient.
3. Changes in contrast may result in contrast images that are higher or lower than desired.

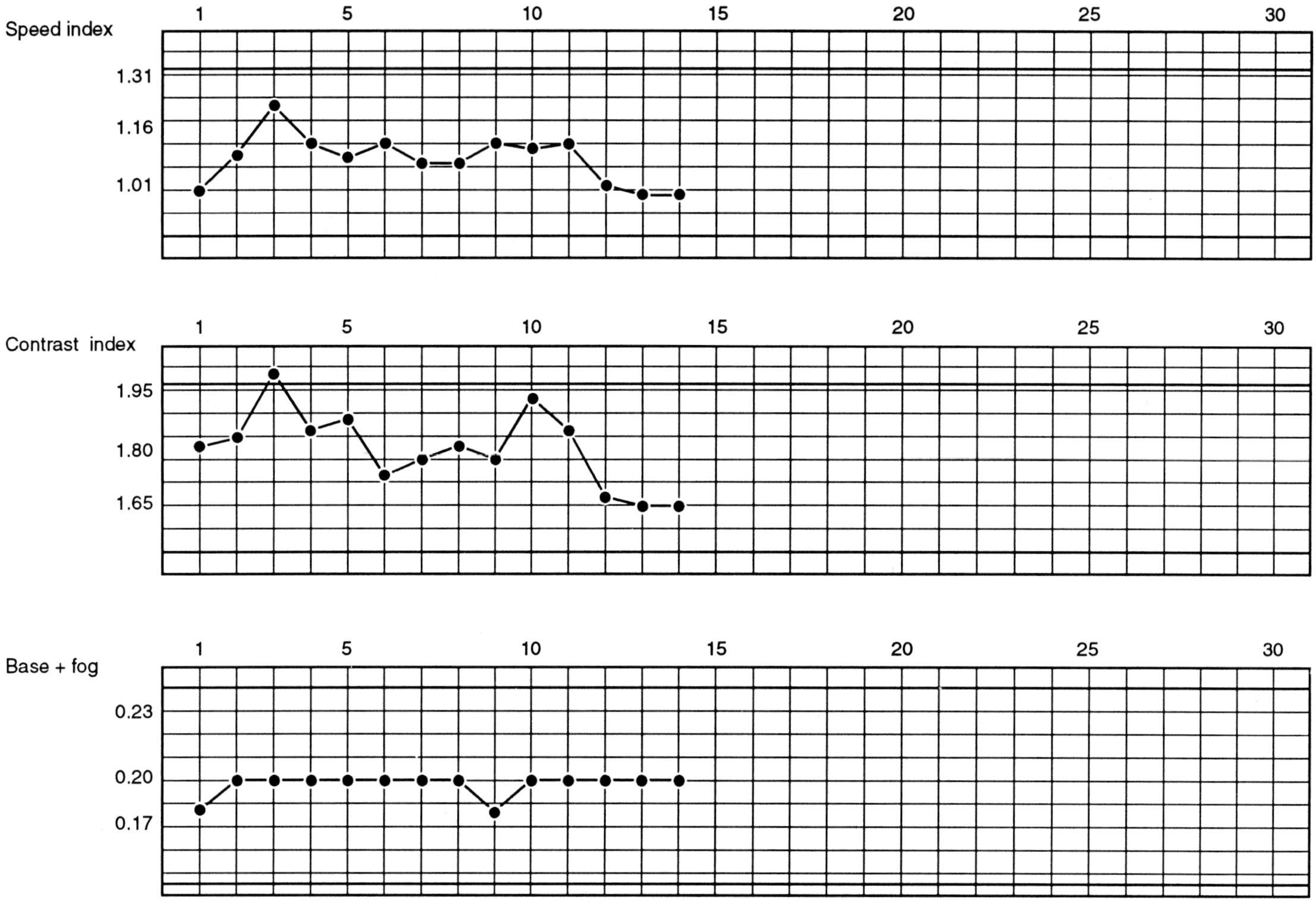

Figure 8.4. Sample processor trend chart, 2 weeks worth of data. *Note*: Solid horizontal lines indicate levels of unacceptability.

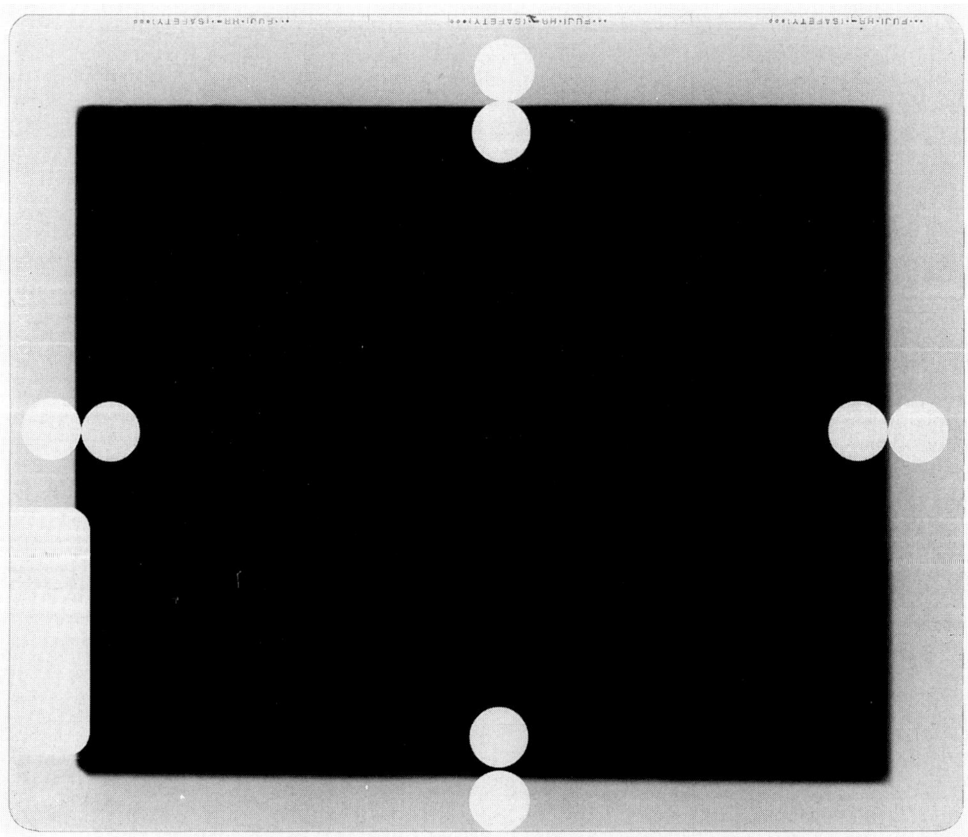

Figure 8.5. Eight-penny test.

Other Simple QC Test Procedures

mAs Reciprocity—Step-Wedge

All combinations of mA and time that produce the same mAs should produce the same exposure with all other variables held constant. Use of a step-wedge at different combinations of mA and time that all provide the same mAs (e.g., 100 mA and 0.1 second; 200 mA and .05 second; and 400 mA and 0.025 second) will indicate whether such mAs reciprocity exists.

Potential Problems If Parameters Are Out of Alignment

1. Overexposure or underexposure.
2. Incorrect mA stations or timers.

X-Ray Beam–Light Beam Congruence

Collimating tightly to the anatomy of interest is usually desirable from the standpoint of film quality and radiation protection. The congruence of the x-ray beam and projected collimator beam light can be checked by a variety of means; the simplest is the eight-penny test (Fig. 8.5).

Potential Problems If Parameters Are Out of Alignment

1. Excessive radiation exposure to the patient.
2. Excessive scatter leading to a degradation of image quality.

X-Ray Beam–Bucky Tray Alignment

The beam must also be in alignment with the Bucky tray. Using a metallic O in the center of the film determines whether the beam and tray are in alignment; a 0.4-inch (1-cm) misalignment is allowed (Fig. 8.6).

Potential Problems If Parameters Are Out of Alignment

1. May cause visual cutoff of the anatomic part to be imaged.
2. On phototimed exposures, may cause part of interest to not appear in middle of photocell, increasing or decreasing image density.

Routine Physical or Visual Evaluations

Two simple visual evaluations should be performed: the accuracy of the focal-film distance/source- to–image receptor distance (FFD/SID) measure(s), which can be evaluated using a tape measure; and the accuracy of the angle indicators, which can be evaluated using a carpenter's level and a protractor.

Potential Problems If Parameters Are Out of Alignment

1. Changes in SID may lead to overexposure or underexposure; however, a change in SID will also change geometric factors such as magnification and sharpness.
2. Incorrect angle indicators will necessitate repeats at the correct angle.

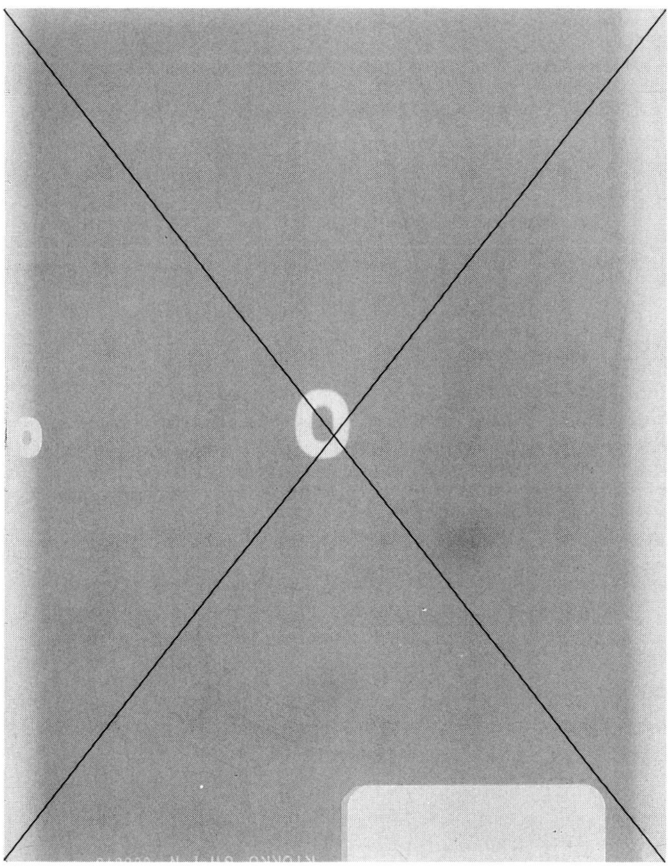

Figure 8.6. X-ray beam—Bucky tray alignment.

ADVANCED GENERATOR AND X-RAY TUBE PERFORMANCE STANDARDS

Digital Dosimeter

A digital display ionization chamber (dosimeter) is a device that allows for more accurate measurements in the QC program.

mAs Reciprocity

mAs reciprocity uses different sets of exposure factors to produce the same mAs. The same mAs, regardless of mA and time chosen, should produce a similar exposure. The variance between the exposures (output measured in mR/mAs) should not be more than 10 percent.

> **Potential Problem If Parameters Are Out of Alignment**
> If different permutations of the same mAs do not give approximately equal exposures, then film density will vary, causing potential overexposures, underexposures, and repeats.

Timer Linearity

Time is assumed to be approximately linear with exposure; that is, as time is doubled, so is exposure. Timer linearity uses the same time values as in the test just described, but keeps the mA constant. The variance (average mR/mAs) should not be more than 10 percent.

> **Potential Problem If Parameters Are Out of Alignment**
> Malfunctioning timers may cause overexposures, underexposures, and repeats.

mA Linearity

It is assumed that every time an mA station is selected (e.g., 400 mA), it produces approximately the same number of electrons. mA is assumed to be approximately linear with exposure; that is, as mA is doubled, so is exposure. mA linearity uses one of the time values from the timer test and the same mA values from the mAs reciprocity test. The variance (average mR/mAs) should not be more than 10 percent.

> **Potential Problem If Parameters Are Out of Alignment**
> Malfunctioning mA stations may cause overexposures, underexposures, and repeats.

Reproducibility

Reproducibility is a test used to document erratic or inconsistent exposures. If a radiographer chooses 400 mA at 0.1 second (40 mAs) routinely for abdomens that measure 21 cm, then that exposure should consistently provide approximately the same exposure and density. In a series of exposures, the resulting variance should be less than 10 percent.

> **Potential Problem If Parameters Are Out of Alignment**
> Erratic exposures will cause repeats; if the cause of the incorrect exposure is not known, the technologist may change technical factors, possibly resulting in additional repeats.

Beam Quality

Beam quality is monitored through the half-value layer (HVL). The HVL is the thickness of any material placed in the beam that reduces intensity to one half the original value. The HVL is a reference point for kVp calibration or tube aging.

> **Potential Problems If Parameters Are Out of Alignment**
> 1. kVp settings do not match kVp produced, resulting in overpenetration or underpenetration and possibly overexposure or underexposure.
> 2. Tube may be due for replacement.

Other Tests Performed by Dedicated Equipment

Kilovolts Peak

Kilovolts peak (kVp) may be measured using a kVp test cassette or a digital kVp test meter. kVp should not vary by more than ± 5 kVp of the set value.

> **Potential Problem If Parameters Are Out of Alignment**
> Overpenetration of the image resulting in images with excessively high or low density or contrast, or both; potential repeats.

Timer Accuracy

Timer accuracy may be checked in one of three ways:

1. On single-phase units, with a spin-top that shows a dot for each pulse produced by the generator (Fig. 8.7).
2. On three-phase or high-frequency units, with a synchronous spin-top that shows an arc corresponding to the exposure time.
3. With a digital timer test tool, giving a direct readout of time. Timers may not be out of alignment more than ± 5 percent.

> **Potential Problems If Parameters Are Out of Alignment**
> 1. Overexposure or underexposure.
> 2. Gross differences (e.g., half the time expected) may indicate rectifier problems.

Focal-Spot Size

Changes in the focal spot may be monitored by the pinhole camera (the most accurate) or the star pattern. National Electric Manufacturers Association standards for new tubes specify that focal spots may be as much as 50 percent greater than the specified value. Management will typically decide in a department the acceptable variance in focal-spot size.

Potential Problem If Parameters Are Out of Alignment
Increased geometric blurring and decreased resolving power.

QC ON ANCILLARY EQUIPMENT

Image Receptors

Screen Cleaning

Proper cleaning of screens removes foreign objects that can show up as artifacts on the film.

Potential Problem If Parameters Are Out of Alignment
Artifacts. Artifacts will obscure information or, in some cases, mask pathology on the film, leading to misdiagnosis.

Screen-Film Contact

The wire-mesh test detects loss of screen-film contact, as illustrated in Figure 8.8.

Potential Problems If Parameters Are Out of Alignment
Areas of poor screen-film contact will cause loss of resolution.

Grids

If grids are misaligned in the Bucky, or are damaged, increased attenuation of the primary beam may occur in certain areas (grid cutoff).

Potential Problems If Parameters Are Out of Alignment
1. Grid cutoff will cause repeats.
2. Unrecognized grid cutoff will cause the radiographer to increase technical factors, increasing patient exposure.

Illuminators

Illuminators are rarely consistent within a department. If one or more bulbs burn out in an illuminator, for example, that film will appear darker than it will on an illuminator in which all bulbs are operational.

Potential Problem If Parameters Are Out of Alignment
A lack of consistency with illuminator intensity may cause the radiographer to produce radiographs that are underexposed or overexposed.

Protective Apparel

If aprons are handled carelessly, the lead in the apron may fold or crack. Also, as many as 20 percent of new aprons may be cracked. Aprons should be periodically checked using fluoroscopy or regular radiography at 100 kVp.

Potential Problem If Parameters Are Out of Alignment
Cracked aprons will allow radiation leaks, increasing the exposure to personnel or patients if they are also used as gonadal shielding.

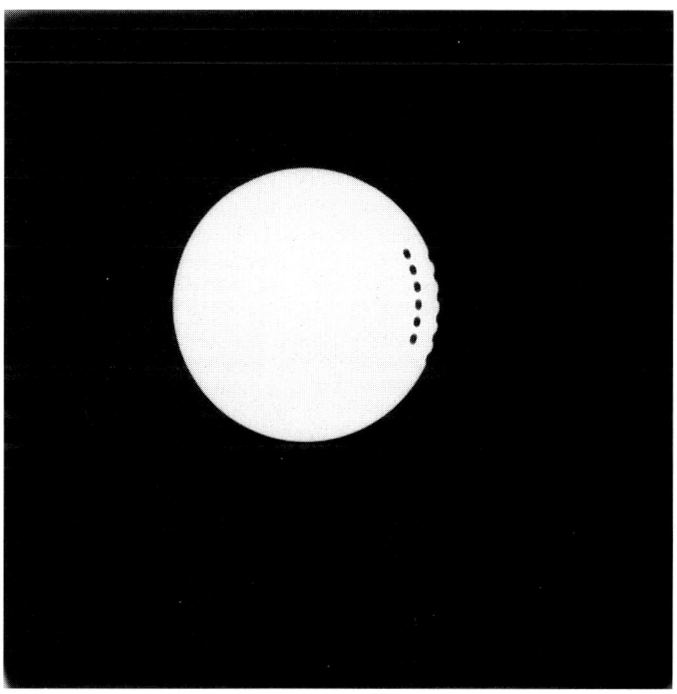

Figure 8.7. Spin-top test, single-phase unit.

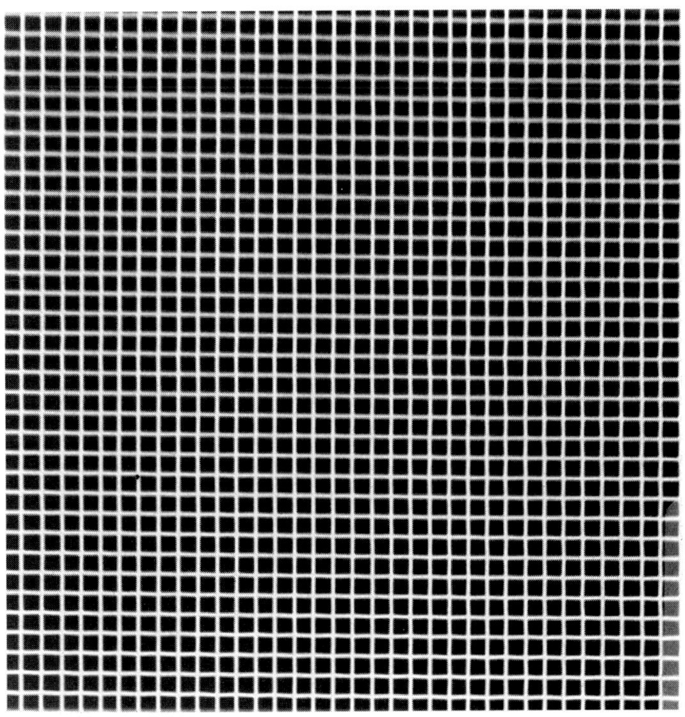

Figure 8.8. Wire-mesh test showing good screen-film contact.

REPEAT ANALYSIS

Repeat analysis is performed to determine the potential cause of repeat exposures. Repeats are saved and, over a period of time (usually 1 month), are classified according to cause (e.g., too dark, too light, centering, positioning, and motion) and room/tube. This allows the department to solve the causes of repeat exposures.

EQUIPMENT AND ACCESSORY MALFUNCTIONS OR MISAPPLICATIONS

Radiographers should be able to determine whether problems that arise are due to equipment or human error (e.g., selecting the wrong technique). This section summarizes some of the more common problems; the problems and their solutions can be found in greater detail in Burns and Dowd (1994a). These problems all assume that a "correct" technique has been set from the technique chart.

Problems of No Exposure

One of the most baffling problems with radiographic equipment is often that of no exposure. Problems of no exposure are summarized here.

PROBLEMS OF NO EXPOSURE

No Power to Generator
Unit not turned on
Circuit breaker tripped

Control Panel Settings or Switches Engaged
One or more control panel settings not set correctly

Automatic Collimator
Bucky/cassette holder tray not pushed in
Incorrect FFD/SID
Both table and upright cassette holder engaged

Rotor Operating but No Exposure
Stator not operating correctly
Filament burned out

Spot-Film Camera
Film magazine loaded incorrectly
Film loaded incorrectly into magazine

Problems of Incorrect Radiographic Density

Six problems of incorrect radiographic density are:

1. Underexposure—Formation of too few latent image centers in the emulsion. **Result: Light films.**
2. Underdevelopment—An insufficient number of silver halide crystals are converted to metallic silver in the developer. **Result: Light Films.**
3. Underpenetration—kVp is too low to provide a sufficient number of photons at the receptor to produce the correct density. **Result: Light films; possibly high contrast.**
4. Overexposure—Formation of too many latent image centers in the emulsion. **Result: Dark films.**
5. Overdevelopment—An excessive number of silver halide crystals are converted to metallic silver in the developer. **Result: Dark films.**
6. Overpenetration—kVp is too high and produces an extremely large number of photons at the receptor. **Result: Dark films; possibly low contrast.**

Insufficient Radiographic Density

Light radiographs (insufficient density) are either underexposed or underdeveloped. Problems of insufficient radiographic density are summarized here.

PROBLEMS OF INSUFFICIENT RADIOGRAPHIC DENSITY (UNDER-EXPOSED OR UNDERDEVELOPED)

Image Receptor
Cassette used upside down
Image receptor slower than specified (e.g., screen-film mismatch)
Correct speed used; incorrect cassette front

Automatic Exposure Control
Incorrect tube selected (e.g., chest tube selected when overhead tube should be)
Incorrect centering of anatomic part
Too-short backup time selected
Incorrect detector selected
Incorrect density setting selected

X-Ray Generator and X-Ray Tube
Failure of timer circuit
Rectifier diode open or broken
Gassy tube
Bad or sticking contacts in mA control circuit
Miscalibrated mA
Filament malfunction
Deposition of tungsten from filament on window

Darkroom/Processing
Decrease in developer activity
Film stops in fixer

Ancillary Equipment
Grid ratio is greater than technique chart calls for
Grid cutoff due to centering or incorrect FFD/SID
Wrong beam size (small) for technical factors
Wrong filtration selected
FFD/SID too long

Excessive Radiographic Density

Dark radiographs (excessive density) are either overexposed or overdeveloped. Problems of excessive radiographic density are summarized here.

PROBLEMS OF EXCESSIVE RADIOGRAPHIC DENSITY (OVEREXPOSED OR OVERDEVELOPED)

Image Receptor
Image receptor faster than specified (e.g., screen-film mismatch)
Correct speed used; incorrect cassette front

Automatic Exposure Control
Exposure goes to backup time (possible wrong detector selected)
Incorrect density setting selected
Technical factors not compensated for beam size

X-Ray Generator and X-Ray Tube
Timer circuit fails
Multiple (machine-gun) exposures are made
Calibration of mA or kVp has drifted
Arc or power surge making timer run longer
Poor contacts in mA control circuit

Darkroom/Processing
Developer activity increased
Film fog (e.g., white light leaks, heat, radiation)

Ancillary Equipment
Grid ratio is less than technique chart calls for
No grid
Beam size inappropriate for technique
FFD/SID less than specified

Problems of Unsharp Images

The most common causes of image blur and subsequent unsharp images are motion and poor geometry. Problems of unsharp images are summarized here.

PROBLEMS OF UNSHARP IMAGES

Motion Blur
Patient moves
Loose Bucky
Tube crane continues to move after radiographer adjustment
Focal spot blur due to worn rotor bearings

Geometric Blur
Incorrect focal spot selected
Object-film distance (OFD) too long

Image Receptor
Poor screen-film contact
Too-fast image receptor

Pseudoblur
Low-contrast will cause an image that *appears* to be blurred (pseudoblur)

Problems of Low Contrast

In general, images with high contrast (also called short-scale contrast; this refers to images with primarily blacks and whites) are preferred in terms of image quality. Problems of low contrast are summarized here.

PROBLEMS OF LOW CONTRAST

Technical Factors
Low density places majority of densities in toe section of H and D curve*
kVp too high for part or pathology

Processing
Developer activity altered (e.g., exhausted, oxidized, low temperature)
Fixer exhausted or contaminated
Unit stops with film in fixer

Image Receptor
Improper storage increases base plus fog of film
Screen not spectrally matched to film
Low-attenuation front cassette used with high kVp

Ancillary Equipment
Grid contrast improvement factor too low (e.g., too low ratio)

*H and D curve, Hurter and Driffield curve; called also D = log E curve and characteristic curve; a plot of a series of known exposures against resulting densities; used to investigate speed, contrast, and fog exhibited on a radiograph.

Problems of Misalignment of Part and Image Receptor

Misalignment of part and image receptor will result in a radiograph in which the anatomy is not centered to the image receptor or is not correctly aligned with the receptor. Problems of misalignment of part and image receptor are summarized here.

PROBLEMS OF MISALIGNMENT OF PART AND IMAGE RECEPTOR

Bucky tray not pushed in
Tube centering and Bucky not in alignment
Central ray not properly centered
Cross-hair template out of position
Collimator improperly seated or loose

CONCLUSION

This chapter has summarized some of the basic QC tests and how they evaluate imaging parameters and the identification of some basic equipment malfunctions. Radiographers, even those not directly involved in QC testing, should have a basic understanding of QC tests and be able to identify basic equipment malfunctions. This will minimize repeat exposures, leading to an increased quality of service at lower cost and lower radiation dose to patients and personnel.

Bibliography

Burns CB, Dowd SB: Equipment and accessory malfunctions or misapplications. *In* Thompson M, Hattaway P, Hall J, Dowd SB (eds): Principles of Imaging Science and Protection. Philadelphia: WB Saunders, 1994a.

Burns CB, Dowd SB. Quality control. *In* Thompson M, Hattaway P, Hall J, Dowd SB (eds): Principles of Imaging Science and Protection. Philadelphia: WB Saunders, 1994b.

Gray JE, Winkler NT, Stears J, et al: Quality Control in Diagnostic Imaging. Rockville, MD: Aspen Publishers, 1981.

McKinney WEJ: Radiographic Processing and Quality Control. Philadelphia: JB Lippincott, 1988.

PART TWO

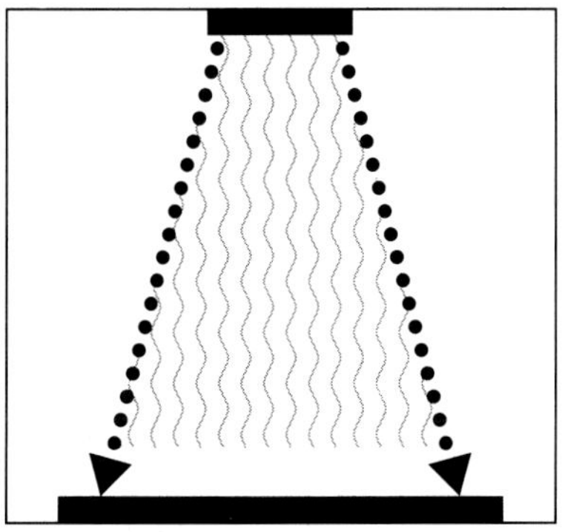

Routine Radiographic Procedures

CHAPTER 9

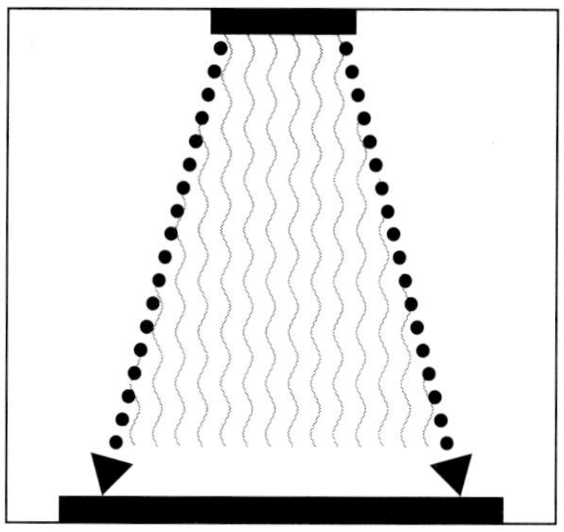

Upper Extremity

Erna Agnarsdottir, B.S.R.T.

Gudrun Fridriksdottir, R.T.

Radiographic Anatomy

Radiographic Positioning

This chapter presents an overview of basic positioning of the upper extremity. The first part reviews basic anatomy and general guidelines for positioning of the upper extremity, whereas the second part describes specific positioning of the upper extremity.

Although upper extremity radiography is often seen as "simple," in fact it requires precise attention to detail to properly radiograph what are often small anatomic parts.

The upper extremities (also called limbs) comprise these portions of the appendicular and the axial skeleton:

- Appendicular skeleton
  - Shoulder (pectoral) girdles
  - Clavicle
  - Scapula
- Axial skeleton
  - Humerus
  - Ulna
  - Radius
  - Carpals
  - Metacarpals
  - Phalanges

SHOULDER, CLAVICLE, AND SCAPULA

Each shoulder (pectoral) girdle consists of a scapula and a clavicle (Fig. 9.1). The shoulder girdle attaches the bones of the upper extremities to the axial skeleton.

The clavicles are long, slender bones with a double curvature. The clavicles lie horizontally in the superior and anterior part of the thorax, superior to the 1st rib.

The scapulae are large, flat, triangular bones, situated in the posterior part of the thorax, between the levels of the 2nd and the 7th ribs. A sharp ridge, the spine, runs diagonally across the posterior surface of the flattened body of scapulae. The end of the spine projects a flattened, expanded body, called the acromion. This process articulates with the clavicle. At the lateral end of the superior border of the scapulae is an anterior surface called the coracoid process. Above and below are two fossa, the supraspinous fossa and the infraspinous fossa.

Inferior to the acromion is the glenoid cavity (fossa). The cavity articulates with the head of the humerus and forms the shoulder joint. The lateral part and the dorsal part of the spine, the coracoid process and the acromion, are commonly used to evaluate positioning of the patient.

HUMERUS

The humerus is the largest and the longest bone of the upper extremity (Fig. 9.2). Proximally it articulates with the scapulae and distally with both the ulna and the radius at the elbow joint. The head of humerus at the proximal end articulates with the glenoid cavity. Distal to the head is the anatomic neck, an oblique groove and the site of the epiphyseal plate. A lateral projection distal to the neck is a palpable bony landmark, the greater tubercle. The lesser tubercle is an anterior projection. Between these tubercles is the bicipital groove (intertubercular sulcus). Distal to the tubercles is the surgical neck.

The shaft (body) of the humerus is cylindrical at its proximal end. It becomes triangular and is flattened at its distal end. At the distal end there is the capitulum, the radial fossa, and the trochlea. The capitulum articulates with the head of radius. The radial fossa is a depression that receives the head of the radius when the forearm is flexed. The trochlea is a surface that articulates with the ulna. The coronoid fossa is an anterior depression that receives part of the ulna when the forearm is flexed. The olecranon fossa is a posterior depression that receives the olecranon of the ulna when the forearm is extended. On either side of the humerus are the medial and the lateral epicondyles to which most muscles of the forearm are attached. The ulnar nerve lies on the posterior side of the medial epicondyle.

ULNA AND RADIUS

The ulna is the medial bone of the forearm (Fig. 9.3). The olecranon (or olecranon process) is at the proximal end of ulna, which forms the prominence of the elbow. The coronoid process is an anterior projection. The olecranon process receives the trochlea of the humerus. Inferior and lateral to the trochlear notch is a depression, the radial notch, which receives the head of the radius. The ulna has a head at the distal end and a styloid process on the posterior side.

The radius is the lateral bone of the forearm. Its proximal end articulates with the capitulum of the humerus and the radial notch of the ulna. A muscle attachment on the medial side is called the radial tuberosity. Distally, the radius articulates with two bones of the wrist, the scaphoid and the lunate.

At the distal end of the radius is a styloid process, and on the medial and lateral side an ulnar notch, which articulates with the distal end of the ulna.

CARPALS, METACARPALS, AND PHALANGES (Fig. 9.4)

The carpals consist of eight small bones, named after their shapes. The proximal row of carpals from the medial to the lateral position consists of the triquetrum (has three articular surfaces), the lunate (resembles a crescent moon in an AP view), and the scaphoid (resembles a boat). The distal row of carpals from the lateral to medial position consists of the trapezium (four-sided), the trapezoid (also four-sided), the capitate (a rounded projection), and the hamate (named for the large hook on its anterior surface).

The metacarpals are composed of five bones. The proximal end is called a base, then there is a shaft, and at the distal end a head. The metacarpal bones are numbered 1 to 5 starting with the lateral bone. The distal end of the carpal bones articulates with the bases of the metacarpals. The heads of the metacarpals articulate with the proximal phalanges of the fingers. The bones of the fingers, like the metacarpals, consist of a base at the proximal end, a shaft, and a head at the distal end. There are two phalanges in the 1st digit (the thumb) and three phalanges in digits 2 through 5. The proximal row of the phalanges articulates with the metacarpal bones and the middle row of the phalanges. The middle row eventually articulates with the distal row of the phalanges. The thumb has no middle row.

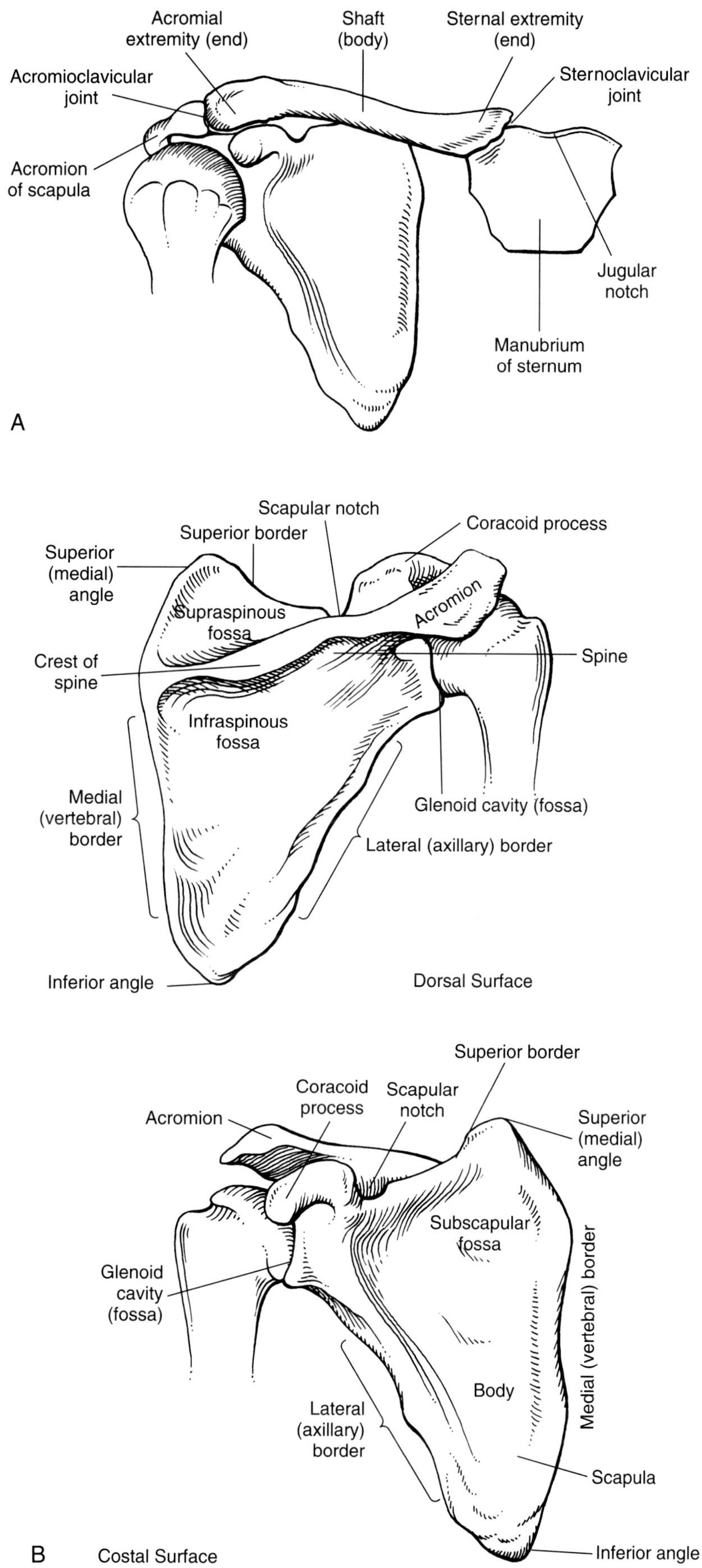

Figure 9.1. Anatomy of the shoulder. A, Clavicle. B, Scapula.

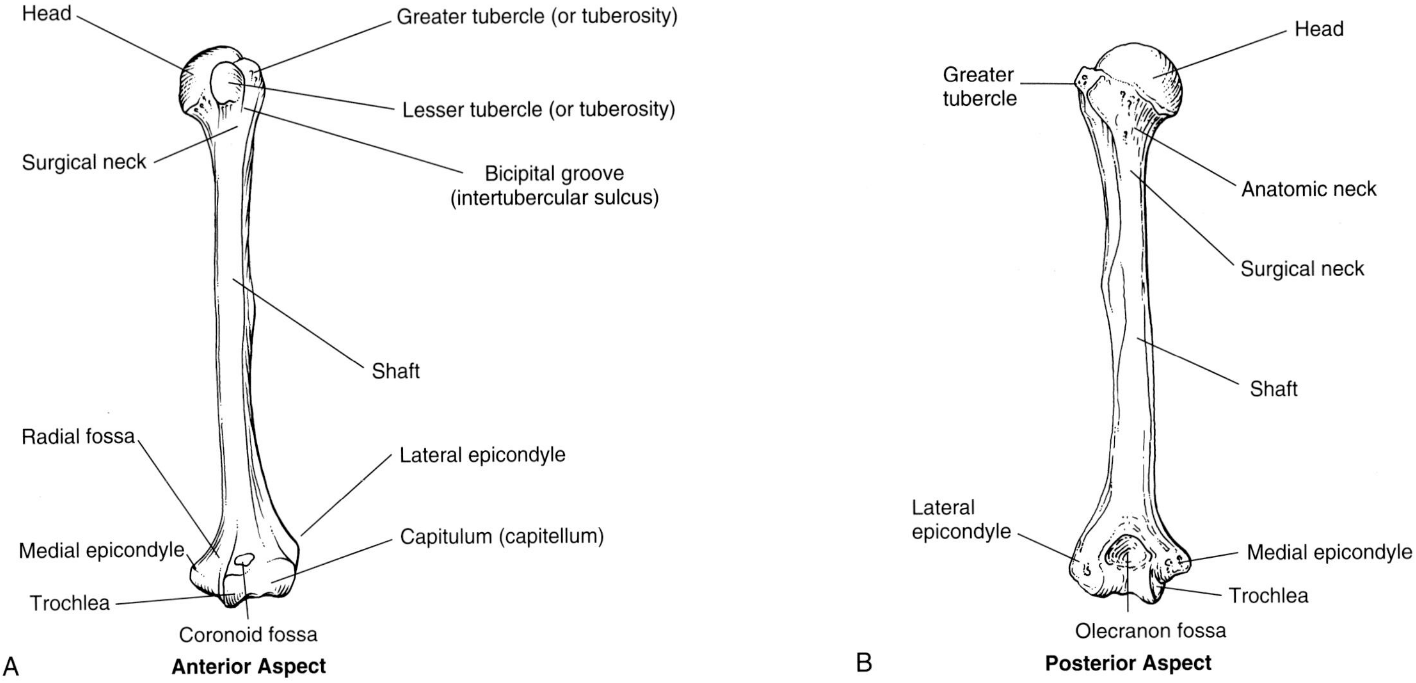

Figure 9.2. Anatomy of the humerus.

RADIOGRAPHY OF THE UPPER EXTREMITIES

General Rules

All skeletal parts should be projected from at least two different directions (angles). These directions are often perpendicular to each other. It is essential to think anatomically and consider principles of projections. To achieve a quality radiograph, several factors must be kept in mind.

Patient Factors

Before all radiographic examinations are performed, the patient's identification must be checked and verified. It is important to explain the procedure to the patient to ensure good cooperation. A patient who is uncomfortable or feels insecure is more likely to move during the exposure. All radiopaque objects, such as rings and bracelets, must be removed. Immobilization devices, pillows, sandbags, compression bands, sponges, and radiolucent pads must be used for support and comfort to minimize motion blurring (motion unsharpness).

Radiation Protection

Adequate radiation protection shall be provided. The most effective way to minimize radiation dose to the patient is the correct use of the tools and techniques available:

- Collimation.
- Proper immobilization.
- Proper use of shielding and patient positioning.
- Proper exposure factors.
- High-speed imaging system.
- As few repeated radiographs as possible.

Positioning procedures (including alternate projections such as PA instead of AP) should be used to reduce radiation doses to sensitive organs, such as breasts, thyroid gland, and gonads. For example, the patient should be seated at the side or at the end of the examining table with the lower part of the body away from the primary beam. It is a good rule to place a rubber sheet under the cassette to absorb the radiation that goes through the cassette. Contact shields (lead rubber of 0.5 mm Pb eq.) on the patient are effective only if they are placed at the edge of the radiation field. They become completely useless when the distance from the edge of the field is 2.5 inches (6 cm) or more. However, radiographers may still wish to provide the patient with such shielding for good public relations and professional appearance.

Exposure Factors

Exposure factors depend on the overall speed of the imaging system (film-screen combination and processing system), characteristics of the grids being used, and the focal-film distance (FFD). Differential absorption in bones and soft tissue is the fundamental characteristic of radiographic imaging. Radiographic contrast is governed by the subject contrast and the imaging systems contrast (film-screen combination and processing system). Subject contrast depends on the patient (e.g., thickness, density) and selected peak kilovoltage (kVp). For the upper extremities, a kVp in the range of 45 to 70 is usually appropriate for good radiographic contrast and detail. The highest possible milliampere (mA) value and lowest exposure time value are selected to produce a density of 1.6 to 2.0 at the darkest point of the film showing anatomy. If these factors are not appropriate, there could be a loss of contrast and detail in the image.

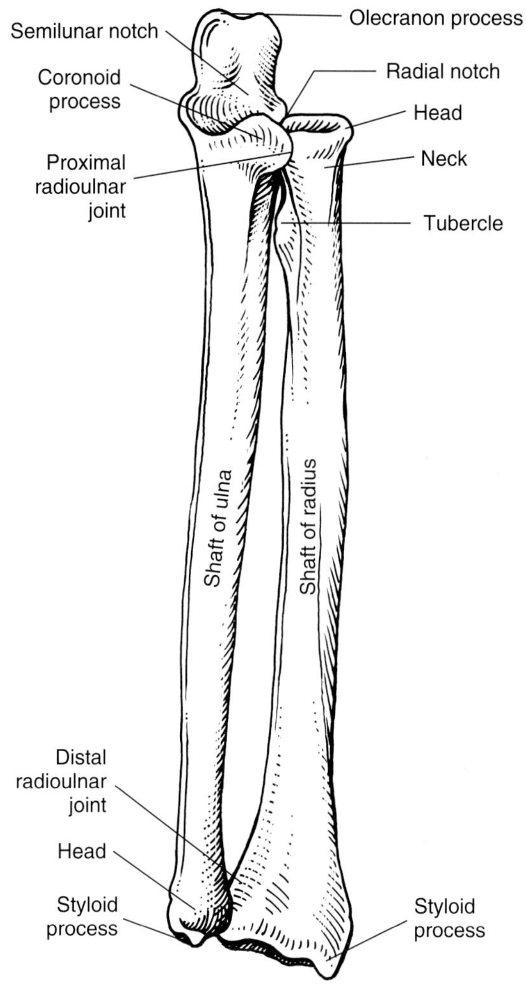

Figure 9.3. Anatomy of the ulna and radius.

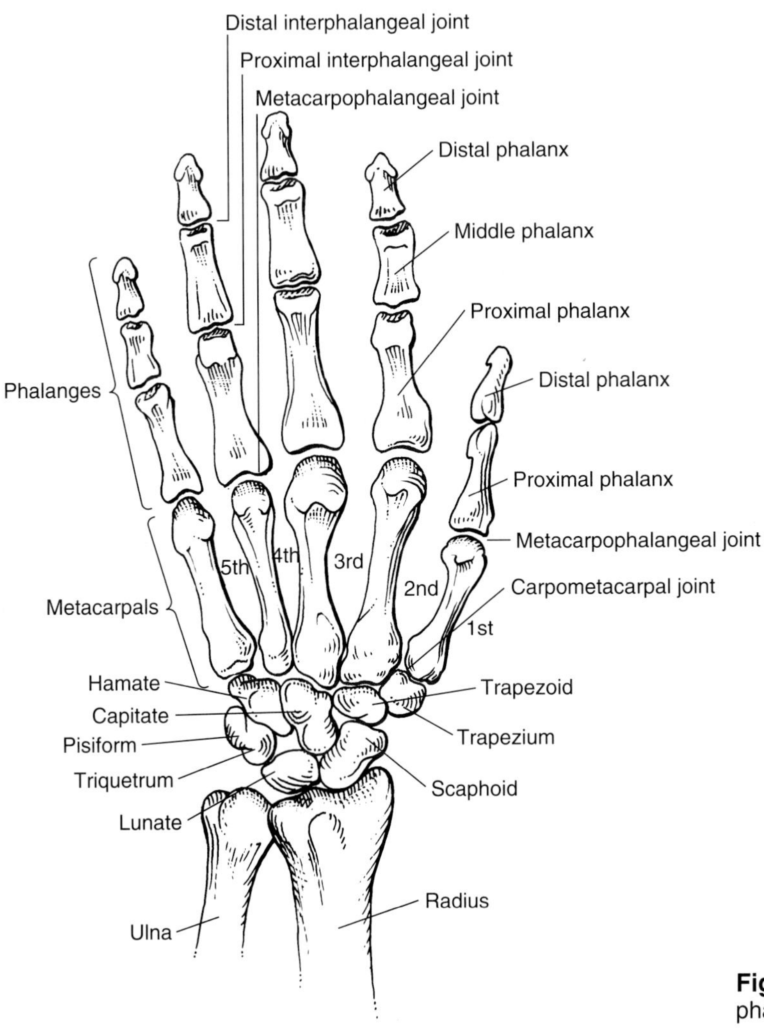

Figure 9.4. Anatomy of the carpals, metacarpals, and phalanges.

Intensifying Screens, Films, and Processing

The general rule is to choose screen-film combinations that give optimum recording of detail and contrast. This is achieved with slow speed systems in which the speed is 100 to 200 (some sources recommend a speed of 100 or less in radiography of the extremities). Recorded detail is a concern in orthopedic radiography owing to the possibility of small fractures or subtle changes in the trabeculae of the bone that may otherwise be missed.

To reduce exposure time and radiation dose, the use of rare-earth screens and film combinations with higher speed is recommended if recorded contrast and detail are acceptable. Low-speed systems require more radiation but give images with more detail and sharpness. Regular daily quality control must be maintained for the film processor to ensure optimum operation. Image quality and patient radiation dose are dependent on optimum processing of radiographic film.

Grids

Moving or stationary grids are necessary for thicker (denser) parts and higher kVp, in which scatter radiation is likely to reduce the quality of the image. Grids are not used for radiographing the hand, forearm, and elbow but are often used for the humerus, shoulder, scapula, and acromioclavicular joints. In general, a grid is used when patient thickness exceeds 4 to 5 inches (10 to 13 cm) and when 60 kVp or greater is used. However, this depends on the preferences of the radiologist, and is part of departmental routine. The recommended ratio for upper extremities is usually an 8:1 grid, with ranges of 6:1 to 10:1 being acceptable. This grid should also be linear (rather than crossed) and focused (rather than parallel), and it allows a range of FFDs. This will provide sufficient improvements in contrast, will require only moderate increases in exposure technique (important in limiting patient exposure), and will be sufficiently easy to use.

Focal-Spot Size

A focal-spot size of 0.6 to 1.2 mm is best suited for examinations of the upper extremity. In general, one can say that the smaller the focal spot the better, as this results in less geometric unsharpness. This is especially true when magnification procedures are used, as long object-to-film distances (OFDs) will reduce geometric unsharpness.

Focal-Film Distance

The FFD should be 40 to 44 inches (102 to 112 cm) when no grid is chosen (i.e., when the cassette is placed on the table). An FFD of 48 inches (122 cm) is often used when the cassette is under the table in the Bucky tray. In general, longer FFDs result in less patient entrance skin exposure and also reduce magnification. When unusually long or short FFDs are used, this should be noted in the patient history for the radiologist. FFDs are typically standardized within the departmental routine.

Soft Tissue Radiography

Soft tissue radiography of the upper extremities is often used in cases of bursitis of the shoulder, calcification in tendons, and foreign body localization. Also, following dislocation or subluxation of the acromioclavicular joints, soft tissue signs can be detected. When radiographing soft tissue, the kV is set 10 kV lower than for standard technique, which greatly increases the subject contrast between bones and soft tissue.

Pathological Conditions of the Skeletal System

Variation from standard exposure technique is sometimes necessary because of pathological conditions or differing tissue composition that can affect the radiographic density and contrast. Most pathological conditions can be divided into additive pathology and destructive pathology. As the name implies, additive pathology indicates that something has been added to the anatomy, and thus, more technique is required; whereas destructive pathology indicates that the anatomy has been eroded or destroyed, and thus, less technique is required. Destructive pathology usually requires lower kV (5 to 10 percent) but additive pathology requires higher kV (5 to 10 percent) or mAs (25 to 50 percent), or both.

Conditions that may require compensation are:

- Additive pathology
  - Acromegaly
  - Exostosis
  - Osteoma
  - Paget's disease
- Destructive pathology
  - Active osteomyelitis
  - Aseptic necrosis
  - Atrophy
  - Carcinoma
  - Degenerative arthritis
  - Gout
  - Osteoporosis

These conditions indicate only in what direction to change the technique. Exact changes depend on the skill of the technologist.

Patients with suspected fractures should never be forced into positions. When this is the case, two possibilities exist: (1) Contact the physician (radiologist), and see if the physician wishes to attempt to move the extremity into position or (2) use alternate projections. In most cases, innovation in the use of equipment will allow the radiographer to secure two projections at 90-degree angles through the use of cross-table and other projections. These projections will not always resemble the "textbook," but should still provide the radiologist or other physician with sufficient information to secure a diagnosis.

Table 9.1 Recommendations for Technique Changes With Various Types of Casts and Splints*

Author	Cast/Splint Type	Recommendation
Carrol, 1993	Dry plaster —medium	2 × mAs or ↑ kVp 15 percent
	Wet plaster —medium	3 × mAs or ↑ kVp 22 percent
	Dry plaster—large	3 × mAs or ↑ kVp 22 percent
	Wet plaster—large	4 × mAs or ↑ kVp 30 percent
	Plaster half cast; fiberglass/plaster mix; plastic cast	+ 50 percent mAs or ↑ kVp 8 percent
	Pure fiberglass	No change
	Wood splint	+ 50 percent mAs or ↑ kVp 8 percent
	Air splint	No change
Watkins and Moore, 1993	Dry plaster	Increase mAs at least 2 ×
	Dry plaster—large	Increase mAs at least 3 ×
	Wet plaster	Increase mAs at least 3 ×
	Wet plaster—large	Increase mAs at least 4 ×
	Pure fiberglass cast	No change
	Wood or aluminum splint	Increase mAs by 50 percent or ↑ kVp by 5
DeVos, 1990	Dry plaster	2 × normal mAs
	Wet plaster	3 × normal mAs
	Fiberglass	Wet, increase kVp by 5 percent; dry, no change
Cullinan and Cullinan, 1994†	Wet plaster	Increase (unspecified)
	Dry plaster	Same increase as above

Based on research by Gratale P, Turner GW, Burns GB: Using the same exposure factors for wet and dry casts. Radiol Technol 1986; 57:325–328.

Key: ↑ = increase.

*If a faster imaging system is used, as recommended in the text, then the increase will be based on that system, not the slower system normally used for extremities. For example, if a 100-speed system is normally used and a 200-speed system is used for casted extremities, then all changes would be based on ½ mAs, since a 200-speed system requires half the mAs of a 100-speed system. For a dry plaster cast, then, the same technique would be used.

The patient may present with a cast or splint. Recommendations from various authors are presented in Table 9.1. Radiographing casts does not usually require the use of slower-speed imaging systems; in fact, it may be contraindicated owing to the artifacts provided by a cast. If possible, splints should be removed prior to radiography to remove potential artifacts; however, this is done only on permission of the physician.

Recommended Routine Projections

The following are recommended routines; this may vary according to physician preferences. The patient's condition may require modification of the routine positions listed. In case of difficult positions, notes should be made for future reference. Make notes if recommended positions cannot be performed. This will assist the radiologist in making an accurate diagnosis. As always, it is vital to indicate the correct right and left marker on the film, and in the case of parts such as fingers, to mark the digit number on the film.

- Fingers—PA and lateral.
- Thumb—AP and lateral.
- Wrist—PA and lateral.
- Hand—PA, oblique, and lateral.
- Pisiform—posterior oblique.
- Carpal tunnel—superoinferior axial.
- Forearm—AP and lateral.
- Elbow—AP and lateral.
- Humerus—AP and lateral.
- Shoulder—AP internal, AP external, AP shoulder joint.
- Acromioclavicular joints—AP with and without weights.
- Clavicle—superoinferior and inferosuperior.
- Scapula—AP and lateral.

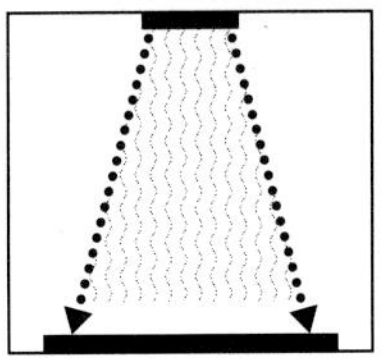

Fingers Two Through Five

Position/Projection

PA projection

Film:
8 × 10 inches (20 × 24 cm) tabletop for two projections crosswise

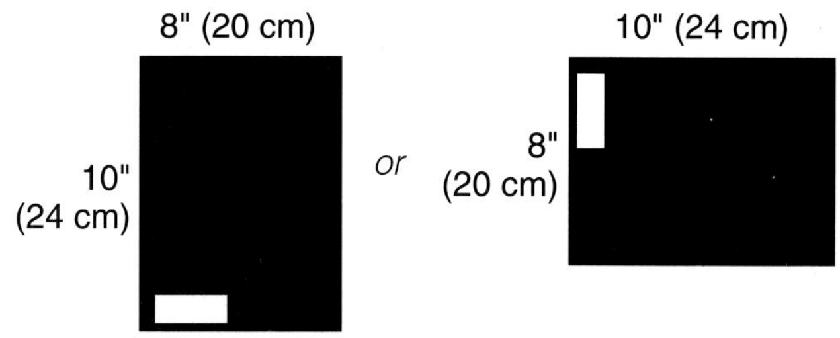

Patient Position

Seated at end or side of table, forearm resting on table, anterior side down. Palm of hand flat against film (Fig. 9.5).

Part Position

Place cassette under palmar side of finger. Separate fingers to isolate digit of interest. Proximal interphalangeal joint centered to film.

Central Ray

Perpendicular to proximal interphalangeal joint. Collimate to area of interest.

Structures Demonstrated

Individual digit (Fig. 9.6).

Evaluation Criteria

1. Phalanges should be clearly visible and phalangeal joints open.
2. Metacarpophalanges should be included. Finger(s) should not be rotated.
3. Radiographic density (1.6 to 2.0 at darkest portion of anatomy) and radiographic contrast (short-scale) should demonstrate both soft tissue and bony trabeculae.
4. Indicate finger number on film.

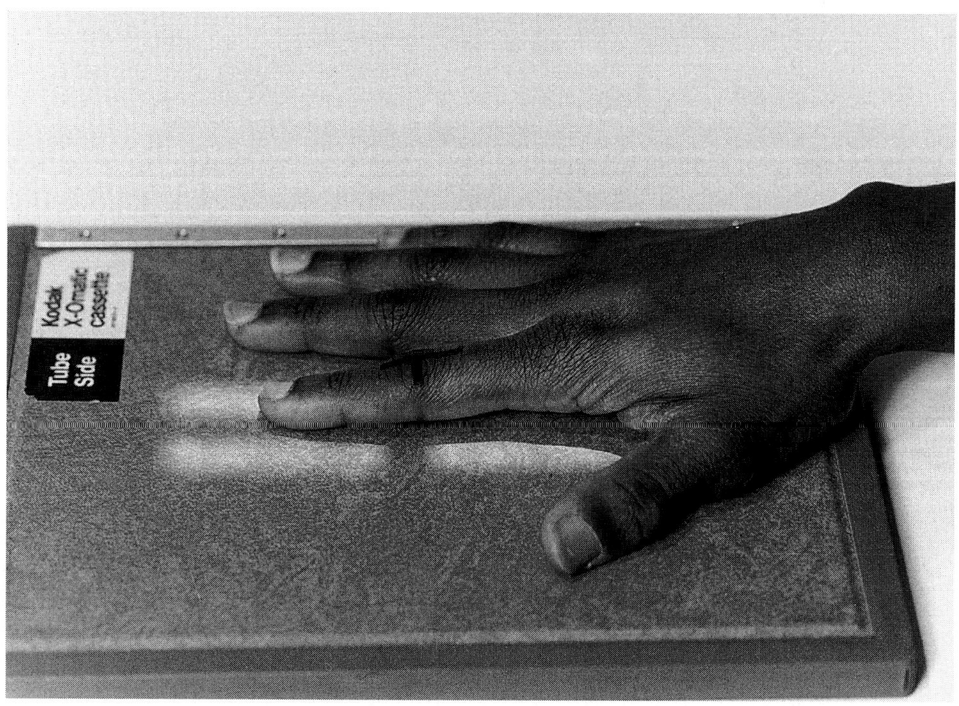

Figure 9.5. PA finger.

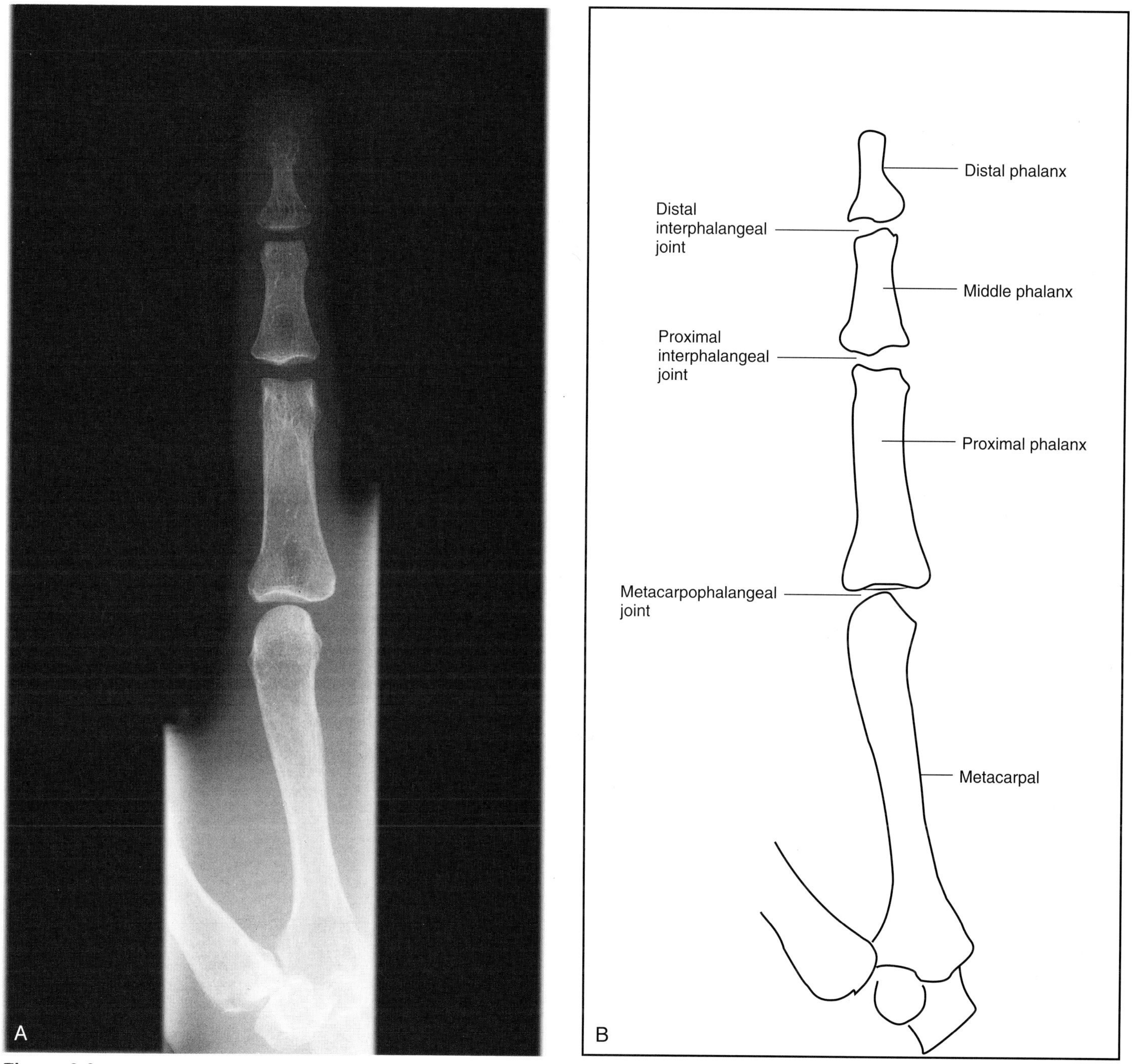

Figure 9.6. A and B, PA finger.

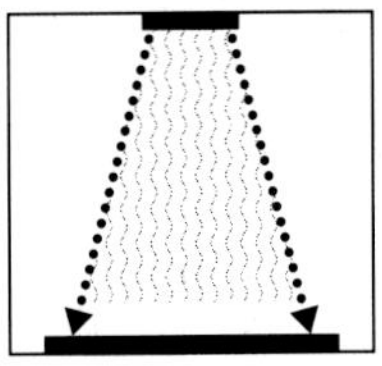

Fingers Two Through Five

Position/Projection

AP projection

Film:
8 × 10 inches (20 × 24 cm)
tabletop for two projections
crosswise

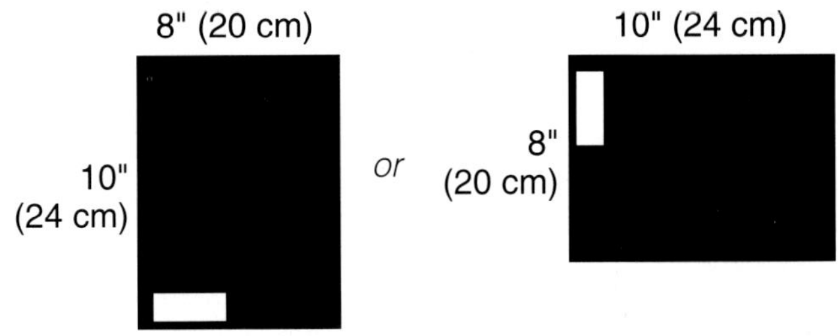

Patient Position

Seated at end or side of table, forearm resting on table, posterior side down (Fig. 9.7).

Part Position

Place cassette under dorsal side of finger. Separate fingers to isolate digit of interest. Proximal interphalangeal joint centered to film.

Central Ray

Perpendicular to proximal interphalangeal joint. Collimate to area of interest.

Structures Demonstrated

Individual digit (Fig. 9.8).

Evaluation Criteria

1. Phalanges should be clearly visible and phalangeal joints open.
2. Metacarpophalanges should be included.
3. Radiographic density (1.6 to 2.0 at darkest portion of anatomy) and radiographic contrast (short-scale) should demonstrate both soft tissue and bony trabeculae.
4. Fingers should not be rotated.
5. This position often gives better possibility than the PA projection to better visualize joint.
6. If fingers cannot be extended, two projections may be needed: with distal part in close contact with cassette and with proximal part in close contact with cassette.
7. Indicate finger number on film.

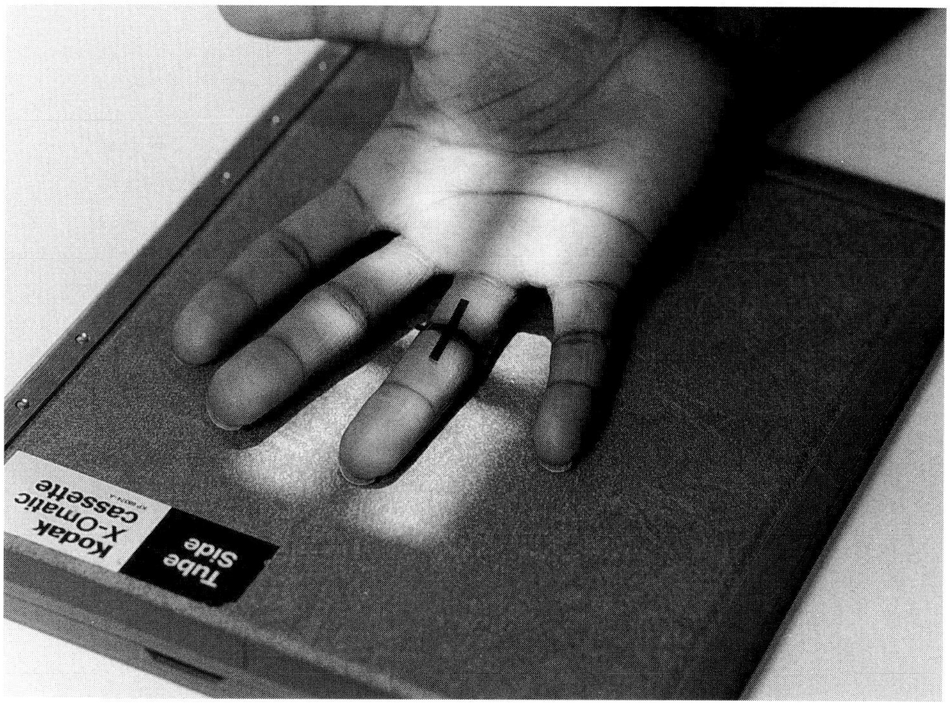

Figure 9.7. AP finger.

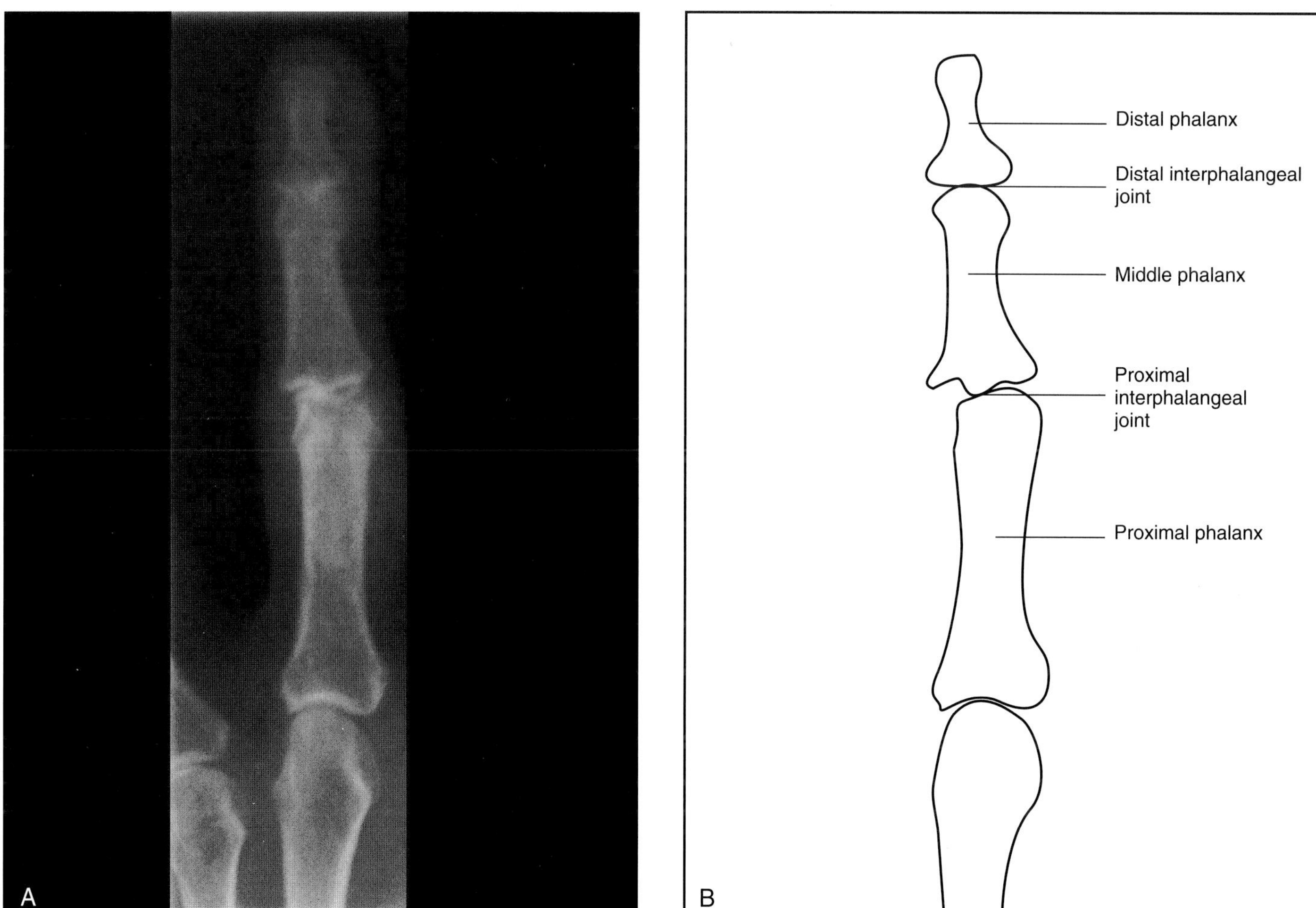

Figure 9.8. A and B, AP finger.

Fingers Two Through Five

Position/Projection

Lateral projection

Film:
8 × 10 inches (20 × 24 cm) tabletop for two projections crosswise

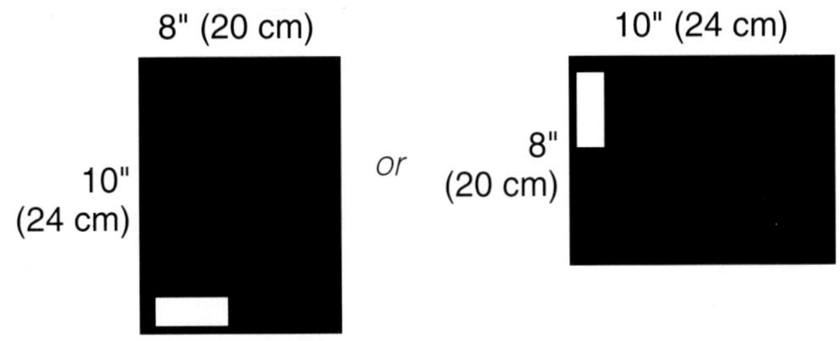

Patient Position

Seated at end or side of table, forearm resting on ulnar side on table (Fig. 9.9).

Part Position

Place cassette under finger—radial side against film in extreme internal rotation when 2nd finger is examined, and ulnar side down for 3rd, 4th, and 5th fingers. For 3rd and 4th fingers, radiolucent sponge is typically necessary to support finger. Finger being examined should be completely extended and other fingers flexed. Proximal interphalangeal joint centered to film.

Central Ray

Perpendicular to proximal interphalangeal joint. Collimate to area of interest.

Structures Demonstrated

Individual finger in profile (Fig. 9.10).

Evaluation Criteria

1. Phalanges should be clearly visible and phalangeal joints open.
2. Proximal aspect of proximal phalanges should be visualized.
3. Radiographic density (1.6 to 2.0 at darkest portion of anatomy) and radiographic contrast (short-scale) should demonstrate both soft tissue and bony trabeculae.
4. If fingers cannot be fully extended, aid such as sponge or radiolucent pad can be used.

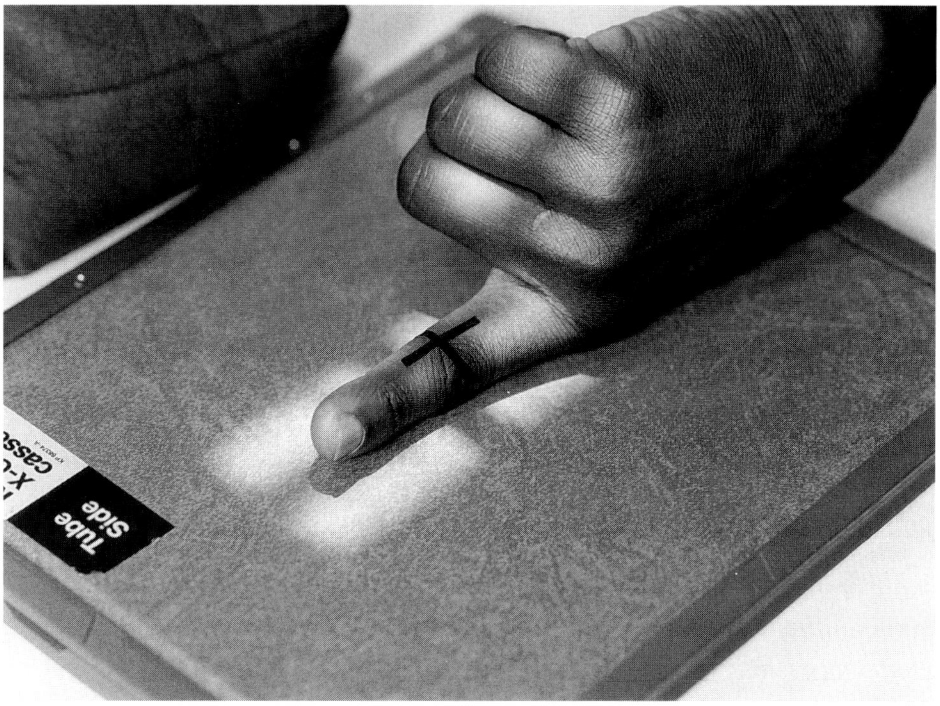

Figure 9.9. Lateral finger.

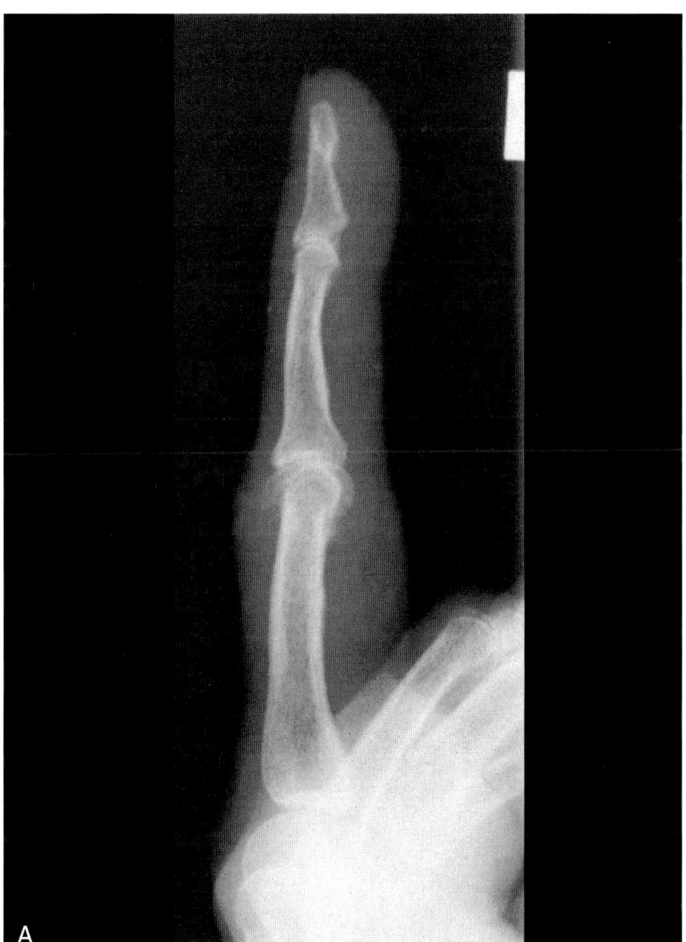

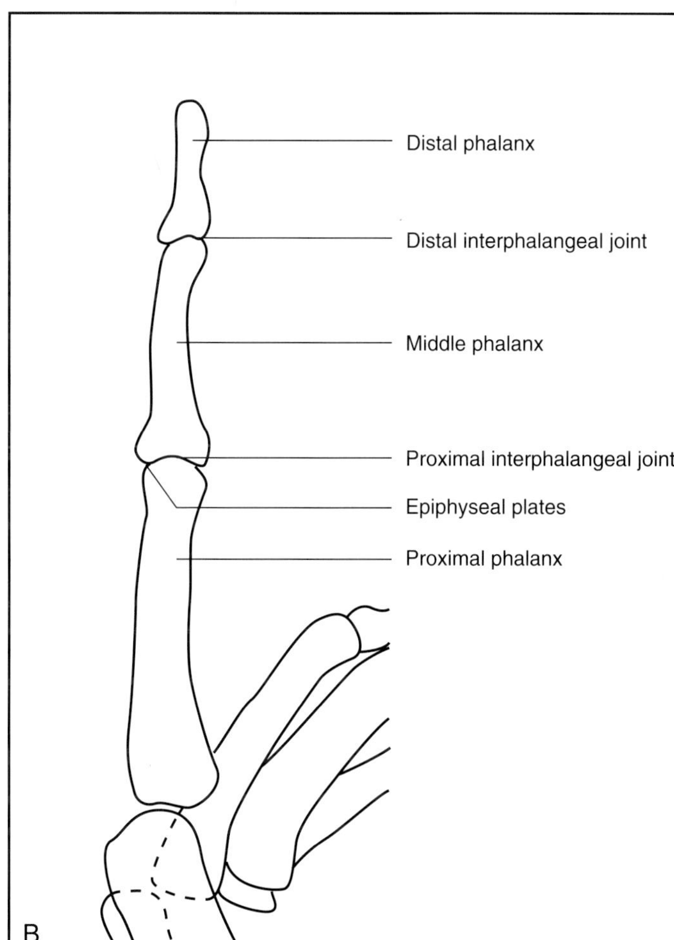

Figure 9.10. A and B, Lateral finger.

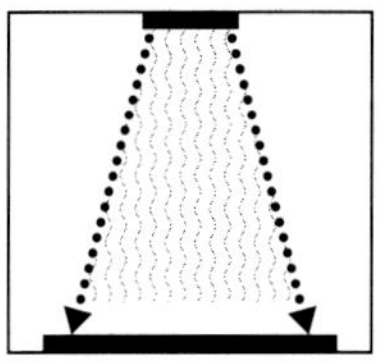

First Metacarpal (Thumb)

Position/Projection

AP projection, ulnoradial position

Film:
8 × 10 inches (20 × 24 cm) tabletop for two projections crosswise

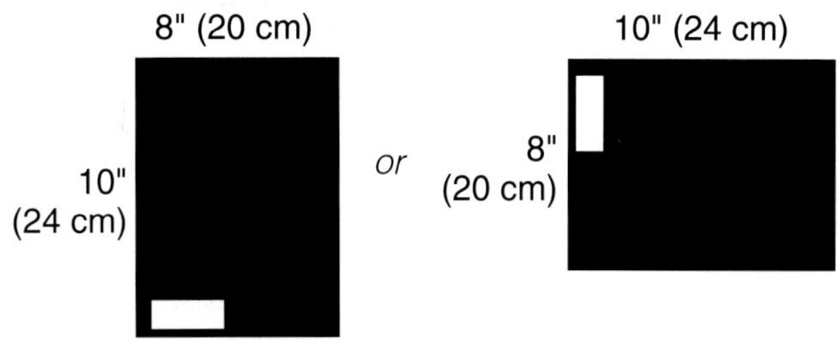

Patient Position

Seated facing away from table, fully extended arm pronated behind back (Fig. 9.11).

Part Position

Place cassette under thumb, dorsal side of thumb in contact with cassette. First metacarpal parallel to cassette. First metacarpophalangeal joint centered to film.

Central Ray

Perpendicular to the 1st metacarpophalangeal joint. Collimate to area of interest.

Structures Demonstrated

First metacarpal and trapeziometacarpal joint (Fig. 9.12).

Evaluation Criteria

1. Phalanges should be clearly visible and phalangeal joints open.
2. Metacarpophalangeal joint should be included, along with trapezium.
3. Radiographic density (1.6 to 2.0 at darkest portion of anatomy) and radiographic contrast (short-scale) should demonstrate both soft tissue and bony trabeculae.
4. Thumb should not be rotated.

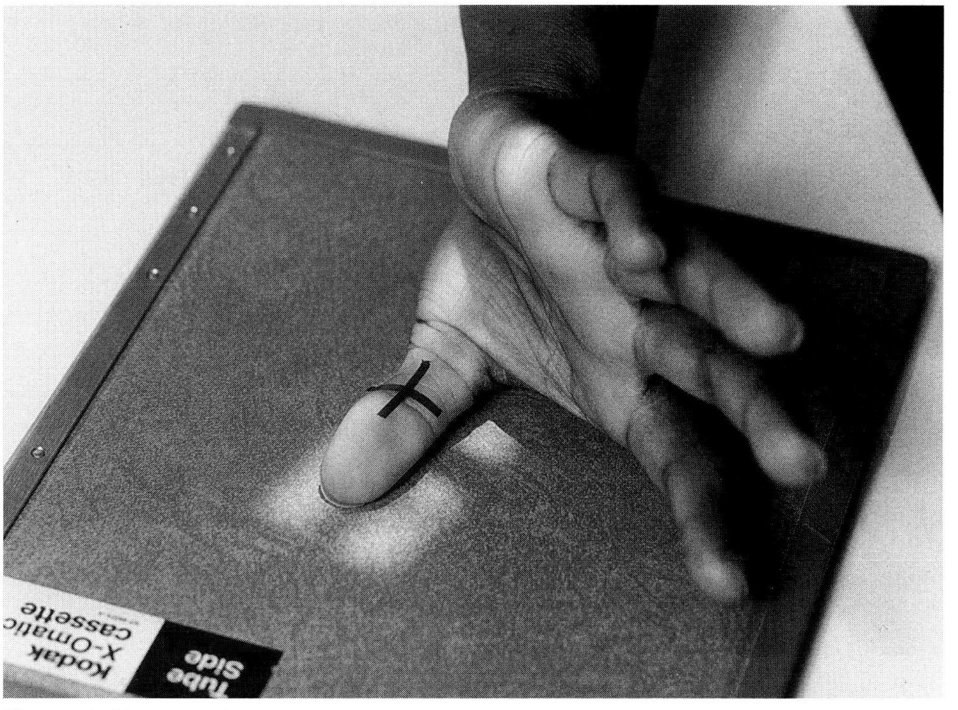

Figure 9.11. AP thumb.

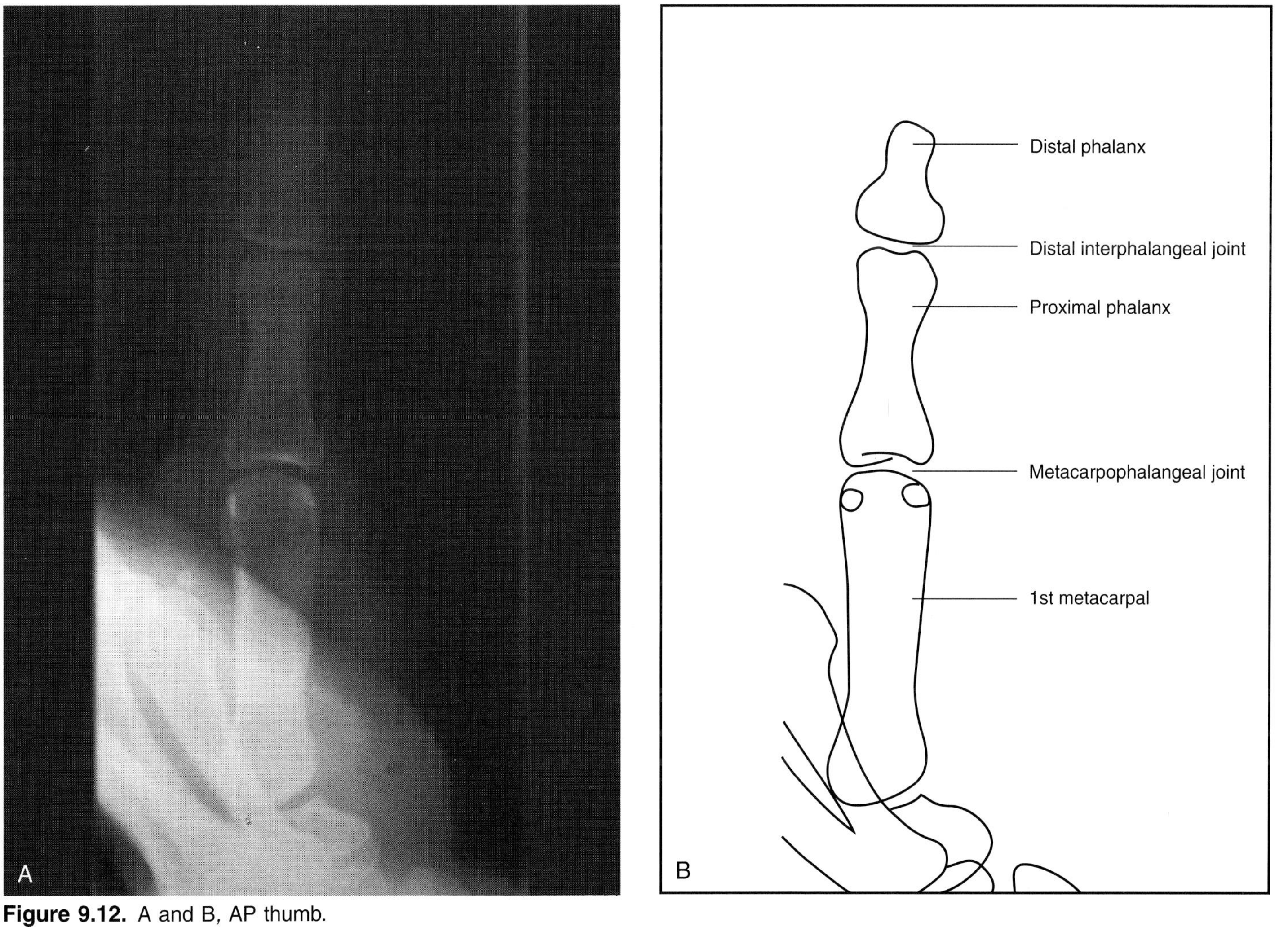

Figure 9.12. A and B, AP thumb.

First Metacarpal (Thumb)

Position/Projection

PA projection, radioulnar position

Film:
8 × 10 inches (20 × 24 cm) tabletop for two projections crosswise

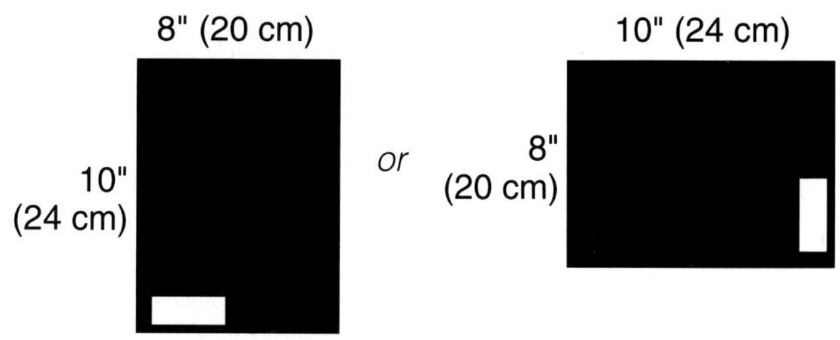

Patient Position

Seated at end or side of table, ulnar side of forearm resting on table (Fig. 9.13).

Part Position

Place cassette under hand. Hand is supinated until extended thumb is parallel to film with palmar surface down. Abduct thumb slightly. Thumb can be supported with sponge or radiolucent pad. First metacarpophalangeal joint centered to film.

Central Ray

Perpendicular to 1st metacarpophalangeal joint. Collimate to area of interest.

Structures Demonstrated

First metacarpal and trapeziometacarpal joint (Fig. 9.14).

Evaluation Criteria

1. Phalanges should be clearly visible and phalangeal joints open.
2. Metacarpophalangeal joint should be included, along with trapezium.
3. Radiographic density (1.6 to 2.0 at darkest portion of anatomy) and radiographic contrast (short-scale) should demonstrate both soft tissue and bony trabeculae.
4. Thumb should not be rotated.

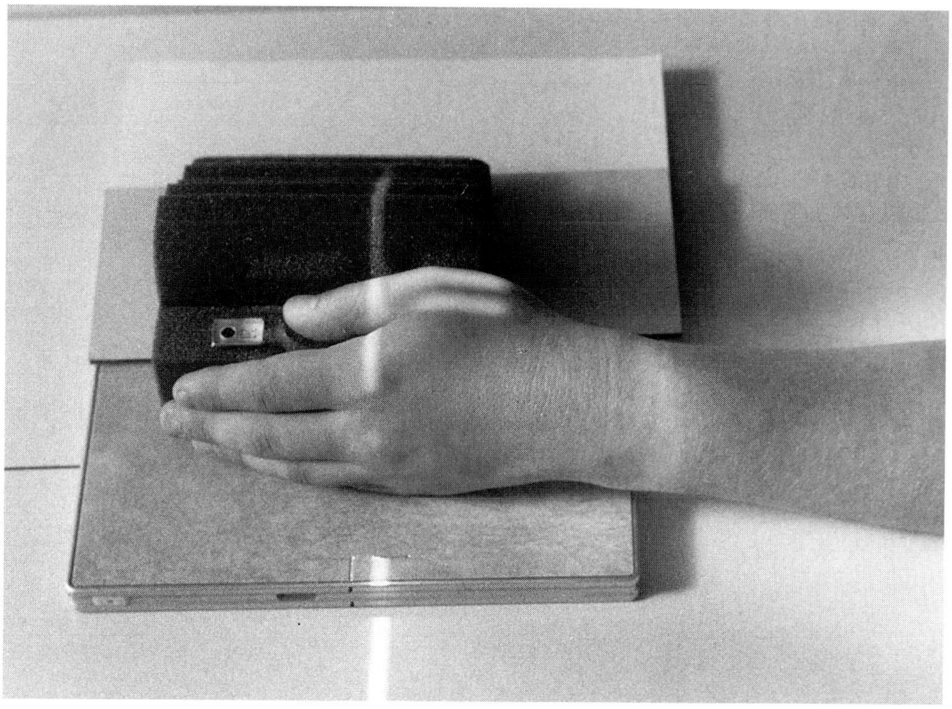

Figure 9.13. PA thumb.

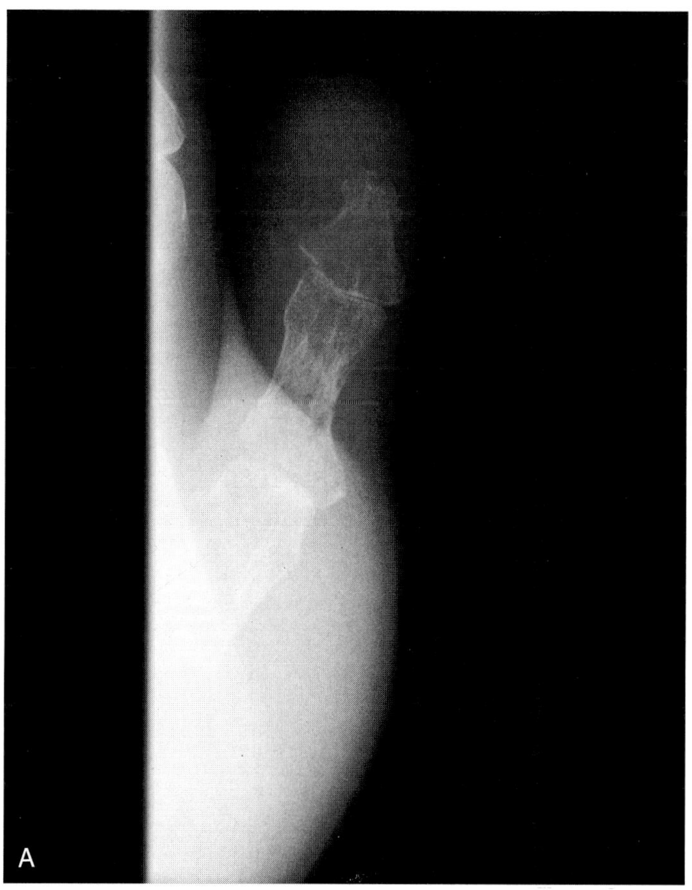

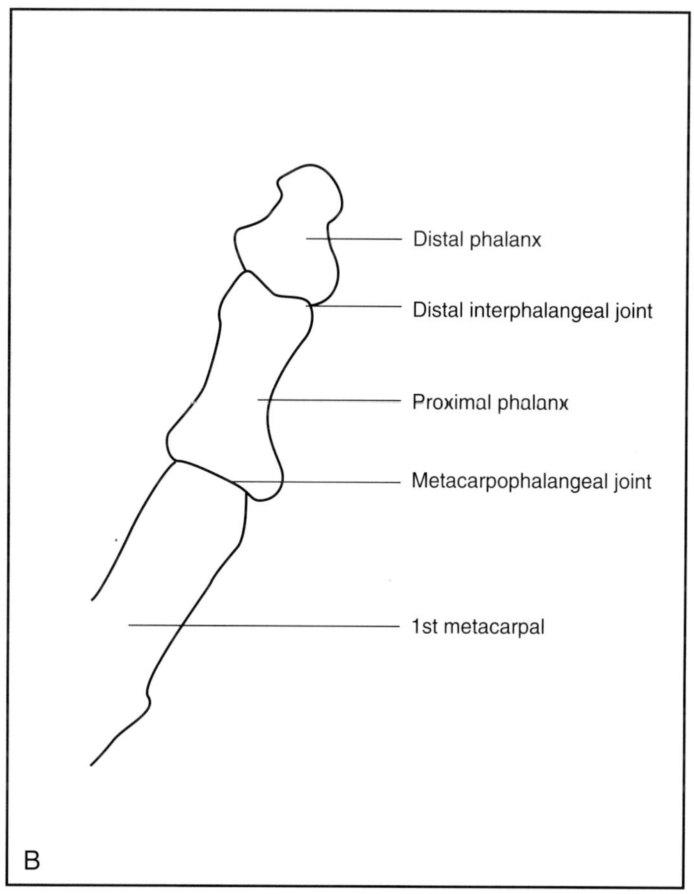

Figure 9.14. A and B, PA thumb.

First Metacarpal (Thumb)

Position/Projection

PA oblique projection, radioulnar position

Film:
8 × 10 inches (20 × 24 cm) tabletop for two projections crosswise

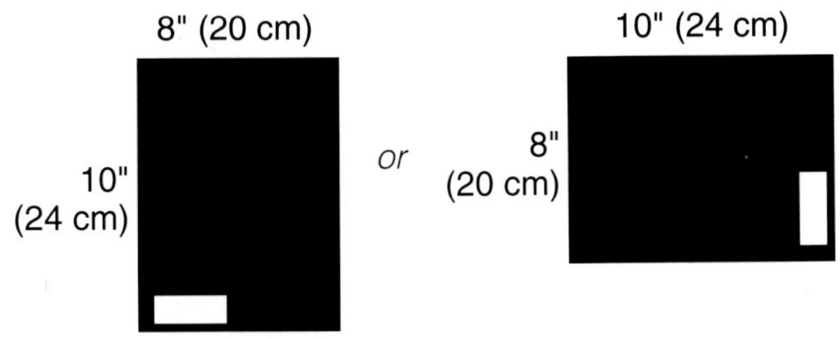

Patient Position

Seated at end or side of table, anterior side of forearm resting on table (Fig. 9.15).

Part Position

Place cassette under hand. Hand is pronated until thumb is in 45° oblique position on cassette. Abduct thumb slightly. First metacarpophalangeal joint is centered to film.

Central Ray

Perpendicular to 1st metacarpophalangeal joint. Collimate to area of interest.

Structures Demonstrated

First metacarpal in obliquity (Fig. 9.16).

Evaluation Criteria

1. Phalanges should be clearly visible and phalangeal joints open.
2. Radiographic density (1.6 to 2.0 at darkest portion of anatomy) and radiographic contrast (short-scale) should demonstrate both soft tissue and bony trabeculae.
3. Metacarpophalangeal joint should be included, along with trapezium.

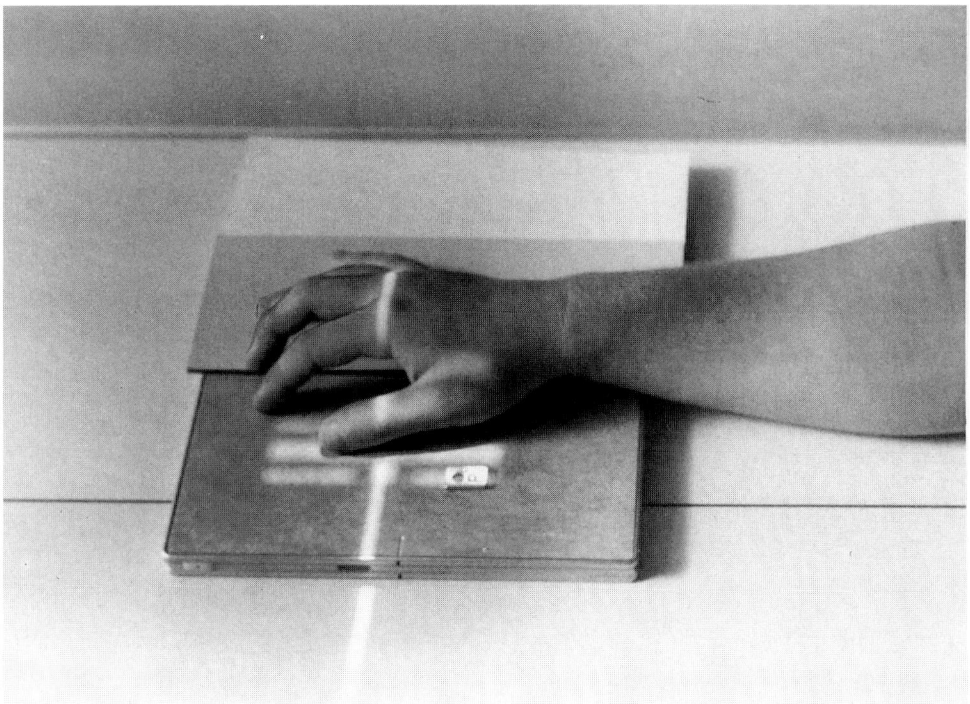

Figure 9.15. PA oblique thumb.

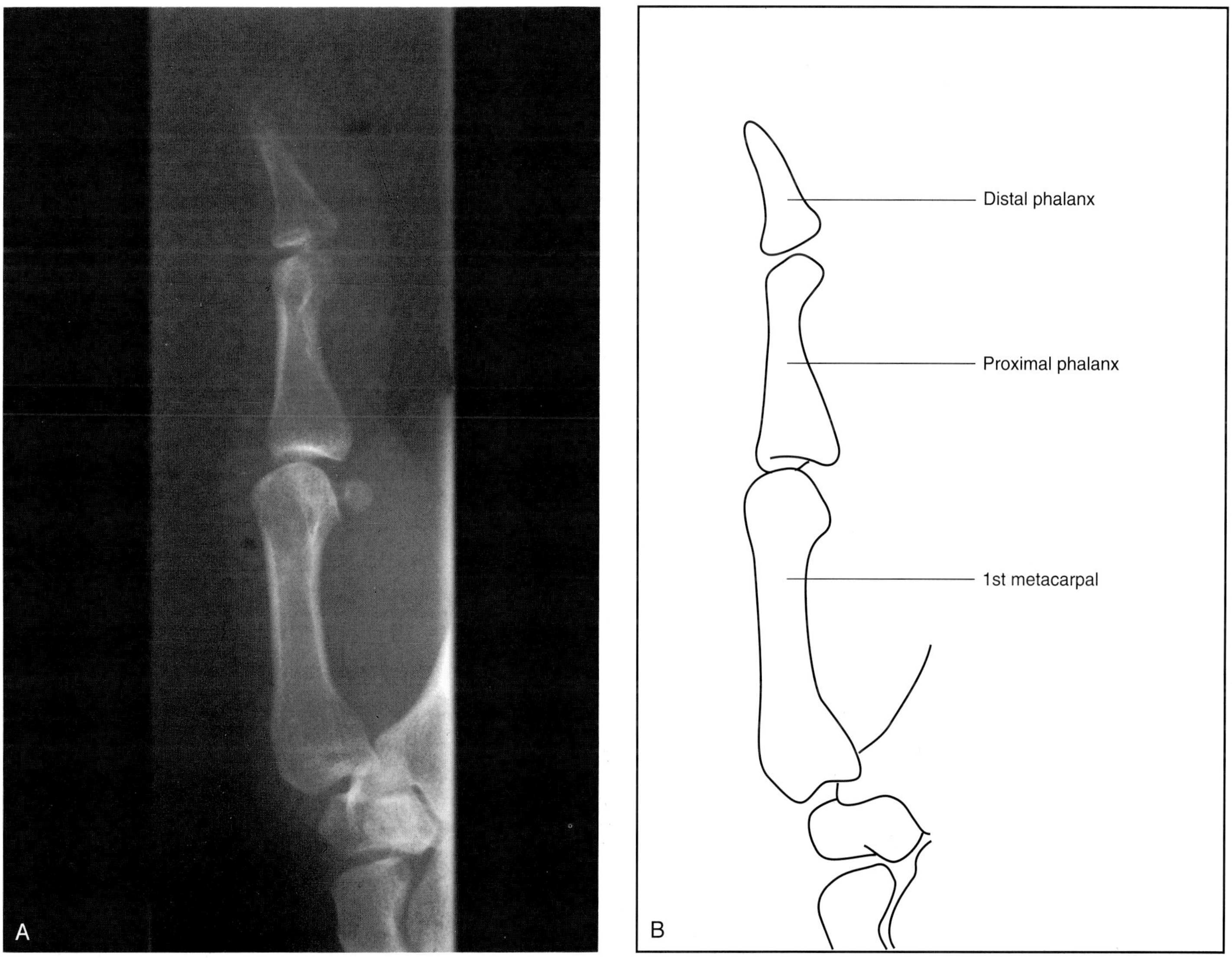

Figure 9.16. A and B, PA oblique thumb.

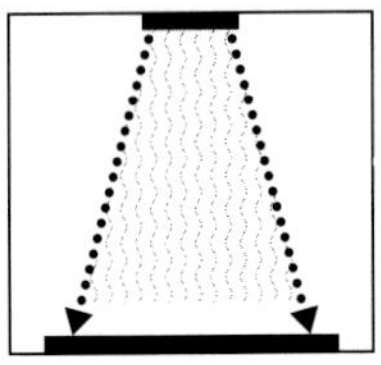

First Metacarpal (Thumb)

Position/Projection

Lateral projection

Film:
8 × 10 inches (20 × 24 cm) tabletop for two projections crosswise

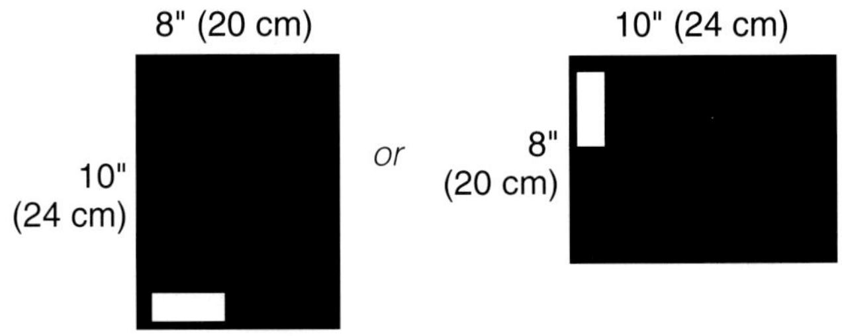

Patient Position

Seated at end or side of table, forearm resting on table, anterior side down (Fig. 9.17).

Part Position

Place cassette under thumb. Hand is pronated slightly until true lateral of thumb is gained. Bend 2nd through 5th fingers. First metacarpophalangeal joint centered to film.

Central Ray

Perpendicular to 1st metacarpophalangeal joint. Collimate to area of interest.

Structures Demonstrated

Anterior and posterior aspects of 1st digit in profile and carpometacarpal (Fig. 9.18).

Evaluation Criteria

1. Phalanges should be clearly visible and phalangeal joints open.
2. Metacarpophalangeal joint should be included, along with trapezium.
3. Radiographic density (1.6 to 2.0 at darkest portion of anatomy) and radiographic contrast (short-scale) should demonstrate both soft tissue and bony trabeculae.
4. Thumb should not be rotated.

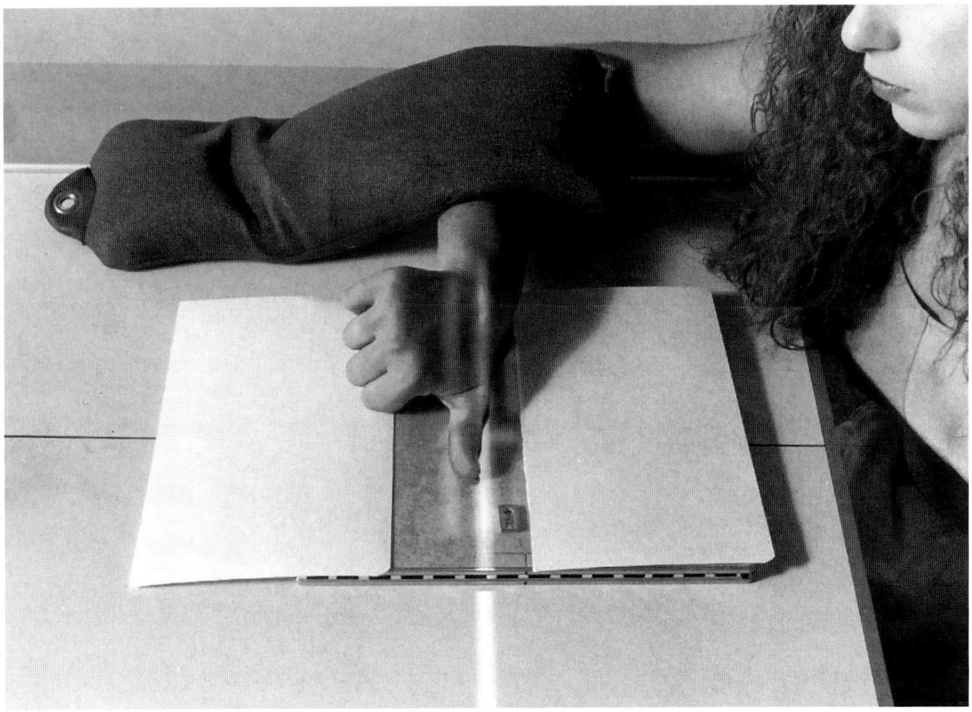

Figure 9.17. Lateral thumb.

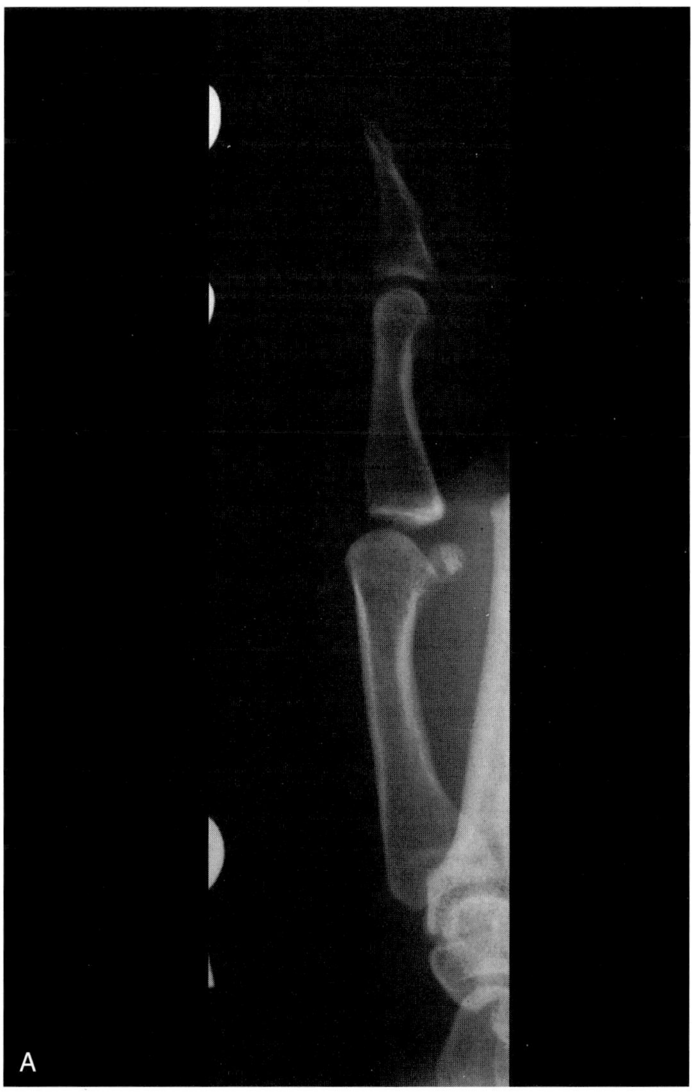

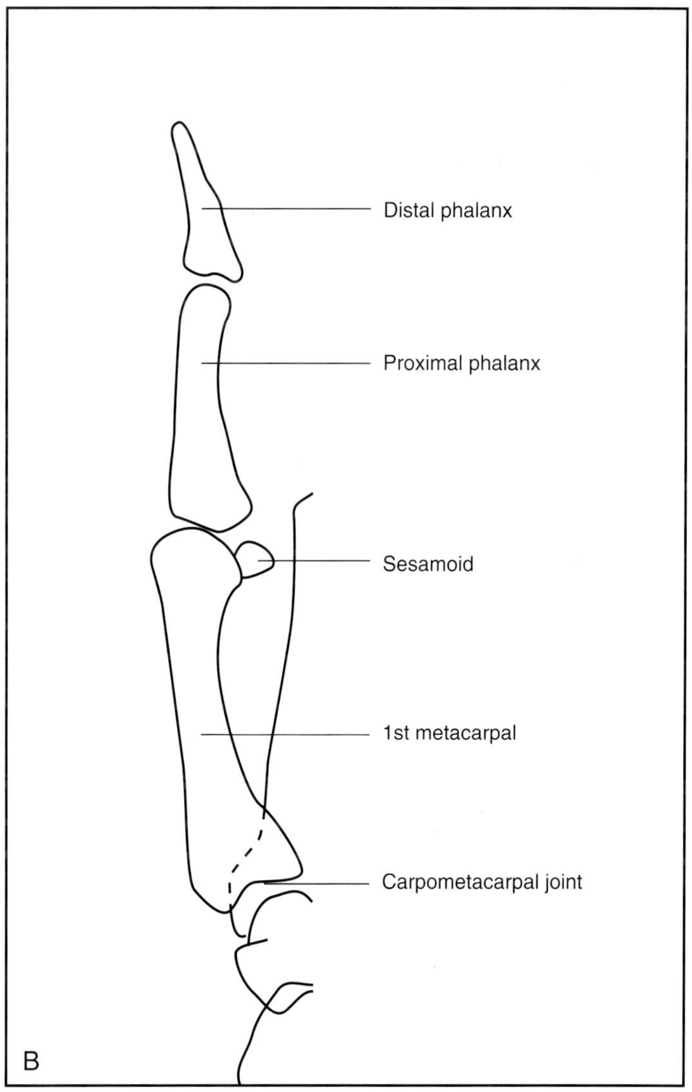

Figure 9.18. A and B, Lateral thumb.

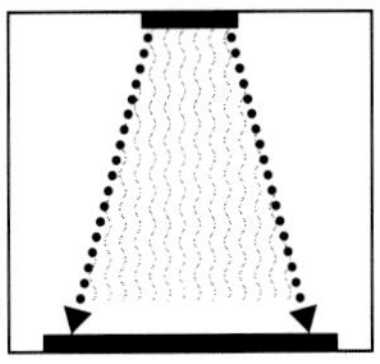

Hand

Position/Projection

PA projection

Film:
8 × 10 inches (20 × 24 cm)
lengthwise, tabletop

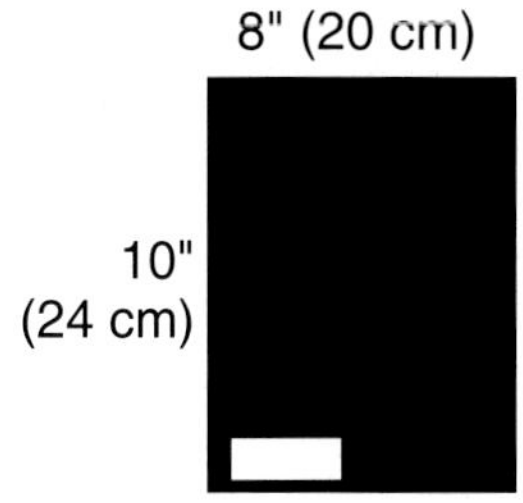

Patient Position

Seated at end or side of table, forearm resting on anterior side (Fig. 9.19).

Part Position

Place cassette under hand, palm down. Fingers are extended and slightly separated. Third metacarpophalangeal joint centered to film.

Central Ray

Perpendicular to 3rd metacarpophalangeal joint. Collimate to area of interest.

Structures Demonstrated

Metacarpals, phalanges, and carpals. Thumb is seen with obliquity (Fig. 9.20).

Evaluation Criteria

1. Anatomy from end of fingers to radial and ulnar styloid processes should be visualized.
2. Fingers should be slightly separated.
3. Metacarpophalangeal and interphalangeal joints should be open.

NOTE: This position is often easier for the patient than the AP position.

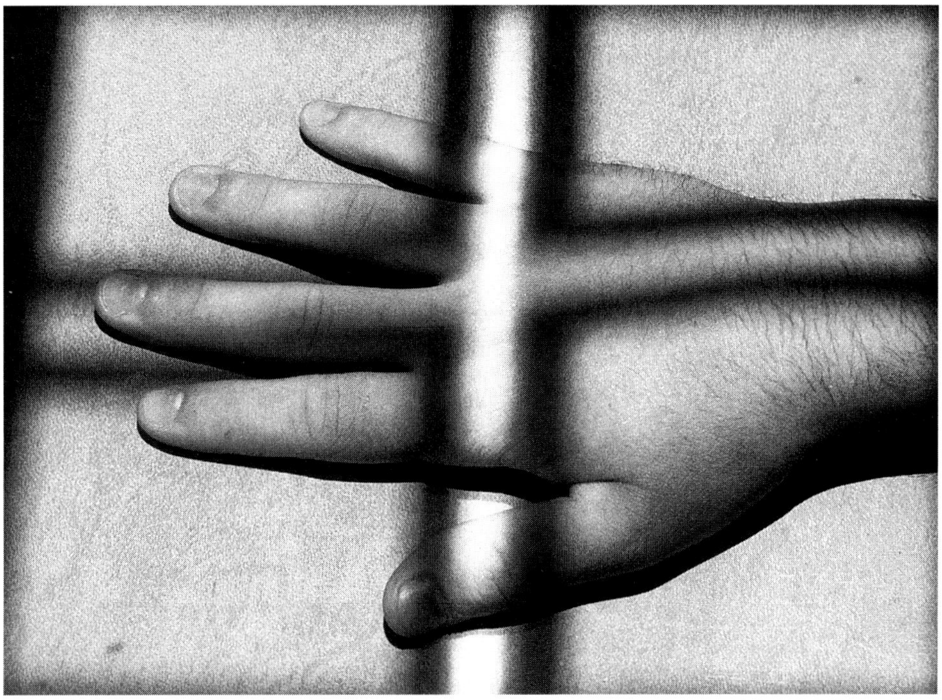

Figure 9.19. PA hand.

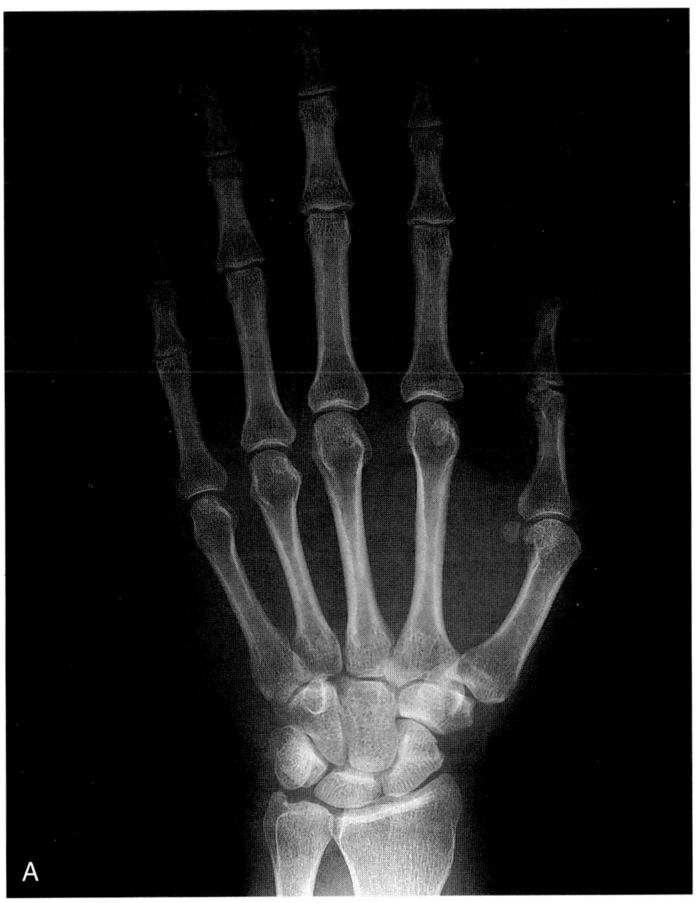

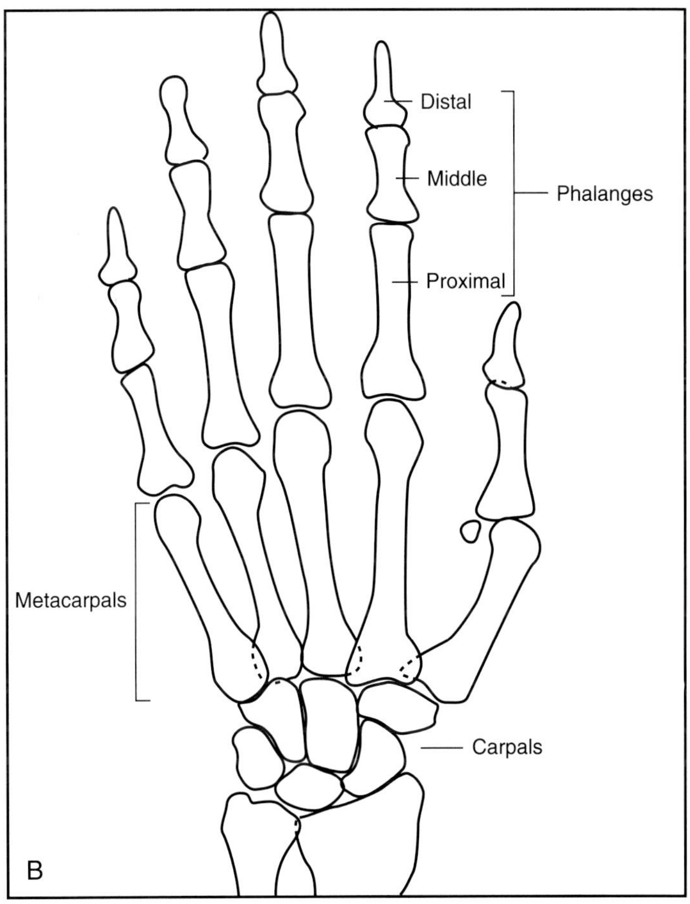

Figure 9.20. A and B, PA hand.

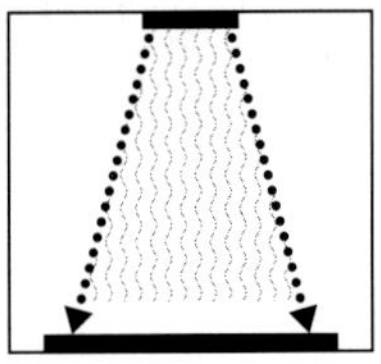

Hand

Position/Projection

AP projection

Film:
8 × 10 inches (20 × 24 cm)
lengthwise, tabletop

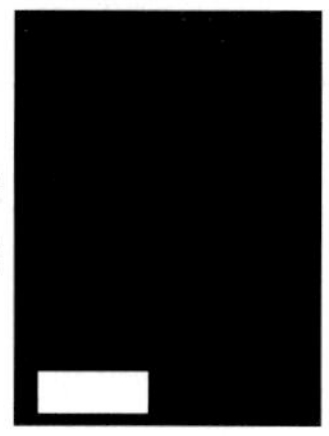

Patient Position

Seated at end or side of table, forearm resting on posterior side (Fig. 9.21).

Part Position

Place cassette under hand, dorsal side down. Fingers are extended and slightly separated. Third metacarpophalangeal joint centered to film.

Central Ray

Perpendicular to 3rd metacarpophalangeal joint. Collimate to area of interest.

Structures Demonstrated

Metacarpals, phalanges, and carpals. Thumb is seen with obliquity (Fig. 9.22).

Evaluation Criteria

1. Anatomy from end of fingers to radial and ulnar styloid processes should be visualized.
2. Fingers should be slightly separated.
3. Radiographic density (1.6 to 2.0 at darkest portion of anatomy) and radiographic contrast (short-scale) should demonstrate both soft tissue and bony trabeculae.
4. Metacarpophalangeal and interphalangeal joints should be open.

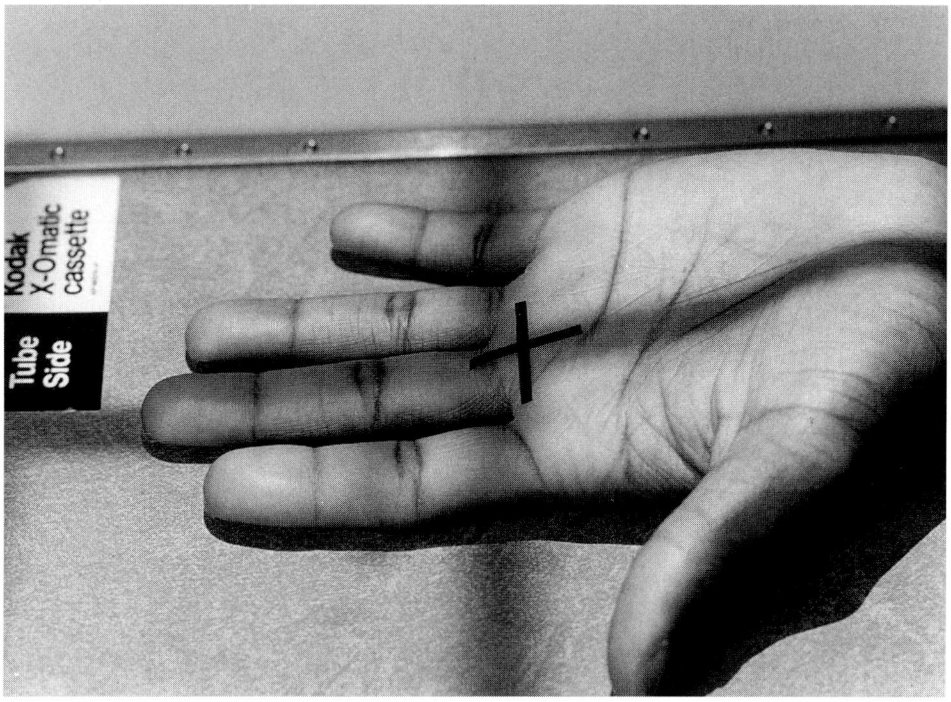

Figure 9.21. AP hand.

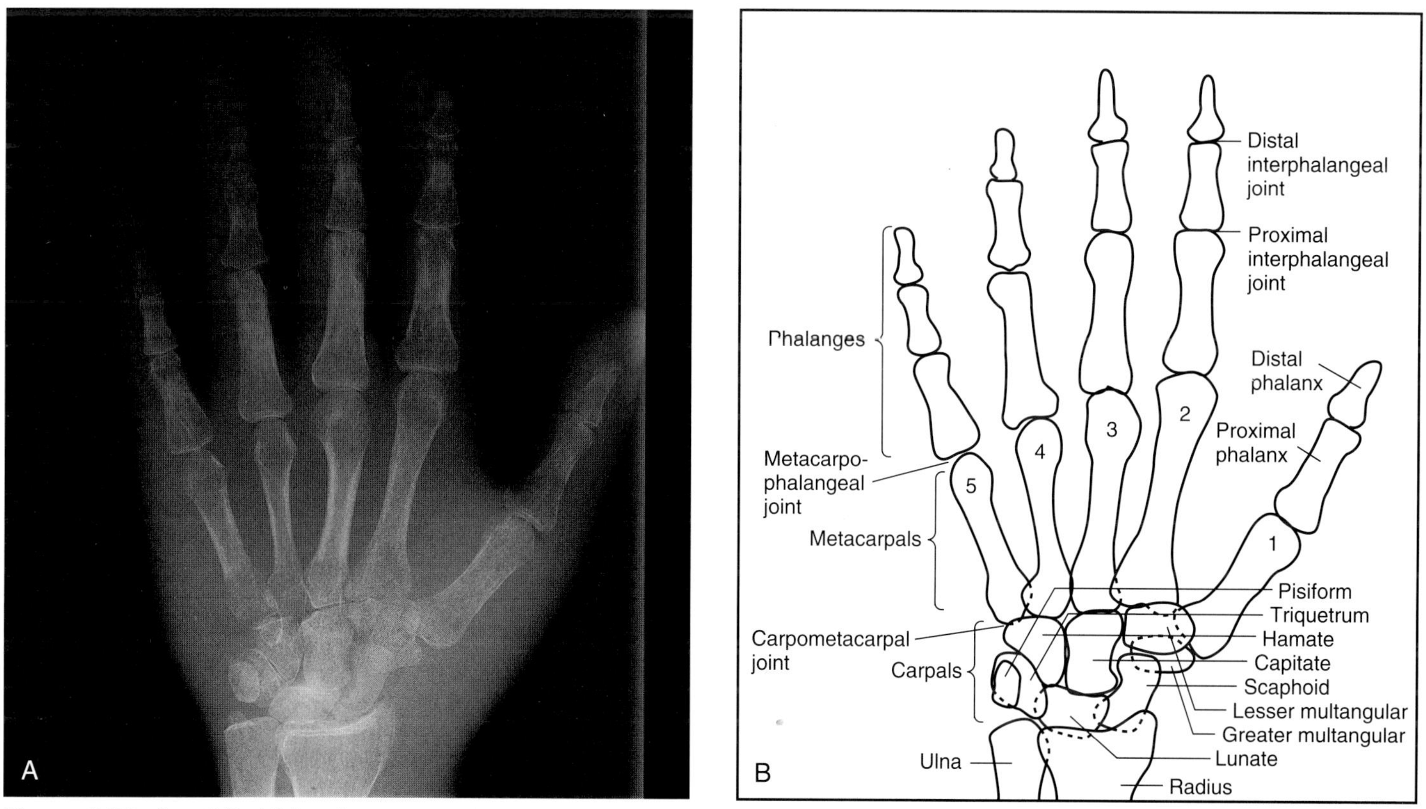

Figure 9.22. A and B, AP hand.

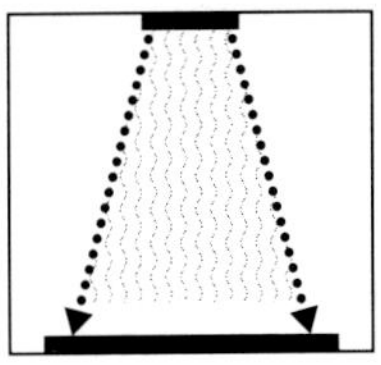

Hand

Position/Projection

PA oblique projection

Film:
8 × 10 inches (20 × 24 cm)
lengthwise, tabletop

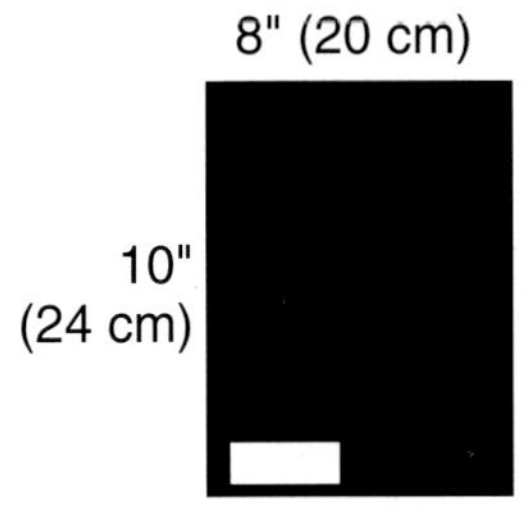

Patient Position

Seated at end or side of table, forearm resting on anterior side (Fig. 9.23).

Part Position

Place cassette under hand, ulnar side down. Hand is pronated 45°. Fingers are slightly flexed so that tips touch film. Third metacarpophalangeal joint centered to film.

Central Ray

Perpendicular to 3rd metacarpophalangeal joint. Collimate to area of interest.

Structures Demonstrated

Metacarpals with corresponding phalanges (Fig. 9.24).

Evaluation Criteria

1. Anatomy from end of fingers to radial and ulnar styloid processes should be visualized.
2. Fingers should not superimpose one another.
3. Radiographic density (1.6 to 2.0 at darkest portion of anatomy) and radiographic contrast (short-scale) should demonstrate both soft tissue and bony trabeculae.
4. First and 2nd are projected clear, and 3rd through 5th metacarpals are superimposed only at bases and slightly at heads.

NOTE: This projection is useful when fracture is suspected.

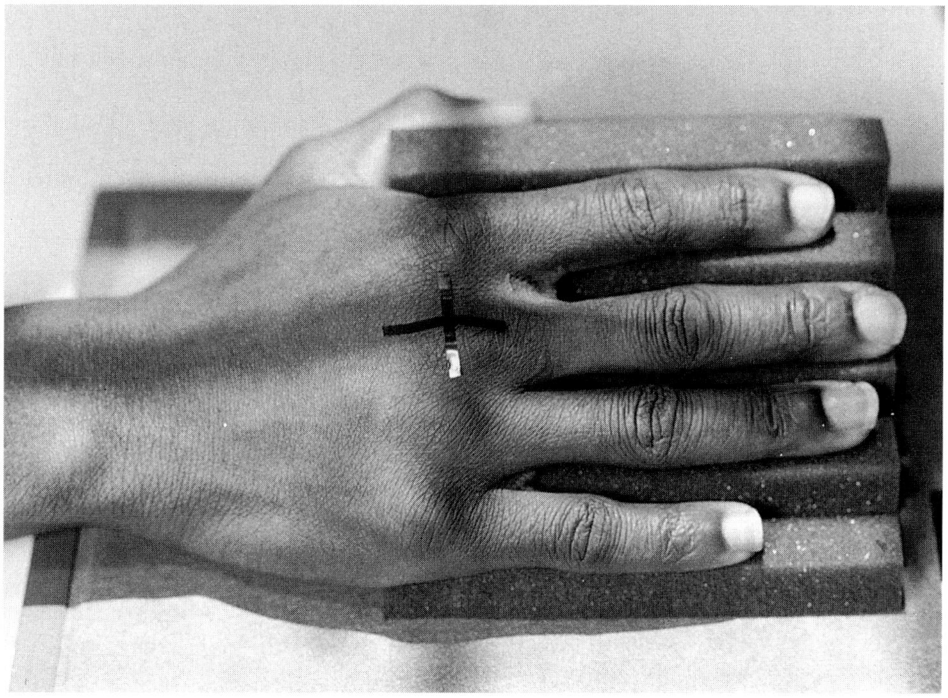

Figure 9.23. PA oblique hand.

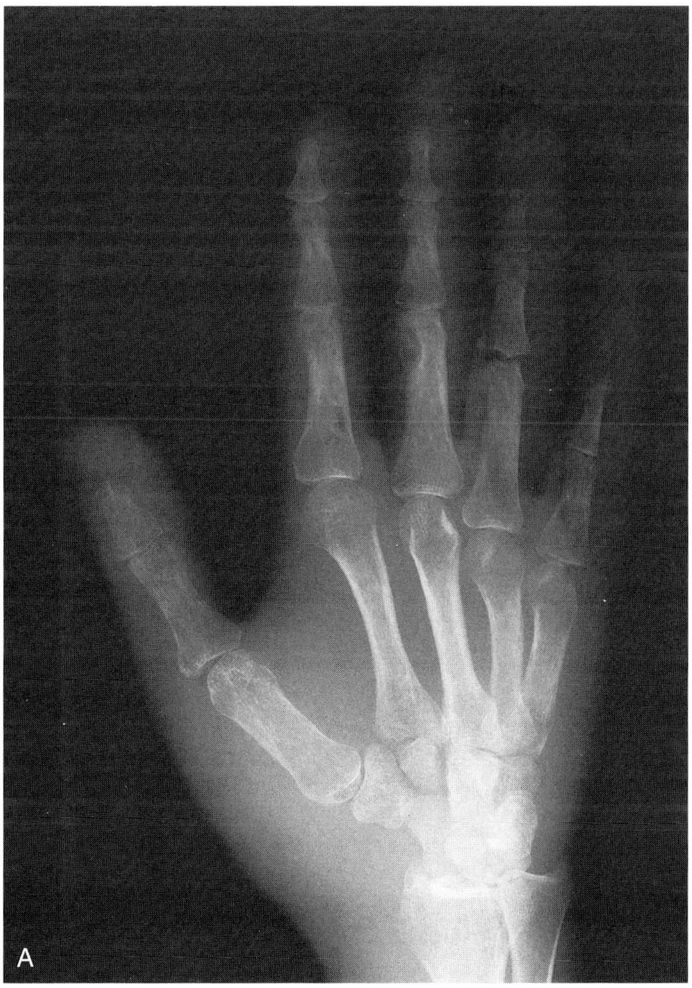

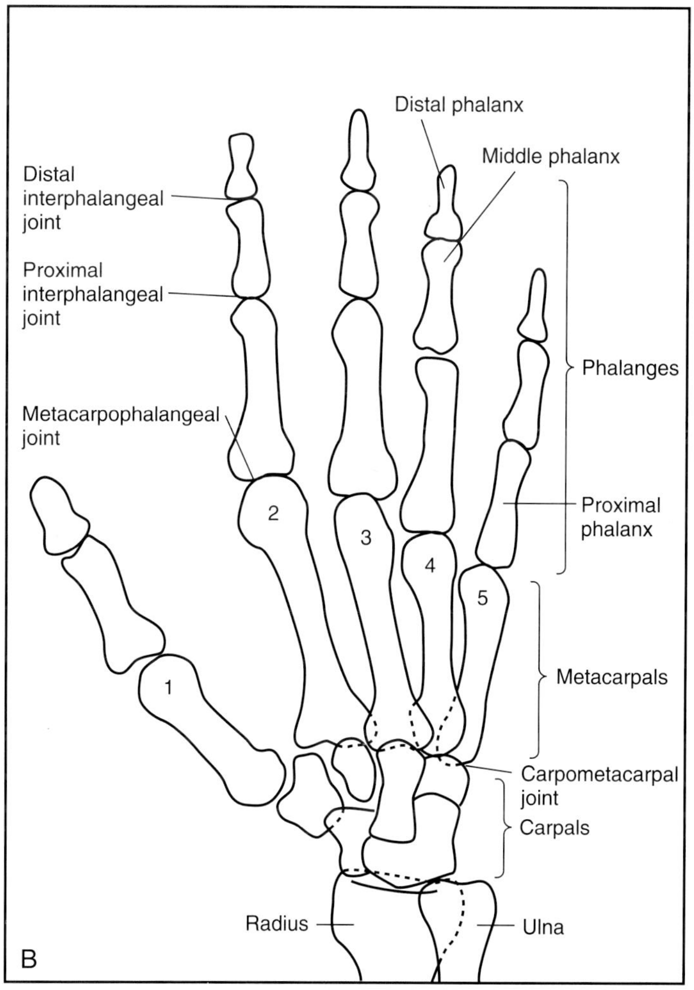

Figure 9.24. A and B, PA oblique hand.

Hands

Position/Projection

PA projection (both hands)

Film:
10 × 12 inches (24 × 30 cm) crosswise, tabletop

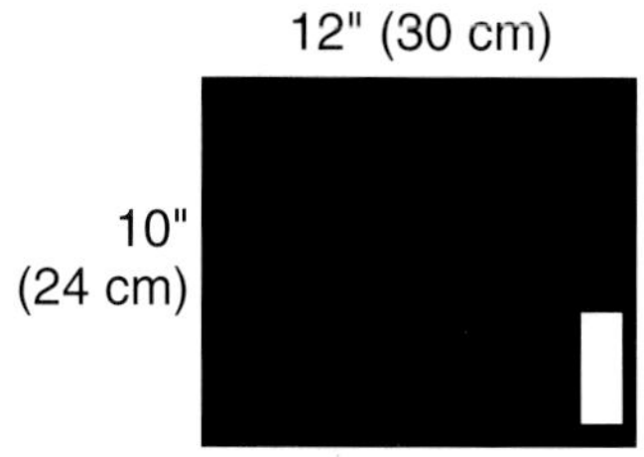

Patient Position

Seated facing table, anterior side of both forearms resting on table (Fig. 9.25).

Part Position

Place cassette under palms. Fingers are extended and separated.

Central Ray

Perpendicular to interphalangeal joints of thumbs. Collimate to area of interest.

Structures Demonstrated

Phalanges, metacarpals, and carpals (Fig. 9.26).

Evaluation Criteria

1. Anatomy from end of fingers to radial and ulnar styloid processes should be visualized.
2. Radiographic density (1.6 or 2.0 at darkest portion of anatomy) and radiographic contrast (short-scale) should demonstrate both soft tissue and bony trabeculae.
3. Fingers should be extended and separated.

NOTE: This projection is used when rheumatoid arthritis or demineralization is suspected.

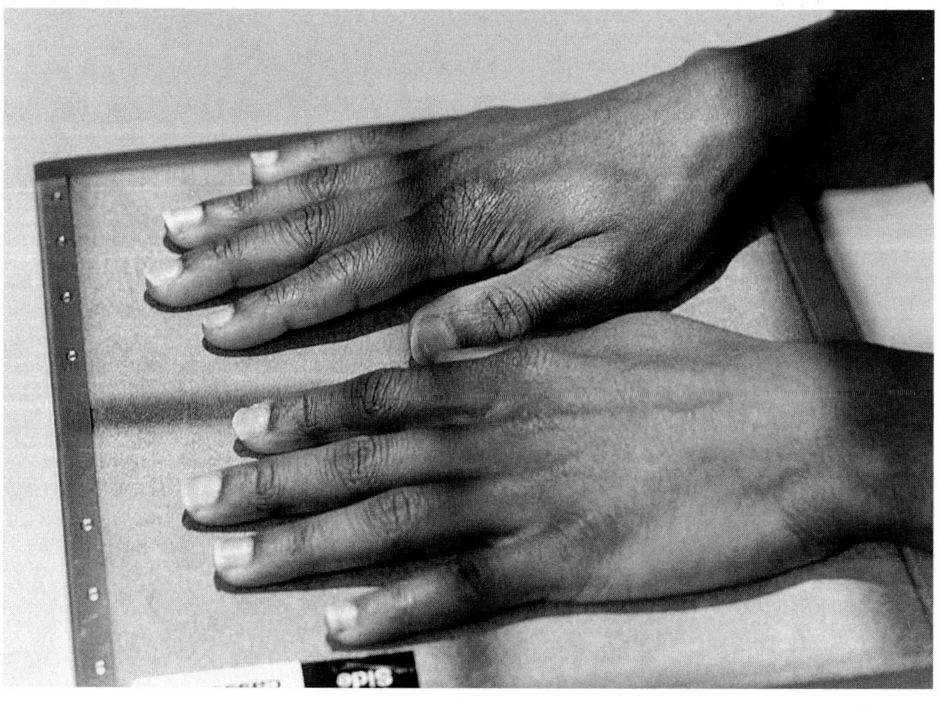

Figure 9.25. Bilateral PA hands.

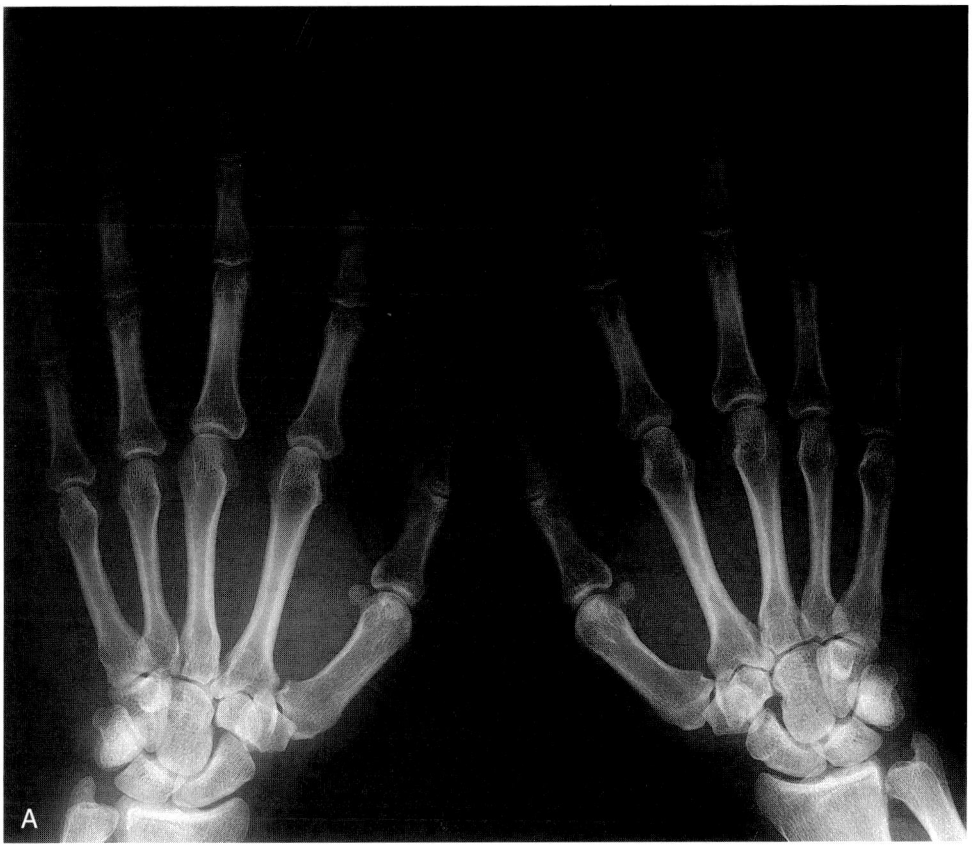

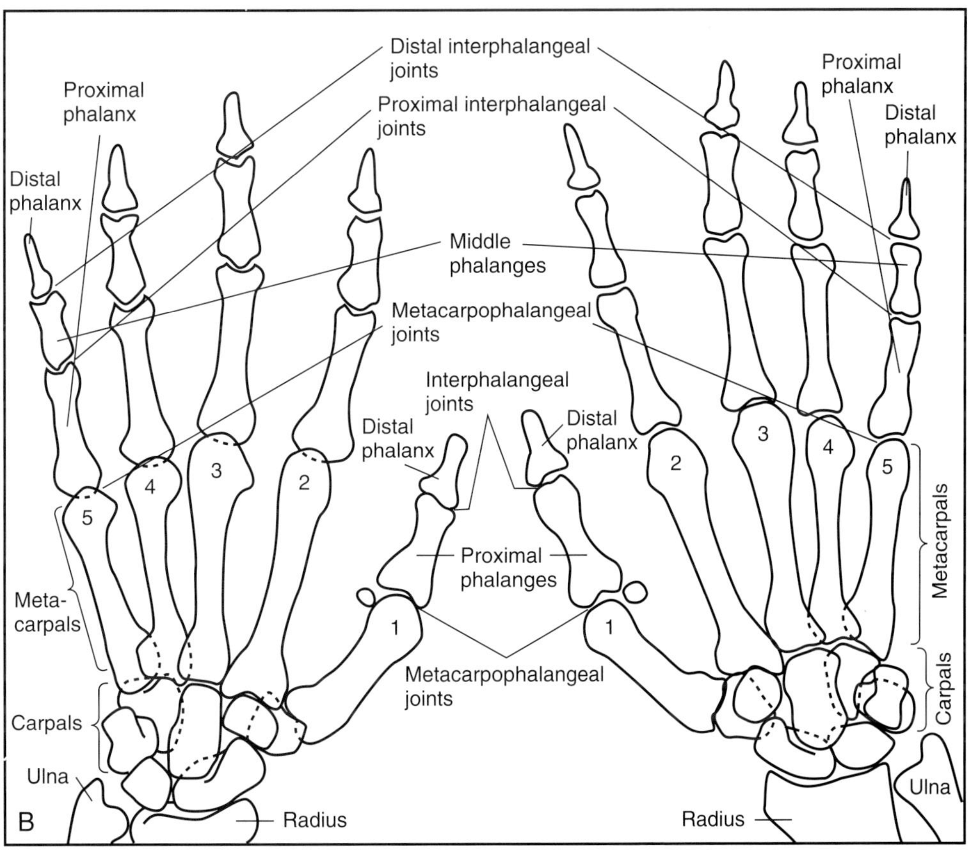

Figure 9.26. A and B, Bilateral PA hands.

Hands

Position/Projection

AP oblique projection (both hands), ballcatcher's position or Norgaard's method

Film:
10 × 12 inches (24 × 30 cm) crosswise, tabletop

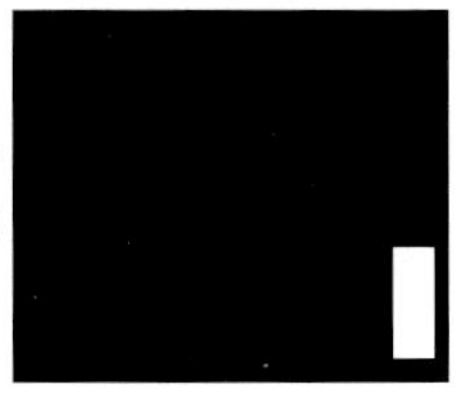

Patient Position

Seated facing table, posterior side of both forearms resting on table (Fig. 9.27).

Part Position

Place cassette under hands, dorsal side down. Fingers are slightly flexed and separated. Rotate hands 45° medially. Ulnar sides of hands touching film. Thumb is slightly abducted. Hands are supported with sponges or radiolucent pads. Fifth metacarpophalangeal joint is centered to film.

Central Ray

Perpendicular to midway between hands at level of 5th metacarpophalangeal joint.

Structures Demonstrated

Phalanges, metacarpals, and carpals (Fig. 9.28).

Evaluation Criteria

1. Anatomy from end of fingers to radial and ulnar styloid processes should be visualized.
2. Fingers should be slightly flexed and separated.
3. Radiographic density (1.6 to 2.0 at darkest portion of anatomy) and radiographic contrast (short-scale) should demonstrate both soft tissue and bony trabeculae.
4. Metacarpal bones should not superimpose one another.

NOTE: This projection is useful when rheumatoid arthritis or possible demineralization is suspected.

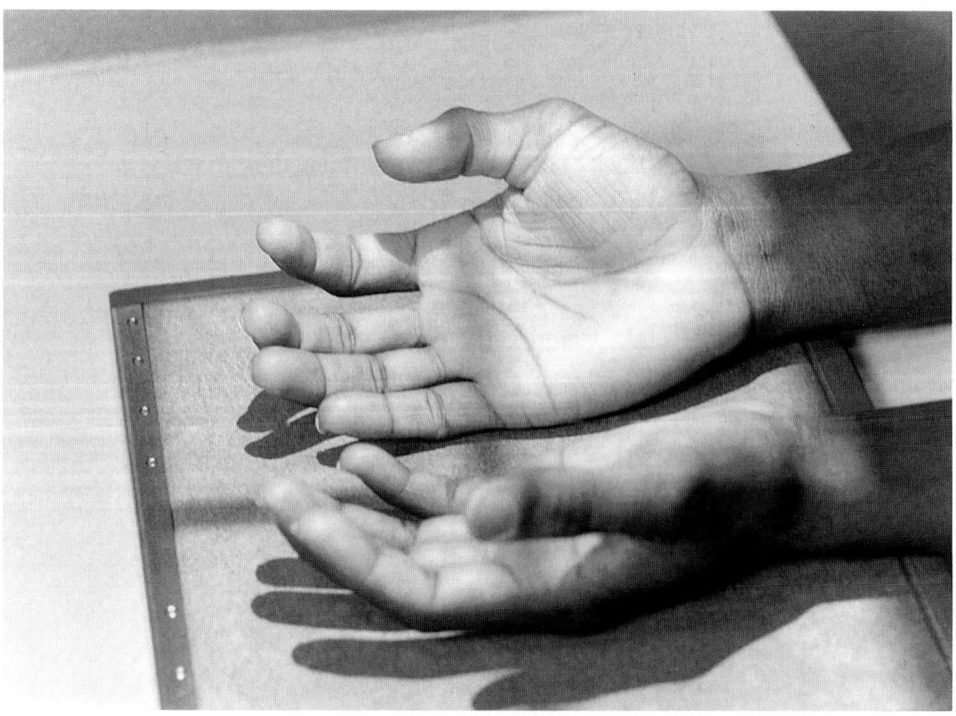

Figure 9.27. Bilateral AP oblique hands.

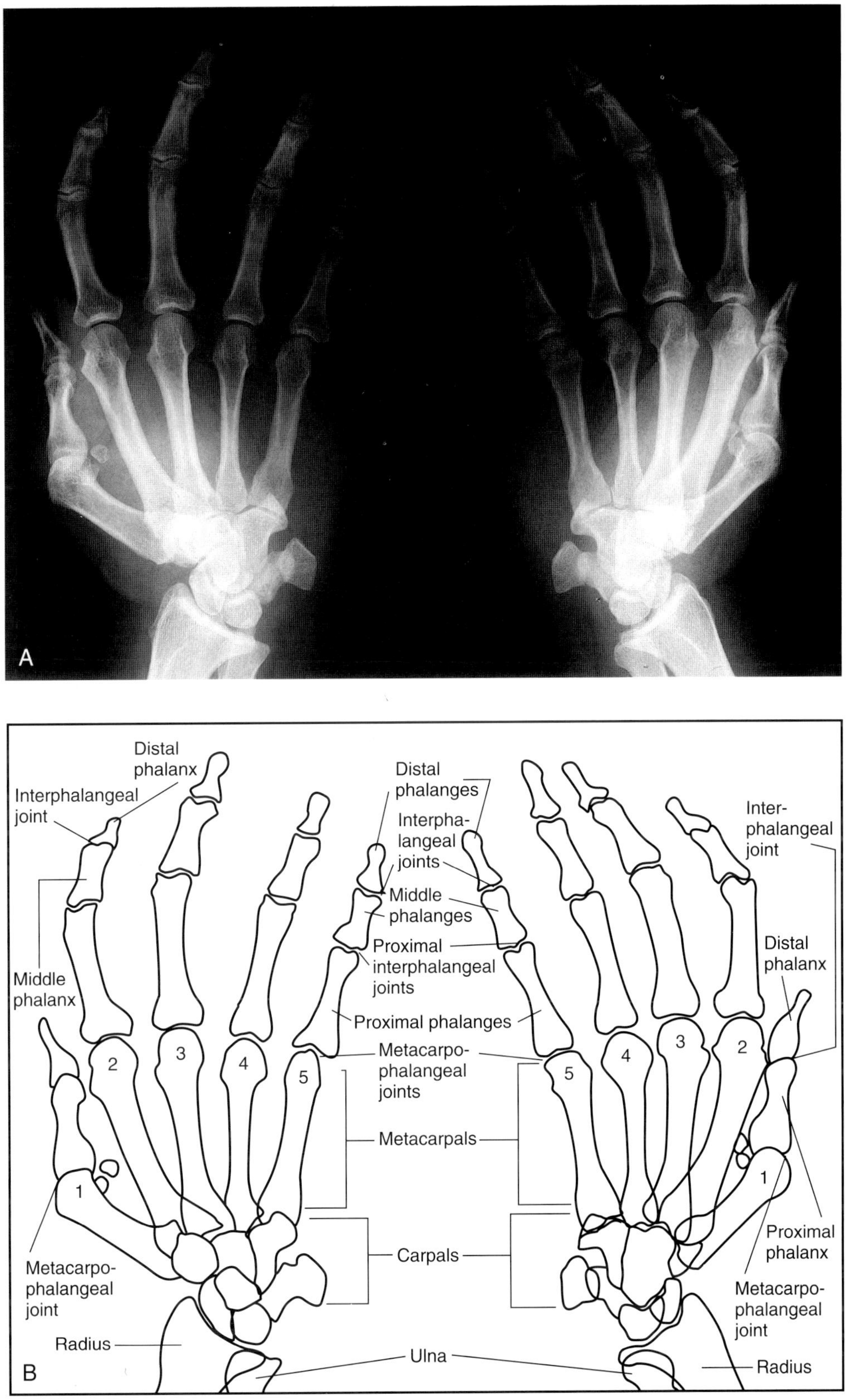

Figure 9.28. A and B, Bilateral AP oblique hands.

Hand

Position/Projection

Lateral projection

Film:
8 × 10 inches (20 × 24 cm) tabletop for one projection lengthwise

or

10 × 12 inches (24 × 30 cm) for two or three projections crosswise

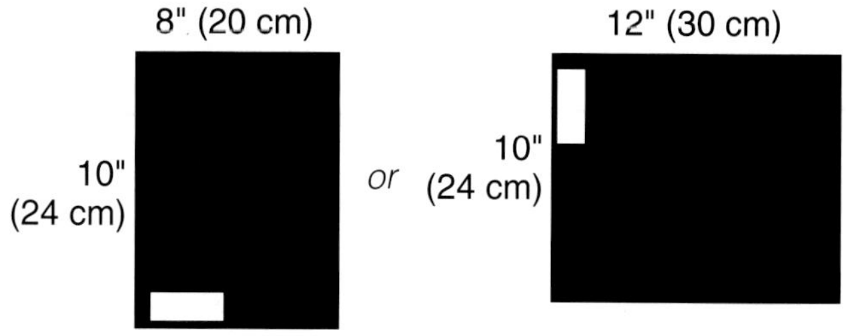

Part Position

Place cassette under hand. Fingers can be flexed or fully extended or fanned to include study of digits. Center of 2nd metacarpal centered to film (Fig. 9.29).

Central Ray

Perpendicular to middle of 2nd metacarpal.

Structures Demonstrated

Displacement of suspected fracture (Fig. 9.30).

Evaluation Criteria

1. Proximal end of fingers, distal end of carpal bones, should be included.
2. Metacarpophalangeal joint should form 90° angle with plane of film.
3. Metacarpals should superimpose one another.
4. Thumb should be abducted and in PA position.

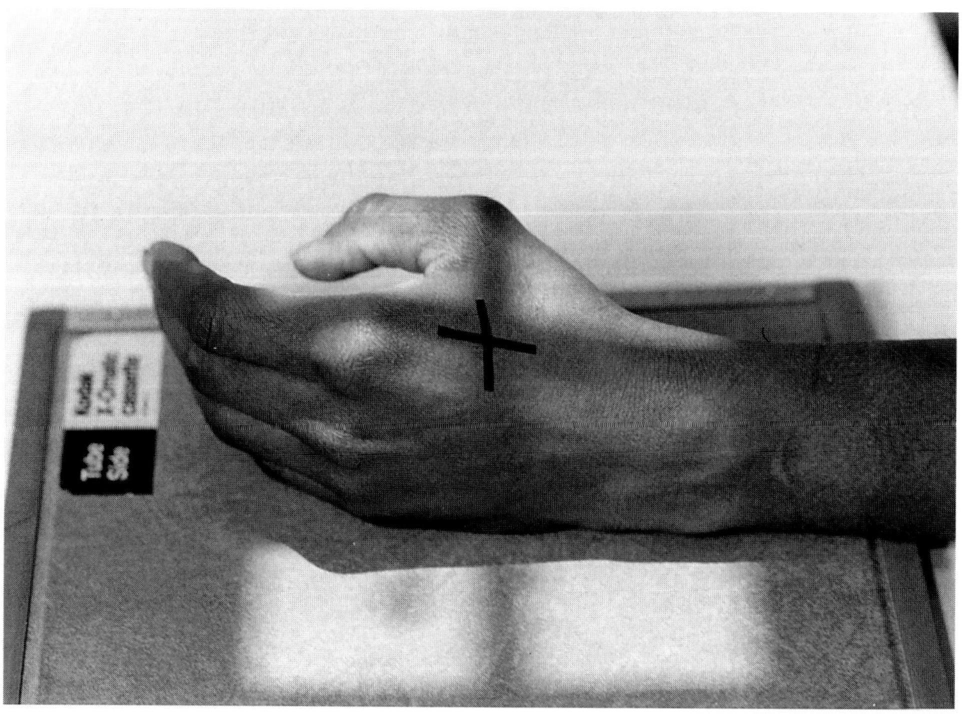

Figure 9.29. Lateral hand.

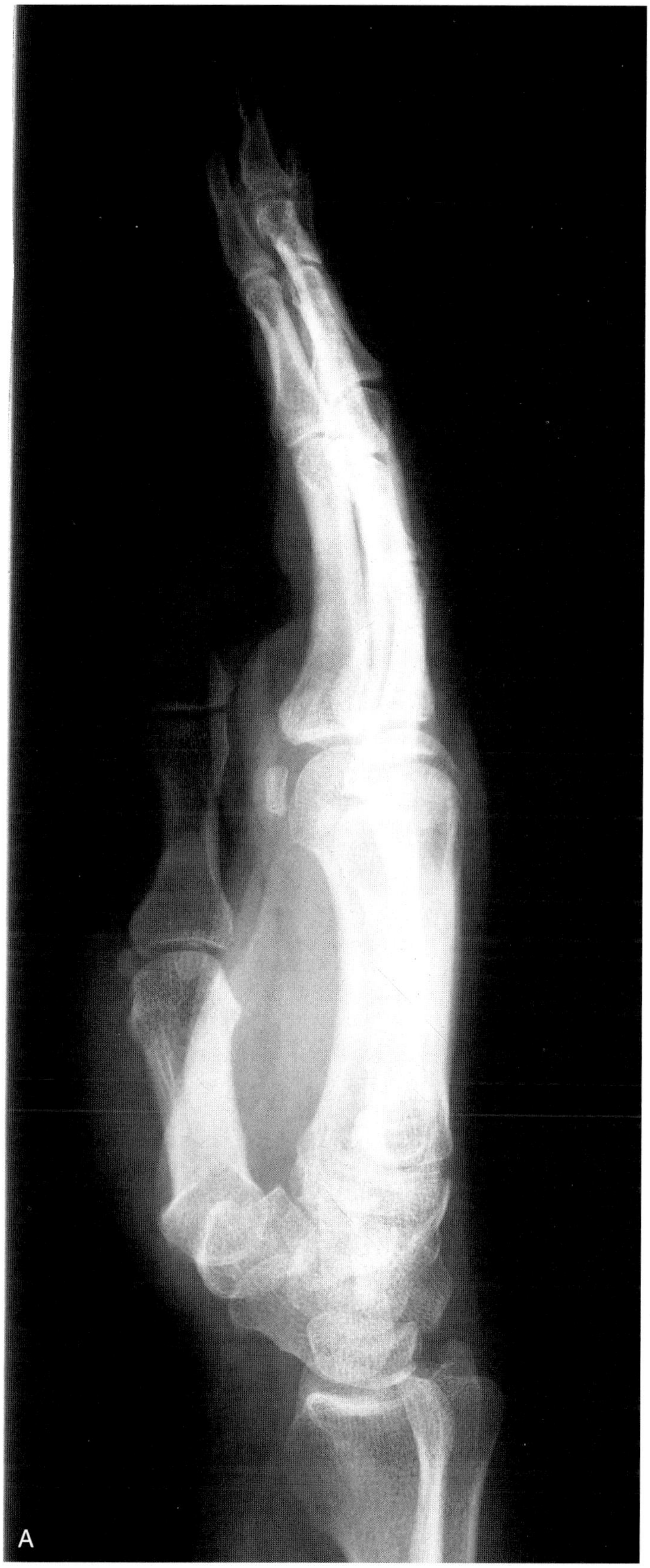

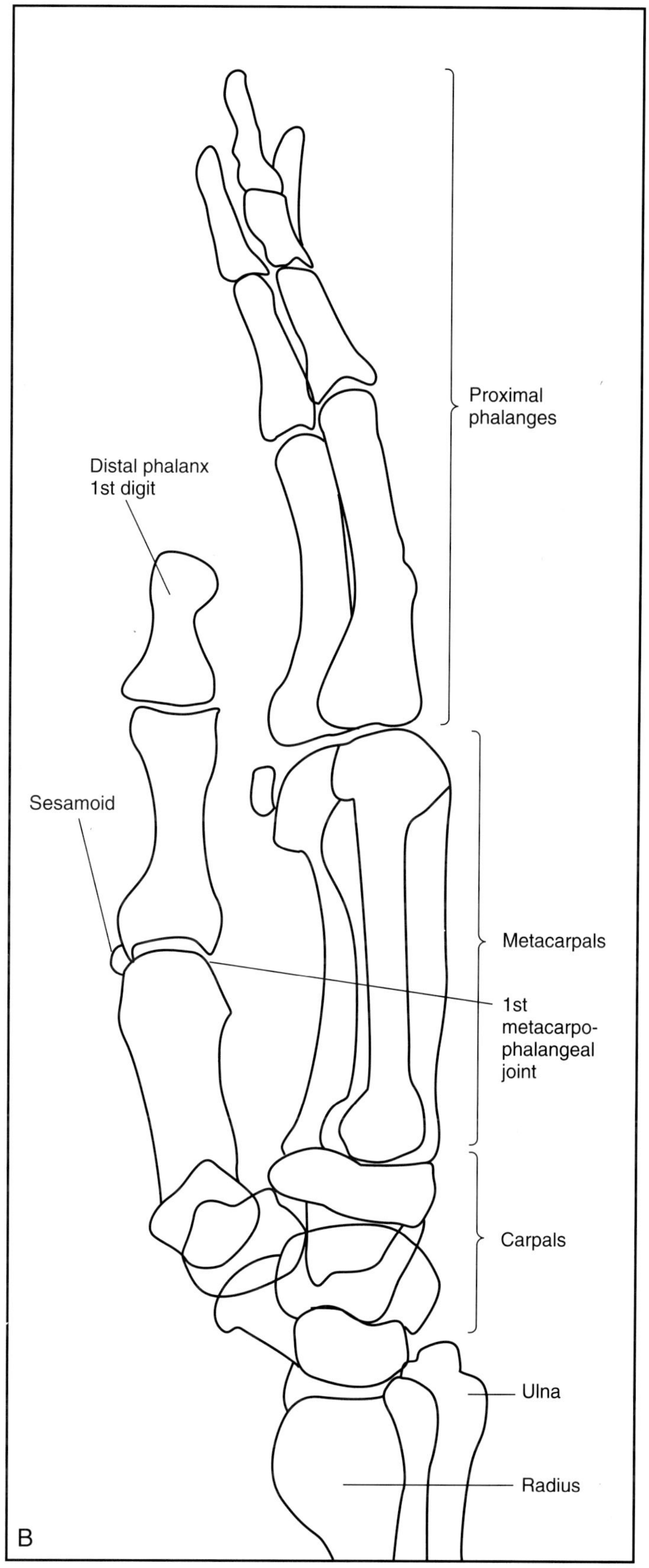

Figure 9.30. A and B, Lateral hand.

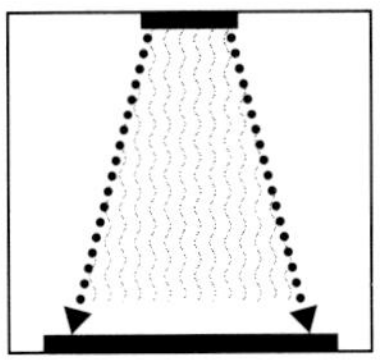

Wrist

Position/Projection

AP projection

Film:
8 × 10 inches (20 × 24 cm) tabletop for one projection lengthwise

or

10 × 12 inches (24 × 30 cm) for two or three projections crosswise

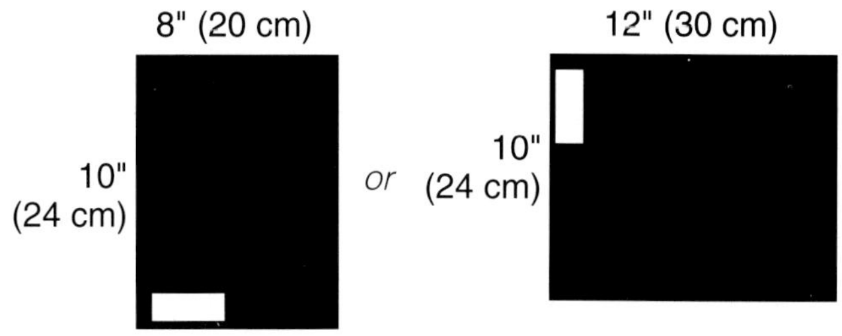

Patient Position

Seated at end or side of table, forearm resting on table, posterior side down (Fig. 9.31).

Part Position

Place cassette under dorsal side of wrist. Patient should lean laterally to achieve ulnar deviation. Area between radial and ulnar styloid processes is centered to film.

Central Ray

Perpendicular between radial and ulnar styloid processes. Collimate to area of interest.

Structures Demonstrated

Carpal joint surfaces (Fig. 9.32).

Evaluation Criteria

1. Proximal metacarpal, carpals, and distal radius and ulna should be included.
2. Bones should not be rotated.
3. Carpus should not be flexed to radial or ulnar side.
4. Ulna should be projected in basic anatomic position.
5. In AP position, divergent beam will graze carpal joint better than PA position.

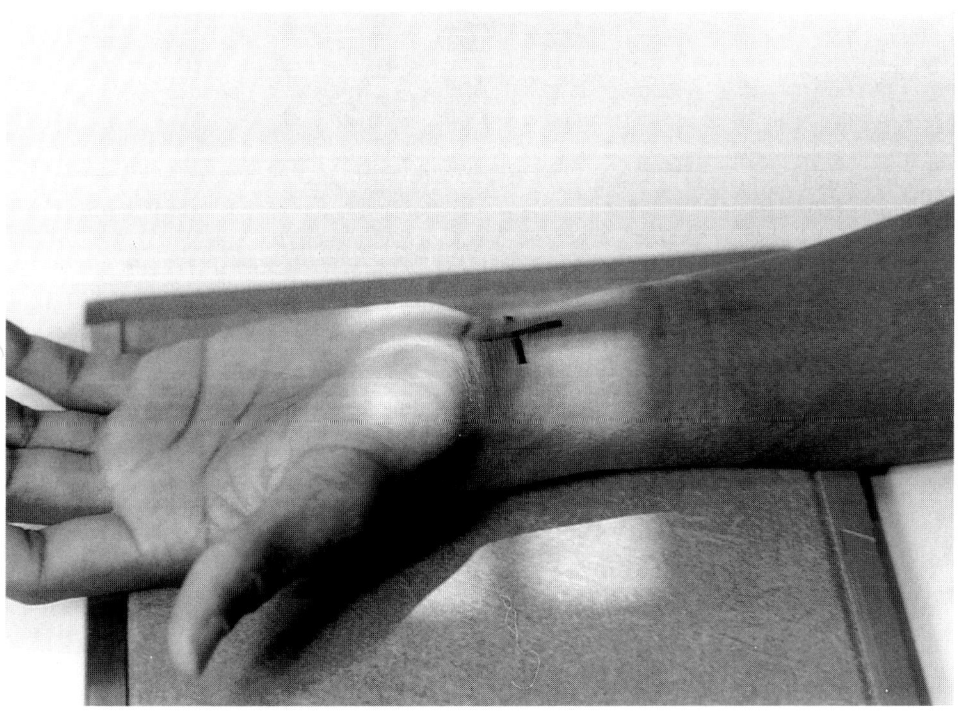

Figure 9.31. AP wrist.

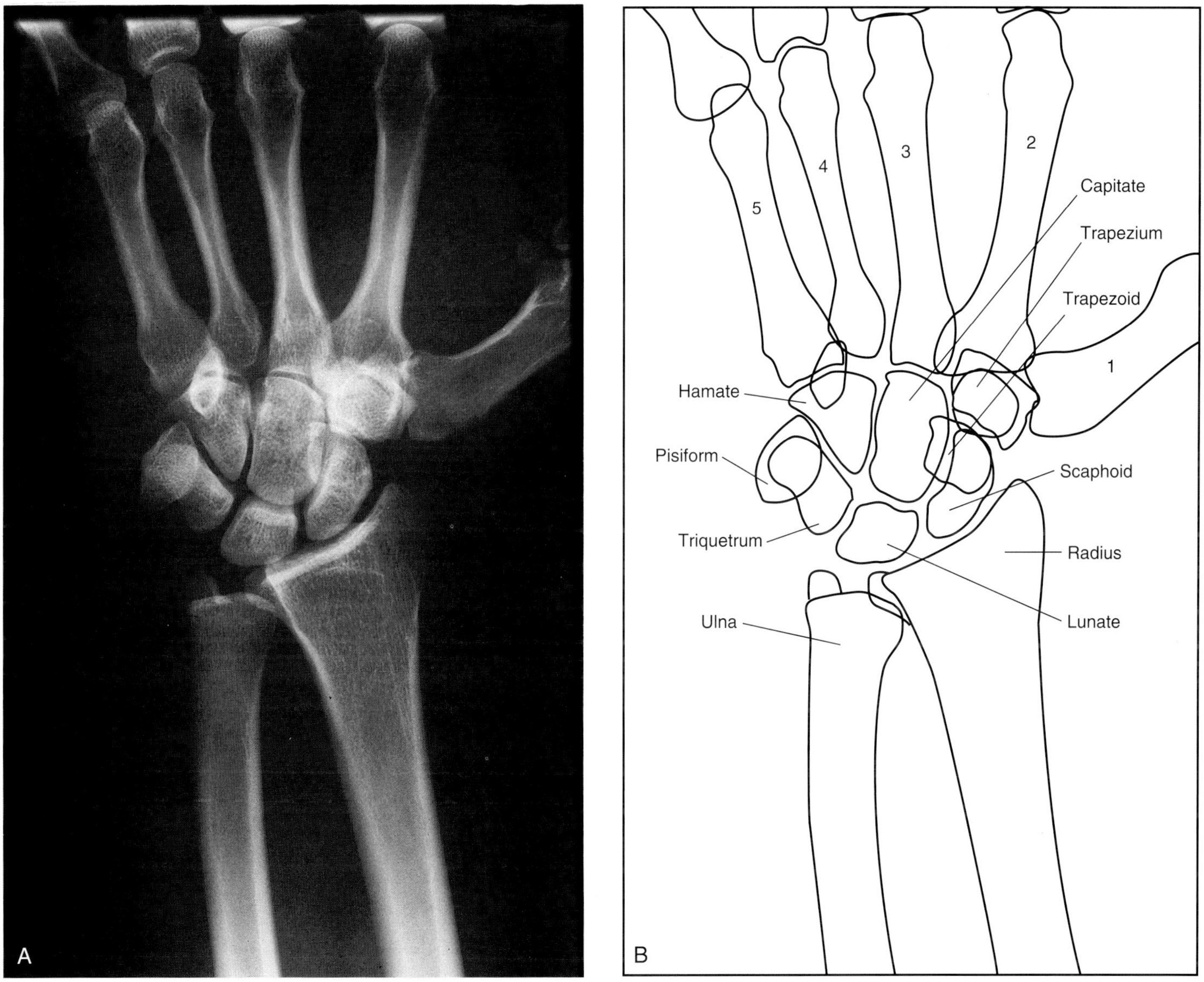

Figure 9.32. A and B, AP wrist.

Wrist

Position/Projection

PA projection

Film:
8 × 10 inches (20 × 24 cm) tabletop for one projection lengthwise

or

10 × 12 inches (20 × 24 cm) for two or three projections

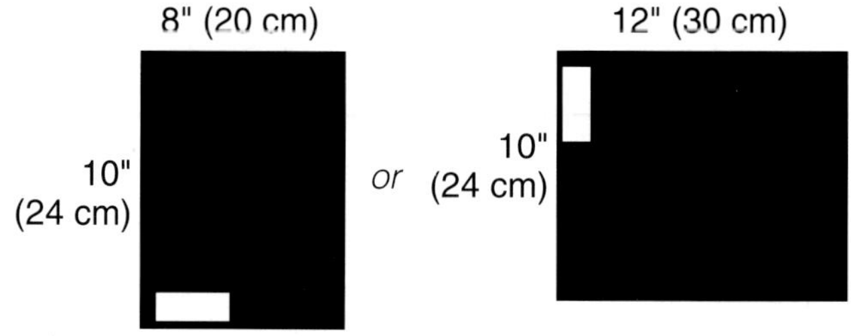

Patient Position

Seated at end or side of table, resting on table, anterior side down (Fig. 9.33).

Part Position

Place the cassette under palmar side of wrist. Fingers are flexed so joint will be in close contact with film. Area between radial and ulnar styloid processes centered to film.

Central Ray

Perpendicular between radial and ulnar styloid processes (midcarpal area). Collimate to area of interest.

Structures Demonstrated

Relationship of carpals, radius, and ulna should be included (Fig. 9.34).

Evaluation Criteria

1. Bones should not be rotated.
2. Carpus should not be deviated to radial or ulnar side.

NOTE: This projection is used after radial fracture is repositioned. An oblique is sometimes also part of departmental routine.

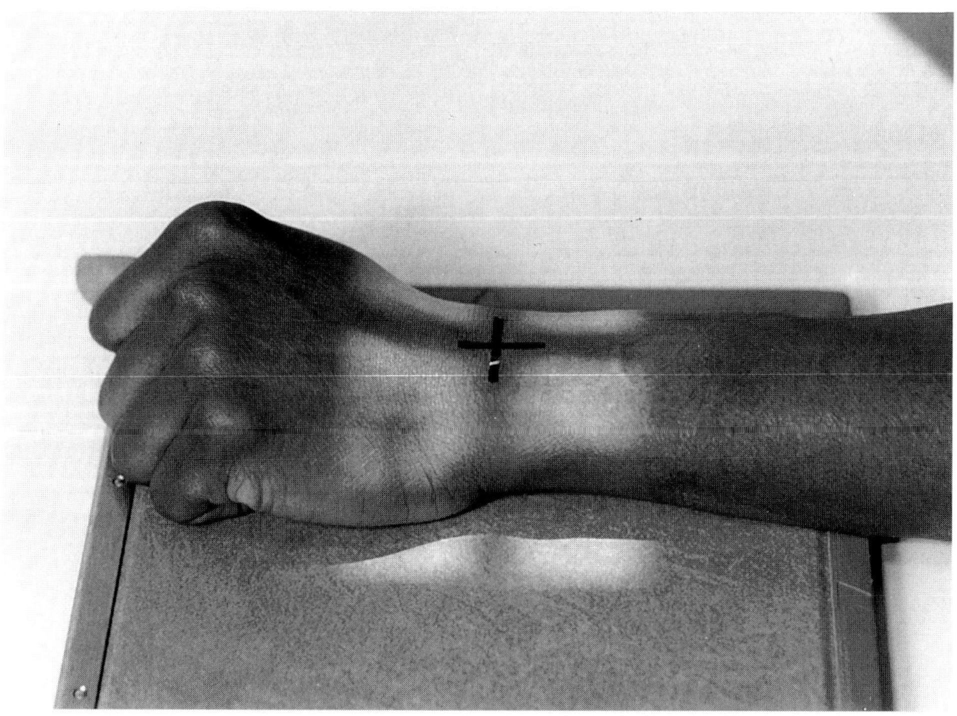

Figure 9.33. PA wrist.

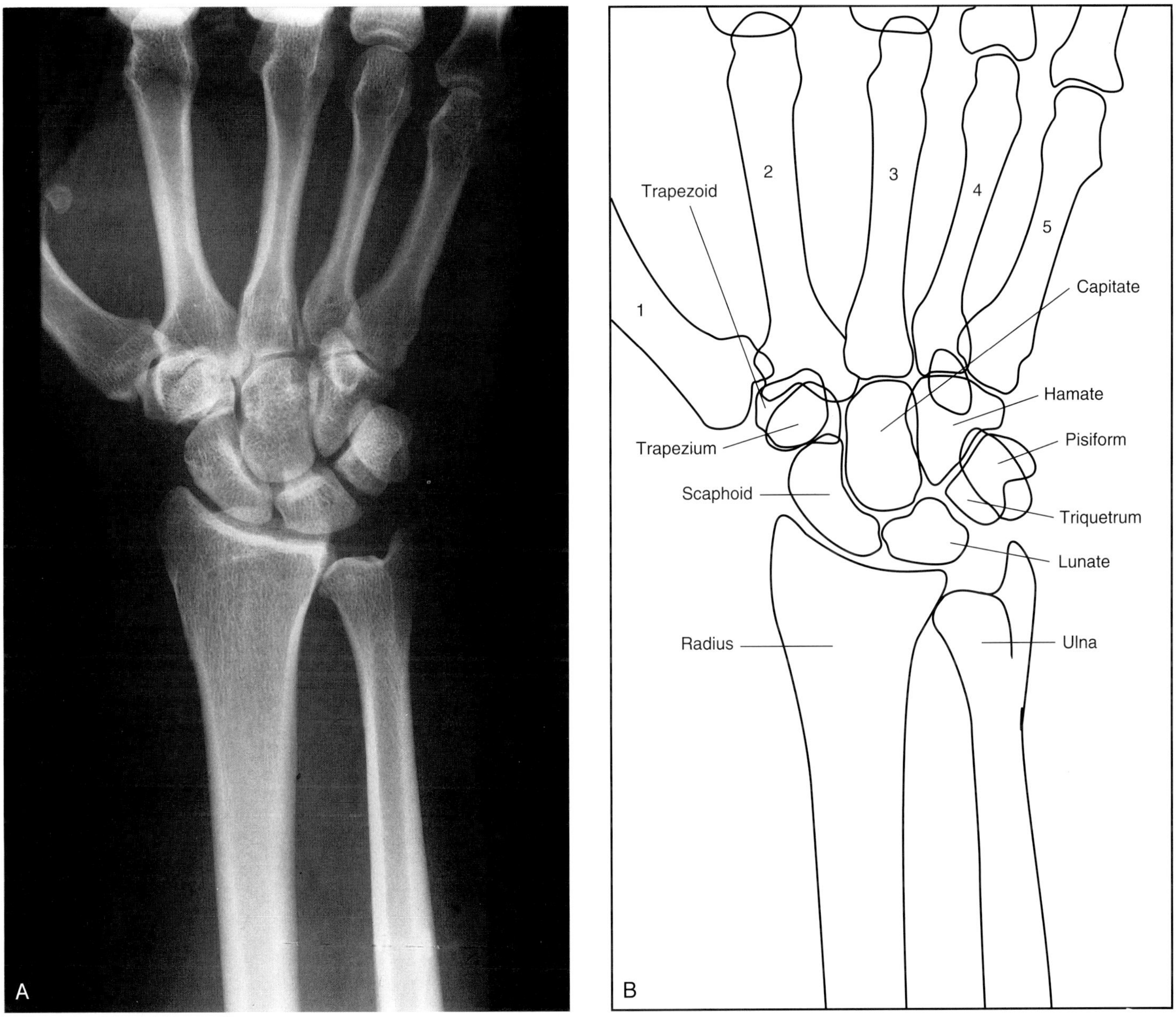

Figure 9.34. A and B, PA wrist.

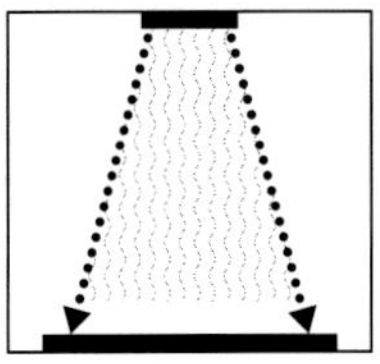

Wrist

Position/Projection

Lateral projection

Film:
8 × 10 inches (20 × 24 cm) lengthwise tabletop for one projection

or

10 × 12 inches (24 × 30 cm) for two or three projections crosswise

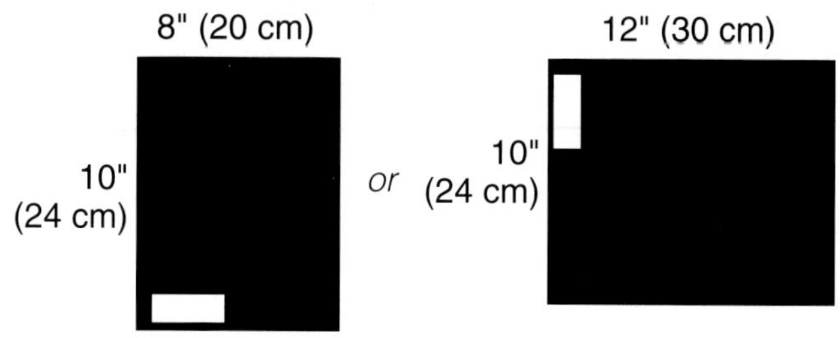

Patient Position

Seated at end or side of table, ulnar side of forearm resting on table (Fig. 9.35).

Part Position

Place cassette under ulnar side of wrist. Middle of wrist is centered to film. Radius and ulna form angle of 90° with plane of film.

Central Ray

Method 1
Perpendicular to the midcarpal area.

Method 2
15° proximal to center of wrist joint. Collimate to area of interest.

Structures Demonstrated

Suspected fracture and joint in lateral aspect (Fig. 9.36).

Evaluation Criteria

1. Distal radius and ulna should be included and superimposed to form true lateral.
2. Metacarpals should be included and superimposed.
3. Method 1 is used when fracture is suspected.
4. In method 2, 15° angulation of central ray is used to graze joint of radius.

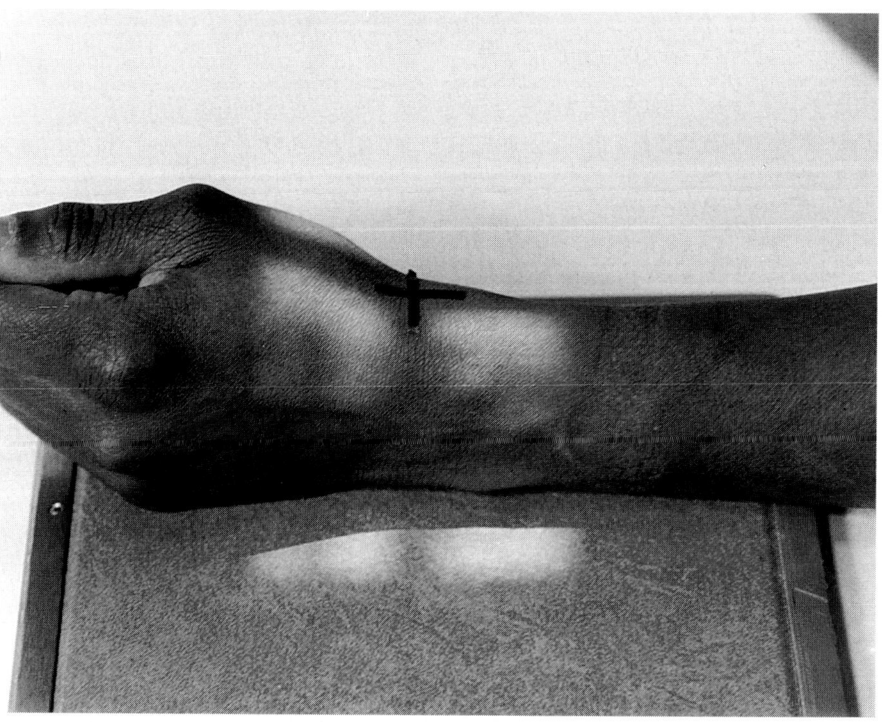

Figure 9.35. Lateral wrist.

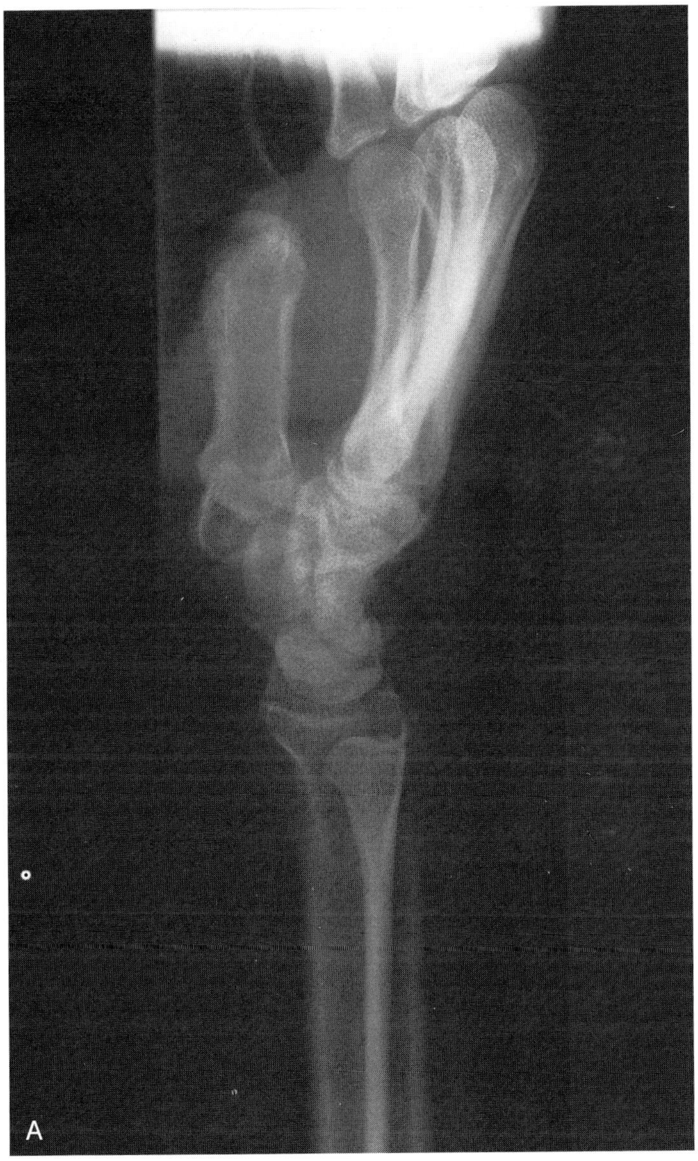

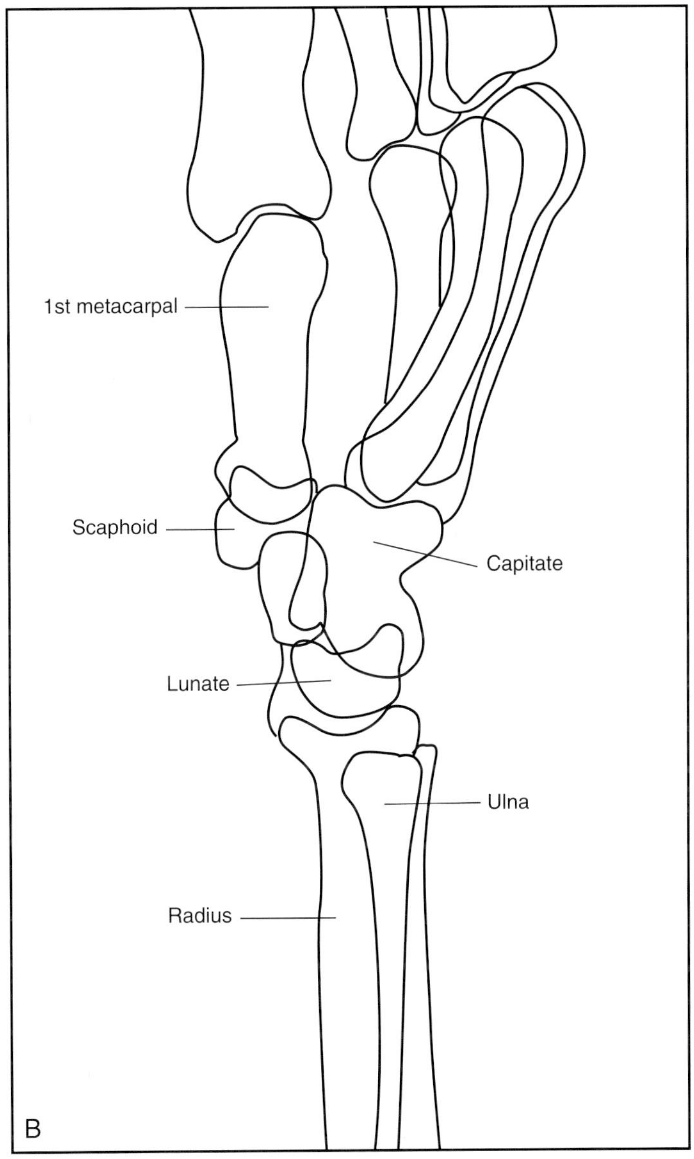

Figure 9.36. A and B, Lateral wrist.

Wrist: Scaphoid

Position/Projection

PA projection, ulnar deviation

Film:
8 × 10 inches (20 × 24 cm) tabletop for one projection crosswise

or

10 × 12 inches (24 × 30 cm) for two or three projections crosswise

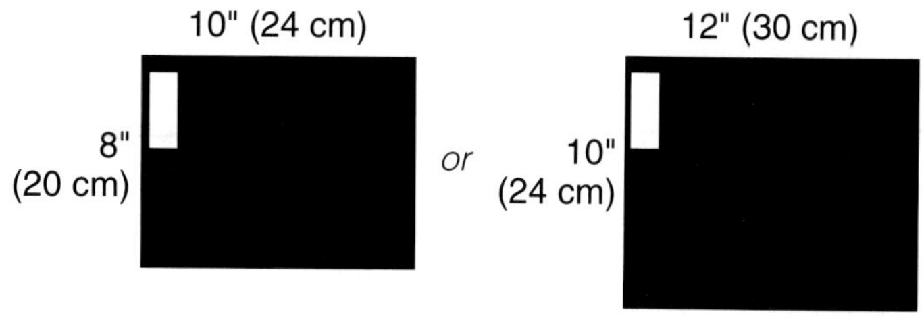

Patient Position

Seated at end or side of table, forearm resting on table anterior side down (Fig. 9.37).

Part Position

Place cassette under palm of hand. Hand is abducted. Scaphoid is centered to film.

Central Ray

Method 1

Perpendicular to exit through scaphoid.

Method 2

10–15° proximal to exit through scaphoid. Collimate to area of interest.

Structures Demonstrated

Joint spaces open (Fig. 9.38).

Evaluation Criteria

Scaphoid should be demonstrated without rotation.

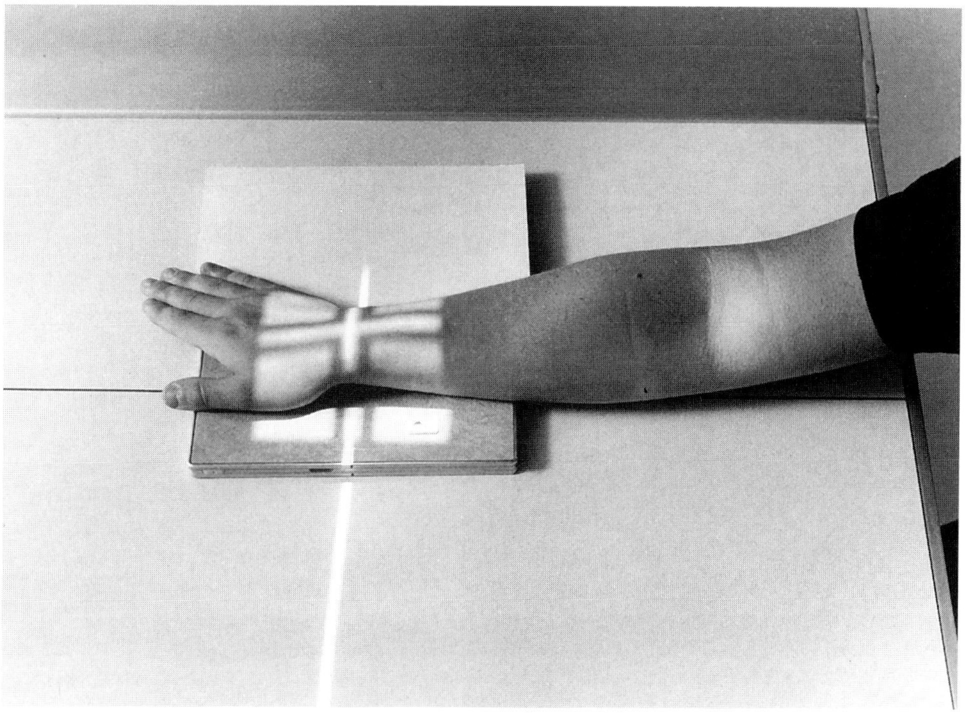

Figure 9.37. PA wrist, ulnar deviation.

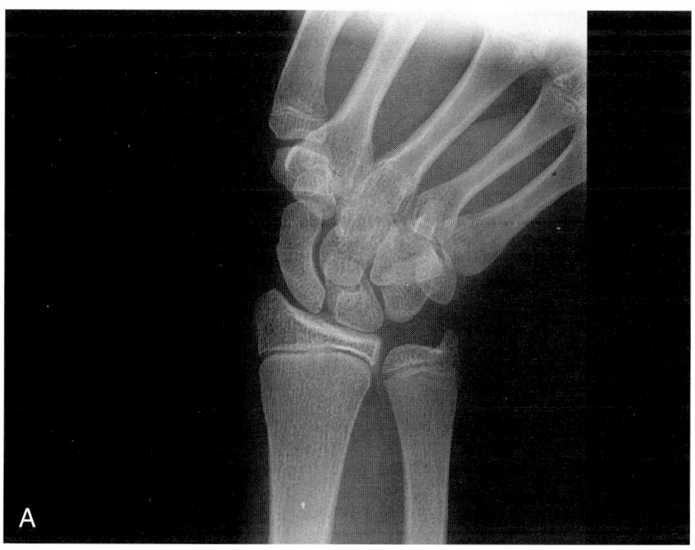

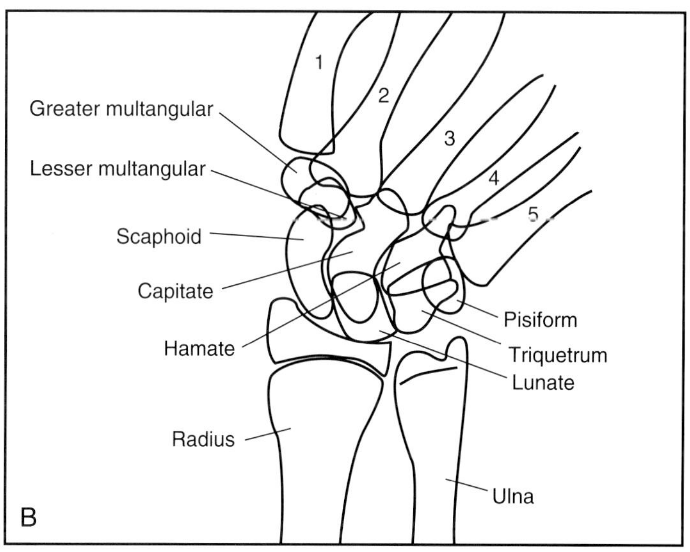

Figure 9.38. A and B, PA wrist, ulnar deviation.

Wrist: Pisiform

Position/Projection

Posterior oblique projection

Film:
8 × 10 inches (20 × 24 cm)
lengthwise, tabletop

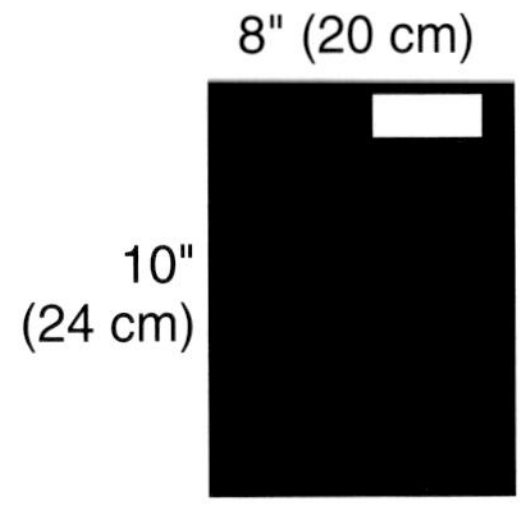

Patient Position

Seated at end or side of table, forearm resting on table ulnar side down (Fig. 9.39).

Part Position

Place cassette under hand. Fingers should be extended and supinated so wrist will form angle of 45° to plane of cassette. Middle of wrist centered to film.

Central Ray

Perpendicular to midpoint of wrist. Collimate to area of interest.

Structures Demonstrated

Entire pisiform (Fig. 9.40).

Evaluation Criteria

1. Pisiform should be projected clear of superimposition.
2. Alternative projection for pisiform: see Carpal Tunnel Projection, Axial.

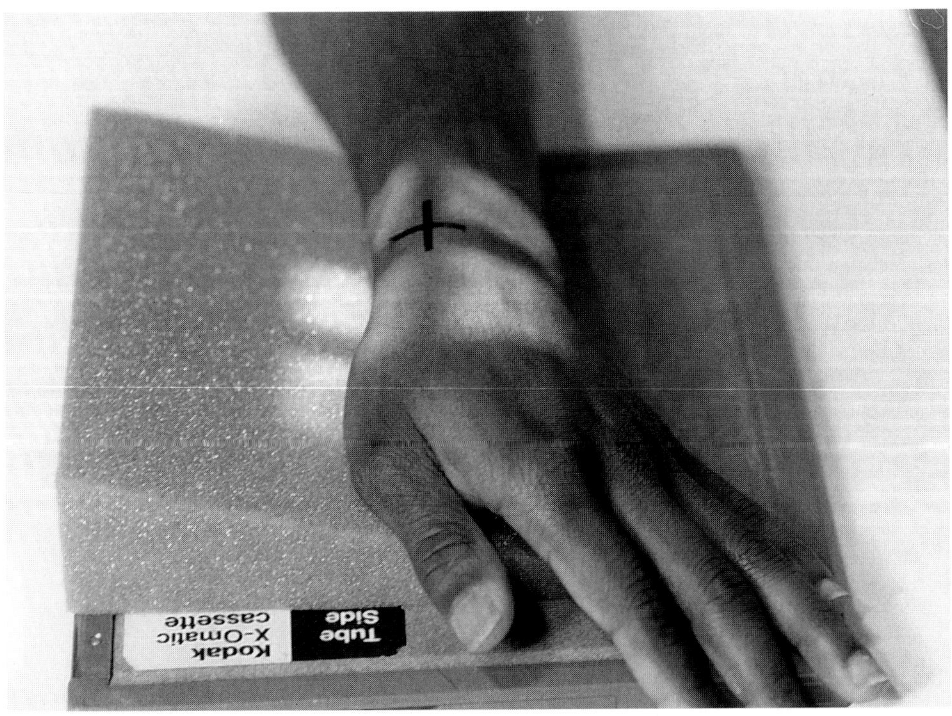

Figure 9.39. PA oblique pisiform.

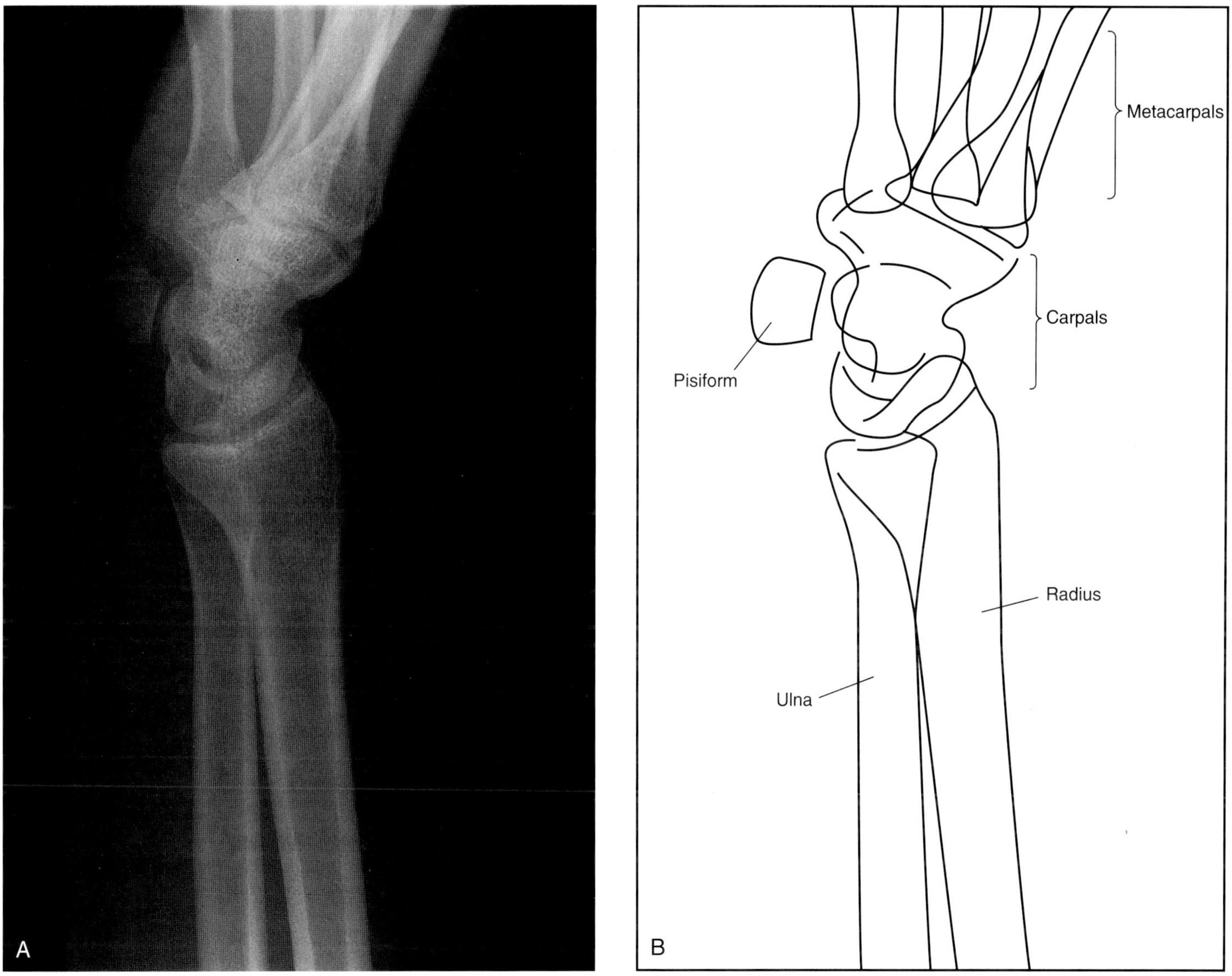

Figure 9.40. A and B, PA oblique pisiform.

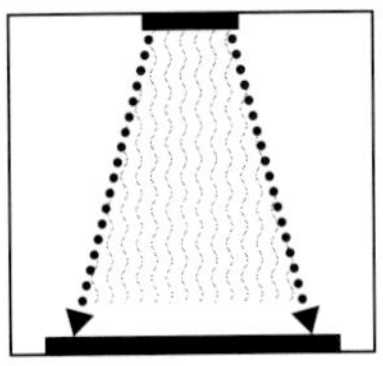

Wrist: Carpal Tunnel

Position/Projection

Axial projection/inferosuperior

Film:
8 × 10 inches (20 × 24 cm)
lengthwise, tabletop

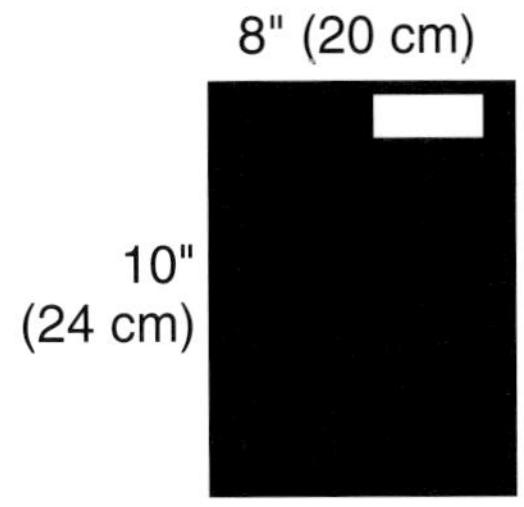

Patient Position

Seated at end of table, forearm resting on table anterior side down (Fig. 9.41).

Part Position

Place cassette under distal part of wrist. Wrist is hyperextended. Patient holds fingers backward with other hand or with bandage. Fourth metacarpal centered to film.

Central Ray

45° proximal to palm of hand. Collimate to area of interest.

Structures Demonstrated

Carpal tunnel (Fig. 9.42).

Evaluation Criteria

Medial and lateral prominences of concavity should be demonstrated.

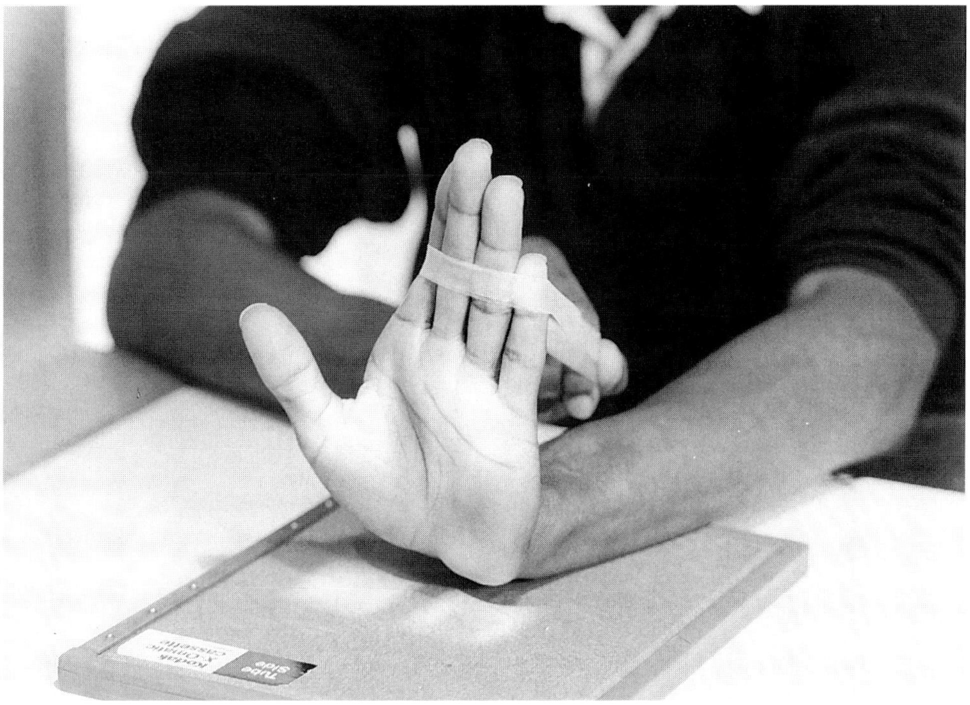

Figure 9.41. Axial inferosuperior wrist (carpal tunnel), central ray angle 45°.

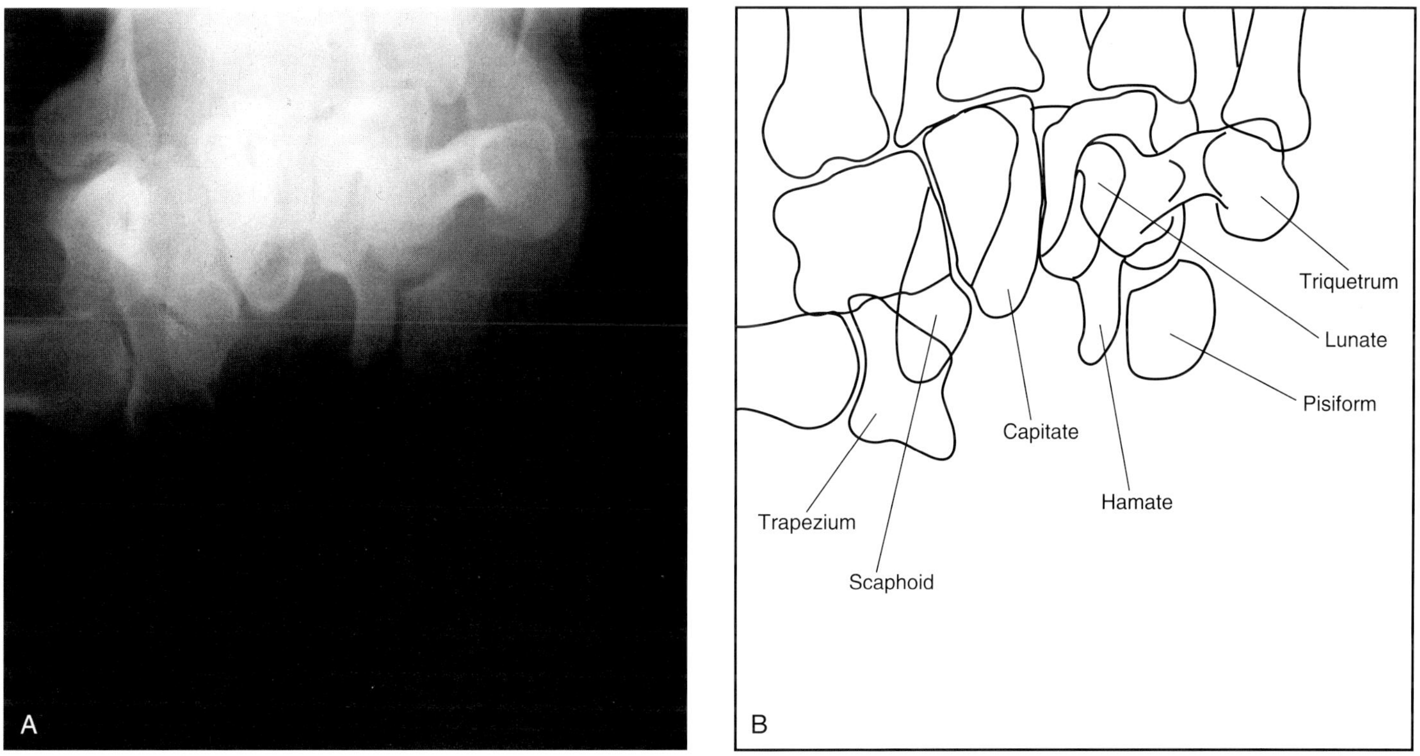

Figure 9.42. A and B, Axial inferosuperior wrist (carpal tunnel)

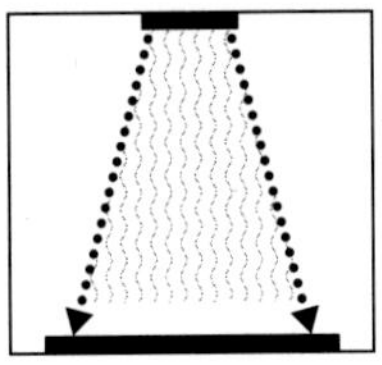

Wrist: Carpal Tunnel

Position/Projection

Axial projection/superoinferior

Film:
8 × 10 inches (20 × 24 cm)
lengthwise, tabletop

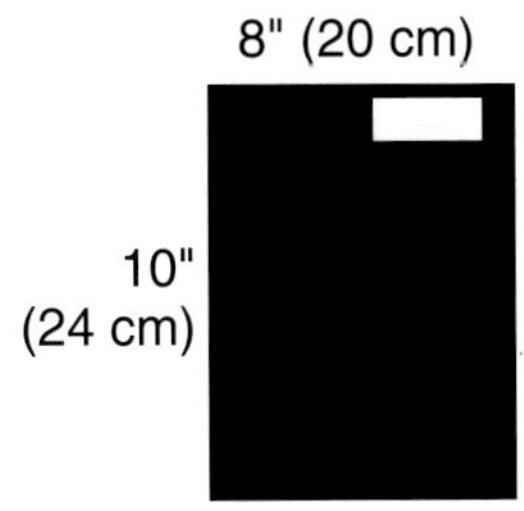

Patient Position

Standing, back to table, forearm approximately 90° against table (Fig. 9.43).

Part Position

Cassette is placed under palm. Wrist is dorsiflexed. Base of 5th metacarpal centered to film.

Central Ray

55° distal through palmar soft tissue of wrist. Collimate to area of interest.

Structures Demonstrated

Carpal tunnel (Fig. 9.44).

Evaluation Criteria

Medial and lateral prominences of concavity should be demonstrated.

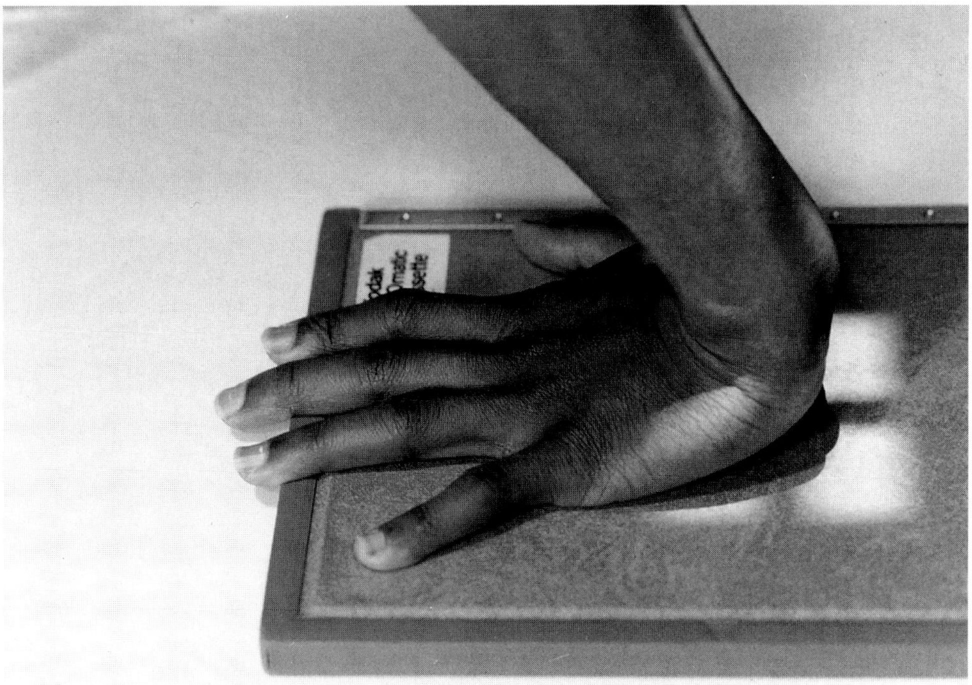

Figure 9.43. Axial superoinferior wrist (carpal tunnel), central ray angle 55°.

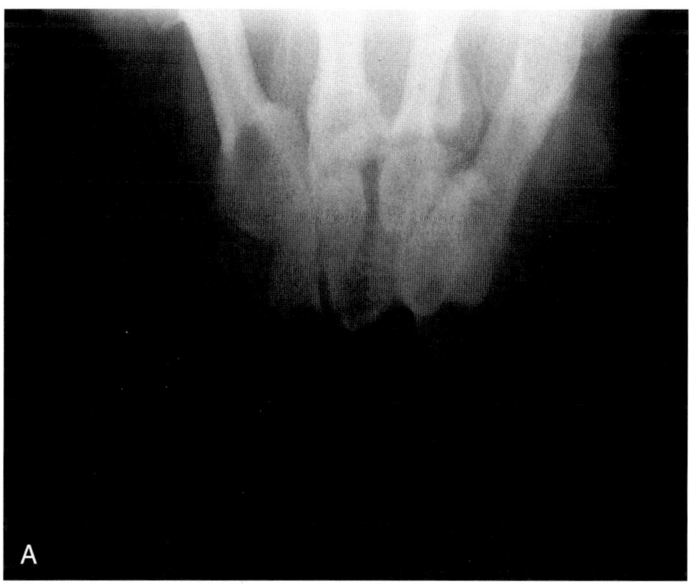

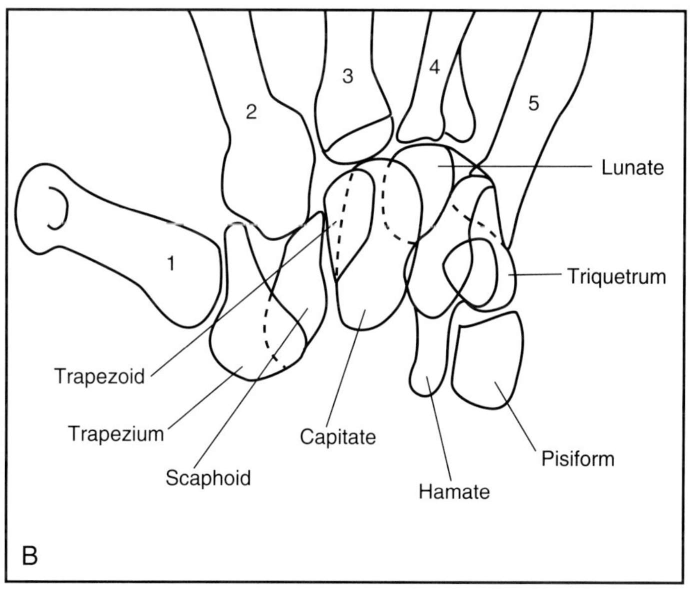

Figure 9.44. A and B, Axial superoinferior wrist (carpal tunnel).

Forearm

Position/Projection

AP projection

Film:
7 × 17 inches (18 × 43 cm) tabletop, lengthwise, or film large enough to include both wrist and elbow joints

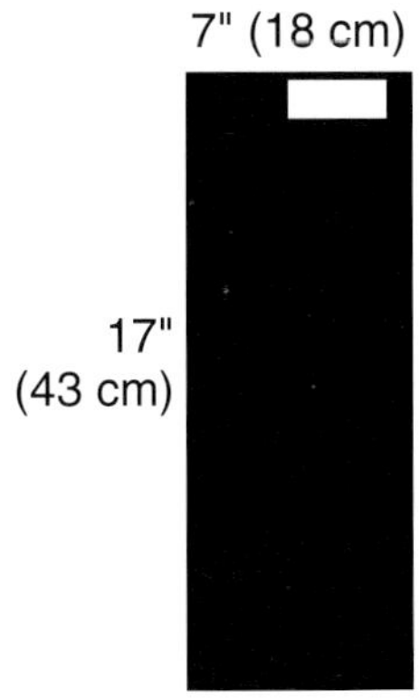

Patient Position

Seated at end or side of table, forearm resting on table posterior side down. Patient should lean laterally to achieve ulnar deviation and true AP position (Fig. 9.45).

Part Position

Place cassette under supinated forearm. Elbow should be extended. Middle of forearm centered to film.

Central Ray

Perpendicular to midpoint of forearm. Collimate to area of interest.

Structures Demonstrated

Entire forearm (Fig. 9.46).

Evaluation Criteria

1. Wrist and distal humerus should be included.
2. Forearm and elbow should be in true AP position.

NOTE: Fractures of the forearm require that modified positions be used. No attempt should be made to rotate the forearm. PA projection may be needed.

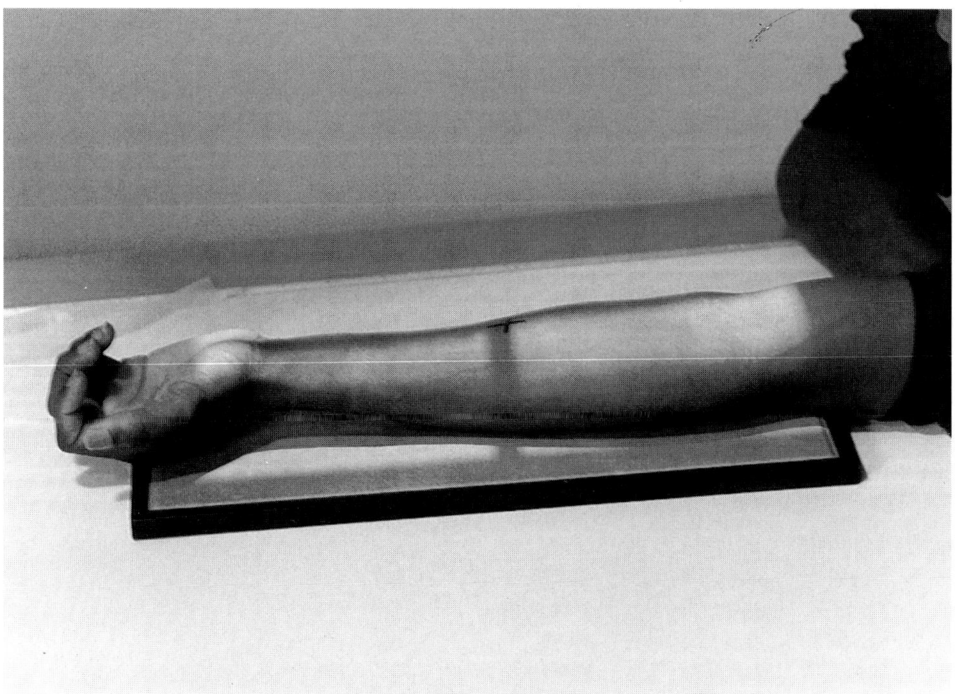

Figure 9.45. AP forearm.

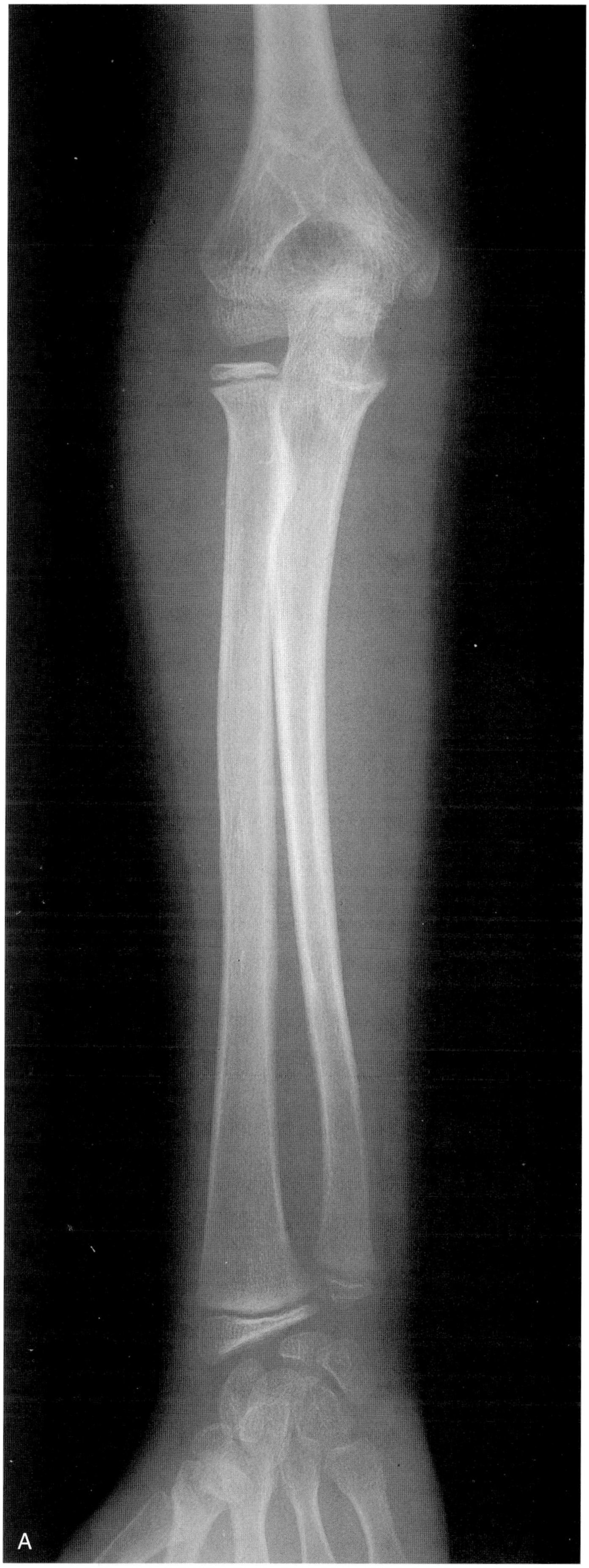

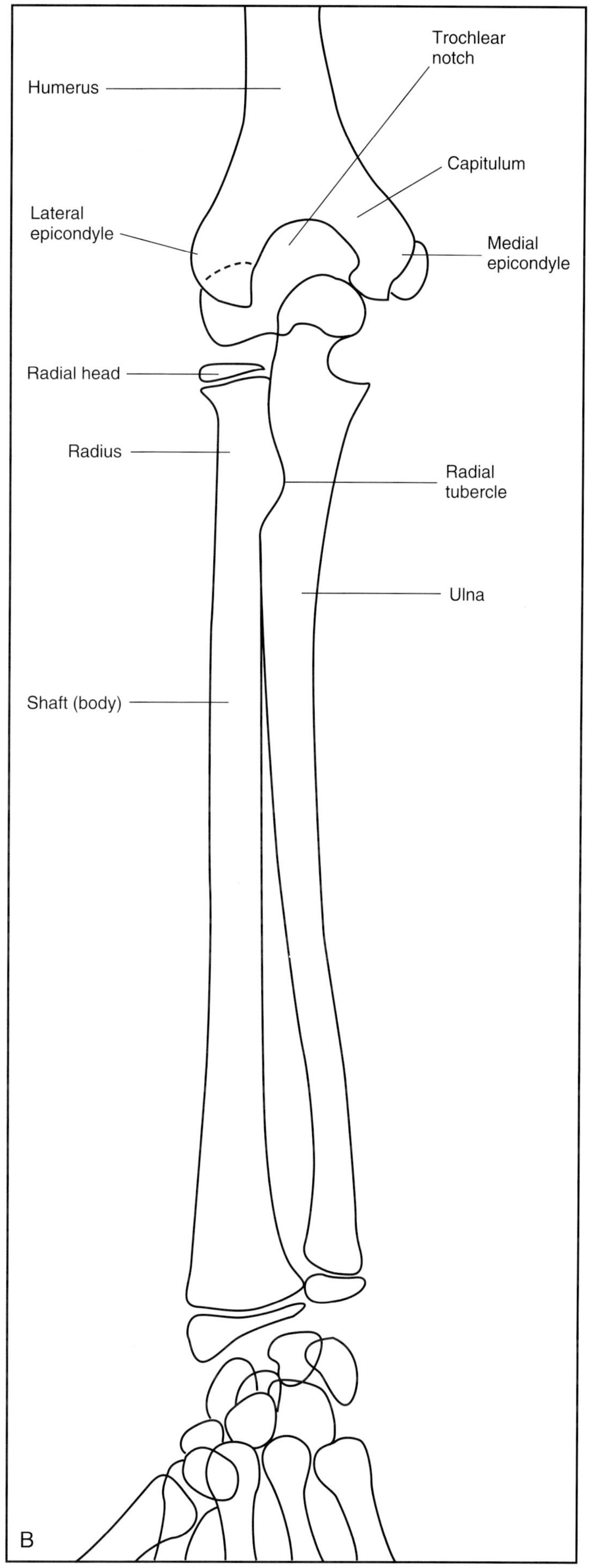

Figure 9.46. A and B, AP forearm.

Forearm

Position/Projection

Lateral projection

Film:
7 × 17 inches (18 × 43 cm) tabletop, lengthwise, or film large enough to include both wrist and elbow joints

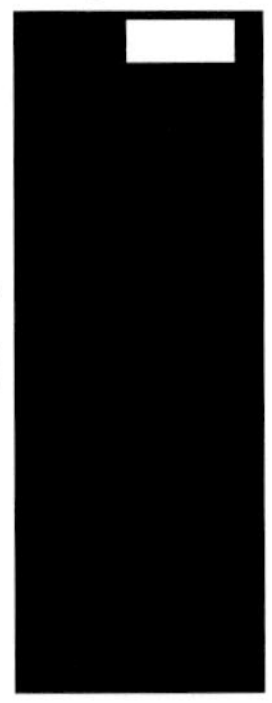

Patient Position

Seated at end or side of table, forearm resting on table, ulnar side down (Fig. 9.47).

Part Position

Place cassette under forearm. Elbow is flexed 90°. Middle of forearm centered to film.

Central Ray

Perpendicular to midpoint of forearm. Collimate to area of interest.

Structures Demonstrated

Forearm in lateral view (Fig. 9.48).

Evaluation Criteria

1. Wrist and distal humerus should be included.
2. Elbow joint must have correct lateral projection.
3. Distal radius and ulna are superimposed.

NOTE: Fractures of the forearm require that modified positions be used. No attempt should be made to rotate the forearm.

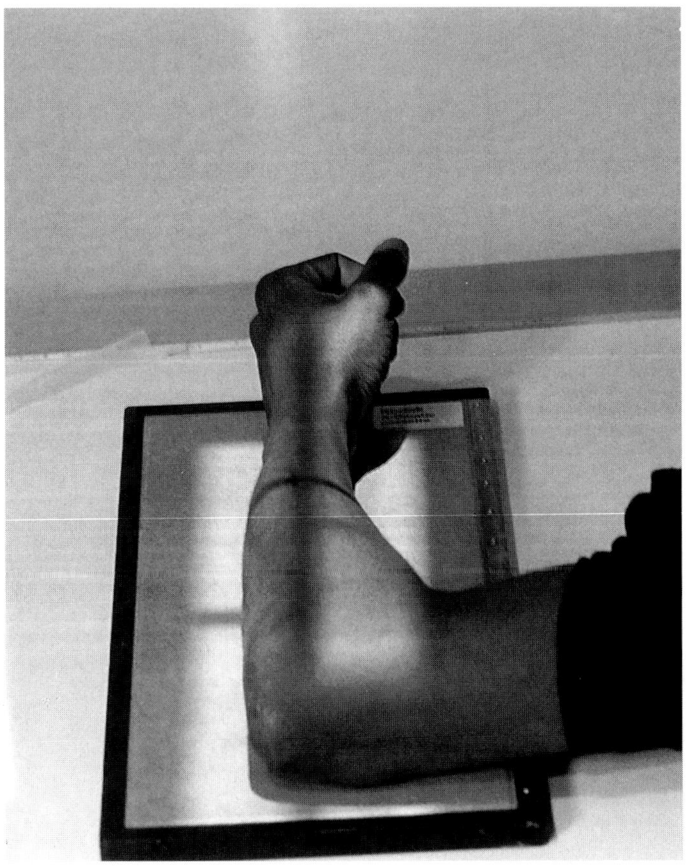

Figure 9.47. Lateral forearm.

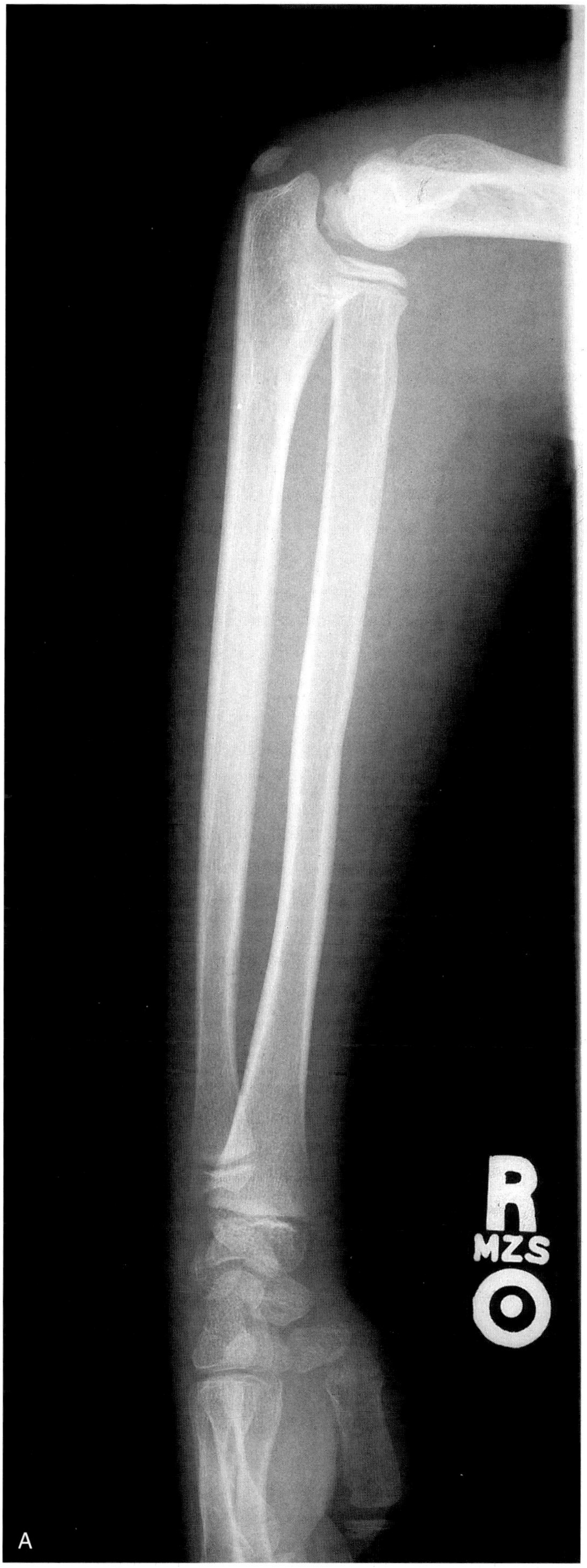

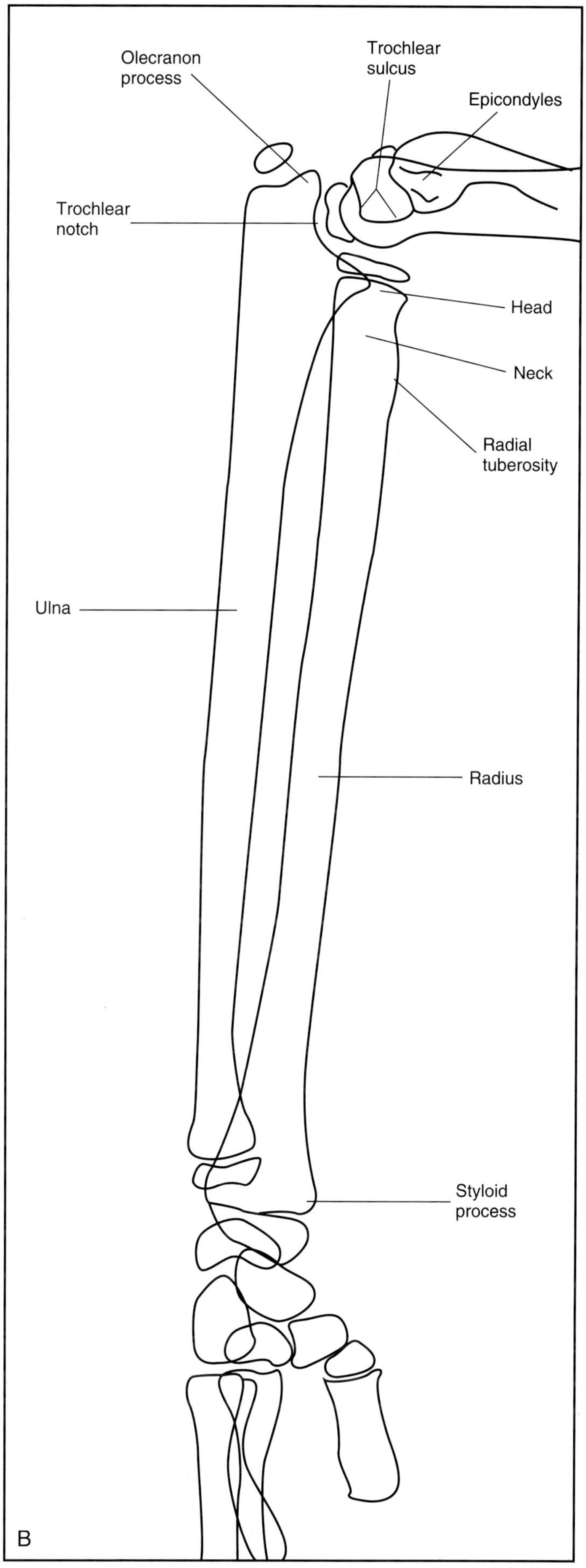

Figure 9.48. A and B, Lateral forearm.

Elbow

Position/Projection

AP projection

Film:
8 × 10 inches (20 × 24 cm) lengthwise, tabletop
or
10 × 12 inches (24 × 30 cm) for two or three projections crosswise

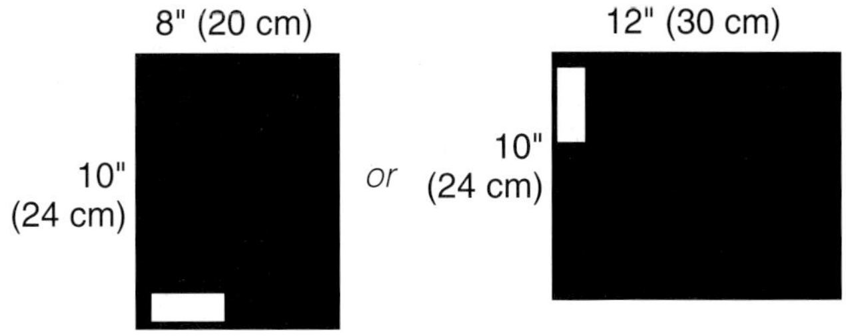

Patient Position
Seated at end or side of table, posterior side of humerus flat against cassette (Fig. 9.49).

Part Position
Place cassette under fully extended elbow. Hand is supinated until palm is facing upward. Shoulder is at same horizontal level as elbow and wrist. Elbow joint centered to film.

Central Ray
Perpendicular to middle of elbow joint. Collimate to area of interest.

Structures Demonstrated
Distal humerus along with proximal radius and ulna (Fig. 9.50).

Evaluation Criteria
1. Elbow joint should be open.
2. Epicondyles of humerus should not be rotated.
3. Joint space between radial head and capitulum is clearly seen.

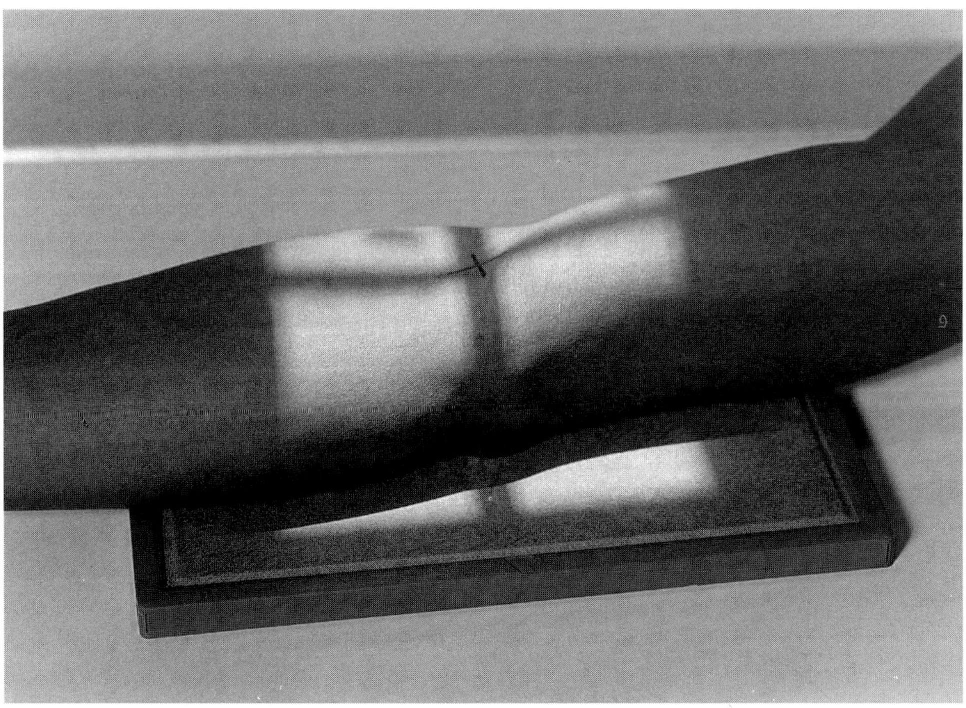

Figure 9.49. AP elbow.

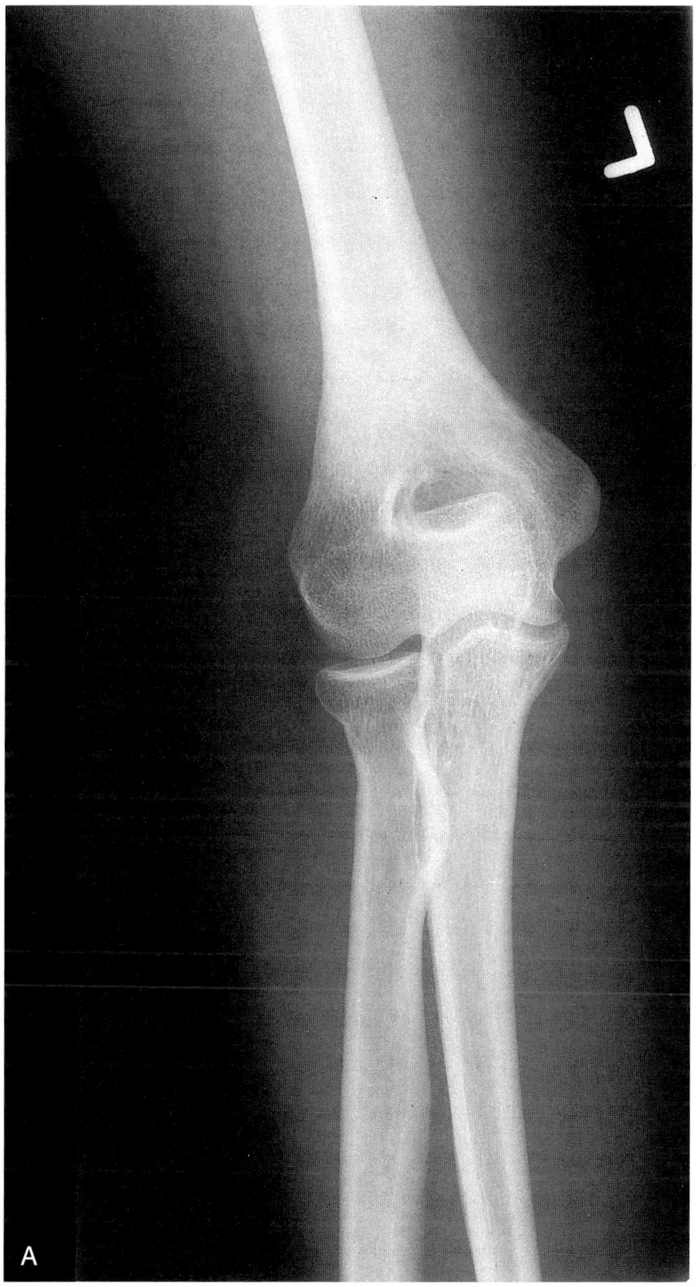

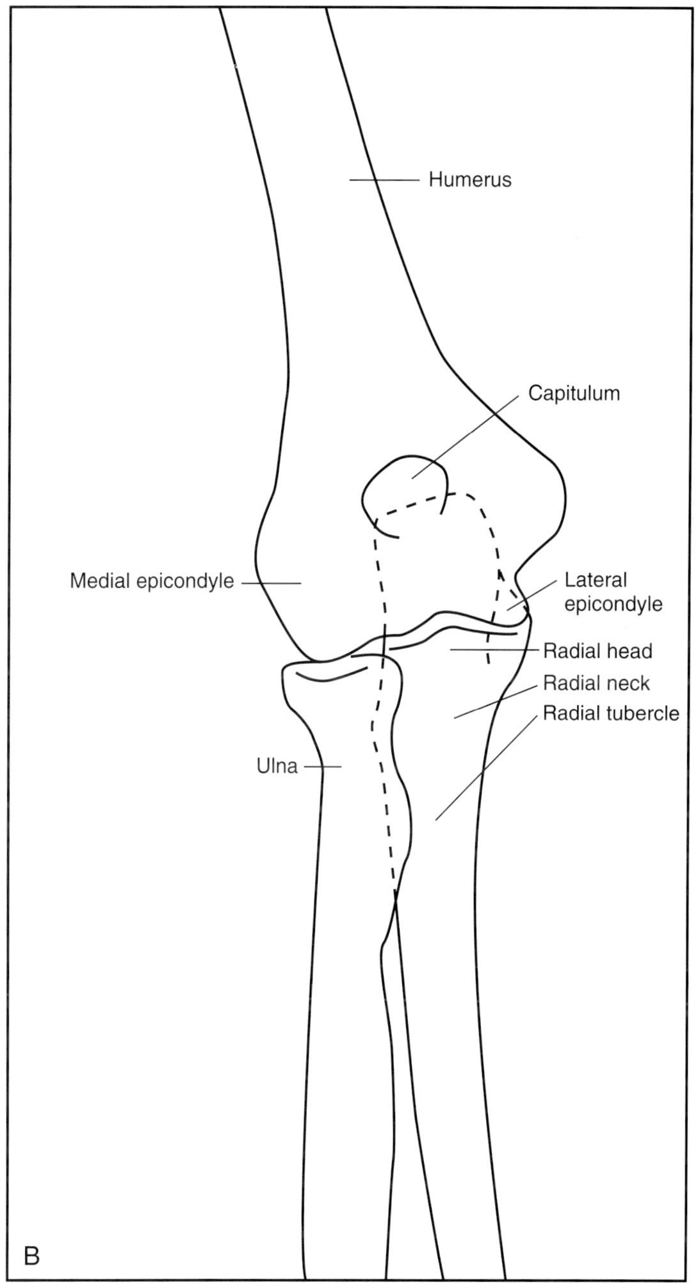

Figure 9.50. A and B, AP elbow.

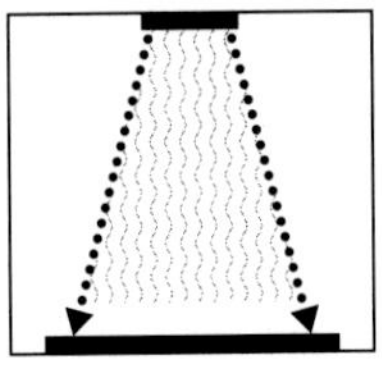

Elbow

Position/Projection

Lateral projection

Film:
8 × 10 inches (20 × 24 cm) lengthwise, tabletop
or
10 × 12 inches (24 × 30 cm) for two or three projections crosswise

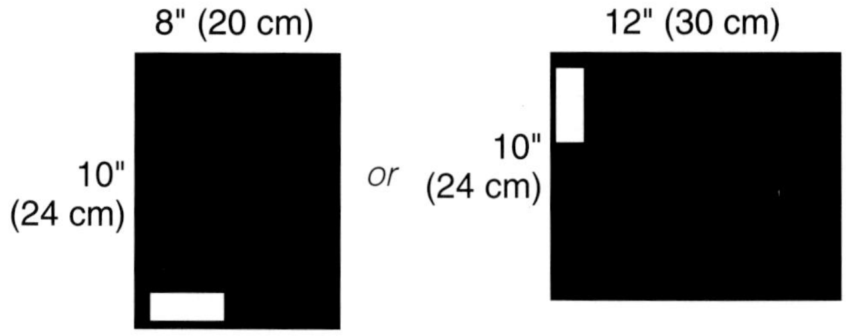

Patient Position

Seated at end or side of table, entire extremity resting on cassette (Fig. 9.51).

Part Position

Place cassette under ulnar side of forearm. Hand and wrist are placed in true lateral position. Shoulder is at same horizontal level as elbow and wrist. Elbow joint centered to film and flexed 90°.

Central Ray

Perpendicular to the joint. Collimate to area of interest.

Structures Demonstrated

Elbow, lower arm, and upper forearm (Fig. 9.52).

Evaluation Criteria

1. Condyles of the distal humerus should be superimposed.
2. Outer two thirds of radial head should be projected clear of superimposition.
3. Olecranon should be in profile.
4. Elevated fat pads should be seen in their most relaxed position. If partial or complete flexion is used, elevation of fat pad may occur, simulating joint pathology.

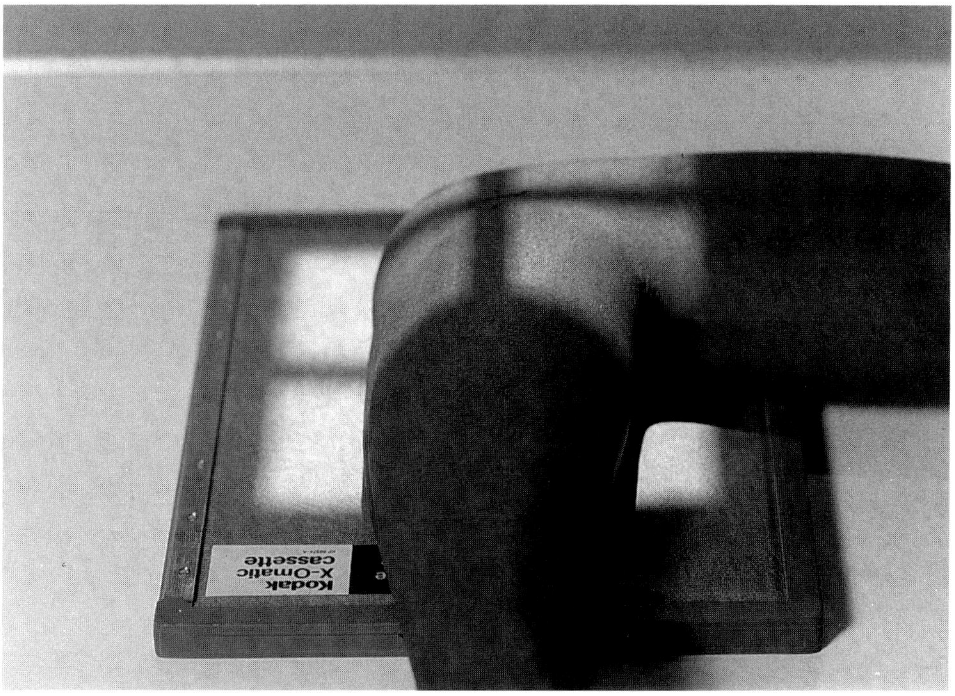

Figure 9.51. Lateral elbow.

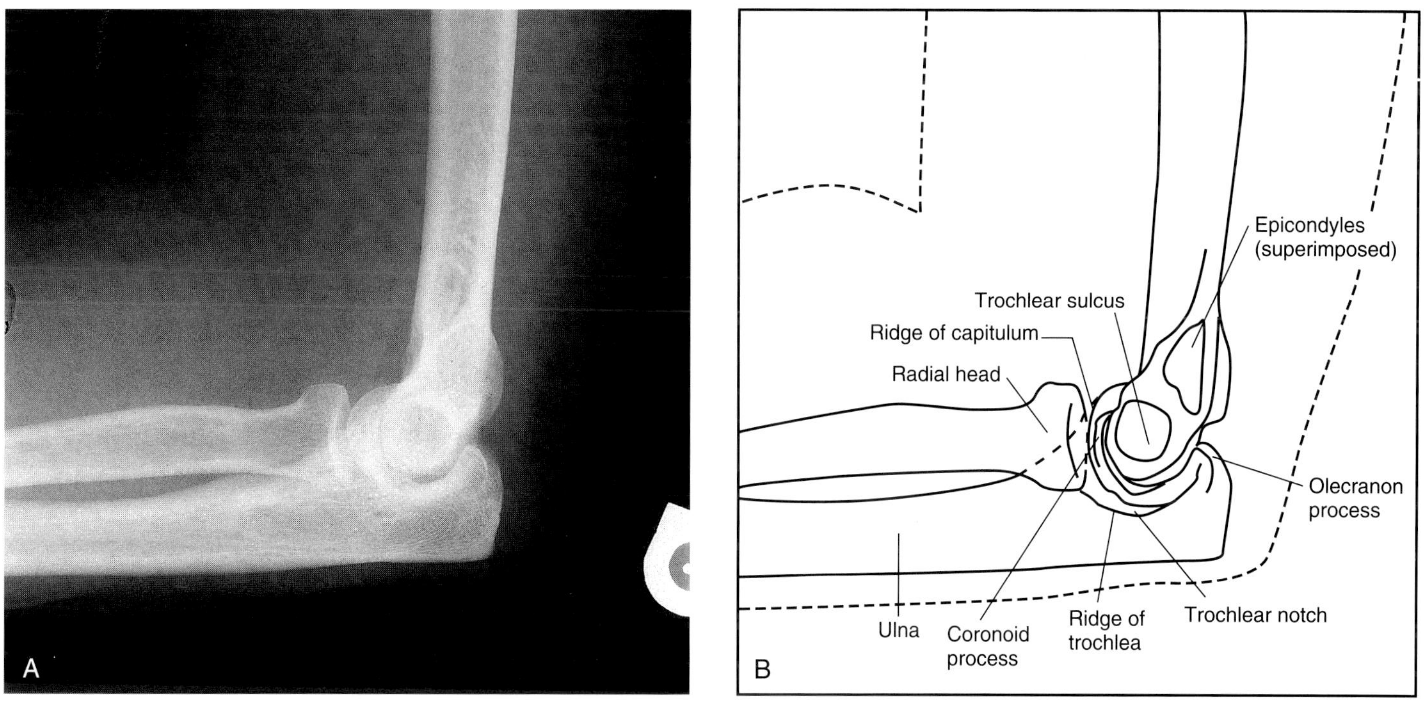

Figure 9.52. A and B, Lateral elbow.

Elbow

Position/Projection

AP projection, external (lateral) oblique

Film:
8 × 10 inches (20 × 24 cm) lengthwise, tabletop

or

10 × 12 inches (24 × 30 cm) for two or three projections crosswise

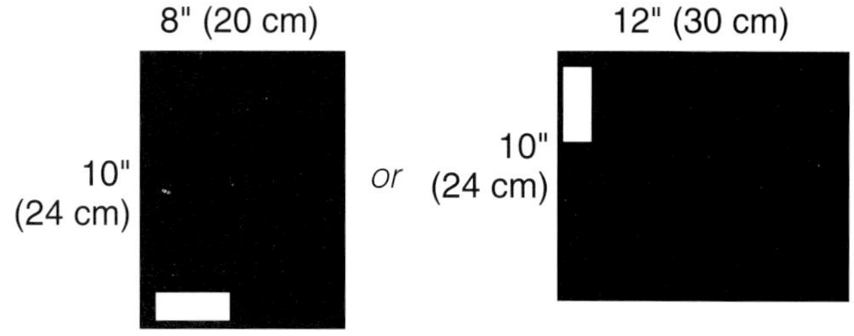

Patient Position

Seated at end or side table, posterior side of entire extremity resting on table (Fig. 9.53).

Part Position

Place cassette under fully extended elbow. Hand is supinated 45° to rotate elbow externally. Shoulder is at same horizontal level as elbow and wrist. Elbow joint centered to film.

Central Ray

Perpendicular to elbow joint. Collimate to area of interest.

Structures Demonstrated

Radial head and capitulum (Fig. 9.54).

Evaluation Criteria

1. Radius projected free of ulna.
2. Elbow joint should be open.

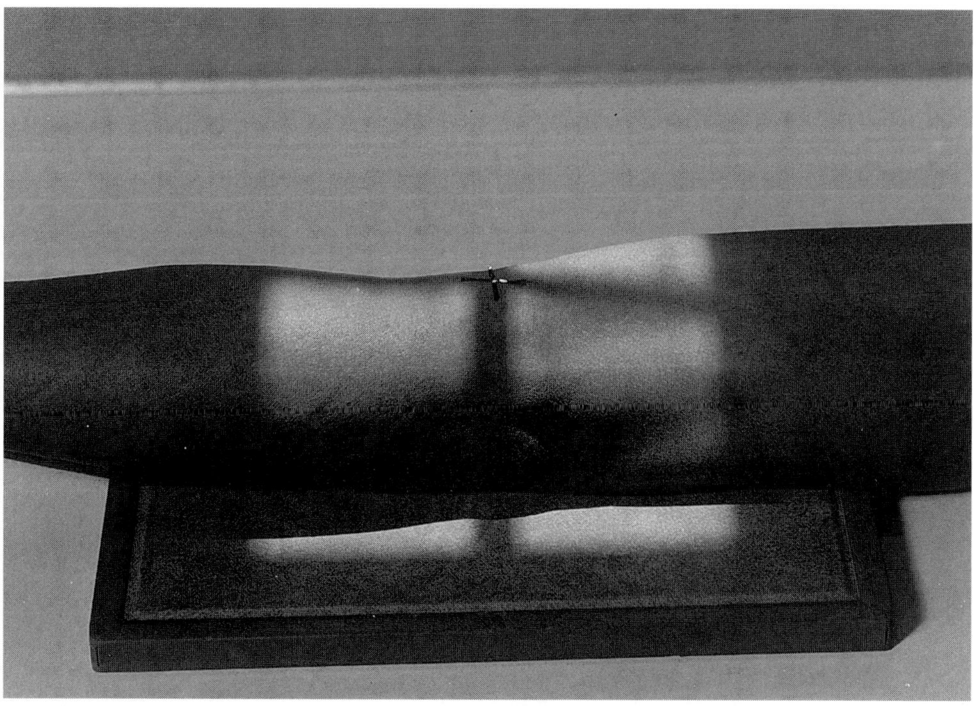

Figure 9.53. AP external oblique elbow.

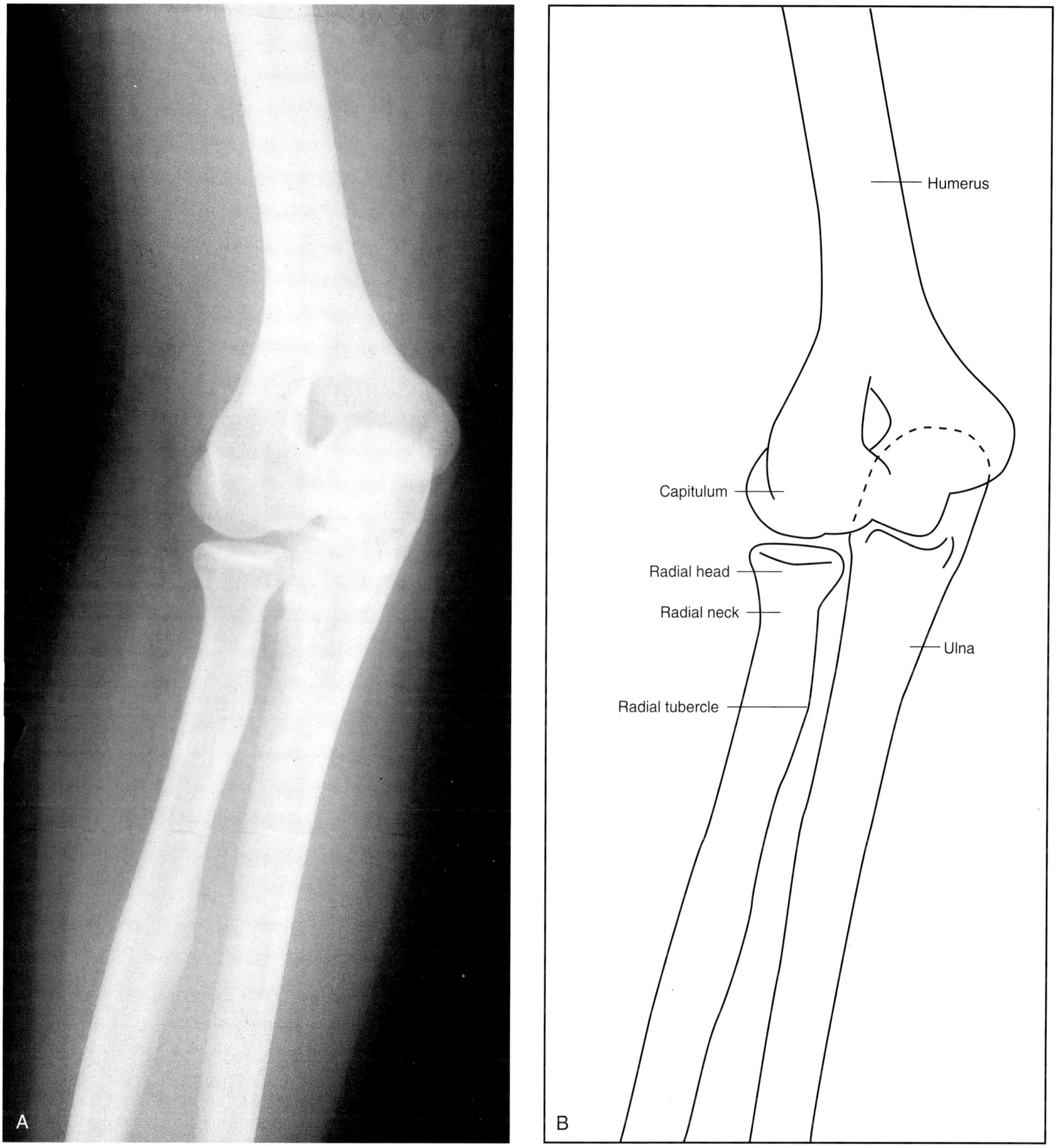

Figure 9.54. A and B, AP external oblique elbow.

Elbow

Position/Projection

AP projection, internal (medial) oblique

Film:
8 × 10 inches (20 × 24 cm) lengthwise, tabletop
or
10 × 12 inches (24 × 30 cm) for two or three projections crosswise

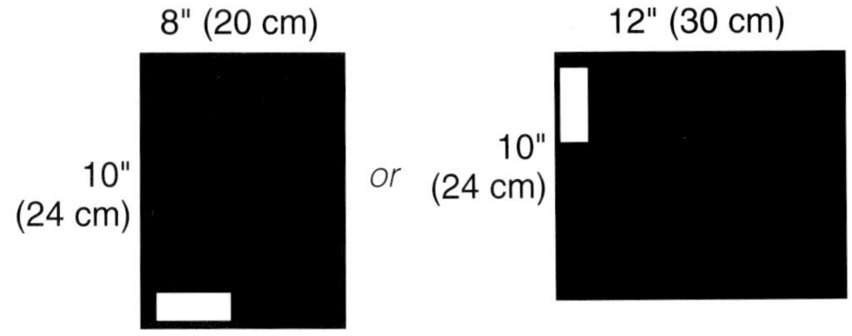

Patient Position

Seated at end or side of table, posterior side of entire extremity resting on table (Fig. 9.55).

Part Position

Place cassette under fully extended elbow. Hand is pronated 45° to rotate the elbow internally. Shoulder is at same horizontal level as elbow and wrist. Elbow joint centered to film.

Central Ray

Perpendicular to elbow joint. Collimate to area of interest.

Structures Demonstrated

Coronoid process, trochlea, and medial epicondyle (Fig. 9.56).

Evaluation Criteria

1. Coronoid process should be demonstrated in profile.
2. Medial epicondyle should be clearly visualized.

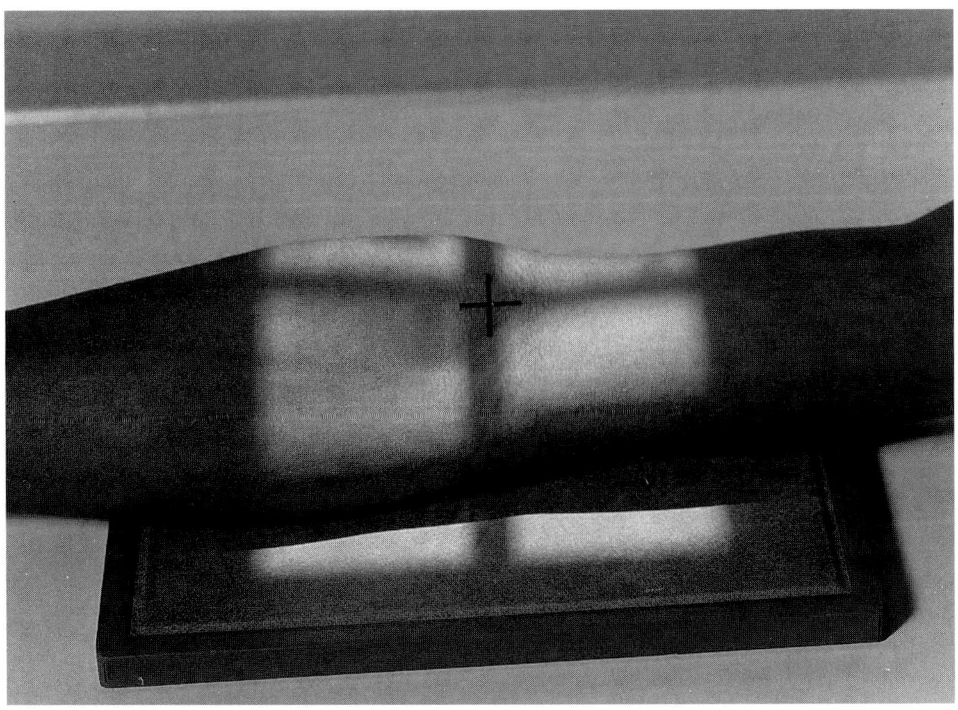

Figure 9.55. AP internal oblique elbow.

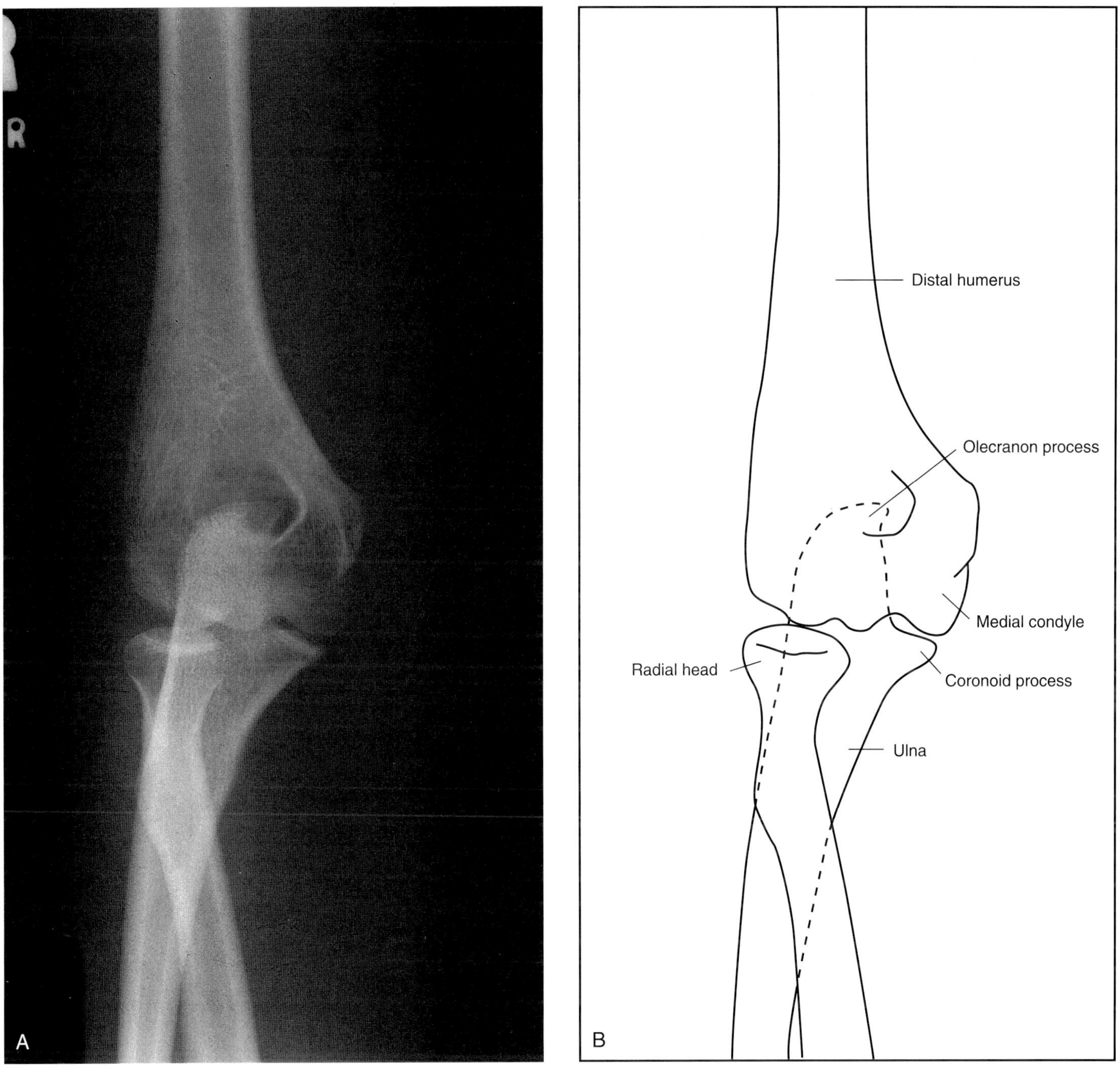

Figure 9.56. A and B, AP internal oblique elbow.

Elbow

Position/Projection

AP projection (to include proximal forearm)

Film:
8 × 10 inches (20 × 24 cm)
lengthwise, tabletop

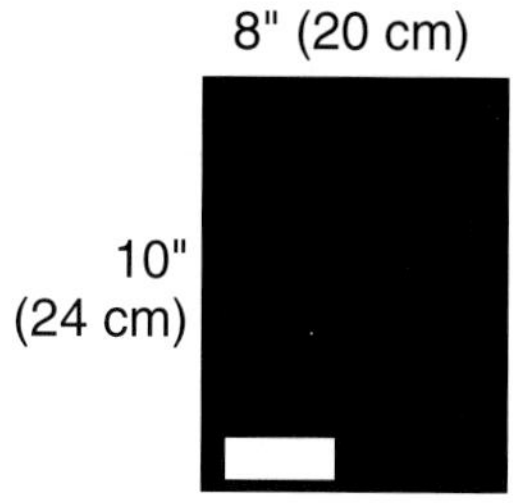

Patient Position

Seated at end or side of table, posterior side of forearm against film (Fig. 9.57).

Part Position

Place cassette under elbow. Elbow is extended as much as possible. Hand is supinated until palm is facing upward, and posterior surface of forearm is parallel to film. Interepicondylar line centered to film.

Central Ray

Perpendicular to elbow joint. Collimate to area of interest.

Structures Demonstrated

Distal end of radius and ulna (Fig. 9.58).

Evaluation Criteria

1. Radius and ulna should have correct AP projection.
2. Elbow joint is partially open. This projection is used when elbow cannot be extended.

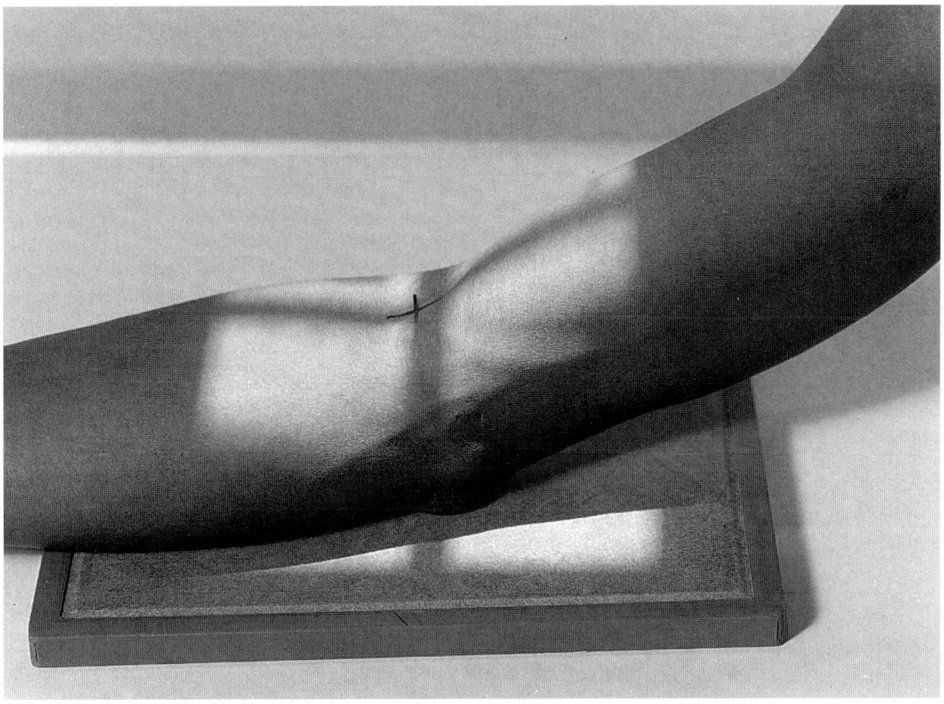

Figure 9.57. AP of elbow for proximal forearm.

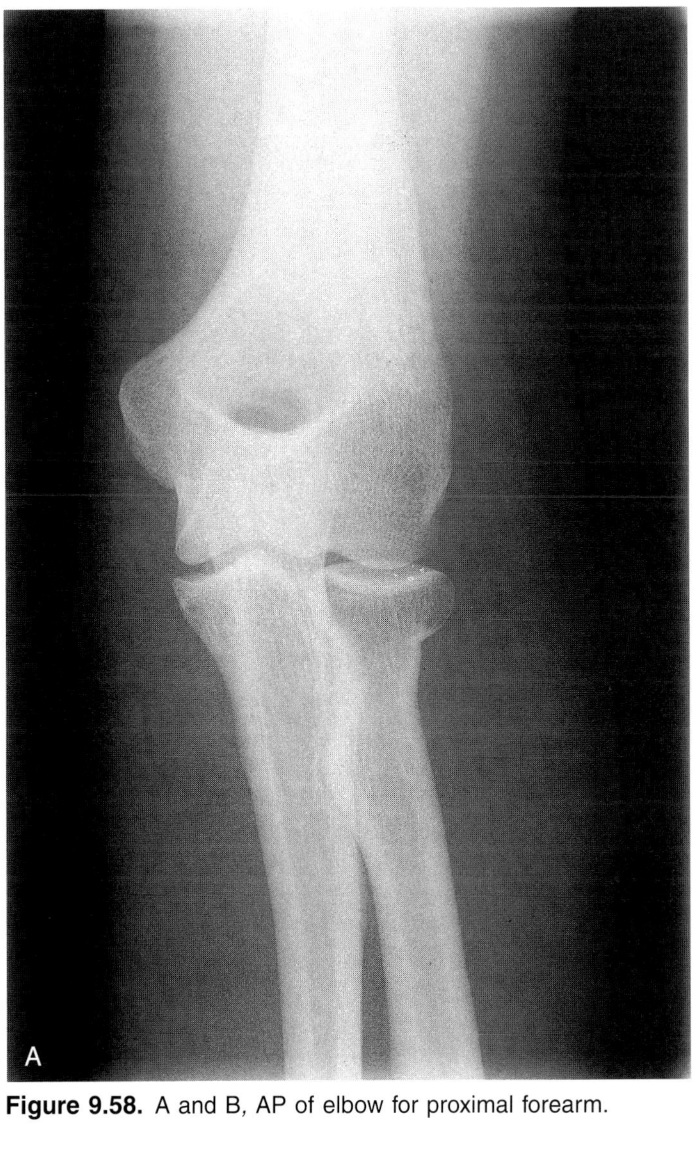

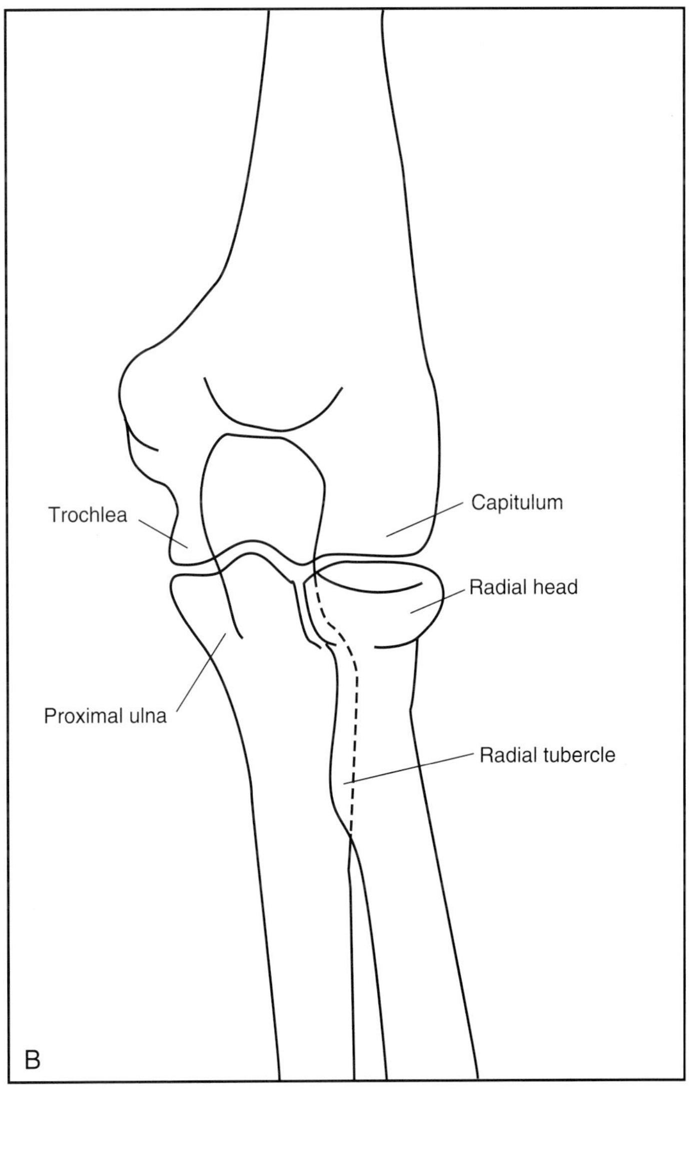

Figure 9.58. A and B, AP of elbow for proximal forearm.

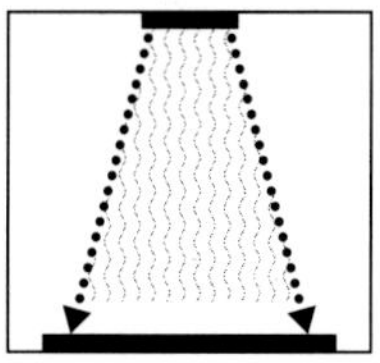

Elbow

Position/Projection

AP projection (to include distal humerus)

Film:
8 × 10 inches (20 × 24 cm)
lengthwise, tabletop

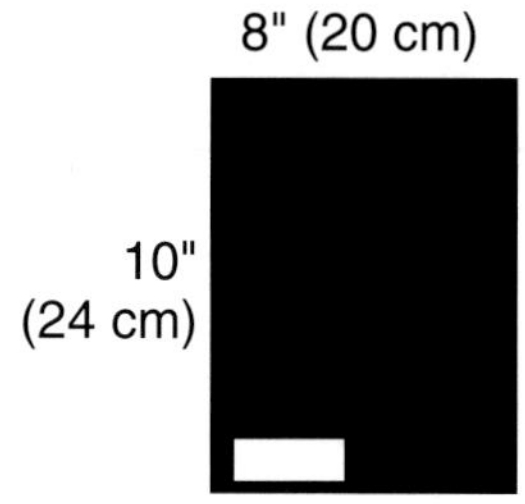

Patient Position
Seated at end or side of table, posterior side of upper arm against film (Fig. 9.59).

Part Position
Place cassette under elbow. Elbow is extended as much as possible. Hand is slightly pronated until posterior surface of upper arm is parallel to film. Elbow joint centered to film.

Central Ray
Perpendicular to elbow joint. Collimate to area of interest.

Structures Demonstrated
Distal end of humerus (Fig. 9.60).

Evaluation Criteria
1. Humerus should have correct AP projection.
2. Elbow joint is closed.

NOTE: This projection is used when elbow cannot be extended.

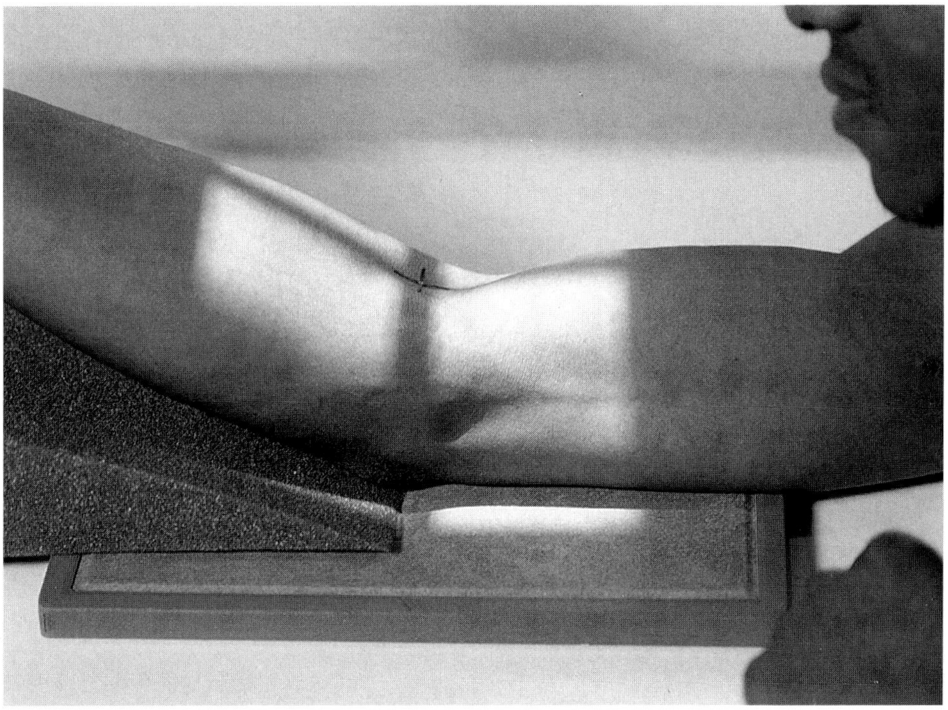

Figure 9.59. AP elbow for distal humerus.

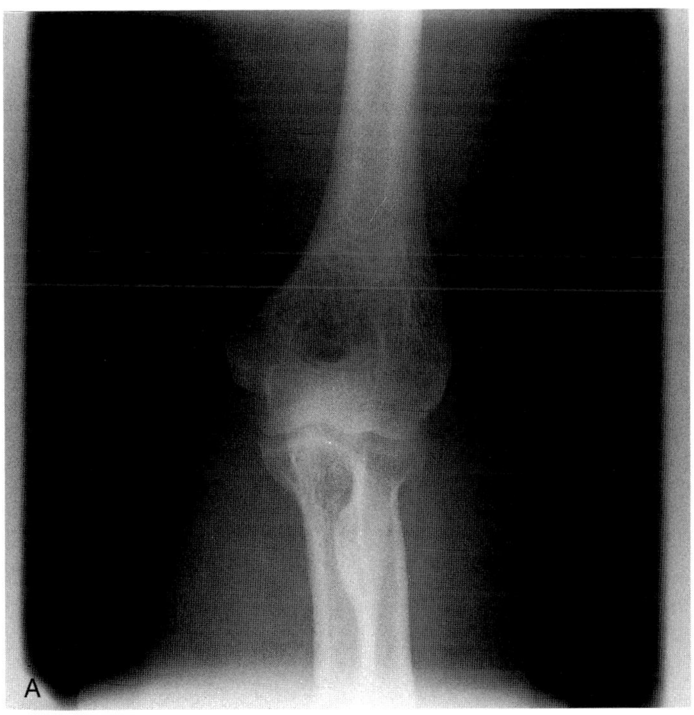

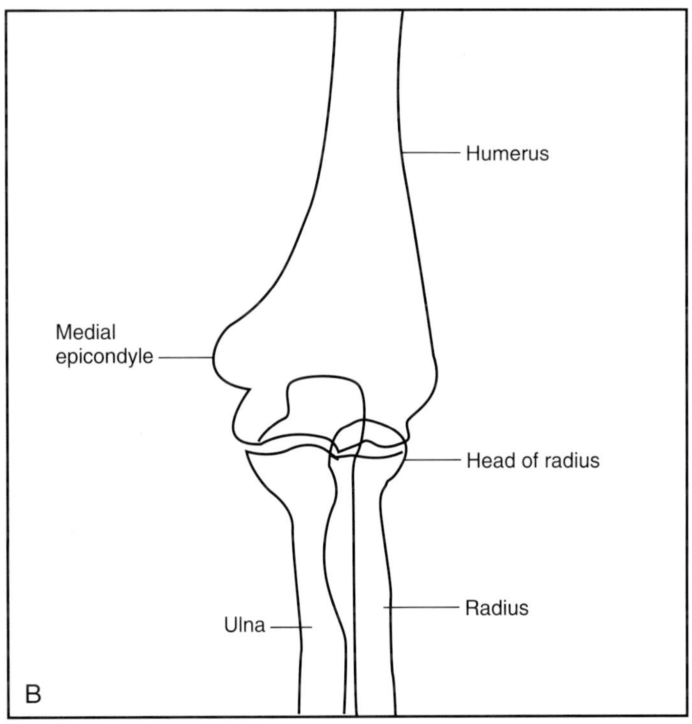

Figure 9.60. A and B, AP elbow for distal humerus.

Elbow

Position/Projection

Axial/distal humerus

Film:
8 × 10 inches (20 × 24 cm)
lengthwise, tabletop

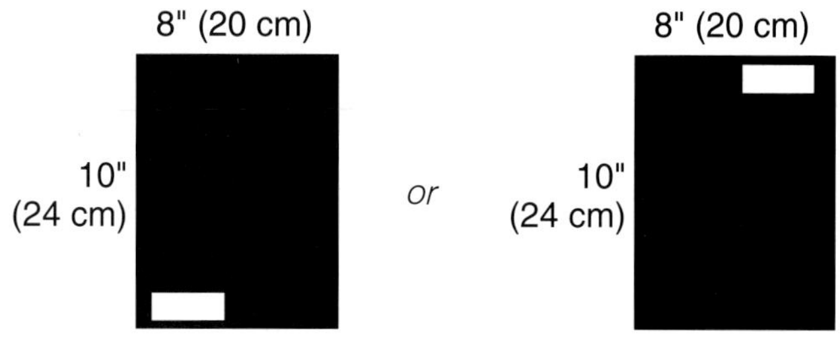

Patient Position

Seated at end of table, posterior side of upper arm resting on table (Fig. 9.61).

Part Position

Place cassette under posterior side of upper arm. Elbow joint is in maximum flexion and palm of hand is facing shoulder. Olecranon process centered to film.

Central Ray

Perpendicular 2 inches (5 cm) distal to olecranon process. Collimate to area of interest.

Structures Demonstrated

Distal humerus (Fig. 9.62).

Evaluation Criteria

1. Humerus and forearm should be superimposed.
2. There should be no rotation.
3. Distal end of humerus and olecranon process should be visualized.

NOTE: This projection is used when the elbow cannot be extended.

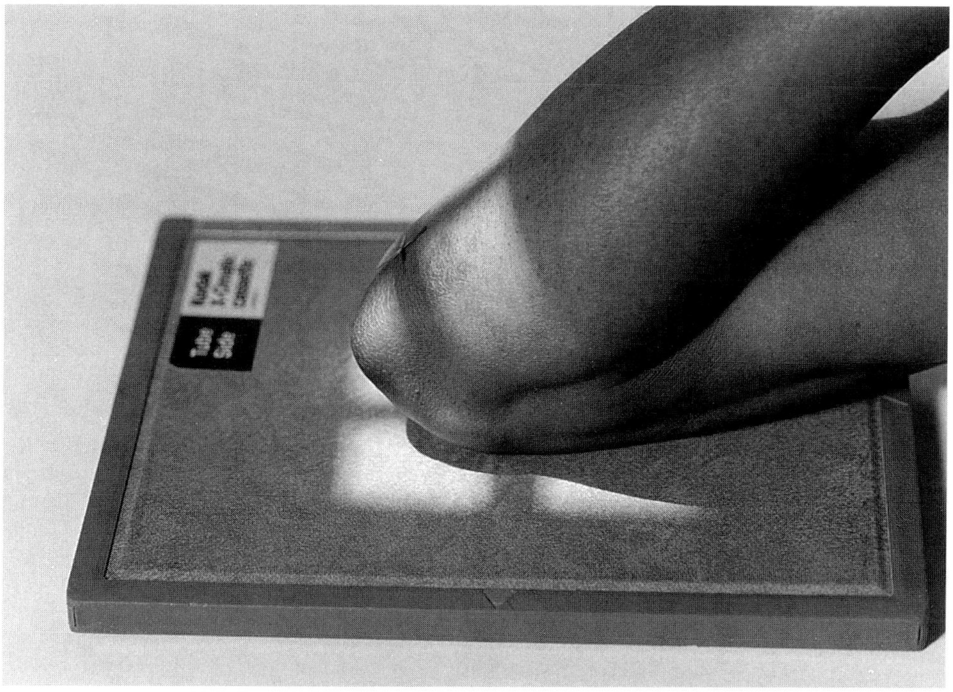

Figure 9.61. Axial elbow for distal humerus.

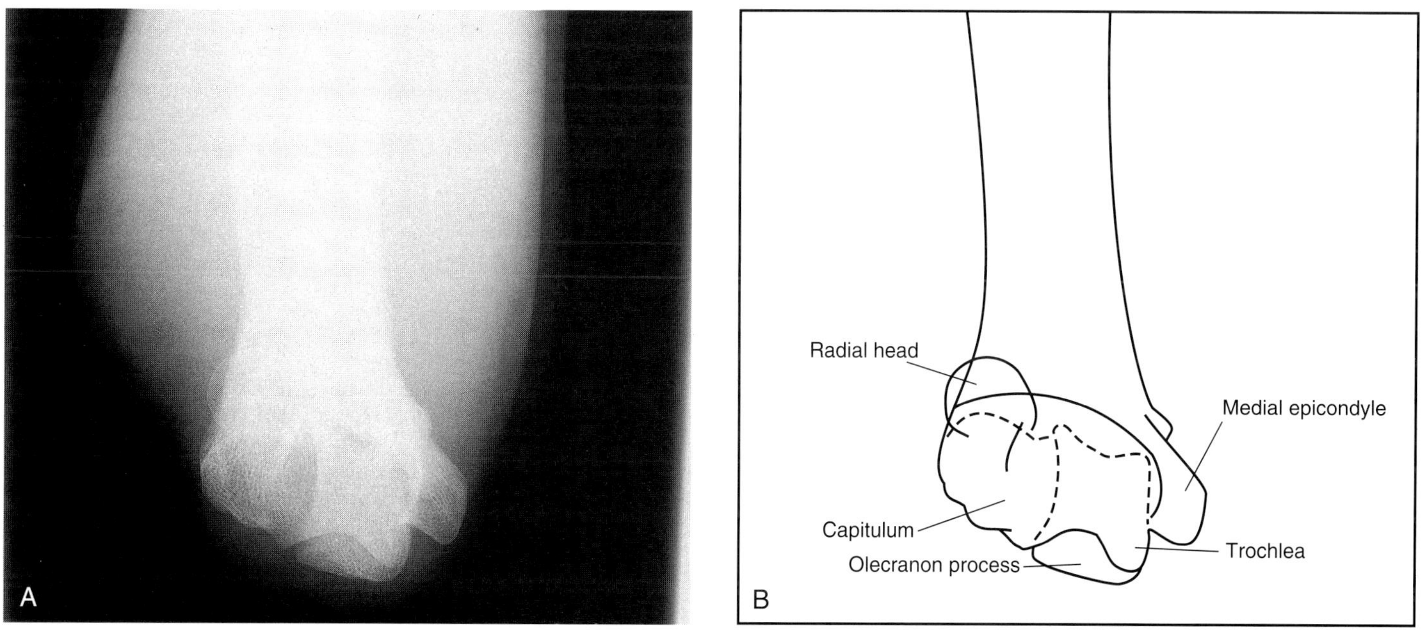

Figure 9.62. A and B, Axial elbow for distal humerus.

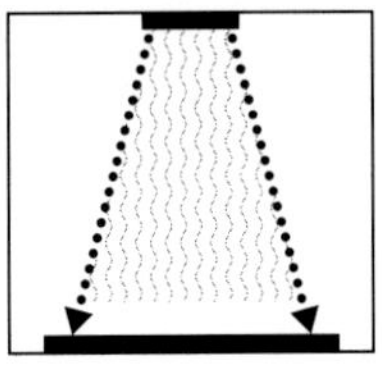

Elbow

Position/Projection

Axial/proximal forearm

Film:
8 × 10 inches (20 × 24 cm)
lengthwise, tabletop

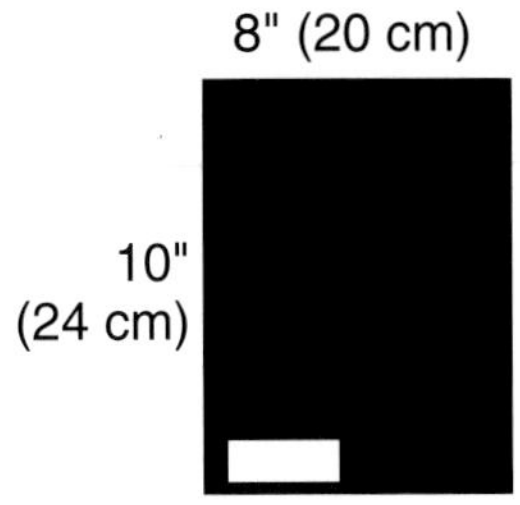

Patient Position

Seated facing away from table, posterior side of forearm resting on table (Fig. 9.63).

Part Position

Place cassette under forearm. Elbow joint is in maximum flexion and palm fully supinated, if possible. Olecranon process centered to film.

Central Ray

Perpendicular 2 inches (5 cm) distal to olecranon process. Collimate to area of interest.

Structures Demonstrated

Proximal part of the forearm (Fig. 9.64).

Evaluation Criteria

1. Proximal end of radius and ulna should be visualized.
2. There should be no rotation.
3. Forearm and humerus superimposed.

NOTE: This projection is used when the elbow cannot be extended.

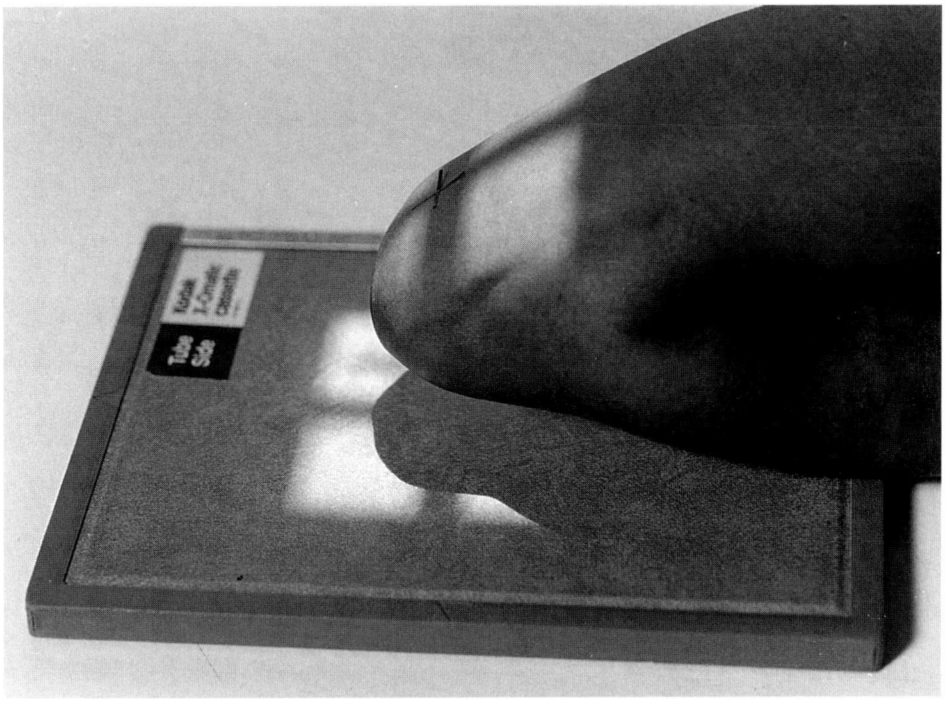

Figure 9.63. Axial elbow for proximal forearm.

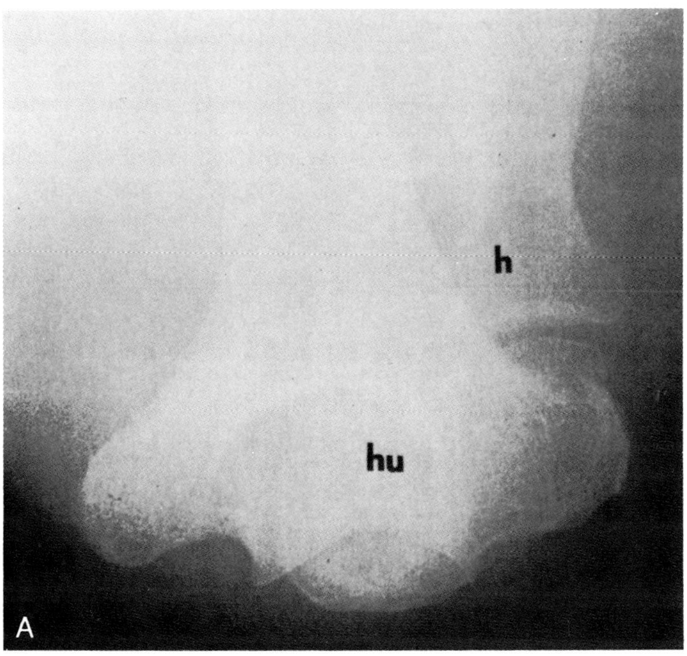

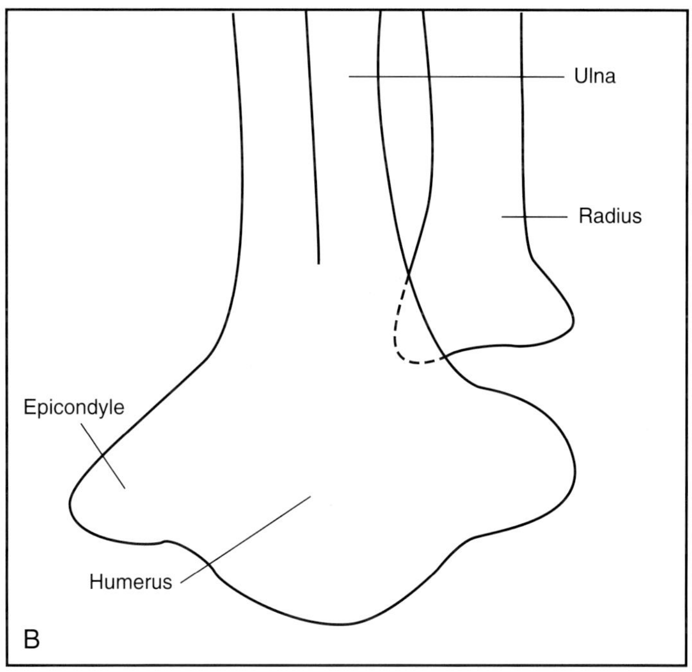

Figure 9.64. A and B, Axial elbow for proximal forearm. h, radial head; hu, humerus. (A, From Sartoris DJ, Resnick D: Plain film radiography: Routine and specialized techniques and projections. *In* Resnick D, Niwayama G [eds]: Diagnosis of Bone and Joint Disorders. Philadelphia: WB Saunders, 1988, vol 1, p 14.)

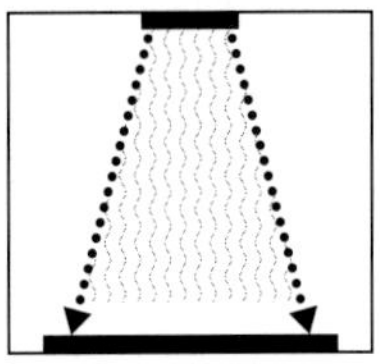

Elbow

Position/Projection

Ulnar nerve sulcus position, olecranon process

Film:
8 × 10 inches (20 × 24 cm)
lengthwise, tabletop

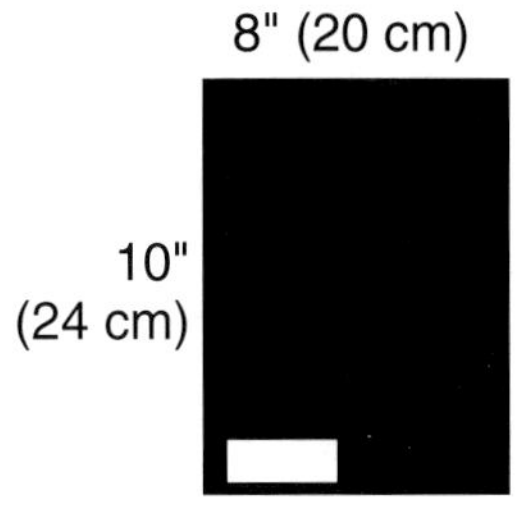

Patient Position

Seated at end or side of table, posterior side of upper arm resting on table (Fig. 9.65).

Part Position

Place cassette under upper arm. Elbow joint is in maximum flexion. Olecranon process centered to film.

Central Ray

30° proximal through ulnar nerve sulcus. Collimate to area of interest.

Structures Demonstrated

Olecranon process and ulnar nerve sulcus (Fig. 9.66).

Evaluation Criteria

1. Olecranon process should be demonstrated.
2. Humerus and forearm should be superimposed.
3. This projection is used when pressure on ulnar nerve is suspected.
4. Inclinations of central ray, such as 20°, 30°, or 40°, are often useful owing to anatomic variations.

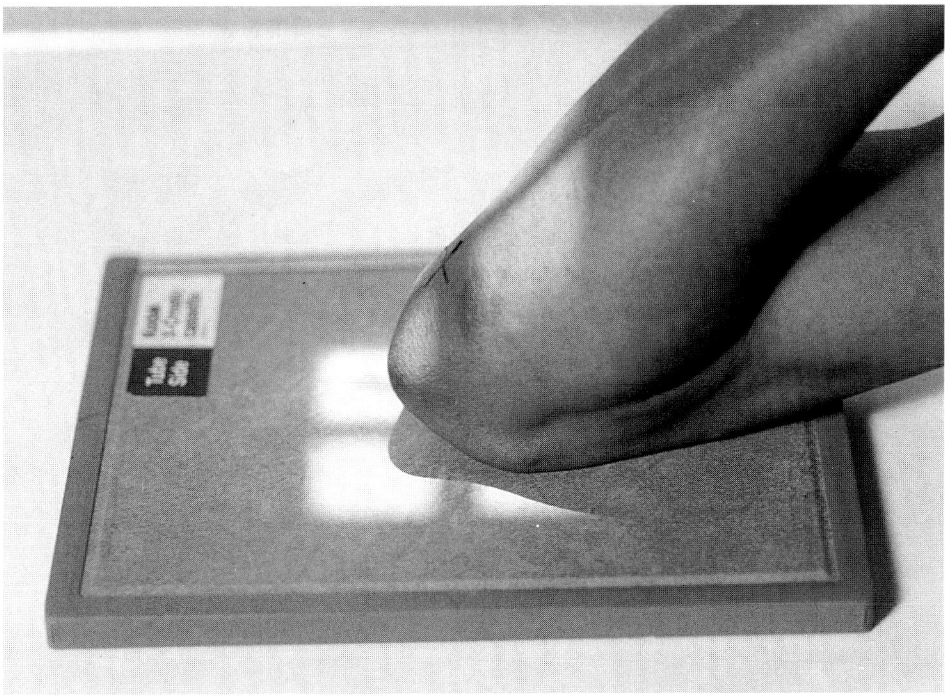

Figure 9.65. Ulnar nerve sulcus position, central ray angle 30° proximally.

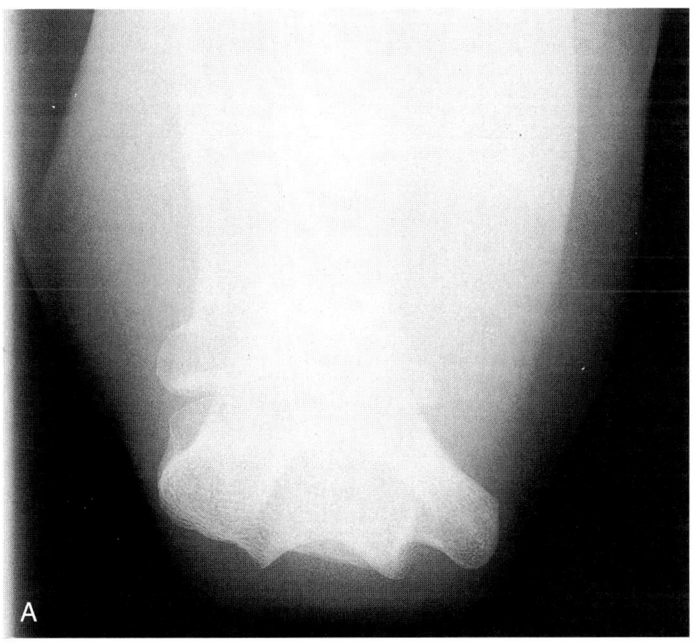

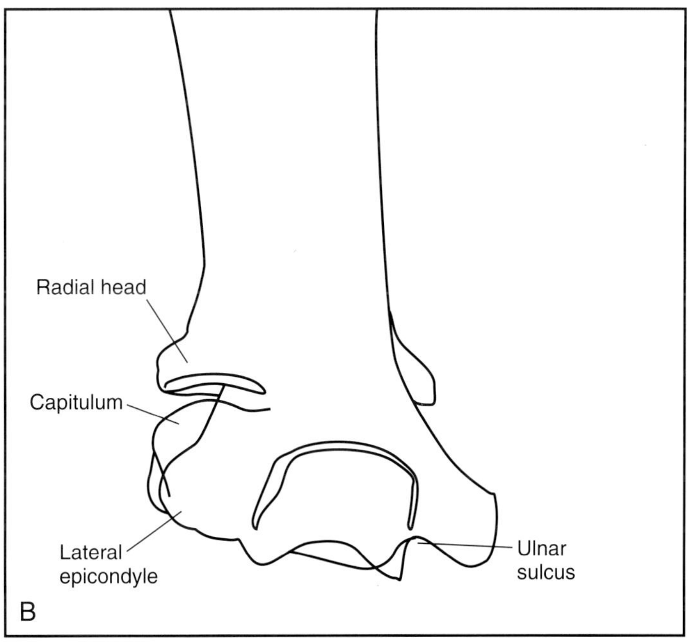

Figure 9.66. A and B, Ulnar nerve sulcus.

Humerus

Position/Projection

AP projection

Film:
11 × 14 inches (30 × 35 cm) lengthwise or film large enough to include both shoulder and elbow joint

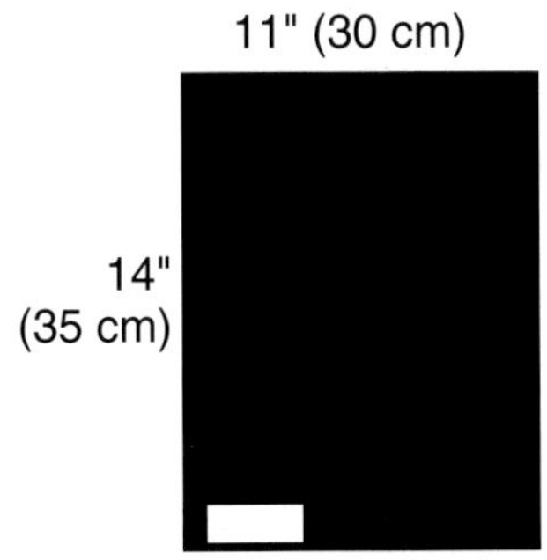

Patient Position

Sitting, standing, or lying supine (Fig. 9.67).

Part Position

Posterior side of upper arm against film. Hand is supinated and entire extremity is placed in true AP position. Long axis of humerus centered to film.

Central Ray

Perpendicular to midshaft of humerus. Collimate to area of interest.

Structures Demonstrated

Entire humerus (Fig. 9.68).

Evaluation Criteria

1. Elbow and shoulder joints should be included.
2. Greater tuberosity should be projected laterally.
3. Humeral condyles should not be rotated.

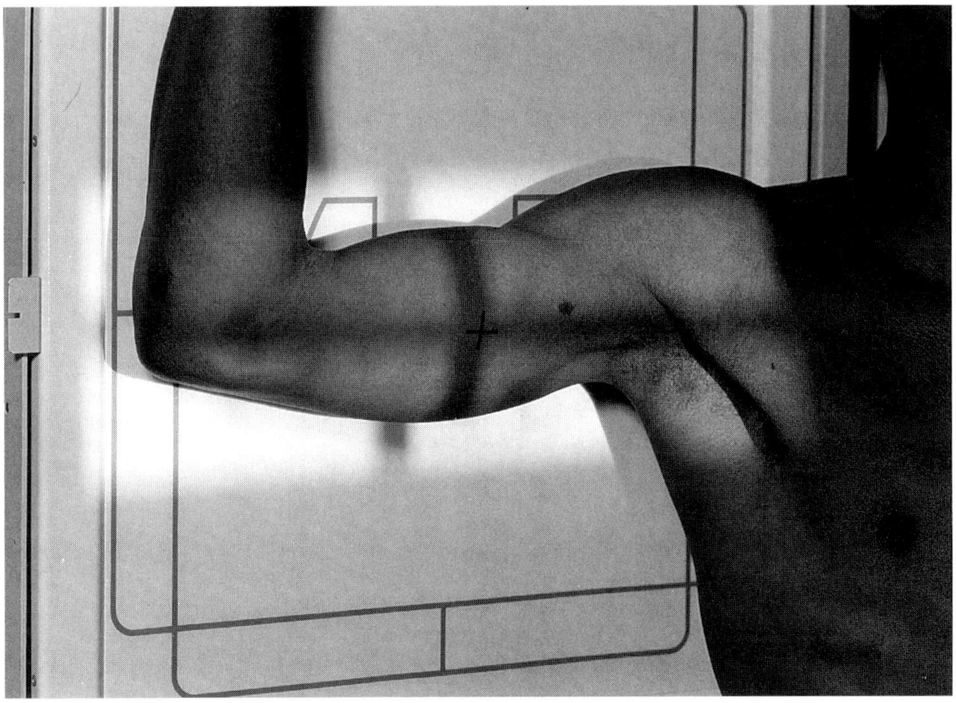

Figure 9.67. AP humerus, standing.

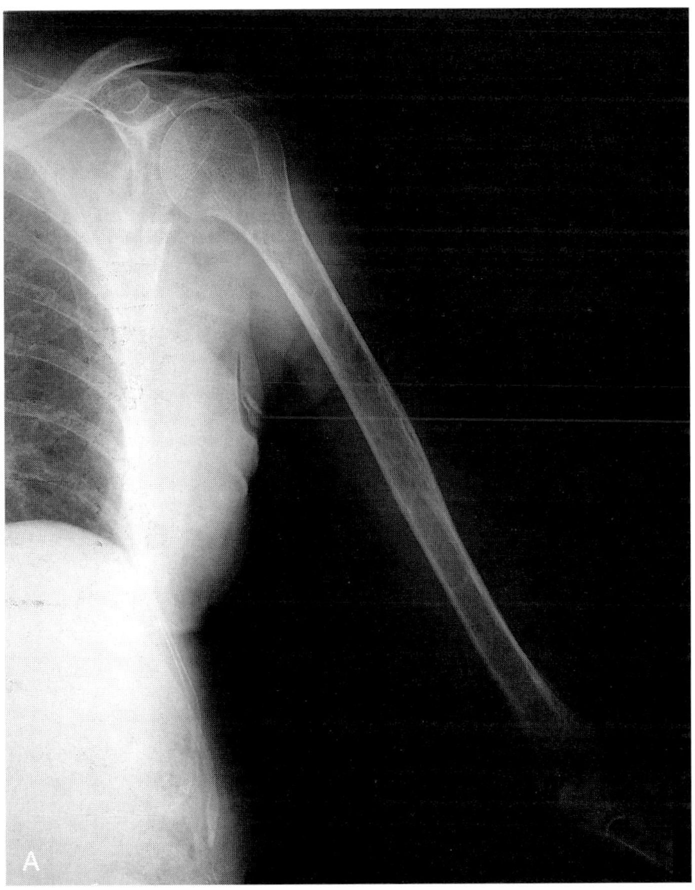

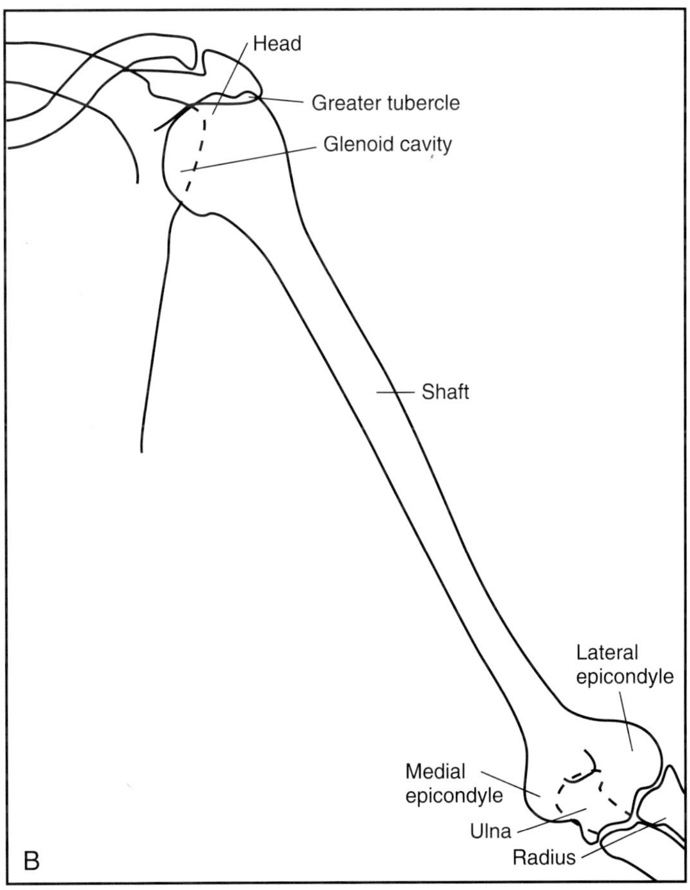

Figure 9.68. A and B, AP humerus, supine.

Humerus

Position/Projection

Lateral projection

Film:
11 × 14 inches (30 × 35 cm) lengthwise or film large enough to include both shoulder and elbow joint; Bucky or grid device

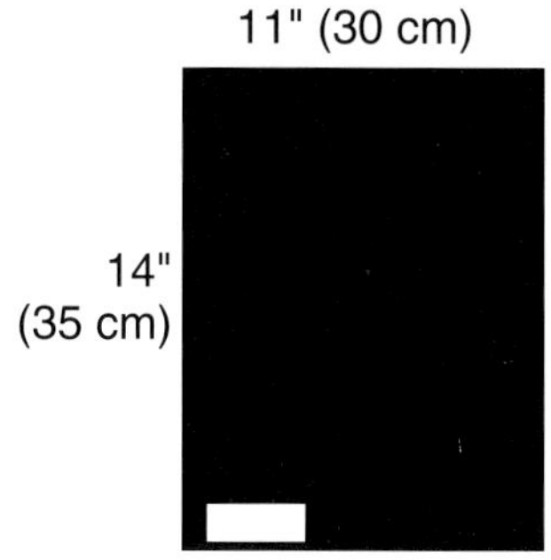

Patient Position

Sitting, standing, or lying supine (Fig. 9.69).

Part Position

Medial side of upper arm against film. Hand is pronated and entire extremity is placed in true lateral position. Long axis of humerus centered to film.

Central Ray

Perpendicular to midshaft of humerus. Collimate to area of interest.

Structures Demonstrated

Entire humerus in lateral view (Fig. 9.70).

Evaluation Criteria

1. Elbow and shoulder joint should be included.
2. Lesser tuberosity should be projected medially.
3. Humeral condyles should be superimposed.

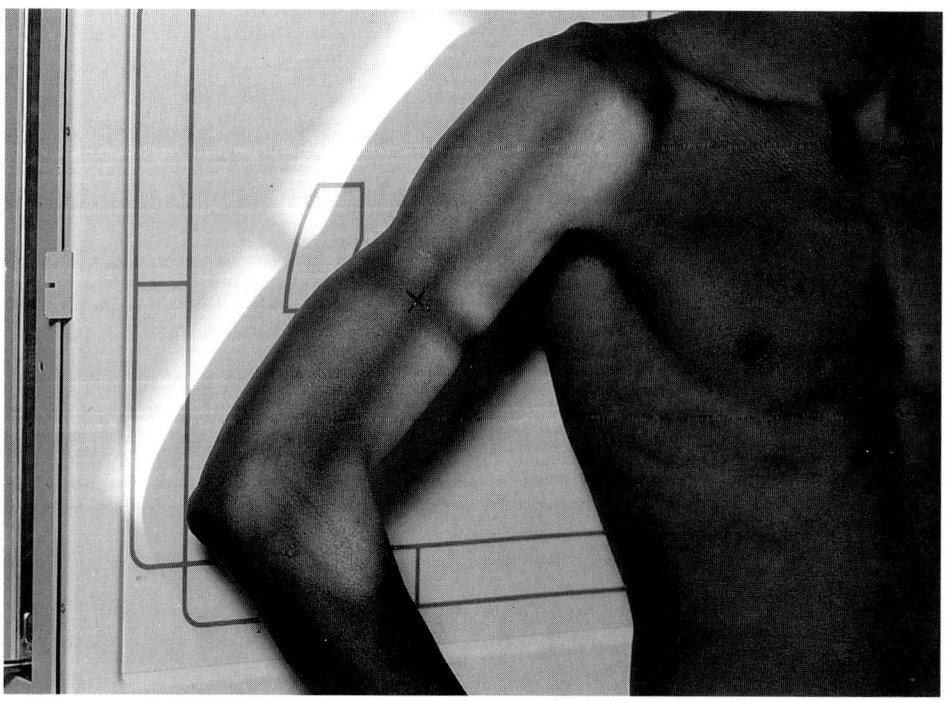

Figure 9.69. Lateral humerus.

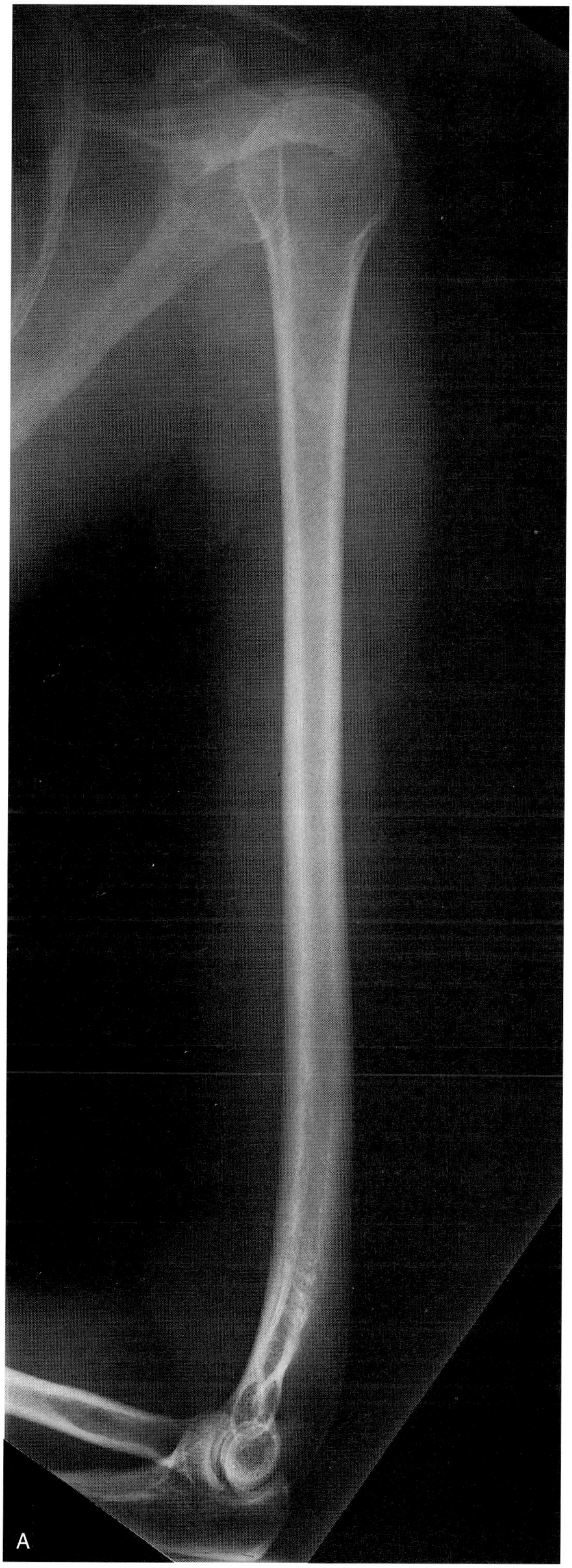

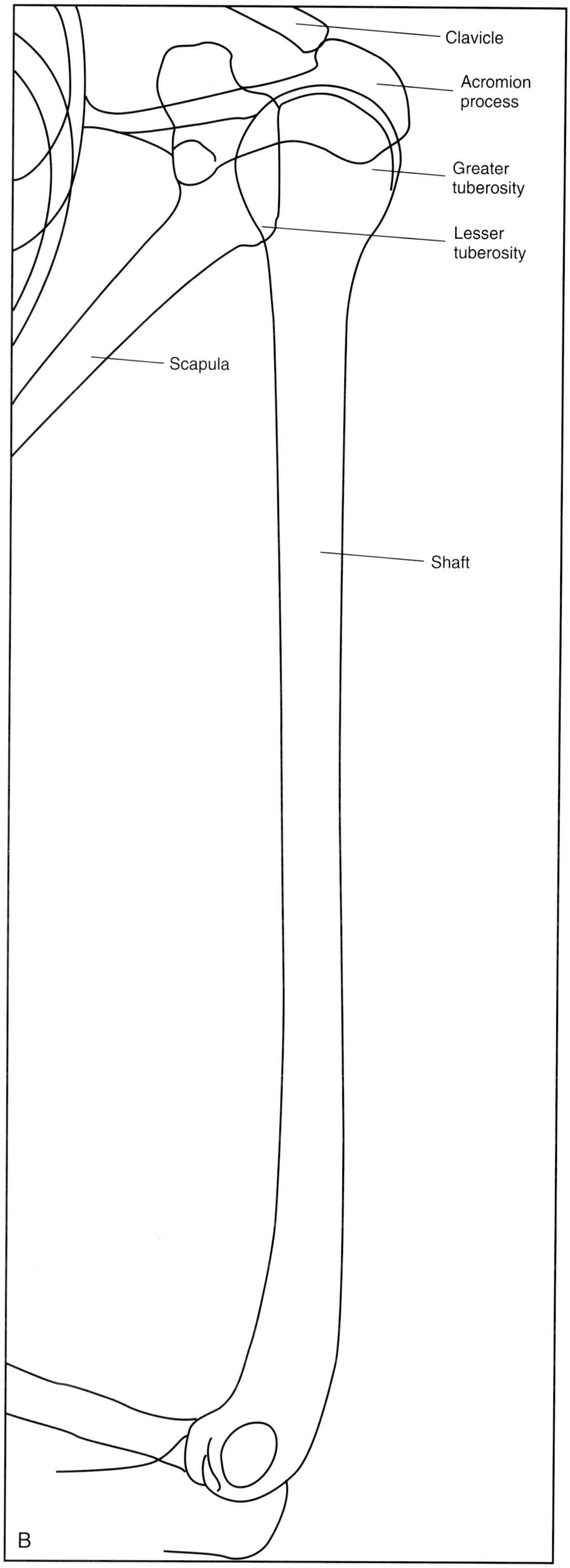

Figure 9.70. A and B, Lateral humerus.

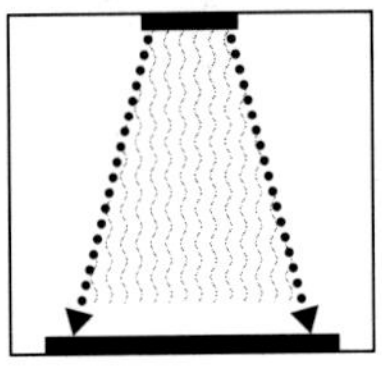

Humerus

Position/Projection

Lateral transthoracic projection

Film:
11 × 14 inches (30 × 35 cm) lengthwise; Bucky or grid device

Patient Position

Ideally erect or seated with side of interest against upright table. Opposite extremity is elevated above patient's head (Fig. 9.71).

Part Position

Extremity being examined is depressed. Long axis of humerus centered to film.

Central Ray

Perpendicular level of surgical neck. Collimate to area of interest.

Breathing Instructions

Usually hold breath in inspiration, although long exposure with breathing technique sometimes used.

Structures Demonstrated

Humeral head and shaft (Fig. 9.72).

Evaluation Criteria

1. Humeral head and shaft are visible through thoracic structures and anterior to spine.
2. Unaffected humerus and shoulder should not overlap area of interest; if so, 10–20° cephalic angle may be necessary.

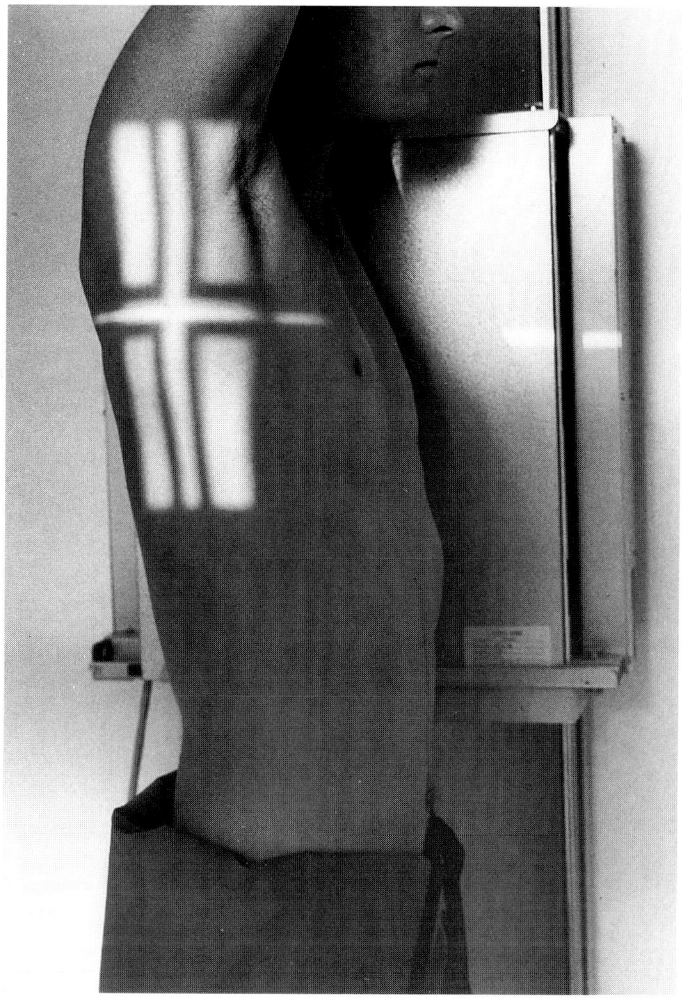

Figure 9.71. Transthoracic lateral humerus.

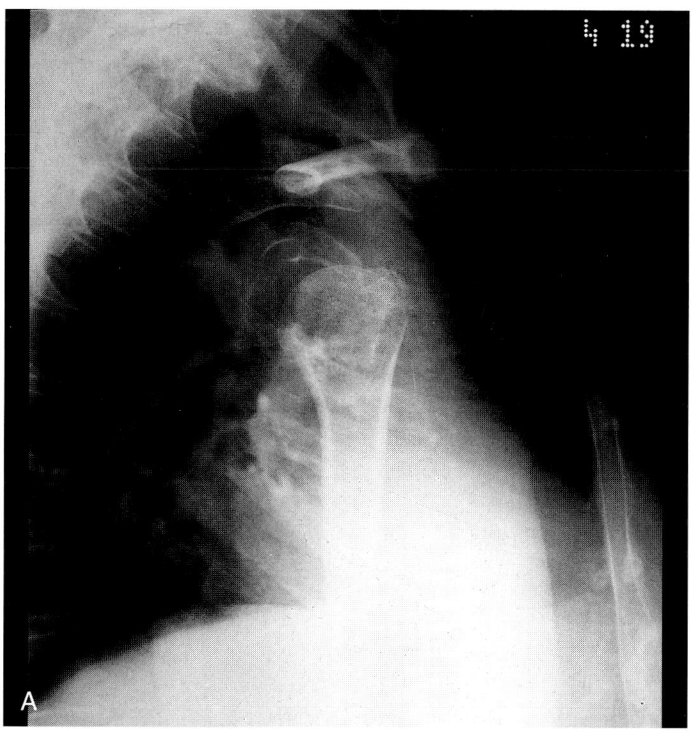

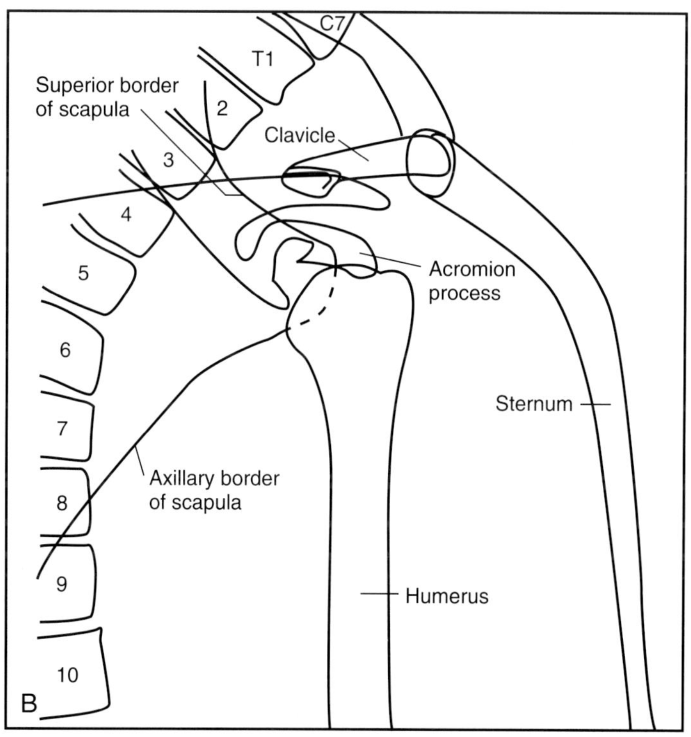

Figure 9.72. A and B, Transthoracic lateral humerus.

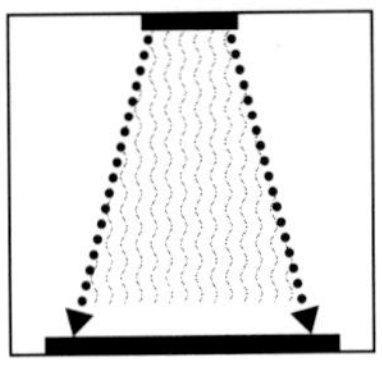

Shoulder

Position/Projection

AP projection, internal rotation

Film:
10 × 12 inches (24 × 30 cm) lengthwise or crosswise; Bucky or grid device

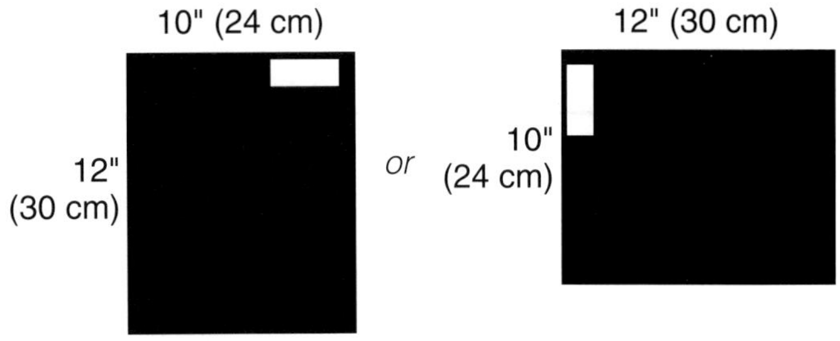

Patient Position

Sitting, standing, or lying supine (Fig. 9.73).

Part Position

Rotated so surface of scapula is parallel to plane of film. Upper arm is held against side of trunk. Elbow joint is flexed 90°. Humerus is rotated laterally 45°. Glenoid cavity centered to film.

Central Ray

Method 1

Perpendicular to coracoid process.

Method 2

10–20° caudad to coracoid process. Collimate to area of interest.

Structures Demonstrated

Shoulder with internal rotation (Fig. 9.74).

Evaluation Criteria

1. Humeral head is projected free.
2. Glenoid cavity should be open.
3. Method 1: When fracture is suspected.
4. Method 2: Gives view of space between acromion and caput. Soft tissue exposure is indicated when infraspinatus and teres minor calcifications are suspected.

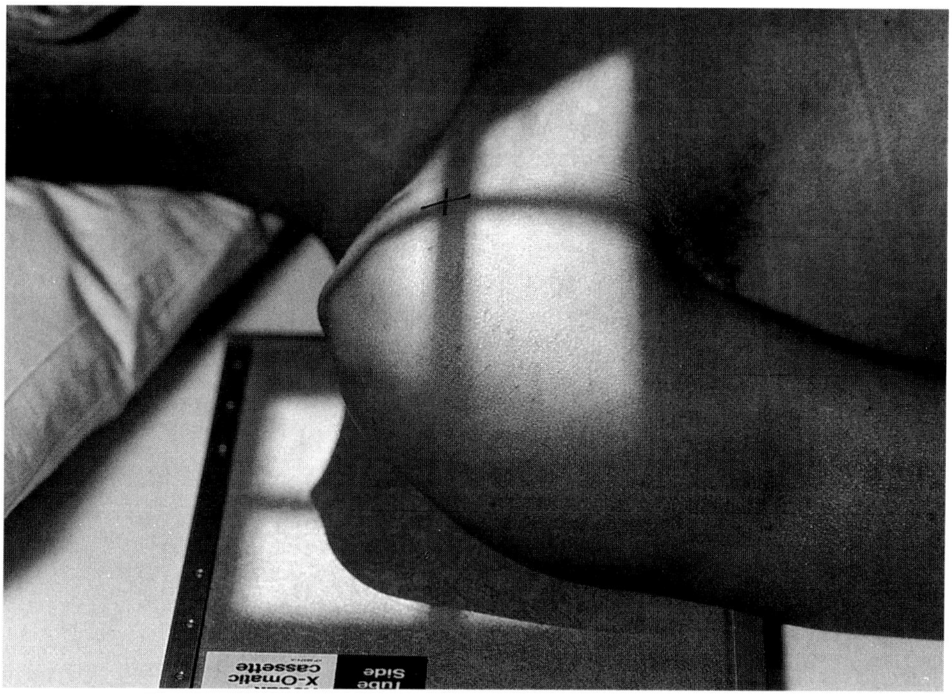

Figure 9.73. AP internal rotation of shoulder.

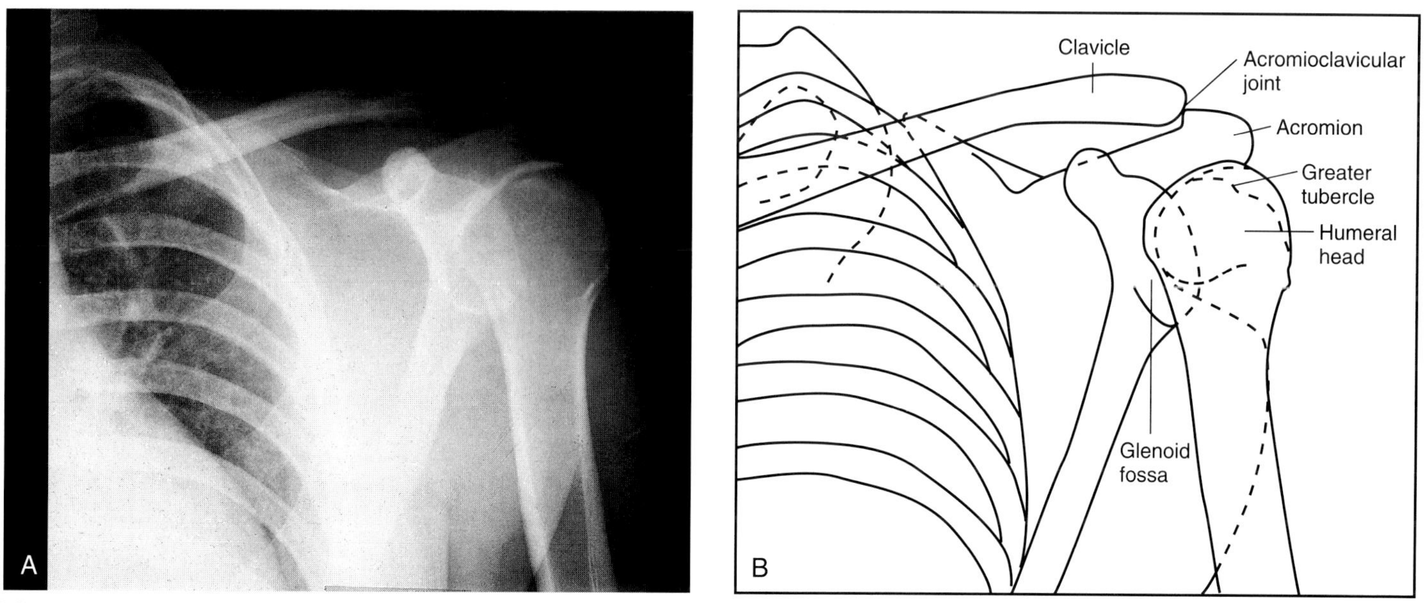

Figure 9.74. A and B, AP internal rotation of shoulder.

Shoulder

Position/Projection

AP projection, external rotation

Film:
10 × 12 inches (24 × 30 cm) lengthwise or crosswise; Bucky or grid device

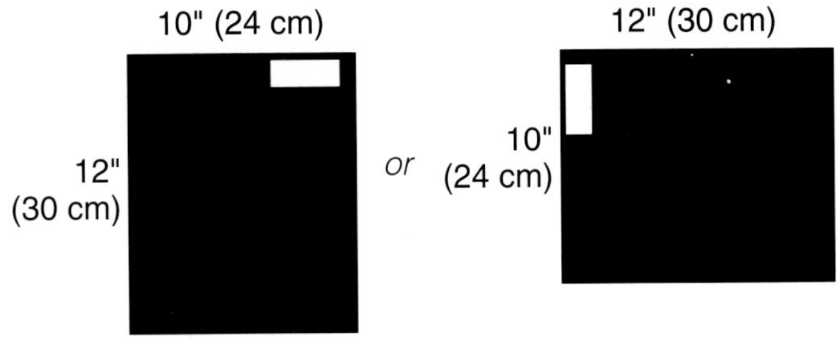

Patient Position

Sitting, standing, or lying supine (Fig. 9.75).

Part Position

Rotated so surface of scapula is parallel to plane of film. Upper arm is held against side of trunk. Elbow joint is flexed 90°. Humerus is rotated laterally 45°. Glenoid cavity centered to film.

Central Ray

1. Method 1: Perpendicular to coracoid process.
2. Method 2: Directed 10–20° caudad to coracoid process. Collimate to area of interest.

Structures Demonstrated

Shoulder with external rotation (Fig. 9.76).

Evaluation Criteria

1. Humeral head is projected free.
2. Glenoid cavity should be open.
3. Humeral head should be in profile.
4. Method 1: When fracture is suspected.
5. Method 2: Gives view of space between acromion and caput. Soft tissue exposure when supraspinatus calcifications are suspected.

NOTE: Many departmental routines also call for an AP projection in a neutral position, which has the patient place the palm of the hand against the thigh. This places the epicondyles at a 45° angle to the plane of the film.

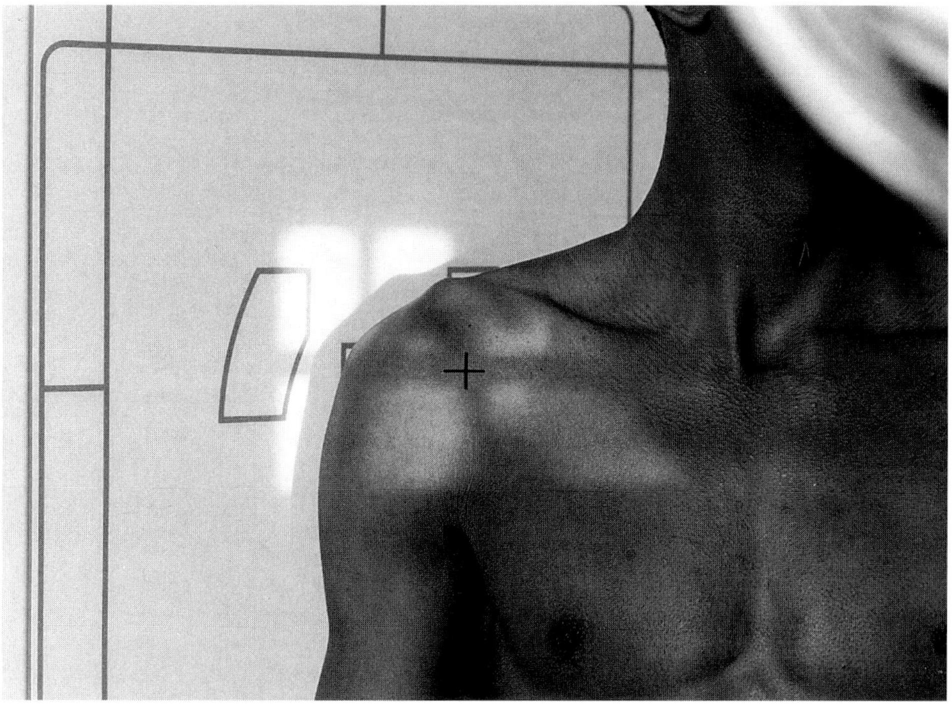

Figure 9.75. AP external rotation of shoulder.

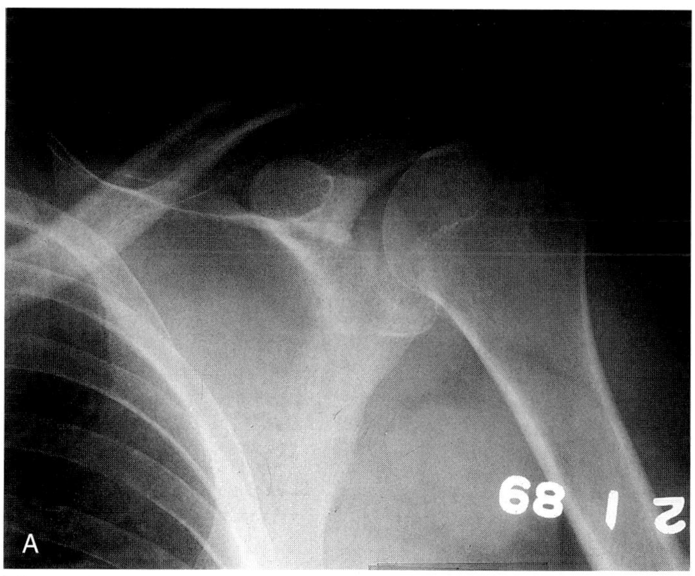

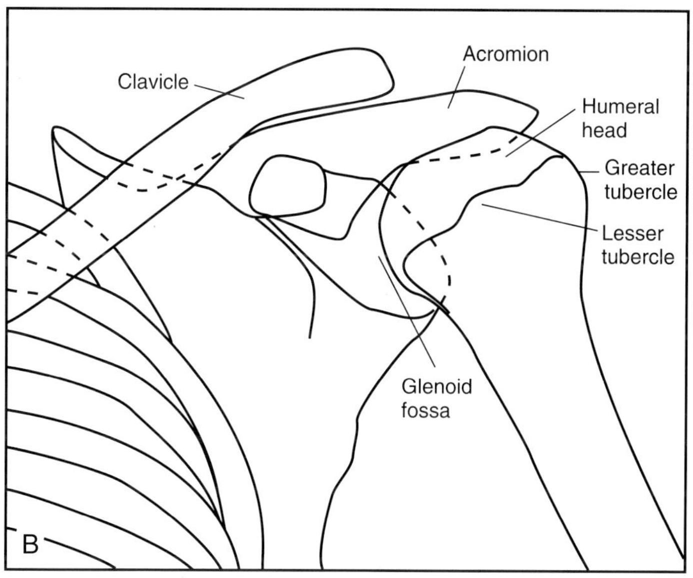

Figure 9.76. A and B, AP external rotation of shoulder.

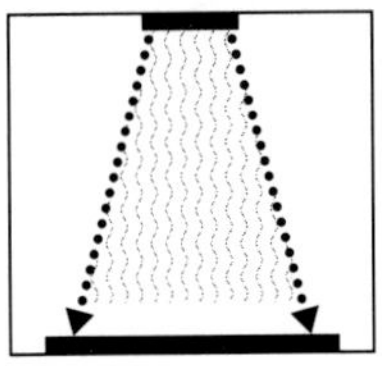

Shoulder

Position/Projection

AP projection, shoulder joint, lateral position of humerus

Film:
10 × 12 inches (24 × 30 cm) lengthwise; Bucky or grid device

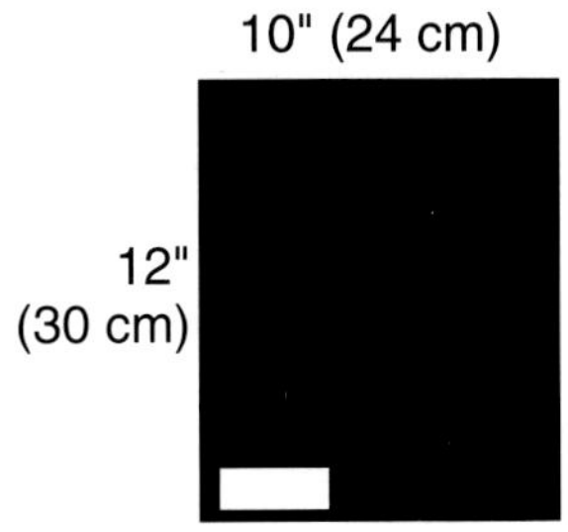

Patient Position

Sitting, standing, or lying supine (Fig. 9.77).

Part Position

Rotated so surface of scapula is parallel to plane of film. Upper arm is abducted 90° and rotated internally 90°. Glenoid cavity centered to film.

Central Ray

10° cranial to glenoid cavity. Collimate to area of interest.

Structures Demonstrated

Humeral head and acromioclavicular joint (Fig. 9.78).

Evaluation Criteria

1. Humeral head should be in profile.
2. Acromioclavicular joint is well projected.

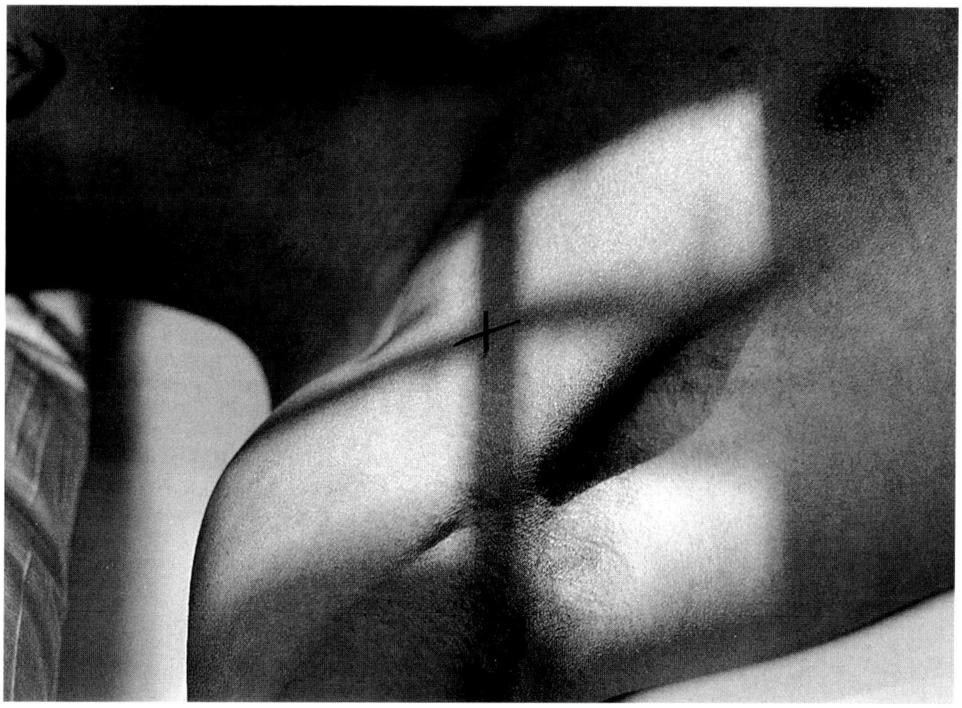

Figure 9.77. AP shoulder joint (lateral position of humerus).

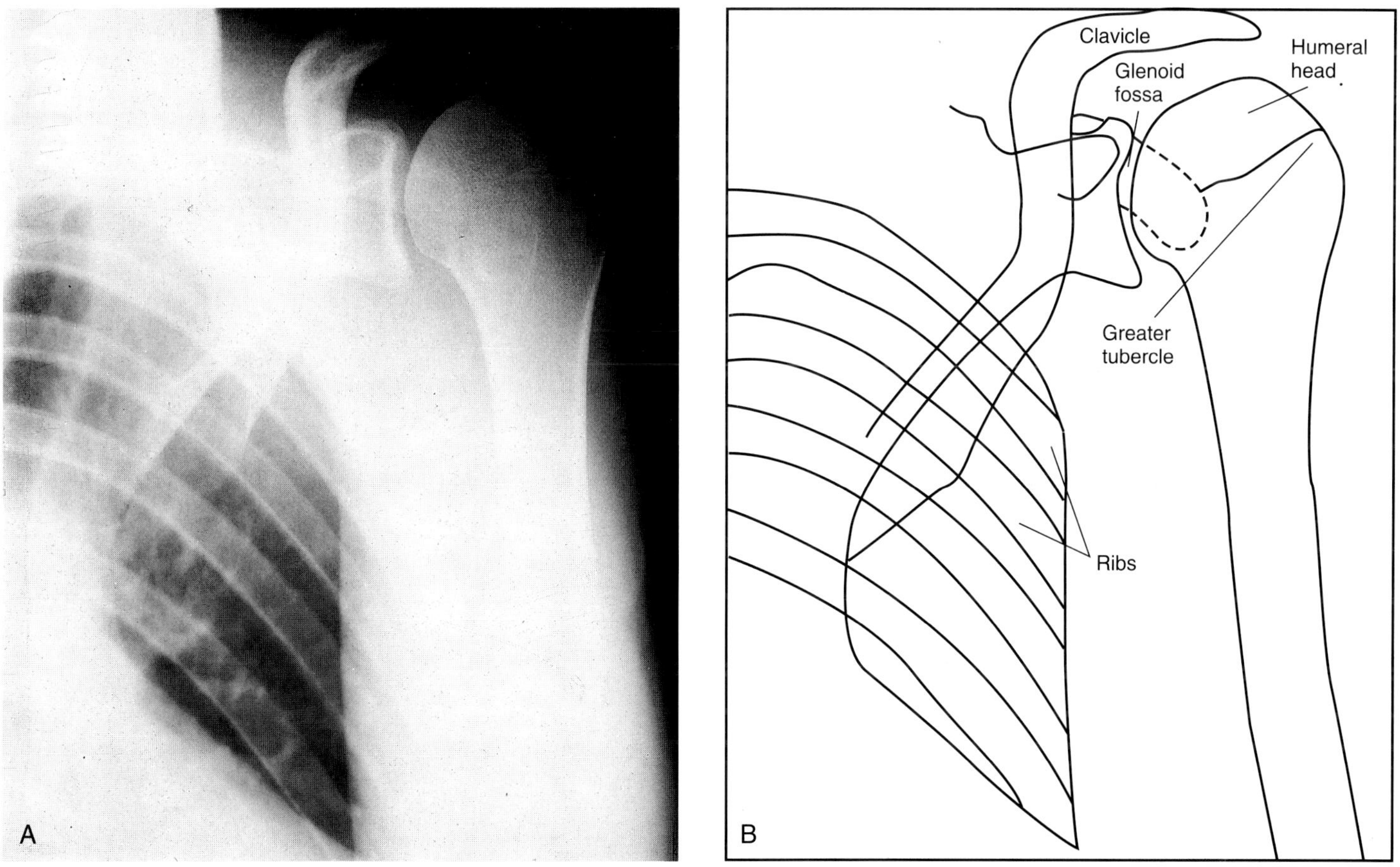

Figure 9.78. A and B, AP shoulder joint (lateral position of humerus).

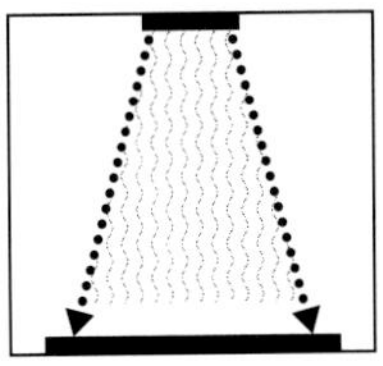

Shoulder

Position/Projection

Lateral oblique (PA oblique)

Film:
10 × 12 inches (24 × 30 cm) crosswise or lengthwise; Bucky or grid device

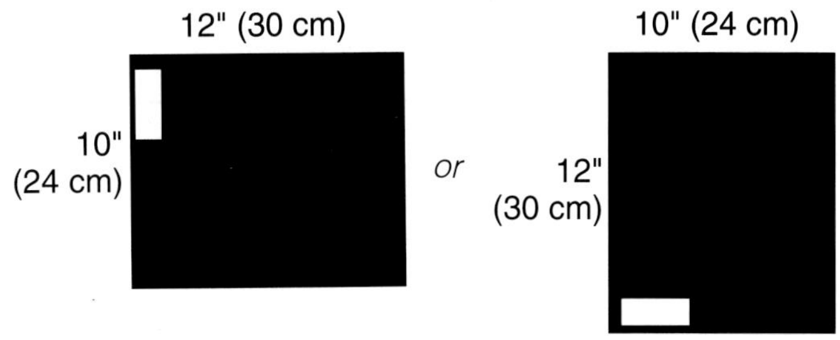

Patient Position

Sitting, standing, or lying prone (Fig. 9.79).

Part Position

Lateral part of shoulder against film. Upper arm is held against side of trunk. Elbow is flexed. Unaffected side of patient is rotated 45° from plane of film. Middle of scapula centered to film.

Central Ray

Perpendicular to middle of scapula. Collimate to area of interest.

Structures Demonstrated

Glenoid fossa (Fig. 9.80).

Evaluation Criteria

1. Humeral axis should be projected free from thorax.
2. Scapula and proximal humerus must be in lateral projection and free from thorax.
3. Glenoidal cavity should be projected in center of head of humerus.

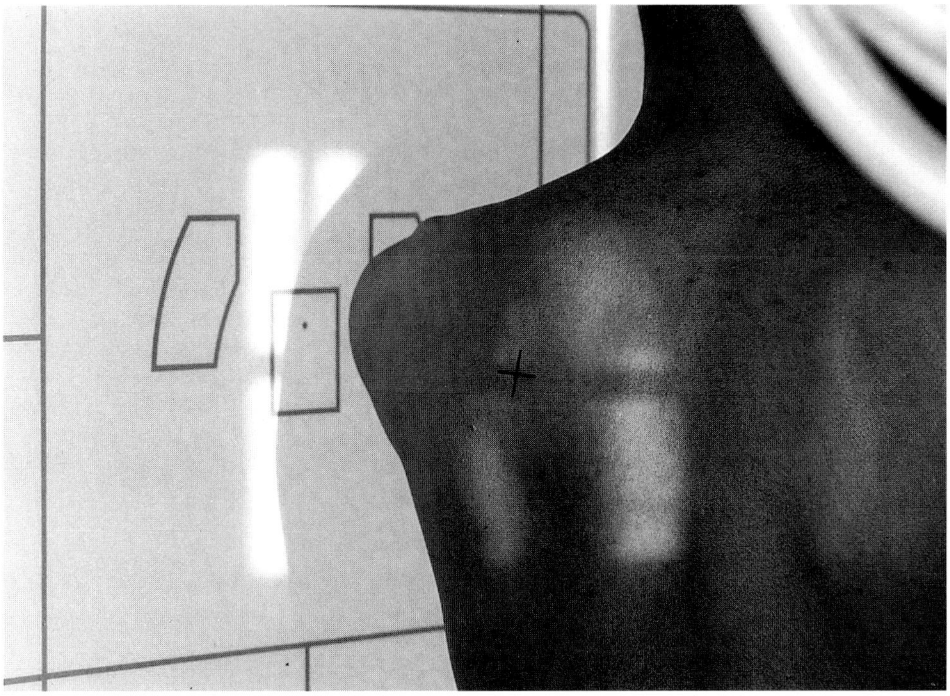

Figure 9.79. PA oblique shoulder.

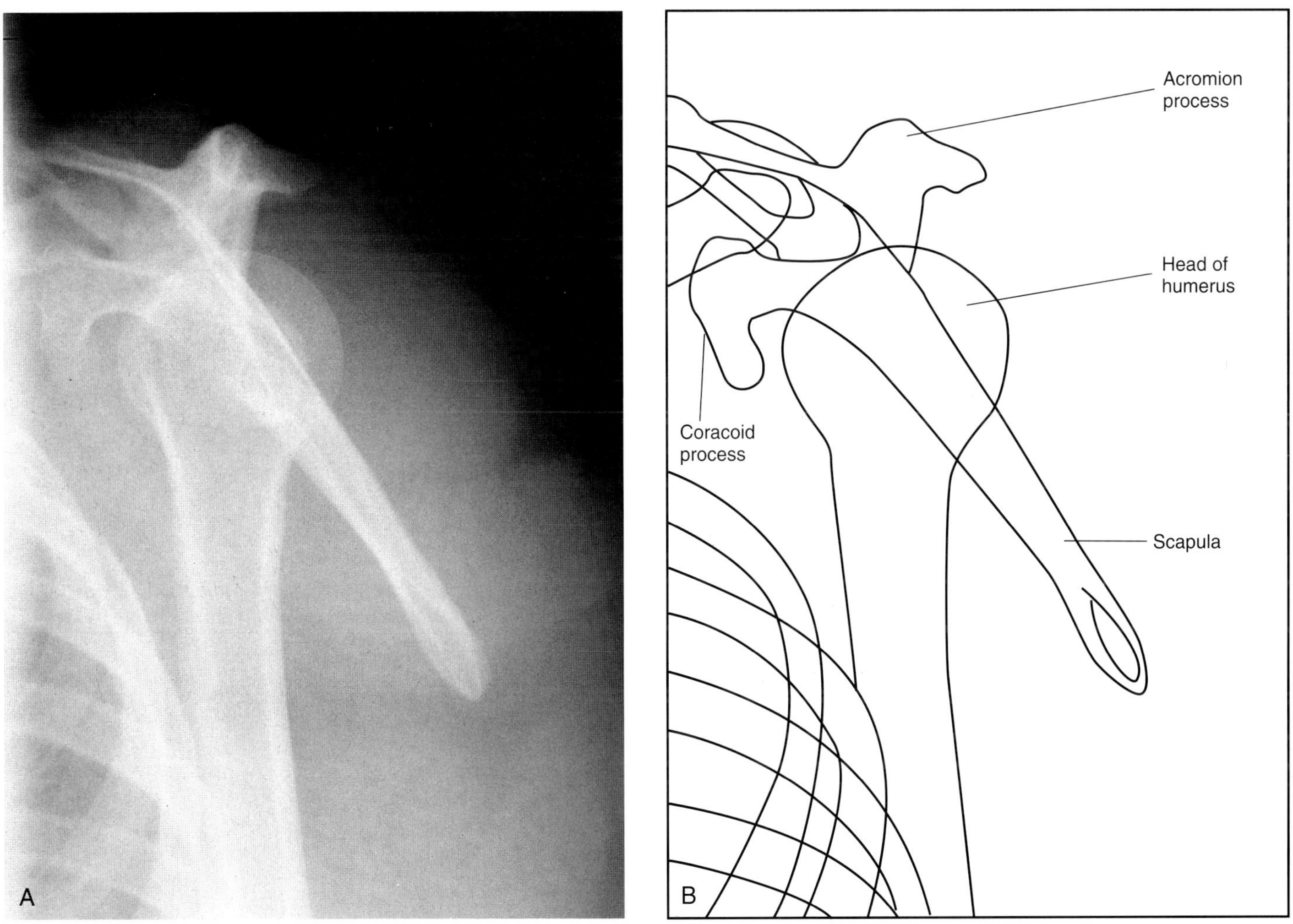

Figure 9.80. A and B, PA oblique shoulder.

Shoulder

Position/Projection

Axial/inferosuperior projection, Epolett

Film:
8 × 10 inches (20 × 24 cm)
crosswise; grid

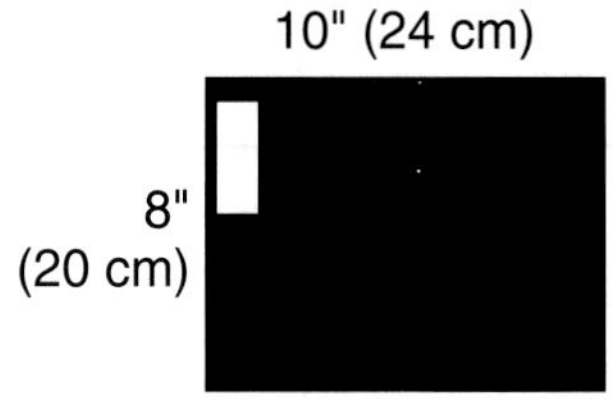

Patient Position

Supine (Fig. 9.81).

Part Position

Cassette is supported vertically against upper border of shoulder as close as possible to neck. Extremity being examined is abducted to form 90° angle with long axis of body. Arm is in external rotation. Axilla centered to film.

Central Ray

Horizontal to center of axilla. Collimate to area of interest.

Structures Demonstrated

Glenohumeral joint (Fig. 9.82).

Evaluation Criteria

1. Glenohumeral joint is well visualized.
2. Lesser tuberosity in profile, directed anterior.
3. Acromion, acromional end of clavicle, and acromioclavicular joint projected through humeral head.

NOTE: An axial projection can also be performed with the patient prone with a double-tube angle of 25° anteriorly and medially (West Point method), or in a lateral recumbent position (Clements' method).

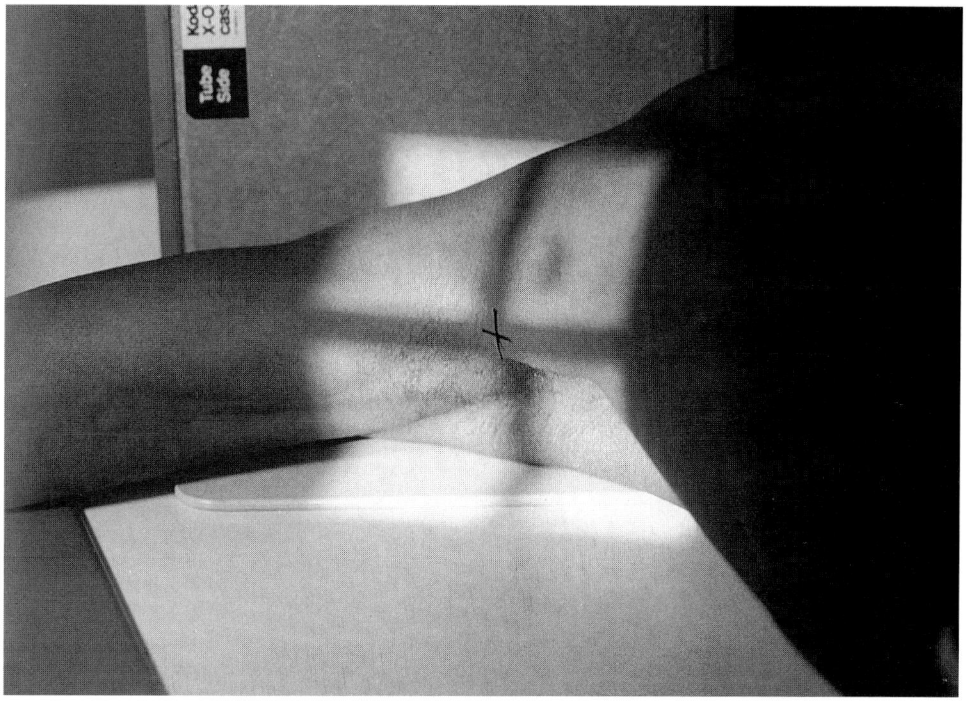

Figure 9.81. Axial inferosuperior shoulder.

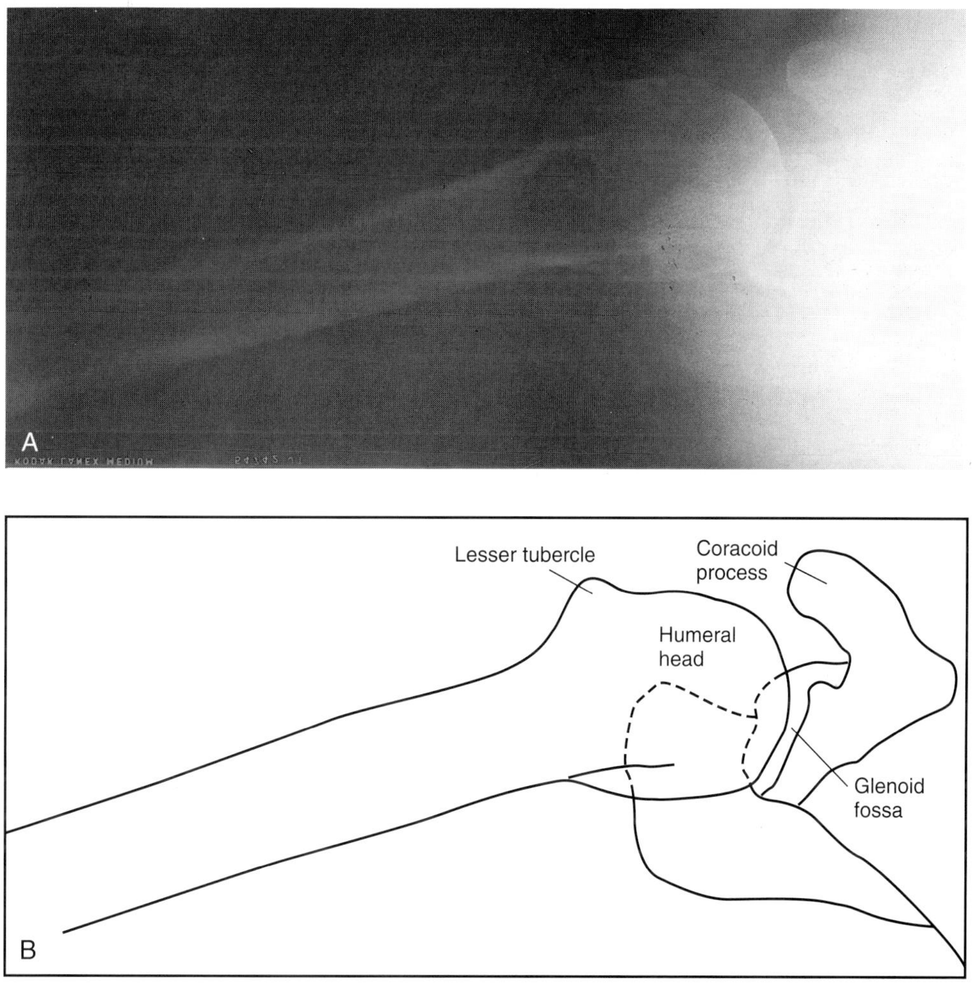

Figure 9.82. A and B, Axial inferosuperior shoulder.

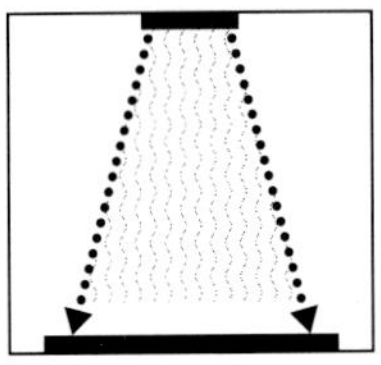

Shoulder: Sulcus

Position/Projection

AP projection, intertuberous sulcus (bicipital groove)

Film:
8 × 10 inches (20 × 24 cm)
lengthwise

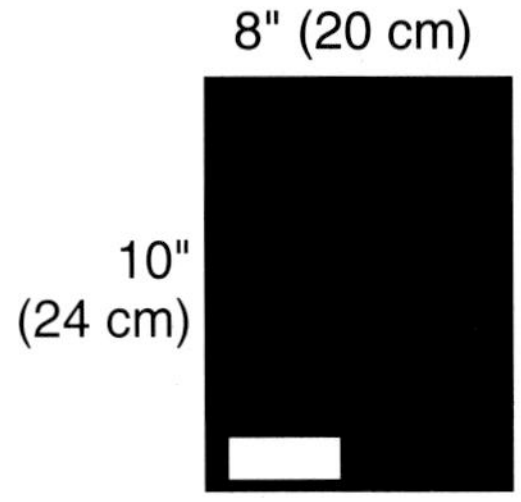

Patient Position

Supine with affected arm by side, slightly abducted (Fig. 9.83).

Part Position

Cassette is supported vertically against upper border of shoulder. Hand is pronated so epicondyles of humerus are at angle of approximately 45° to trunk. Anterior part of head of humerus centered to film.

Central Ray

Almost perpendicular, making angle of about 10° to shaft of humerus and to anterior aspect of head of humerus. Collimate to area of interest.

Breathing Instructions

Suspend respiration during exposure.

Structures Demonstrated

Intertuberous sulcus (bicipital groove) of humerus (Fig. 9.84).

Evaluation Criteria

1. Intertuberous sulcus (bicipital groove) is clearly visible.
2. Glenohumeral joint is well visualized.

NOTE: This position was originally described by Fisk (1965) with the patient standing; the elbow is flexed and the patient holds the cassette, leaning forward to place the posterior surface of the forearm on the table. The central ray is perpendicular to the film.

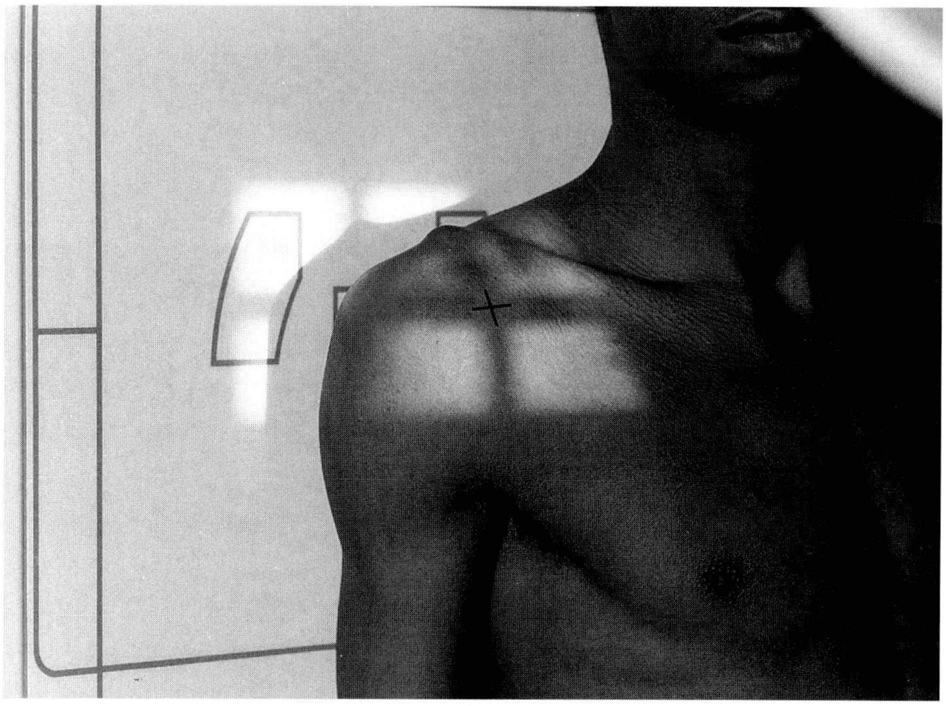

Figure 9.83. AP shoulder—bicipital groove.

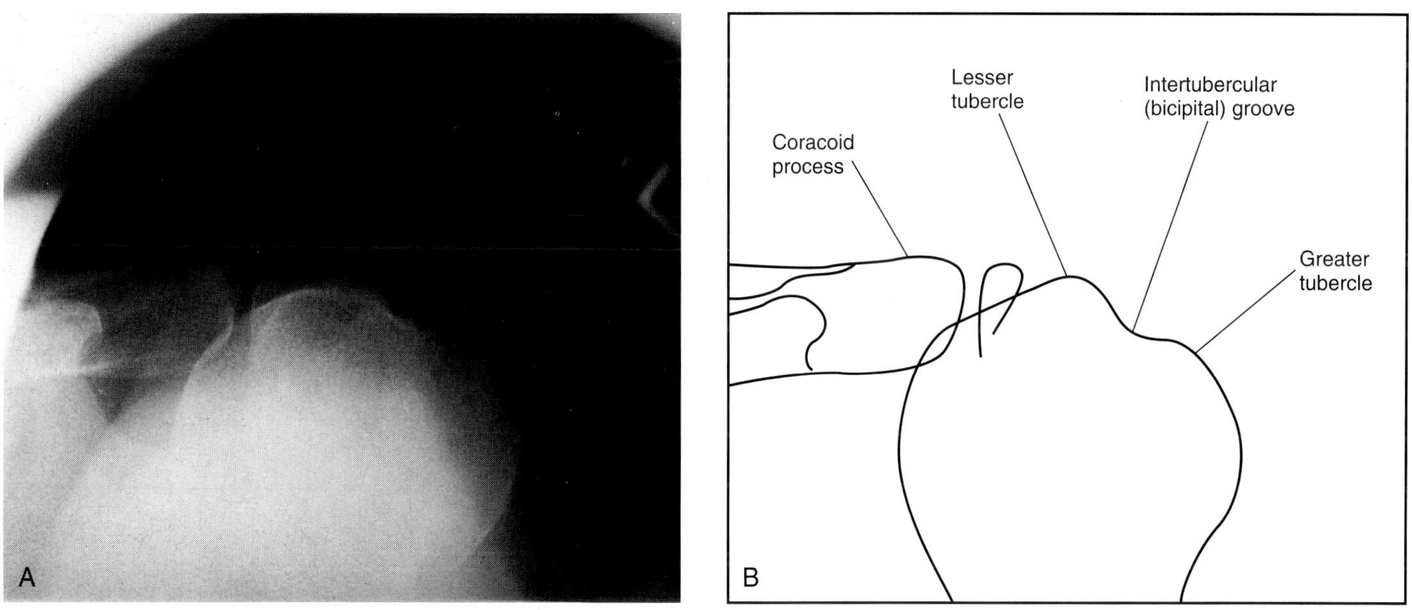

Figure 9.84. A and B, AP shoulder—bicipital groove.

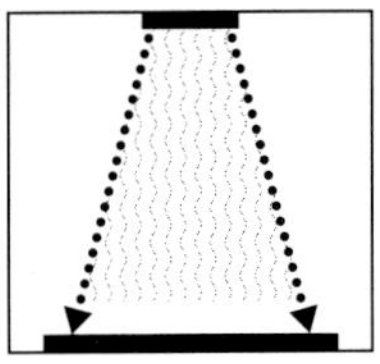

Acromioclavicular Joints

Position/Projection

AP projection

Film:
11 × 14 inches (30 × 35 cm), or larger, crosswise, bilateral; Bucky or grid device

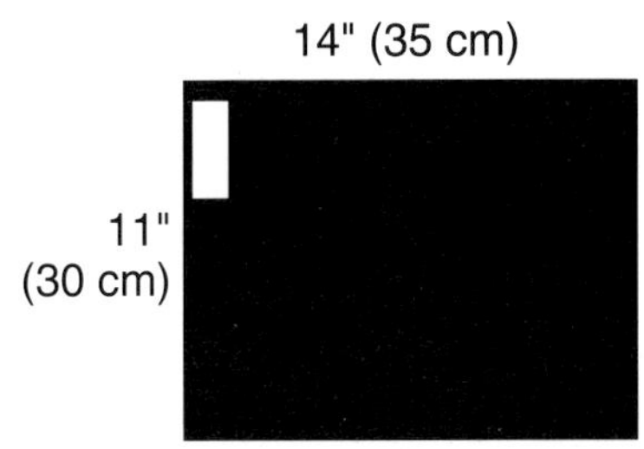

Patient Position

Erect AP position. Extremities are in true AP position. Usually taken with and without weights; weights of 3 to 5 lbs are placed in patient's hands (Fig. 9.85).

Part Position

Place cassette behind patient. Sternoclavicular joints centered to cassette.

Central Ray

Perpendicular to level of sternoclavicular joints. Collimate to area of interest.

Breathing Instructions

Suspend respiration during exposure.

Structures Demonstrated

Acromioclavicular joints, bilateral. If both joints are not seen on film, another must be taken (Fig. 9.86).

Evaluation Criteria

1. Acromioclavicular joints should be visualized.
2. No leaning of patient evident.
3. Lack of rotation.

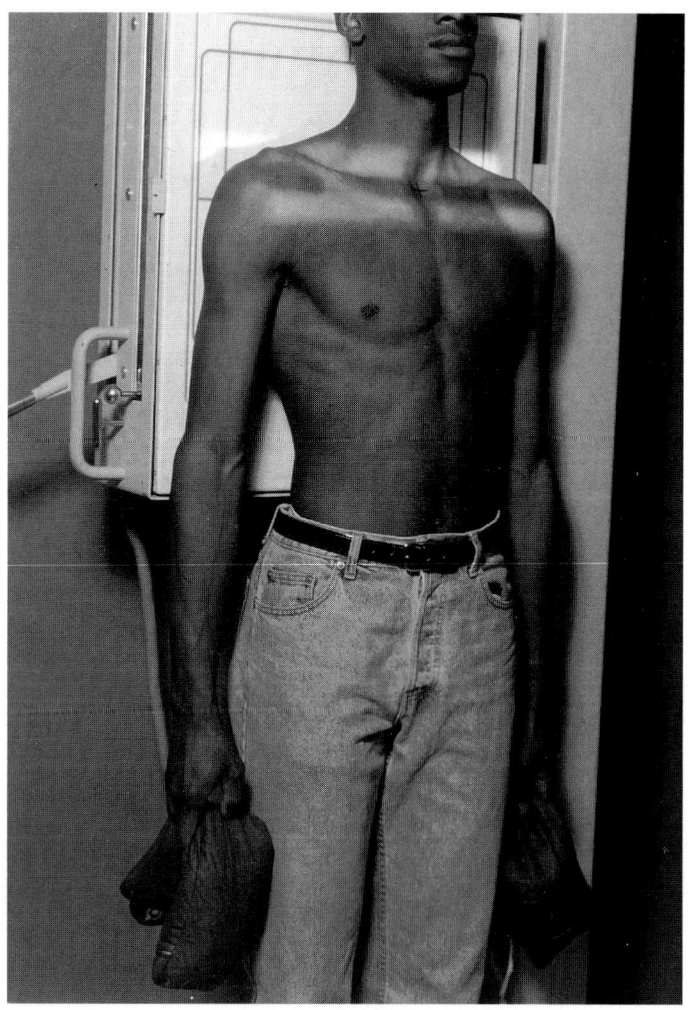

Figure 9.85. Bilateral AP acromioclavicular joints with weights.

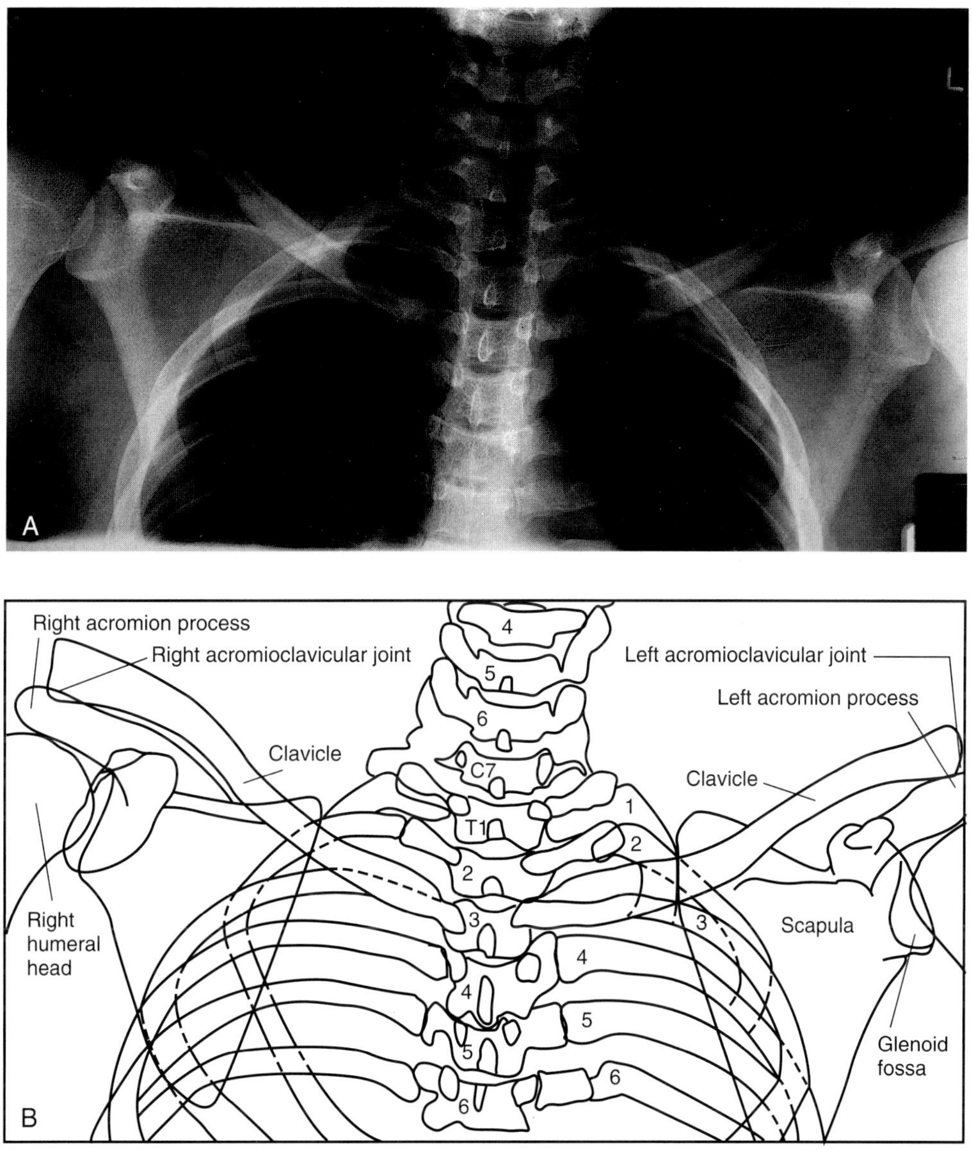

Figure 9.86. A and B, Bilateral AP acromioclavicular joints with weights.

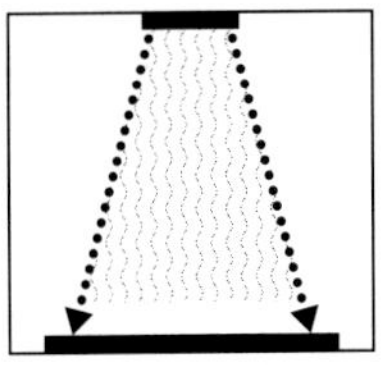

Clavicle

Position/Projection

PA projection, inferosuperior, superoinferior

Film:
8 × 10 inches (20 × 24 cm) crosswise; Bucky or grid device

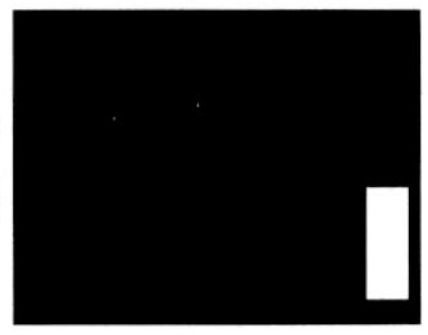

Patient Position

Erect or prone PA position. Head is turned away from affected clavicle (Fig. 9.87).

Part Position

Place cassette against clavicle. Clavicle centered to table.

Central Ray

Method 1
10° cranial to midclavicular area.

Method 2
10° caudal to midclavicular area.

Breathing Instructions

Suspend respiration during exposure.

Structures Demonstrated

Clavicle (Fig. 9.88).

Evaluation Criteria

1. Clavicle, sternoclavicular joint and acromioclavicular joints should be visualized.
2. Two different angulations to visualize clavicle in two positions.

NOTE: An AP position is used if fracture is suspected or the patient cannot be in an erect position. The same basic procedure is used.

Ballinger (1992) describes a PA axial projection using a 25–30° degree caudad angle, with the central ray directed to the supraclavicular fossa. He also gives an AP axial projection, with the patient in a lordotic position, using an angled central ray.

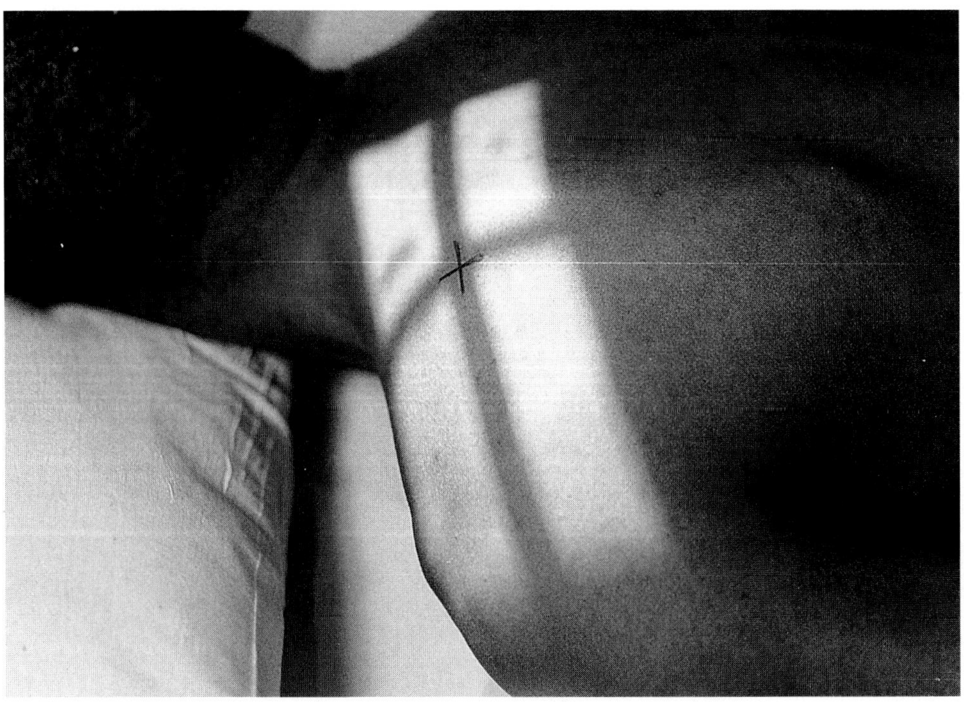

Figure 9.87. PA clavicle (10° angle cranially or caudally).

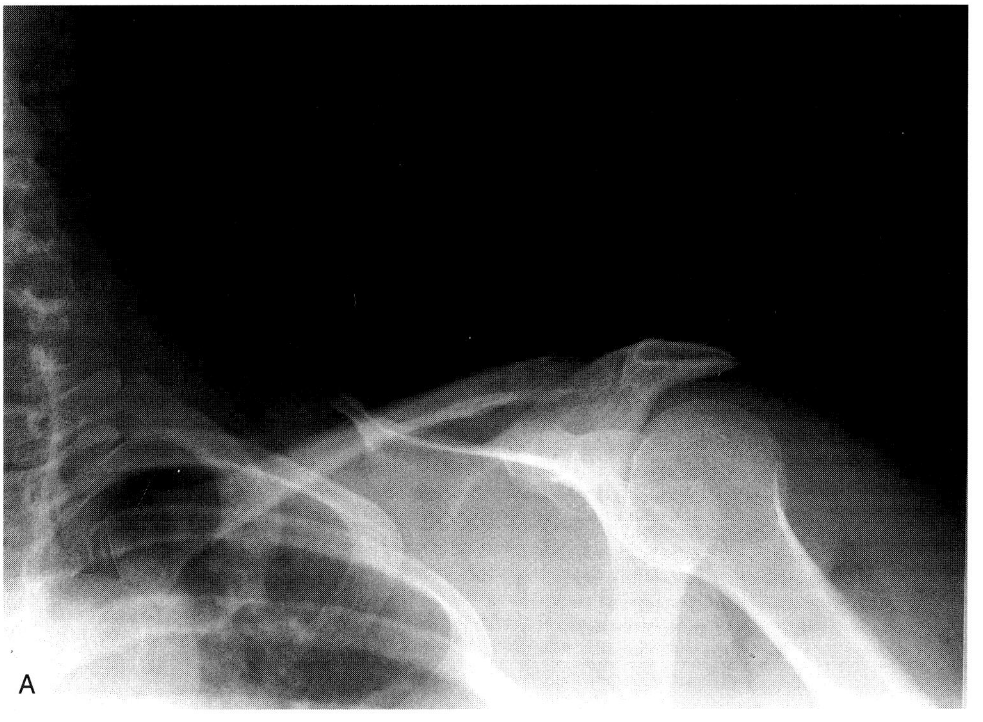

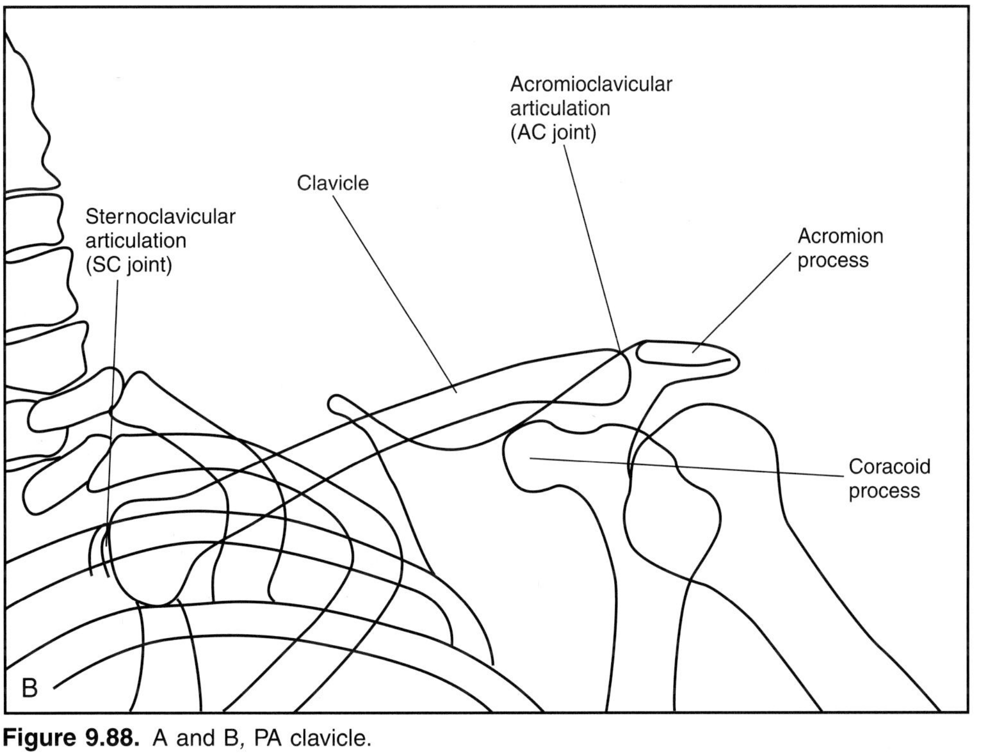

Figure 9.88. A and B, PA clavicle.

Scapula

Position/Projection

AP projection

Film:
10 × 12 inches (24 × 30 cm) lengthwise; Bucky or grid device

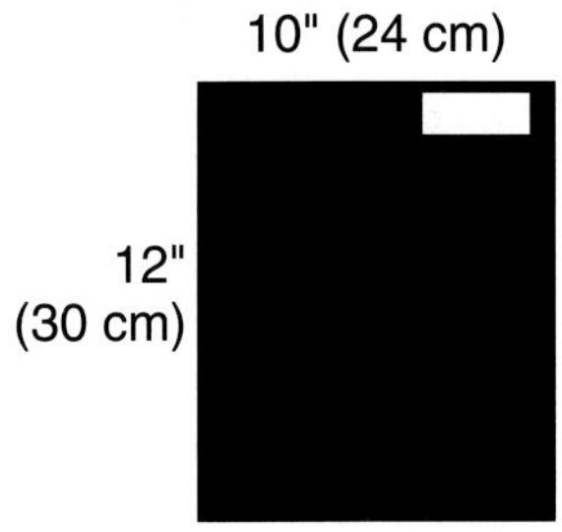

Patient Position

Erect or supine. Patient is rotated 5–10° to affected side (Fig. 9.89).

Part Position

Surface of scapula is against film. Arm is elevated with hand on head. Midpoint of scapula centered to film.

Central Ray

Perpendicular to midscapular area about 2 to 3 inches (5 to 7.6 cm) below coracoid process. Collimate to area of interest.

Structures Demonstrated

Anterior view of scapula (Fig. 9.90).

Evaluation Criteria

1. Scapula horizontal.
2. Scapula visualized through lung and ribs.
3. Lateral portion not superimposed by ribs.

NOTE: An AP position is used if fracture is suspected or if the patient cannot assume an erect position. The same procedure is used.

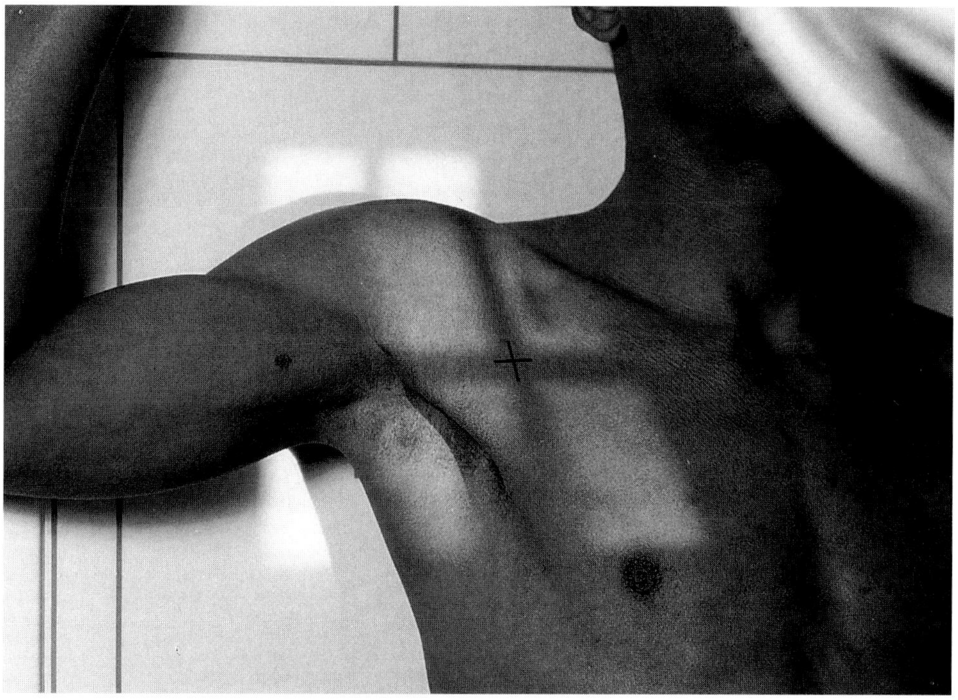

Figure 9.89. AP scapula.

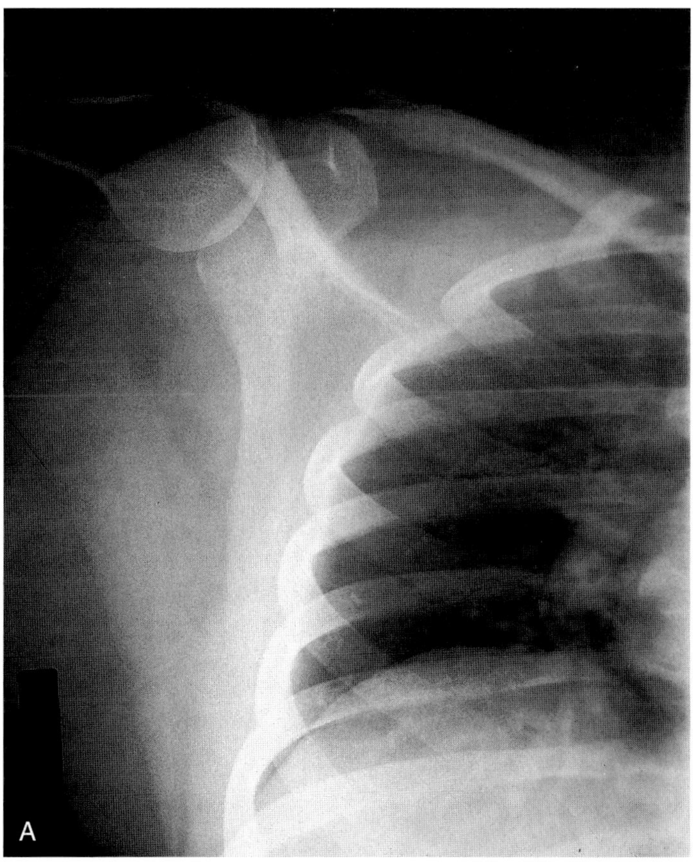

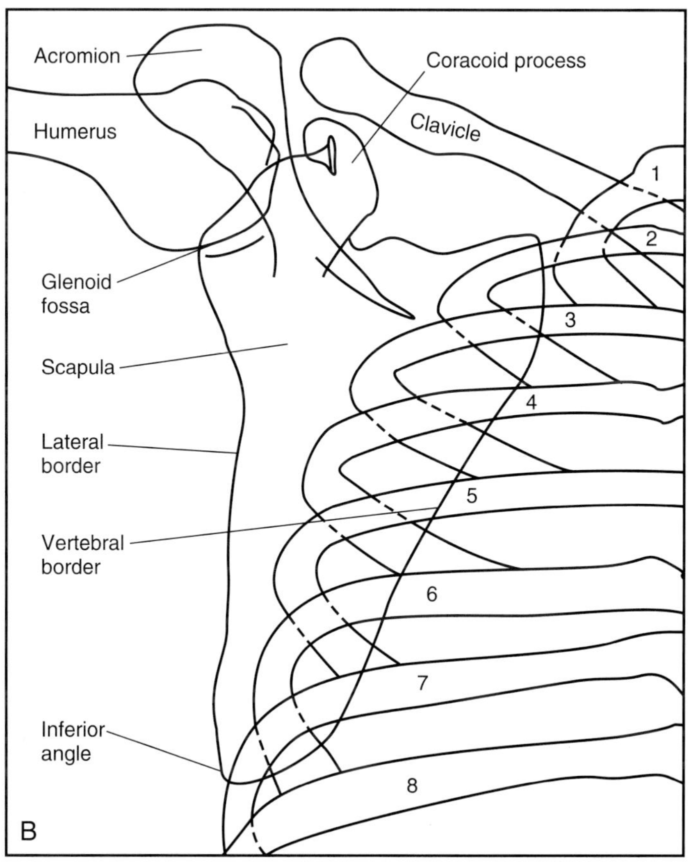

Figure 9.90. A and B, AP scapula.

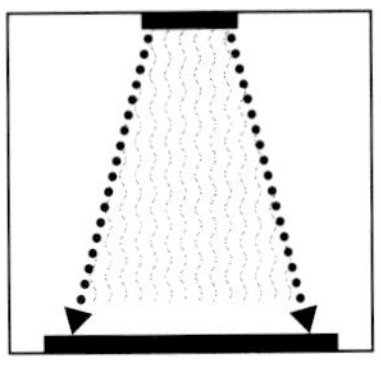

Scapula

Position/Projection

Lateral projection

Film:
10 × 12 inches (24 × 30 cm) lengthwise; Bucky or grid device

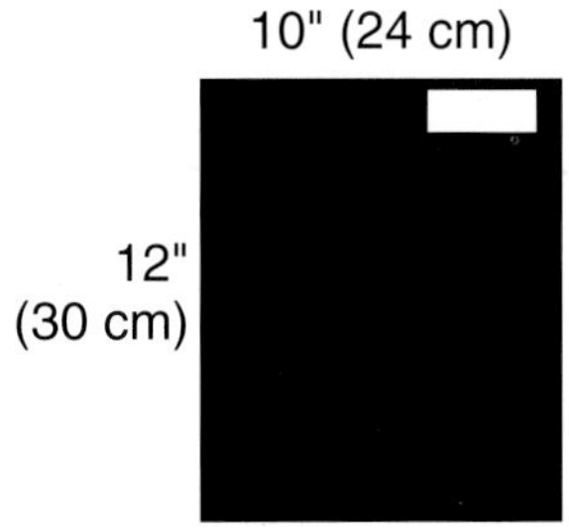

Patient Position

Erect or supine. Place arm of side of interest on opposite shoulder (Fig. 9.91).

Part Position

Body of scapula forms right angle to film. Midpoint of scapula centered to film.

Central Ray

Perpendicular to exit at midpoint of medial border of scapula. Collimate to area of interest.

Structures Demonstrated

Lateral view of scapula (Fig. 9.92).

Evaluation Criteria

1. Arm or ribs should not superimpose scapula.
2. Medial and lateral scapular edges should superimpose.
3. This projection can also be performed in prone position.

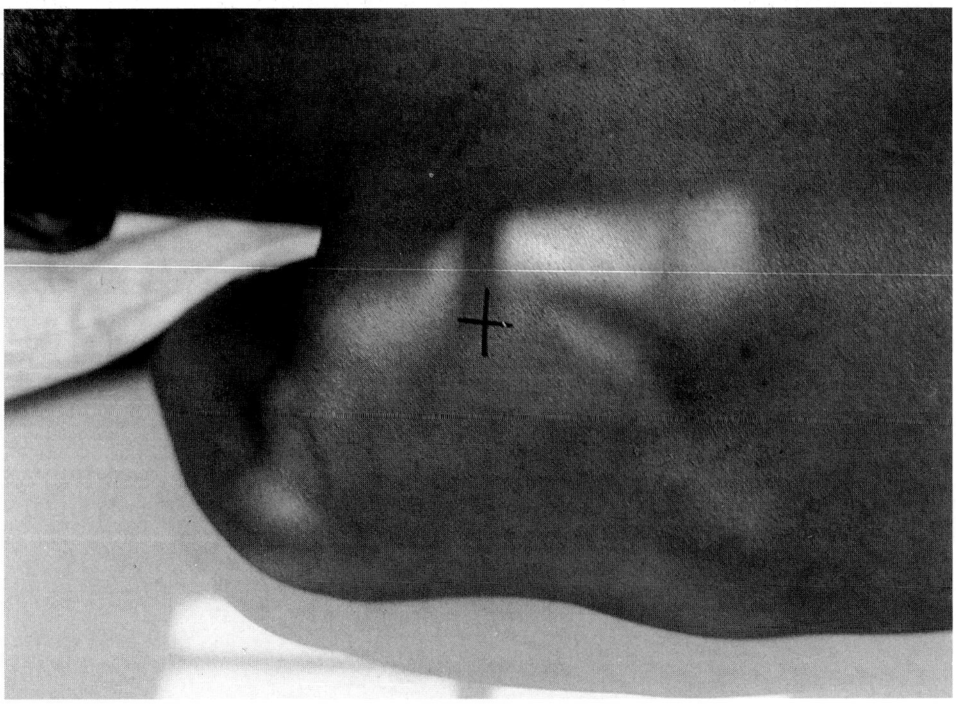

Figure 9.91. Lateral scapula.

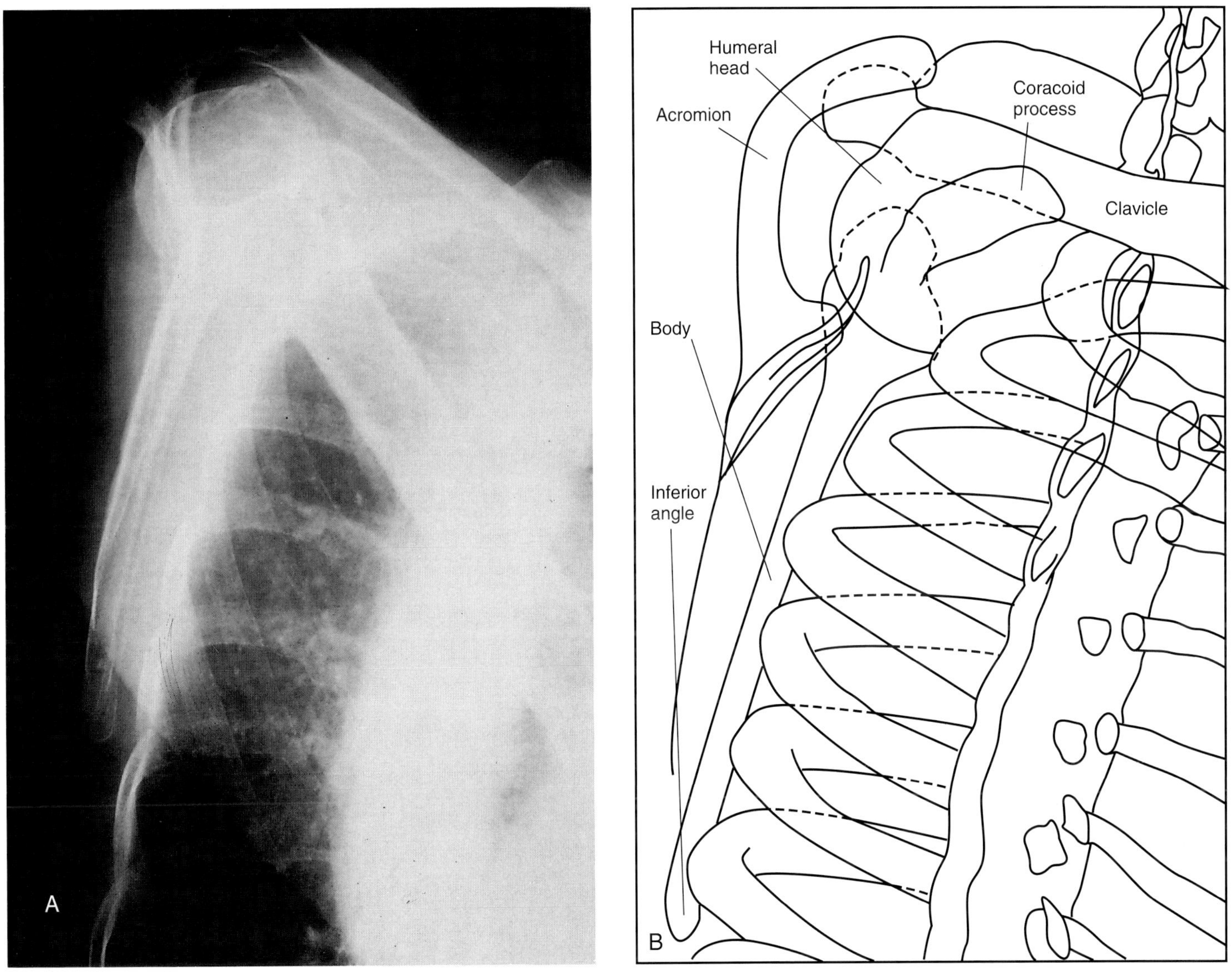

Figure 9.92. A and B, Lateral scapula.

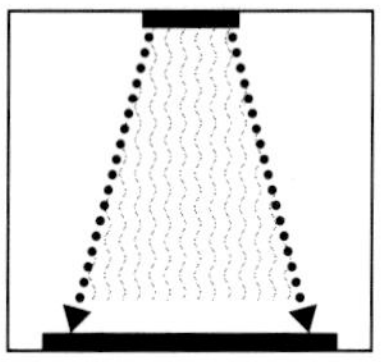

Scapula

Position/Projection

Lateral projection. Y position

Film:
10 × 12 inches (24 × 30 cm) lengthwise; Bucky or grid device

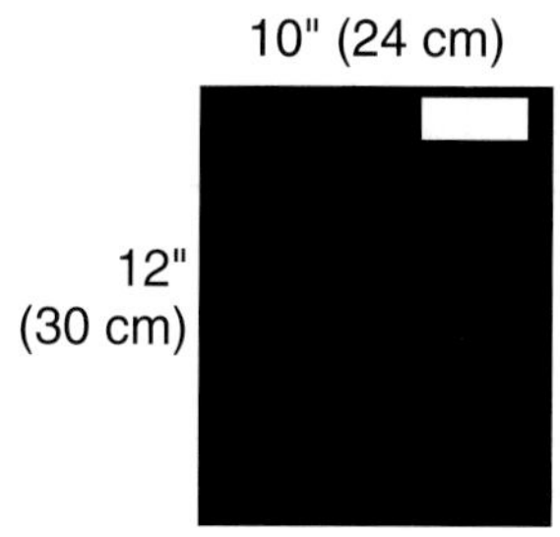

Patient Position

Erect or supine. Place arm of side of interest on opposite hip (Fig. 9.93).

Part Position

Body of scapula forms right angle to film. Midpoint of scapula centered to film.

Central Ray

Perpendicular to midpoint of medial border of scapula. Collimate to area of interest.

Structures Demonstrated

Glenohumeral joint (Fig. 9.94).

Evaluation Criteria

1. Glenoid fossa should be superimposed in center of humeral head.
2. Arm or ribs should not superimpose scapula.
3. Medial and lateral scapular edges should superimpose.
4. Sternoclavicular joint, manubrium, and medial end of clavicle should be demonstrated. Joint should be nearly at right angle to film.
5. Both sides are sometimes taken for comparison.

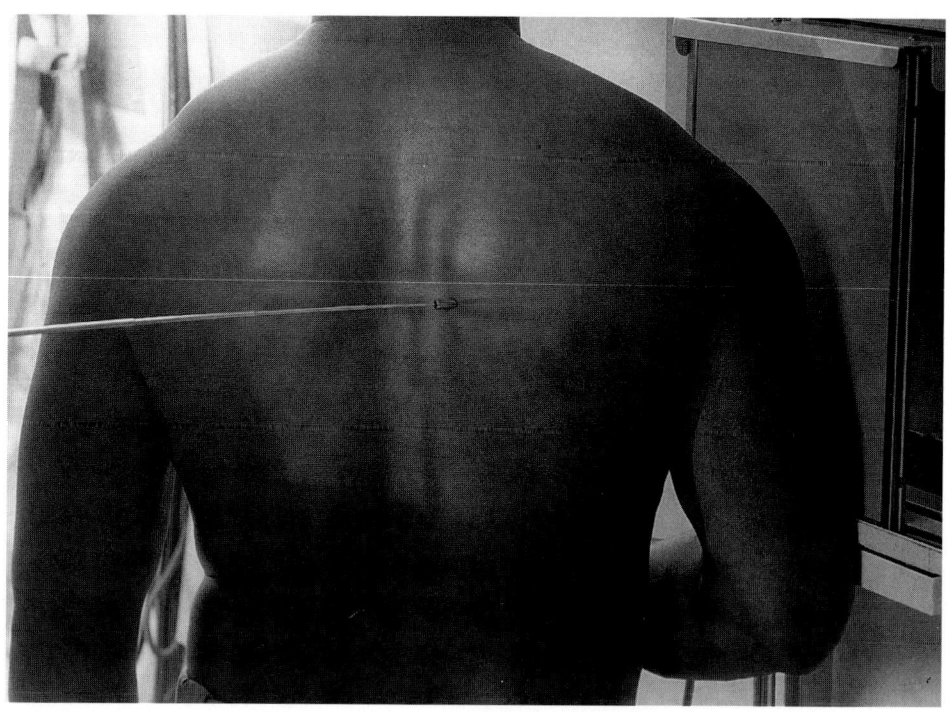

Figure 9.93. Scapula Y position.

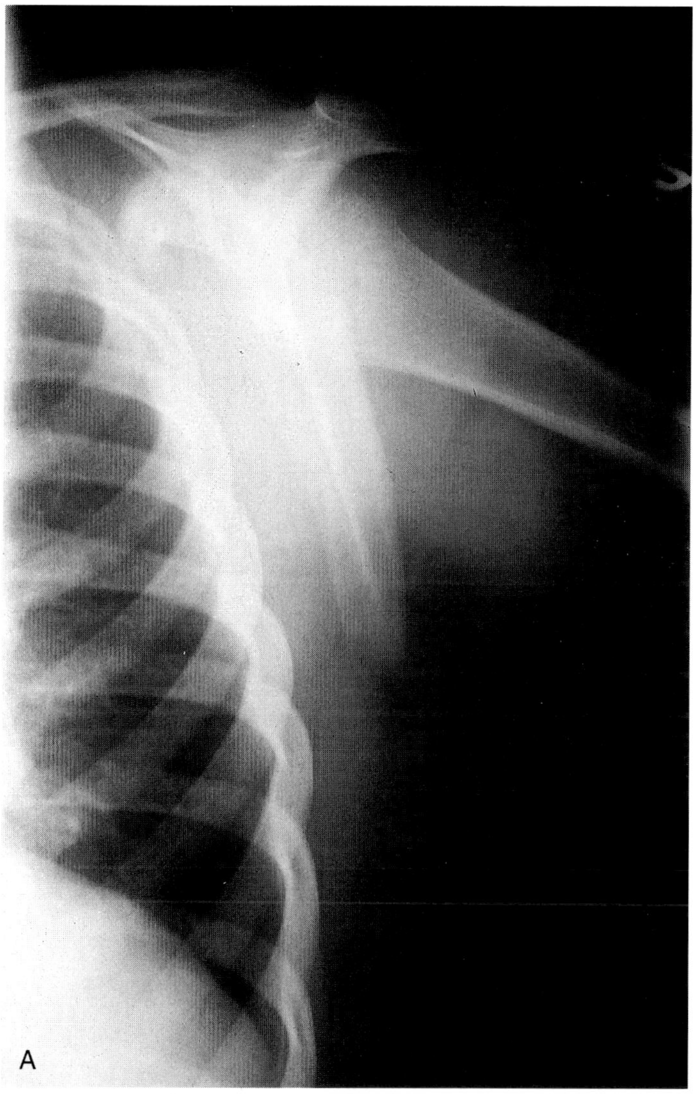

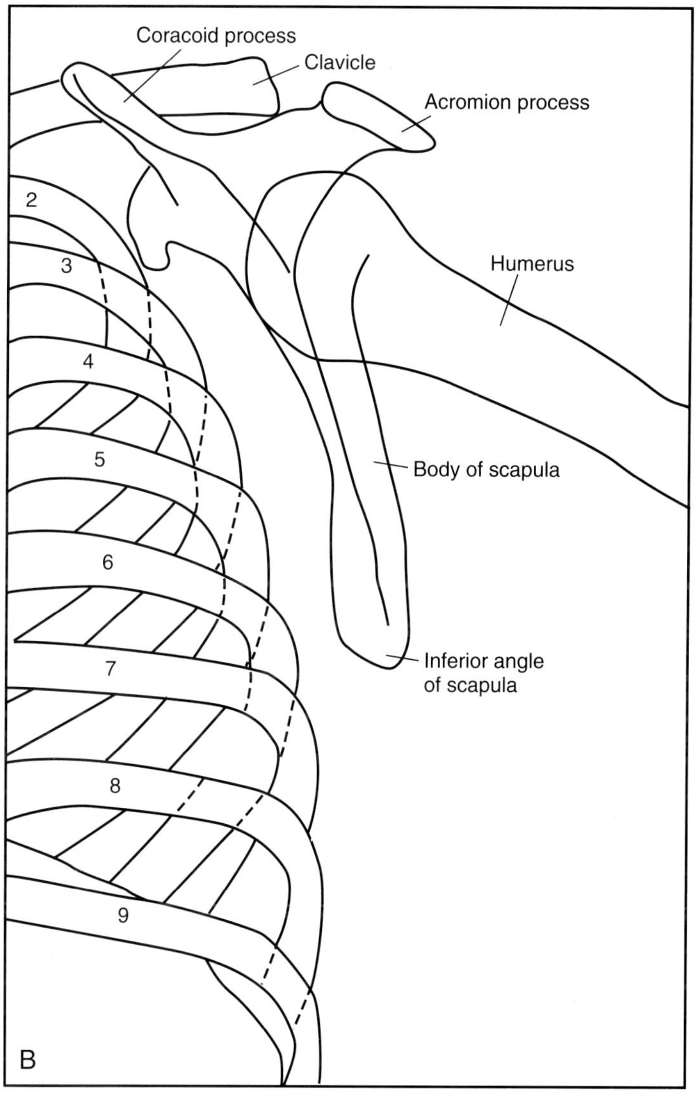

Figure 9.94. A and B, Scapula Y projection.

Bibliography

Ballinger PW: Merrill's Atlas of Radiographic Positions and Radiologic Procedures. 7th ed. St. Louis: Mosby–Year Book, 1992.

Carroll QB: Fuchs' Radiographic Exposure, Processing and Quality Control. 5th ed. Springfield, IL: Charles C Thomas, 1993.

Clements RW: Adaptation of the technique for radiography of the glenohumeral joint in the lateral position. Radiol Technol 1979; 51:305–312.

Cullinan AM, Cullinan JE: Producing Quality Radiographs. 2nd ed. Philadelphia: JB Lippincott, 1994.

DeVos DC: Basic Principles of Radiographic Exposure. Philadelphia: Lea & Febiger, 1990.

Fisk C: Adaptation of the technique of radiography of the bicipital groove. Radiol Technol 1965; 34:47–50.

Griswold R: Elbow fat pads: A radiography perspective. Radiol Technol 1982; 53:303–307.

Hagler M. The Pocket Rad Tech. Philadelphia: WB Saunders, 1993.

Watkins GL, Moore TF. Atypical Orthopedic Radiographic Procedures. St. Louis: Mosby–Year Book, 1993.

C H A P T E R 1 0

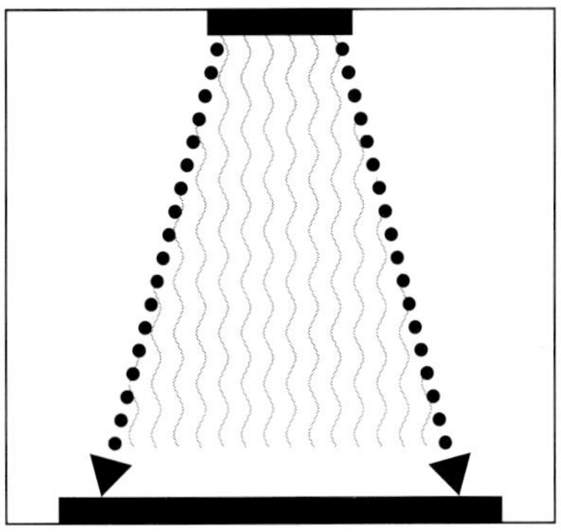

Lower Extremity

Donna F. Burr, M.A.Ed., R.T.(R.)

Radiographic Anatomy

Radiographic Positioning

Lower extremity radiography is one of the most important aspects of radiography owing to the stress and strain we place on our extremities as members of a health-conscious society, as well as for everyday use. The lower extremities carry the body in the upright position and the amount we walk, run, and exercise affects all the bones and joints of these extremities. The lower extremities are more liable to injury than the upper extremities, with the knee being the most susceptible of all extremities. Stress fractures of the bone and pulled tendons of the ankle and knee are common injuries.

This chapter provides a reference for practitioners and students that describes lower extremity positioning and an overview of anatomy shown on lower extremity radiographs.

Radiographers must obtain optimum radiographs so an accurate diagnosis can be made. Sufficient density and contrast are needed for radiographs of the lower extremities. The radiographer is responsible for performing thorough examinations of the bones and joint spaces to assist the radiologist in accurate diagnosis of injuries and diseases.

As a form of orthopedic radiography, two basic factors a radiographer must consider are: (1) the special care required by orthopedic patients and (2) exposure factors (Watkins and Moore, 1993).

Patients may present with possible joint injuries or conditions, possible fractures, or severe trauma. The patient's ability to assume a position must be assessed *before* having the patient assume the position. Although the radiographer can usually make this assessment alone, it may be wise to (1) ask another radiographer to aid in that assessment; and if still unsure, (2) have a physician make that assessment. If joints are immovable and the physician wants to force movement, it is best to have the physician perform that movement.

In terms of exposure factors, an appropriate screen-film combination, peak kilovoltage (kVp) and milliampere-seconds (mAs), and focal-film distance (FFD) and object-to-film distance (OFD) must be selected. In general, "detail" or "extremity" film is used for most lower extremity radiography (exception: pelvis and hip); relatively low kVps provide sufficient image contrast (50 to 70 kVp); FFDs of 40 inches (102 cm) and short OFDs. However, sometimes longer OFDs are used to magnify the image, as with erosive arthropathies and small fractures. Additionally, beam alignment (angulation) is important to minimize distortion.

FOOT

The foot has 26 bones (Fig. 10.1)—the 7 tarsals, or ankle bones; the 5 metatarsals, or instep bones; and the 14 phalanges, or toe bones. The tarsal bones are the talus, calcaneus, navicular, cuboid, and the 3 cuneiform bones. The metatarsal bones connect the cuneiform and the cuboid with the phalanges and form the front part of the instep. The great toe, or 1st toe, has two phalanges (proximal and distal). Each of the other toes has three phalanges (proximal, middle, and distal). The hinge-type diarthrodial joints form the interphalangeal articulations. The 2nd through the 5th toes have a proximal and a distal interphalangeal joint and the great toe has only an interphalangeal joint. The ends of the phalanges meet the underside of the metatarsals to form the ball of the foot.

The metatarsal bones connect the cuneiform and the cuboid with the phalanges and form the front part of the instep. The 1st metatarsal is the thickest of the five. The 2nd metatarsal is the longest and the 5th metatarsal has a very prominent tuberosity at the base on its lateral side. Normally, on the plantar surface of the 1st metatarsal, two sesamoid bones begin appearing between the ages of 8 and 12 years.

The largest of the tarsal bones is the calcaneus, or heel bone. The talus is the second largest tarsal bone; it lies above the calcaneus. The talus supports the tibia and rests on the calcaneus. It articulates anteriorly with the navicular, and at the sides with the malleoli of the tibia and fibula.

The navicular lies on the medial side of the foot between the talus and the cuneiform. The cuboid lies on the lateral side of the foot between the calcaneus and the 4th and 5th metatarsals. The cuneiforms lie in the middle and on the medial sides of the foot. The cuneiforms articulate proximally with the navicular and distally with the bases of the 1st, 2nd, and 3rd metatarsals. The 2nd cuneiform is the smallest.

ANKLE

The ankle joint is a diarthrodial hinge joint (Fig. 10.2), which allows only flexion and extension. The articulation of the talus with the distal tibia and fibula forms the ankle joint.

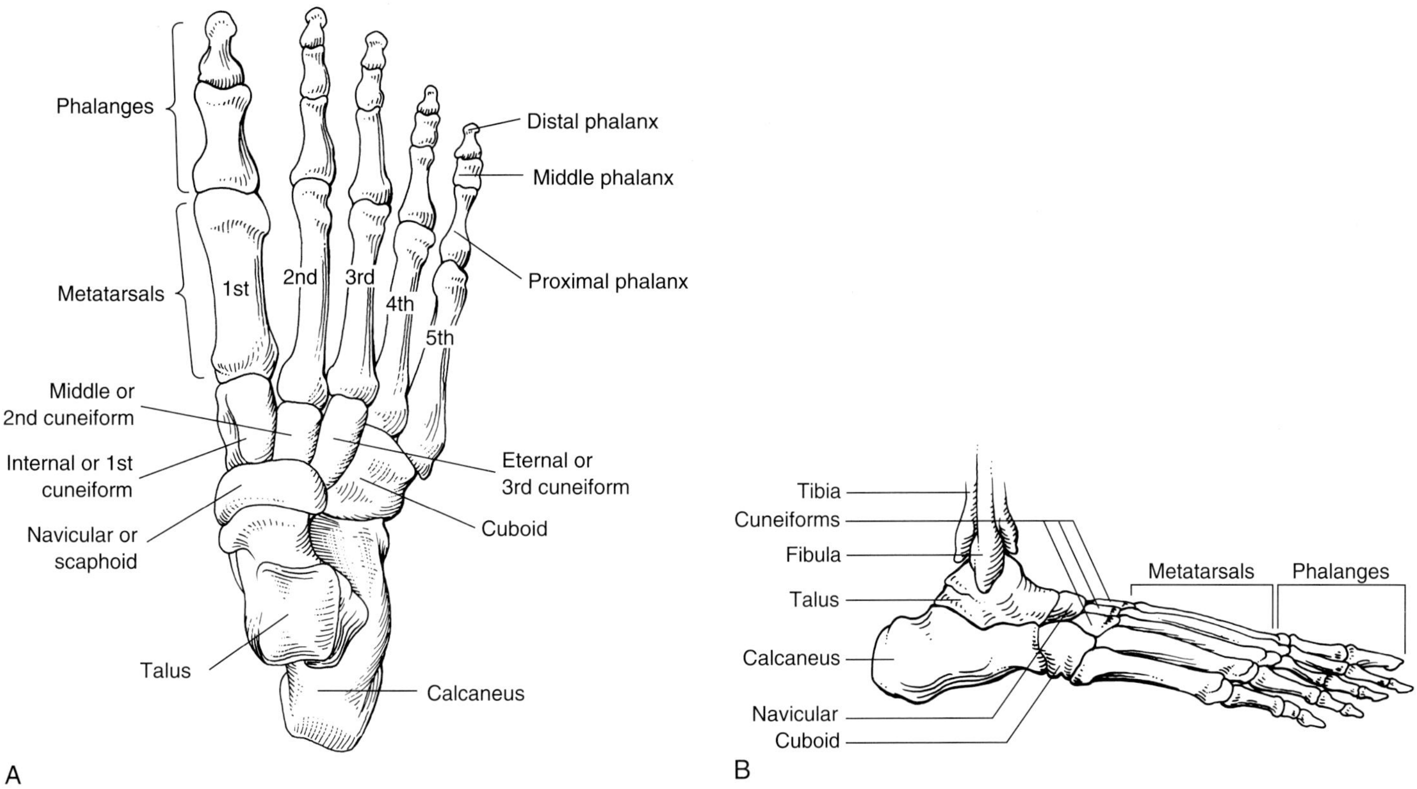

Figure 10.1. A and B, Foot.

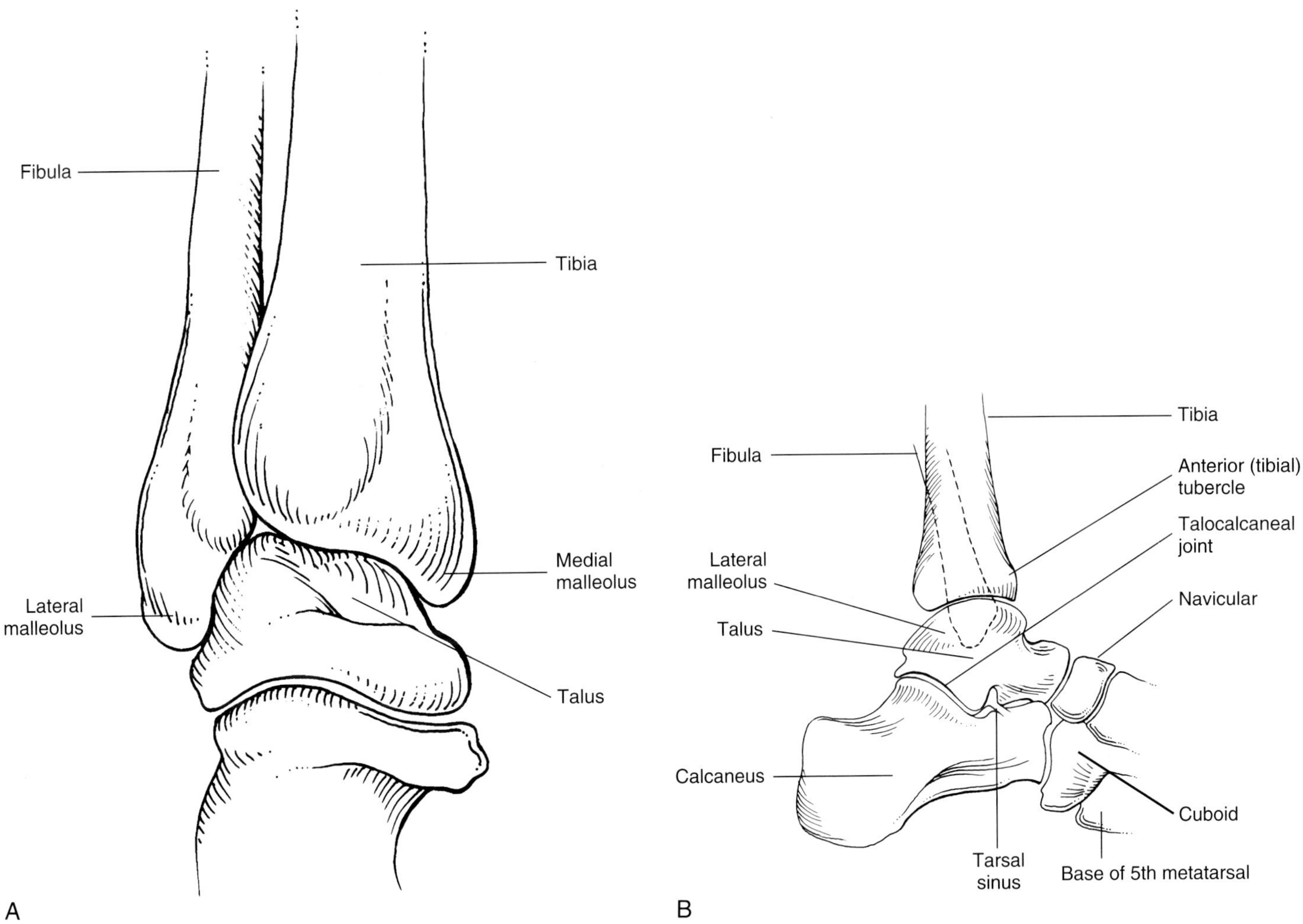

Figure 10.2. A and B, Ankle.

LOWER LEG

The lower leg consists of the tibia and fibula (Fig. 10.3). The tibia is the larger of the two bones and is located on the medial side, anterior to the fibula. The medial condyle, lateral condyle, tibial plateau, and tibial spine make up the proximal end of the tibia. At the knee joint, the medial and lateral condyles articulate with the femoral condyles. The tibial spine is a sharp projection between these two articulators and is also known as the intercondylar eminence. The tibial spine has two pointed processes called tubercles. The tibial plateau is the upper surface of the condyles that articulates with the femur. On the upper anterior portion of the tibial shaft is the tibial tuberosity. On the medial side of the tibia is the large process that is the medial malleolus.

The fibula is the smaller, slender bone located laterally on the leg. The styloid process is at the head of the fibula laterally and posteriorly. The lateral malleolus is the large end of the fibula that articulates with the medial surface of the talus at the ankle.

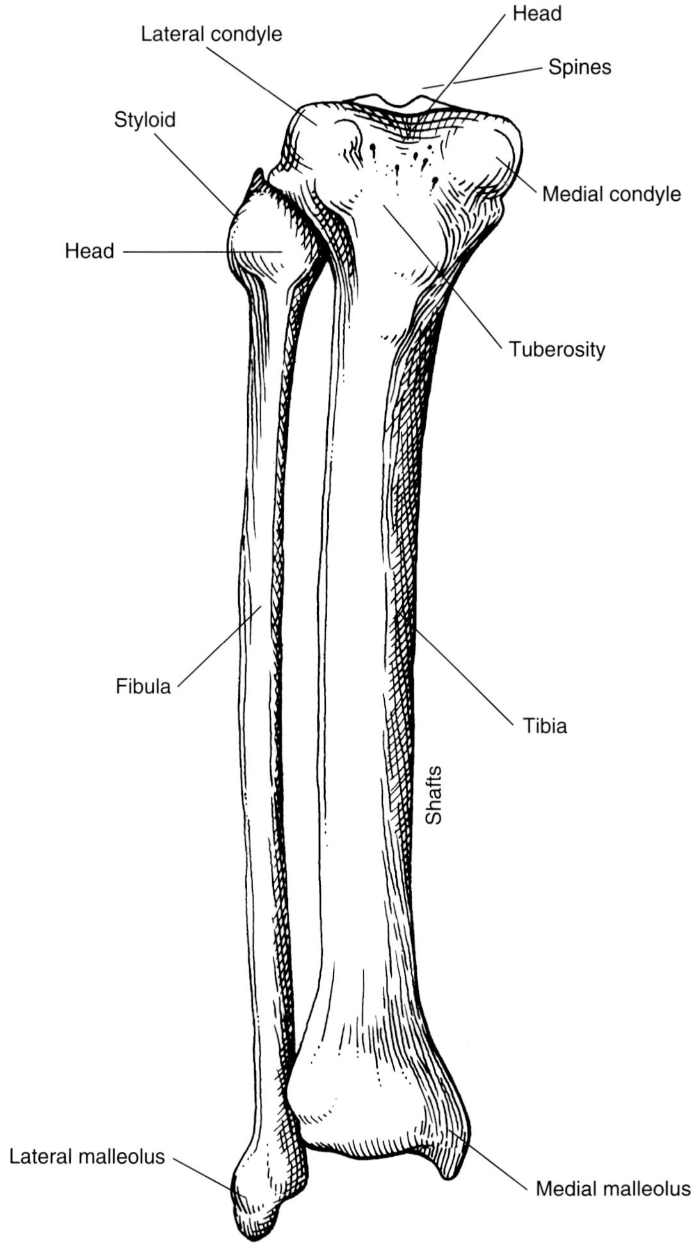

Figure 10.3. Lower leg.

KNEE

The knee is a diarthrodial hinge joint (Fig. 10.4), which allows for flexion and extension only. The popliteal region lies behind the knee joint and the patella lies in front. The patella is the largest sesamoid bone in the body; it provides protection to the anterior aspect of the knee.

FEMUR

The femur is the longest, heaviest, and strongest bone (Fig. 10.5). It has a shaft and articular surfaces at both the distal and the proximal ends. The distal end comprises a large medial condyle and a small lateral condyle, separated by a notch or deep depression—the intercondylar fossa. Two rough prominences at the upper outer margin of the condyles are the medial and lateral epicondyles.

The femoral head is located at the proximal portion of the femur. It comprises a neck and the greater and lesser trochanters. The greater trochanter is located on the upper lateral aspect of the femur and the lesser trochanter is located medially and posteriorly.

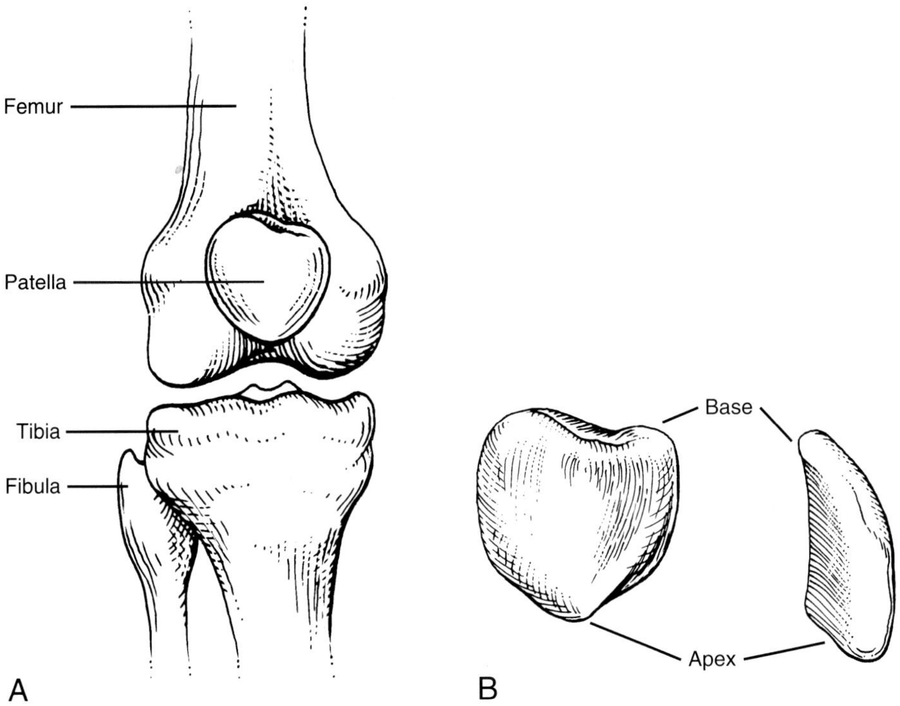

Figure 10.4. A and B, Knee.

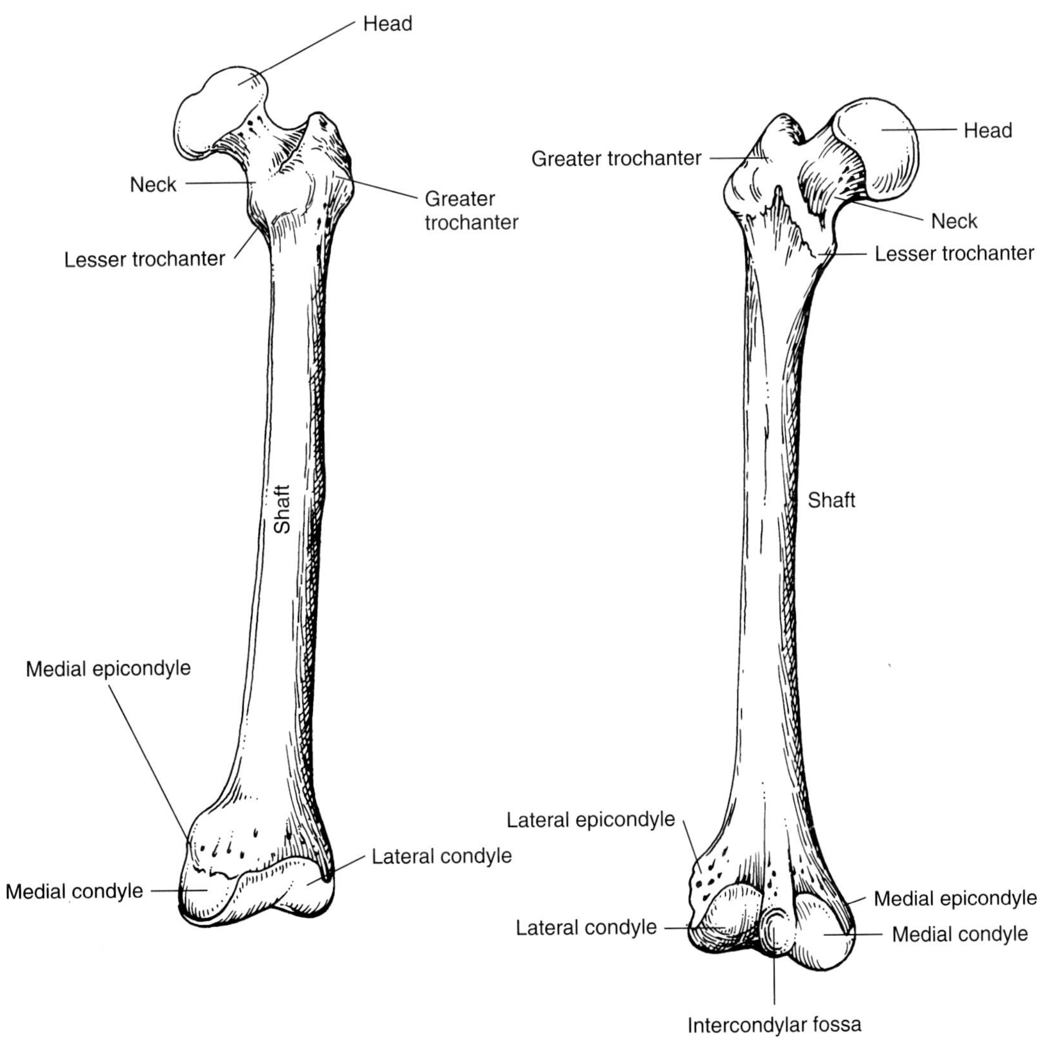

Figure 10.5. Femur.

PELVIS

The pelvis is a strong, basin-shaped bone (Fig. 10.6). Its side walls are formed by two irregular-shaped hip bones called the innominate bones. Each innominate bone has three parts, the ilium, ischium, and pubis. On each side of the pelvis is a socket into which the femora fit. The whole pelvis is supported on the two legs.

The largest of the hip bones is the ilium. The ilium has a body and a curved winged portion called the ala (wing). The iliac crest is the upper portion of the ala. It extends from the anterior superior iliac spine (ASIS) to the posterior superior iliac spine (PSIS).

The ischium is formed by a body and two rami. The ischial tuberosity is located near the junction of the superior and inferior rami. The ischial spine is a bony projection located posterior to the acetabulum.

The pubic bone consists of a body and two rami. The lower anterior portion of the acetabula is formed by the body of the pelvis. The symphysis pubis is formed by the superior pubis rami, which project inferiorly and medially from both acetabula and meet at the midline. The obturator foramen is the largest foramen in the human skeleton; it is the large opening formed by the rami of each ischium and the pubis.

The female pelvis is broader and shallower and the inlet is larger and more rounded than the male pelvis.

SACRUM AND COCCYX

The sacrum and coccyx form the pelvic girdle (Fig. 10.7). Both the sacrum and the coccyx form the posterior portion of the pelvic girdle, and the hip bones form the lateral, anterior, and inferior margins of the pelvic girdle. The sacrum is wider and curves more posteriorly and sharply in the female.

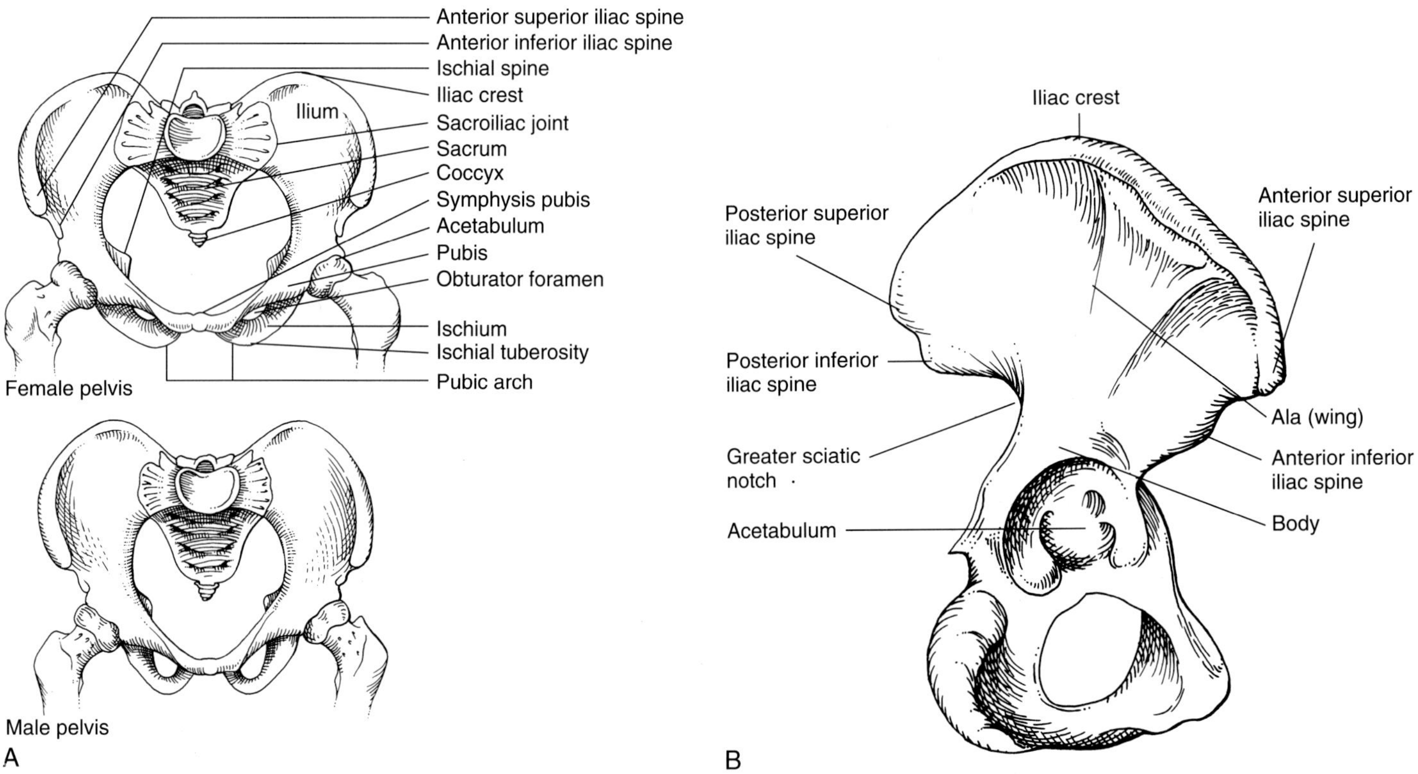

Figure 10.6. A and B, Pelvis.

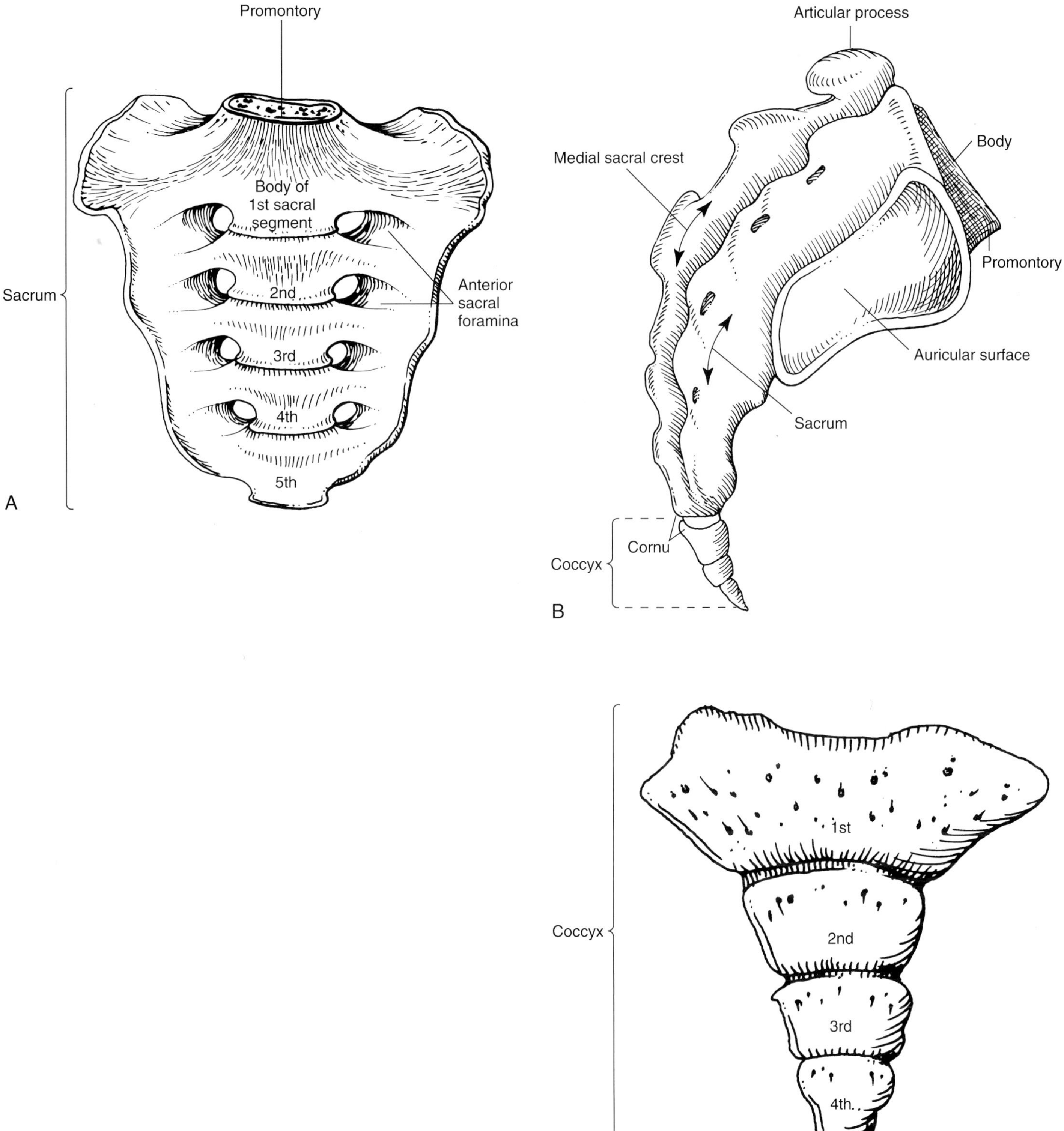

Figure 10.7. A–C, Sacrum and coccyx.

Toes

Position/Projection

Dorsoplantar (AP) projection

Film Size:
8 × 10 inches (20 × 24 cm)
crosswise or lengthwise
tabletop
Divide cassette in halves or thirds

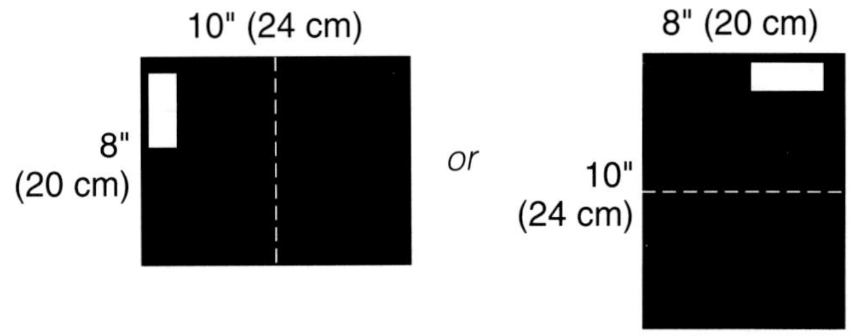

Patient Position

Supine or seated with knee of affected foot flexed and plantar surface of foot resting flat on cassette (Figs. 10.8 and 10.9).

Part Position

Adjust position of toes so their long axis coincides with unmasked portion of cassette. Center base of 3rd metatarsophalangeal joint or metatarsophalangeal joint of affected toe to midpoint of unmasked portion of cassette.

Central Ray

15° cephalic angle toward calcaneus to enter at base of 3rd metatarsophalangeal joint.

or

Perpendicular to base of 3rd metatarsophalangeal joint.

or

Place toes on a 15° wedge and direct central ray perpendicular to base of 3rd metatarsophalangeal joint.

NOTE: The 15° angle of the central ray or the 15° wedge under the toes opens the joint spaces.

Structures Demonstrated

AP projection of phalanges, interphalangeal joints, metatarsophalangeal joints, and distal end of the metatarsals (Figs. 10.10 and 10.11).

Evaluation Criteria

1. Phalanges and distal metatarsals should not be rotated.
2. Interphalangeal joint spaces and metatarsophalangeal joint spaces should be open.
3. Toes should not overlap.

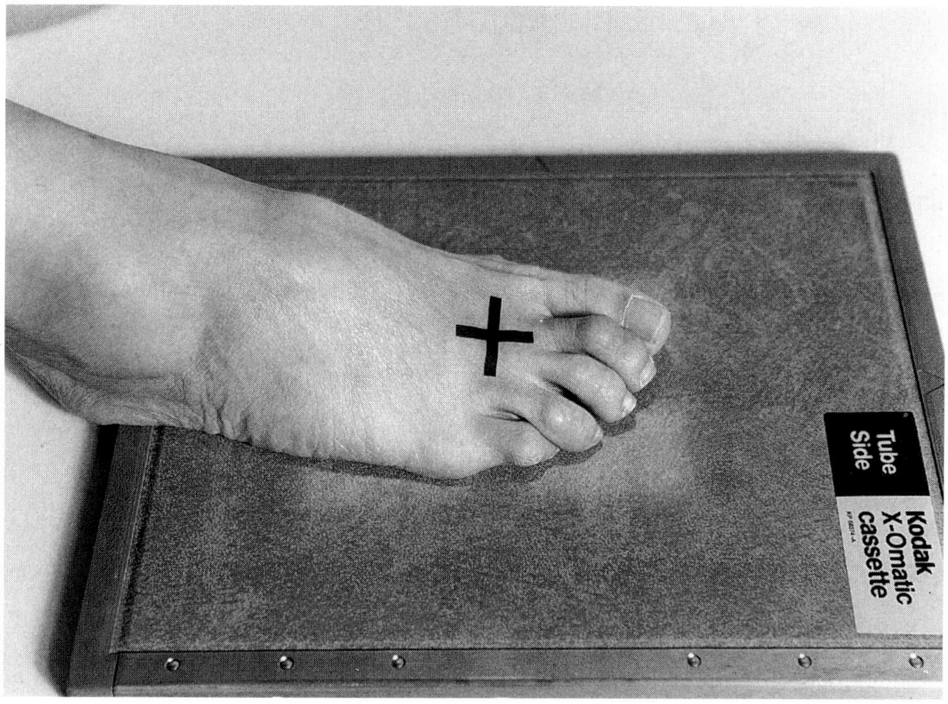

Figure 10.8. AP toes.

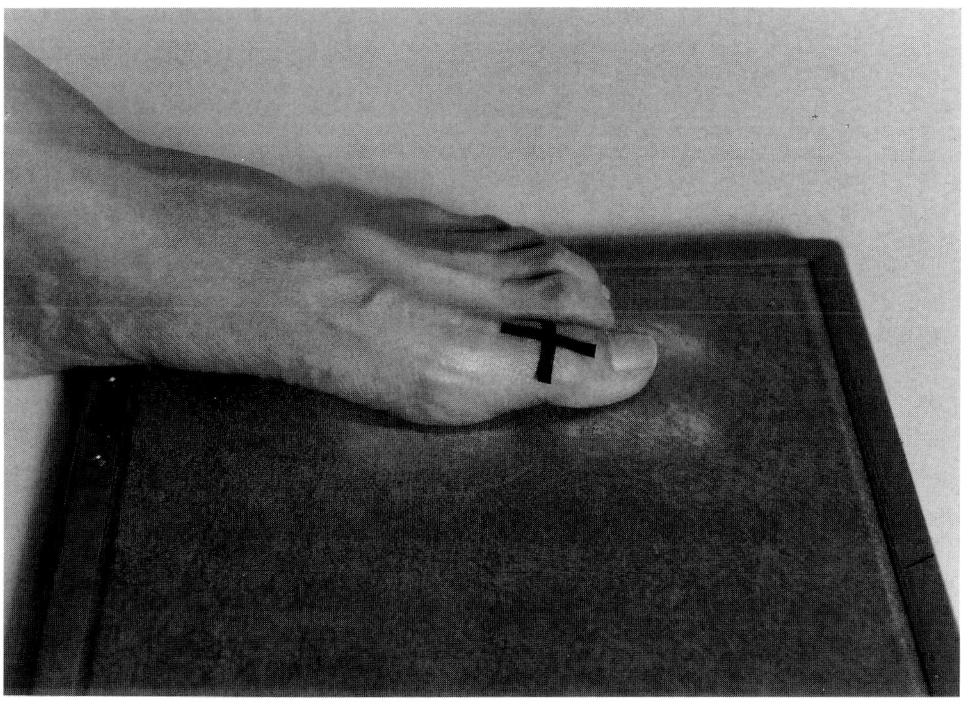

Figure 10.9. AP 1st toe.

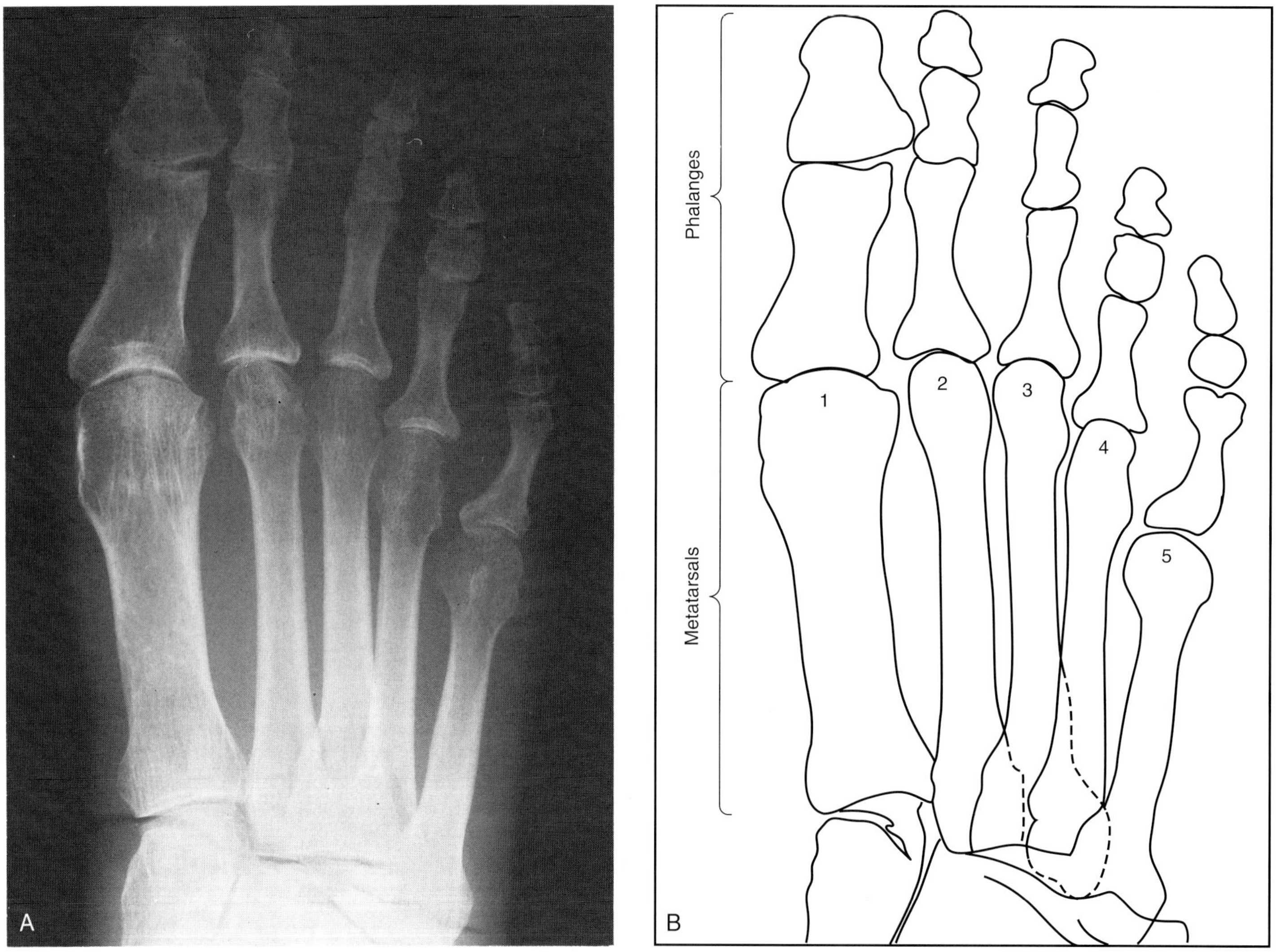

Figure 10.10. A and B, AP toes.

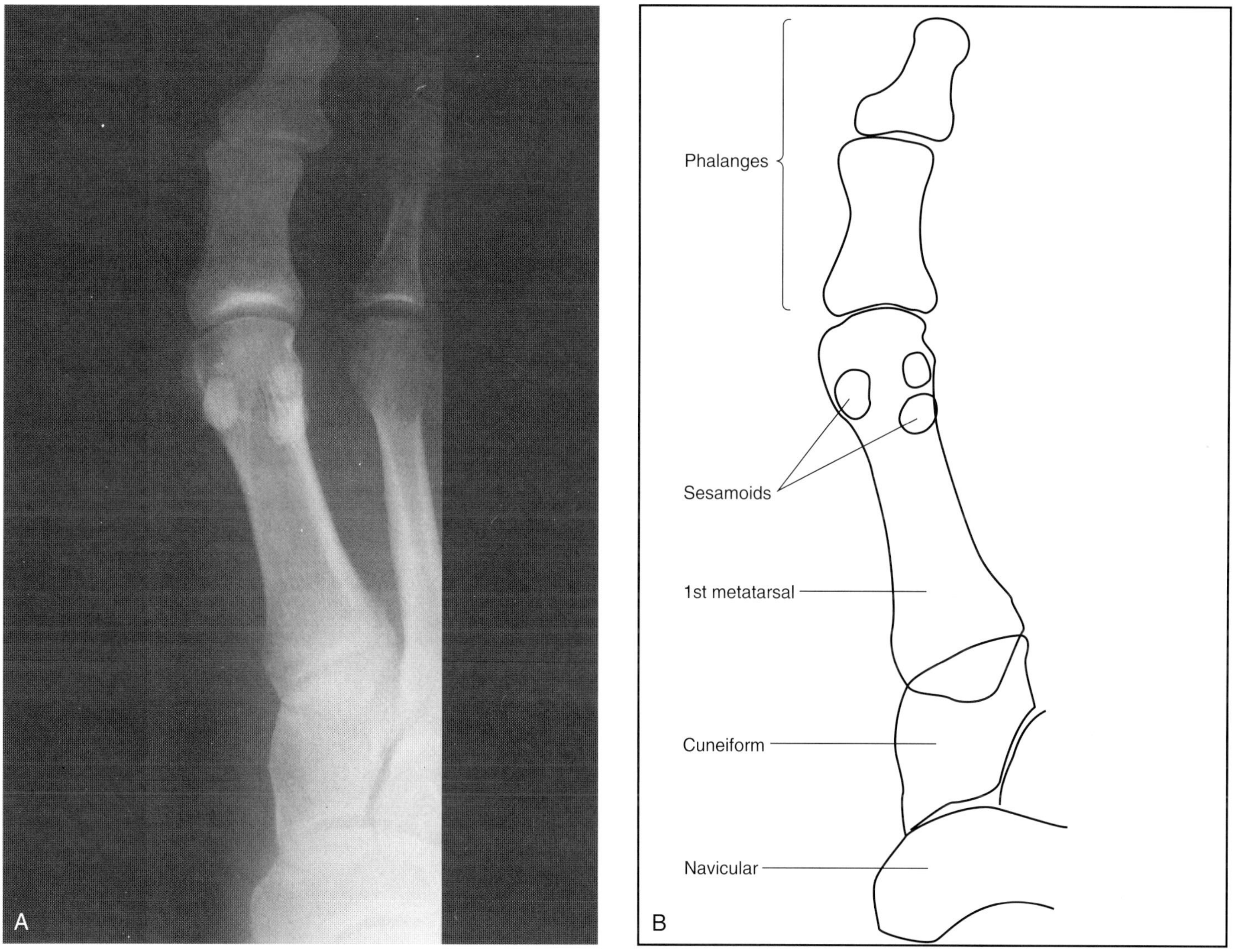

Figure 10.11. A and B, AP 1st toe.

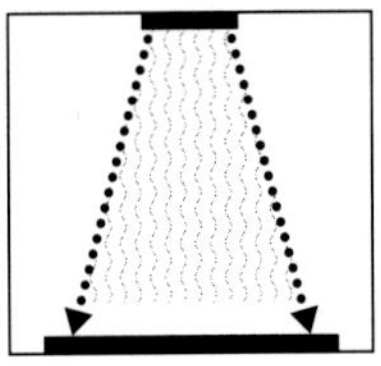

Toes

Position/Projection

Plantodorsal (PA) projection

Film Size:
8 × 10 inches (20 × 24 cm)
crosswise or lengthwise
tabletop
Divide cassette in halves or
thirds

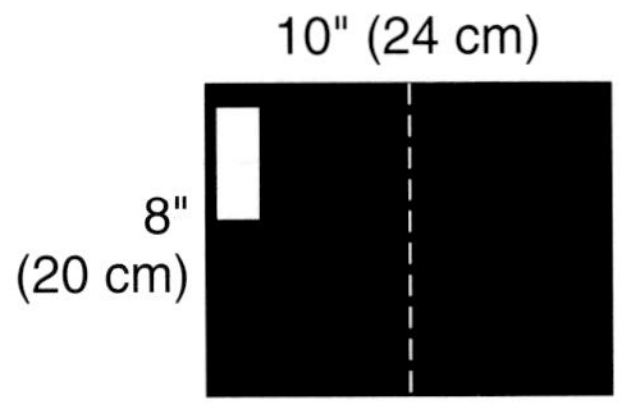

or

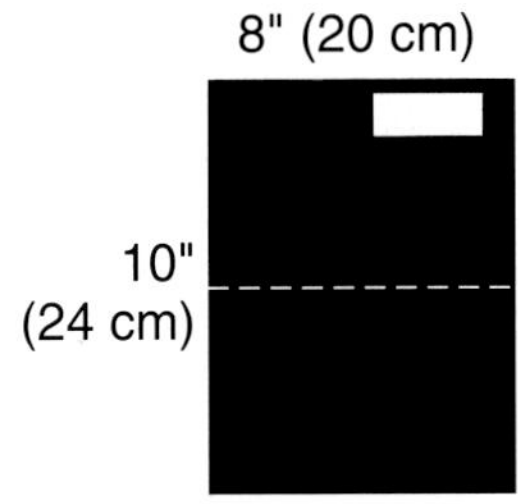

Patient Position

Prone with leg extended (Fig. 10.12).

Part Position

Align long axis of toes to unmasked portion of cassette. Elevate foot to place phalanges parallel to plane of cassette. Center 3rd metatarsophalangeal joint or metatarsophalangeal joint of affected toe to midpoint of unmasked portion of cassette.

Central Ray

Perpendicular through 3rd metatarsophalangeal joint or through metatarsophalangeal joint of affected toe.

Structures Demonstrated

PA projection of phalanges, interphalangeal joints, metatarsophalangeal joints, and distal end of metatarsals (Fig. 10.13).

Evaluation Criteria

1. Phalanges and distal metatarsals should not be rotated.
2. Interphalangeal joint spaces and metatarsophalangeal joint spaces should be open.
3. Toes should not overlap.

NOTE: Some departments require all toes to be included on the radiograph—center at the 3rd metatarsophalangeal joint. Some departments require just the affected toe on the radiograph—center at the metatarsophalangeal joint of the affected toe.

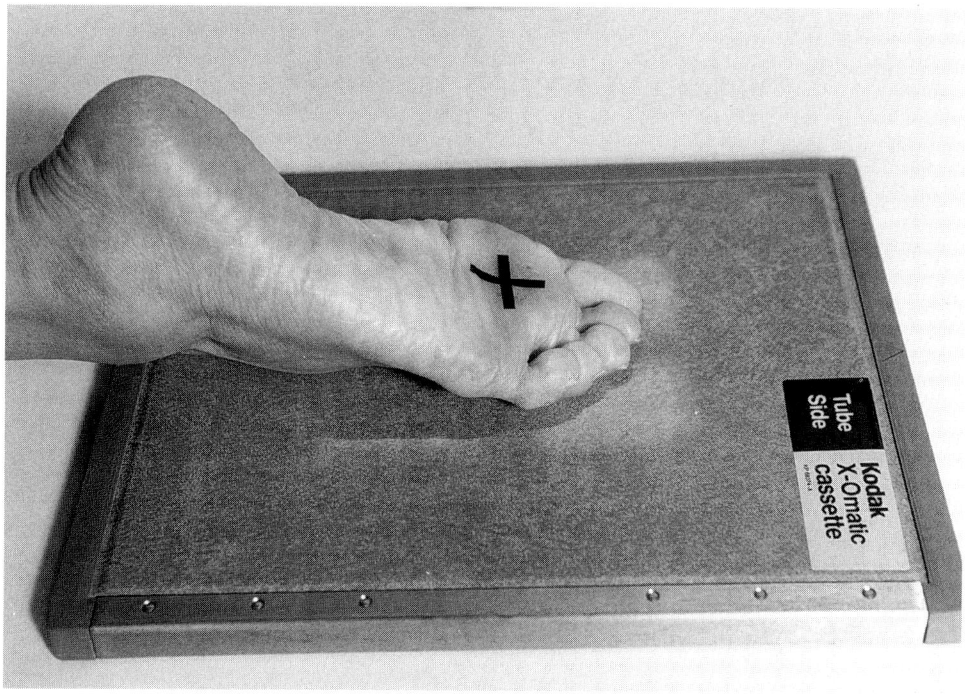

Figure 10.12. PA toes.

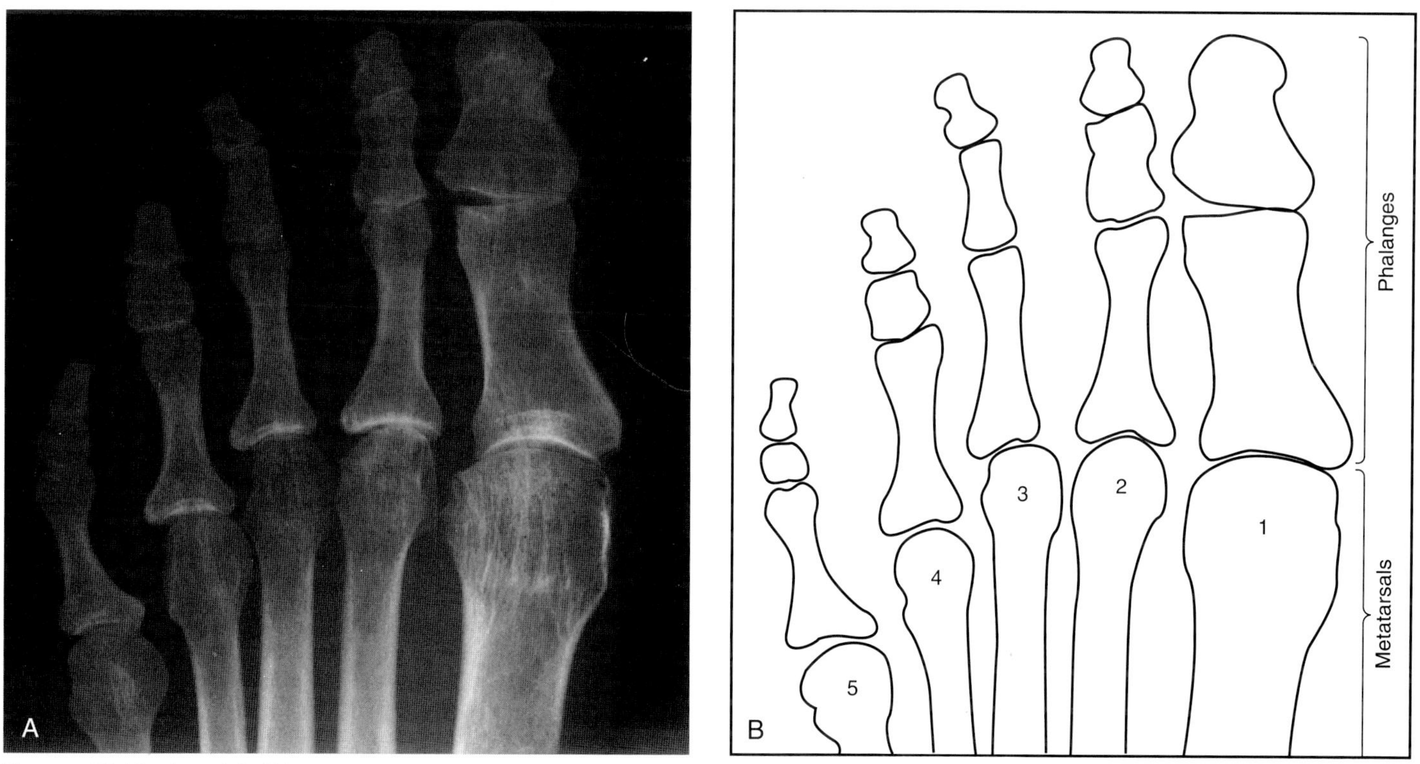

Figure 10.13. A and B, PA toes.

Toes

Position/Projection

Dorsoplantar oblique (AP) projection

Film Size:
8 × 10 inches (20 × 24 cm)
crosswise or lengthwise
tabletop
Divide cassette in halves or thirds

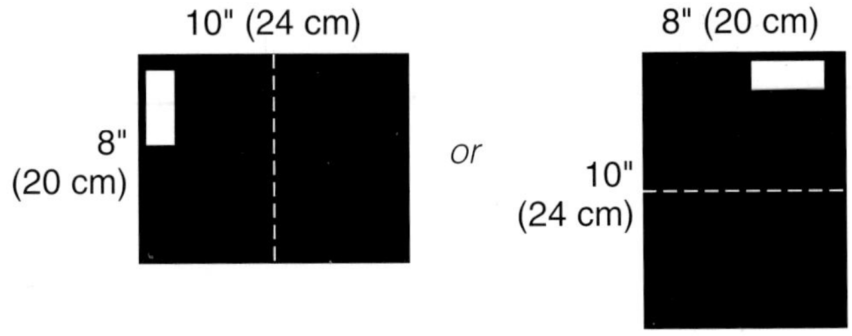

Patient Position

Supine or seated with knee of affected foot flexed and plantar surface of foot resting flat on cassette (Fig. 10.14).

Part Position

Align cassette with long axis of foot. Rotate leg medially to place plantar surface of foot 30° to plane of cassette. Center base of 3rd metatarsophalangeal joint or metatarsophalangeal joint of affected toe to midpoint of unmasked portion of cassette.

Central Ray

Perpendicular to 3rd metatarsophalangeal joint or to metatarsophalangeal joint of affected toe.

Structures Demonstrated

AP oblique projection of phalanges, interphalangeal joints, metatarsophalangeal joints, and distal end of metatarsals (Fig. 10.15).

Evaluation Criteria

1. Phalanx or phalanges should be seen with no overlapping.
2. Distal end of metatarsals should be oblique.
3. Joint space of 2nd through 5th metatarsophalangeals should be open (sometimes not completely opened).

NOTE: Some departments require all toes to be included on the radiograph—center at the 3rd metatarsophalangeal joint. Some departments require just the affected toe on the radiograph—center at the metatarsophalangeal joint of the affected toe.

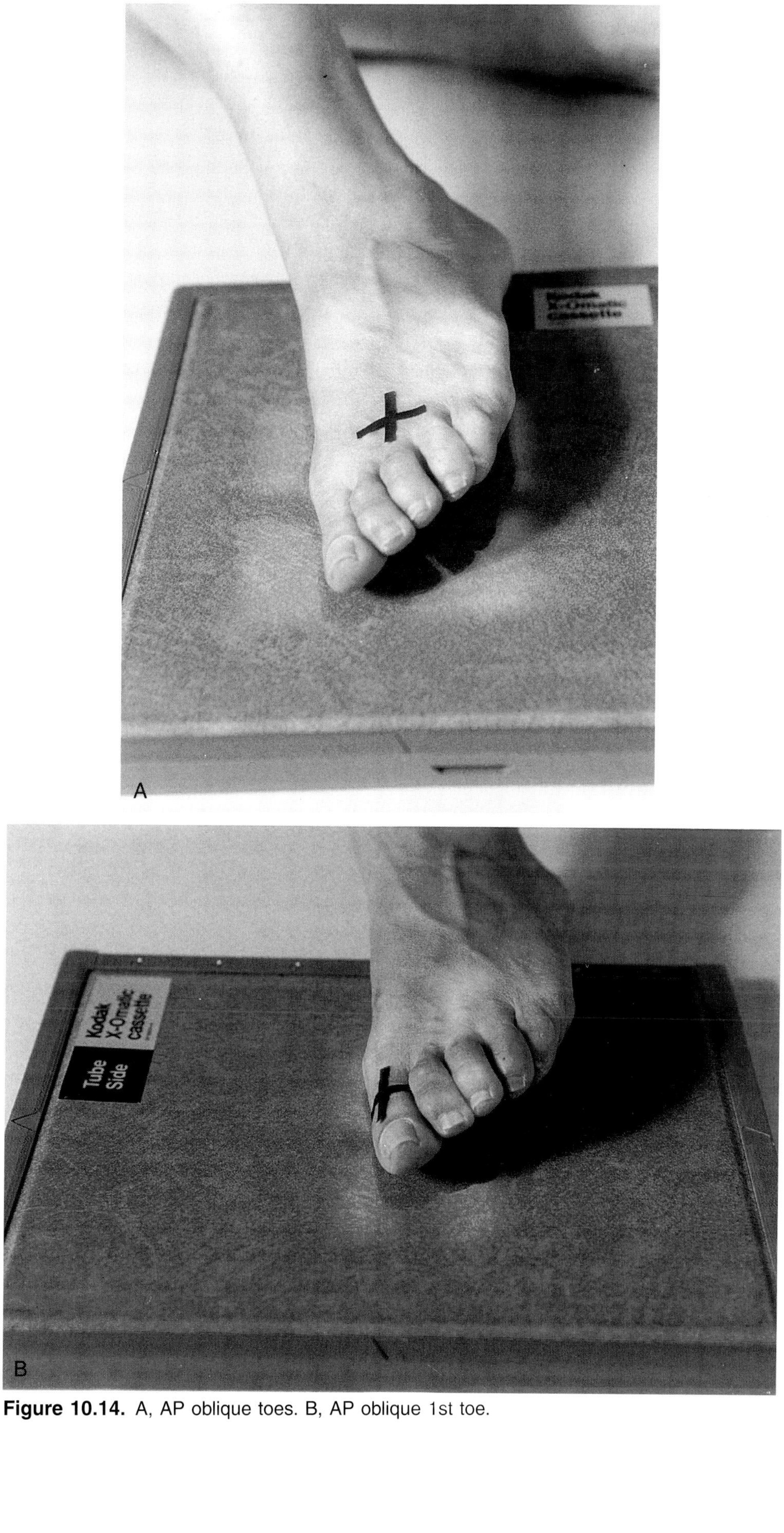

Figure 10.14. A, AP oblique toes. B, AP oblique 1st toe.

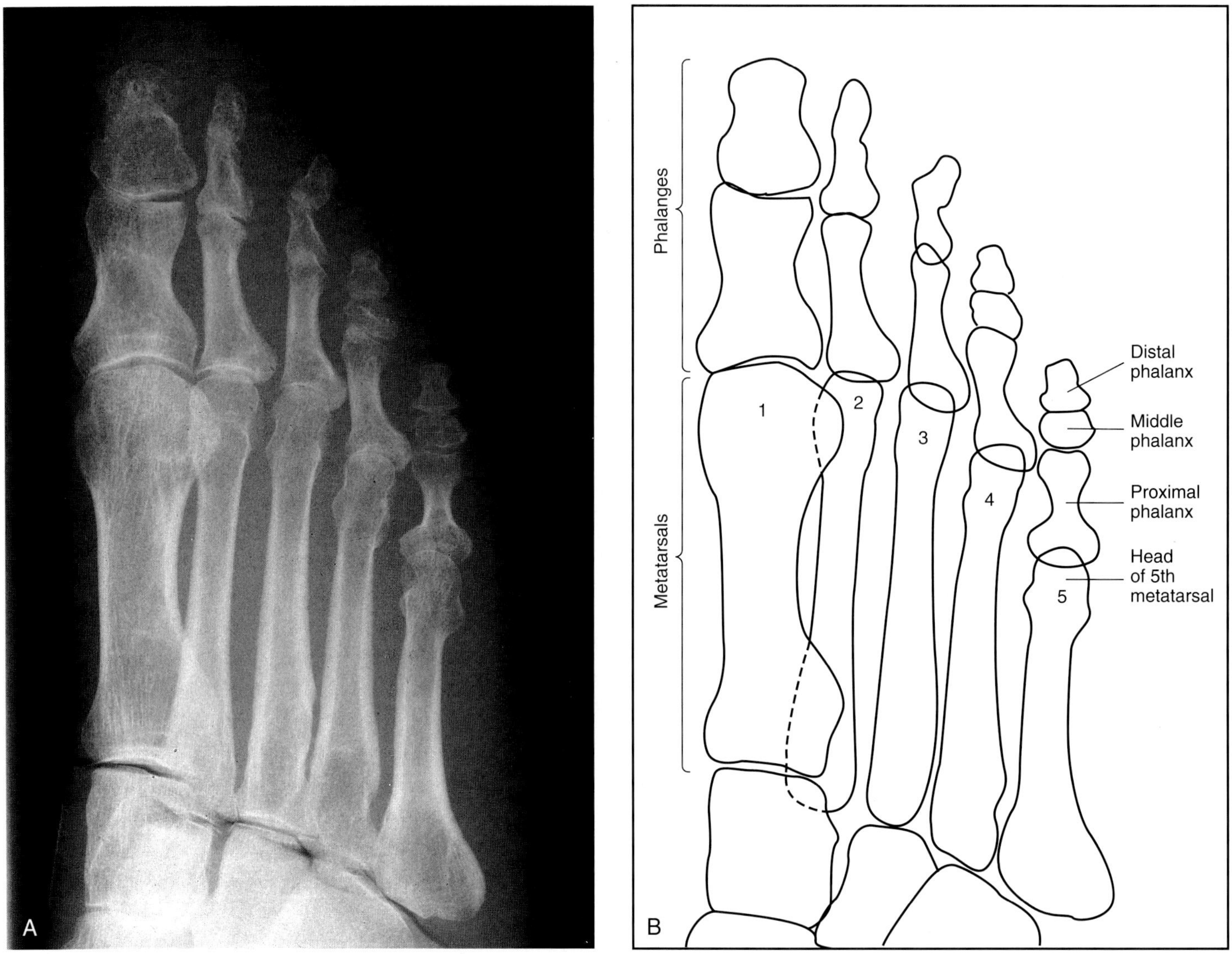

Figure 10.15. A and B, AP oblique toes.

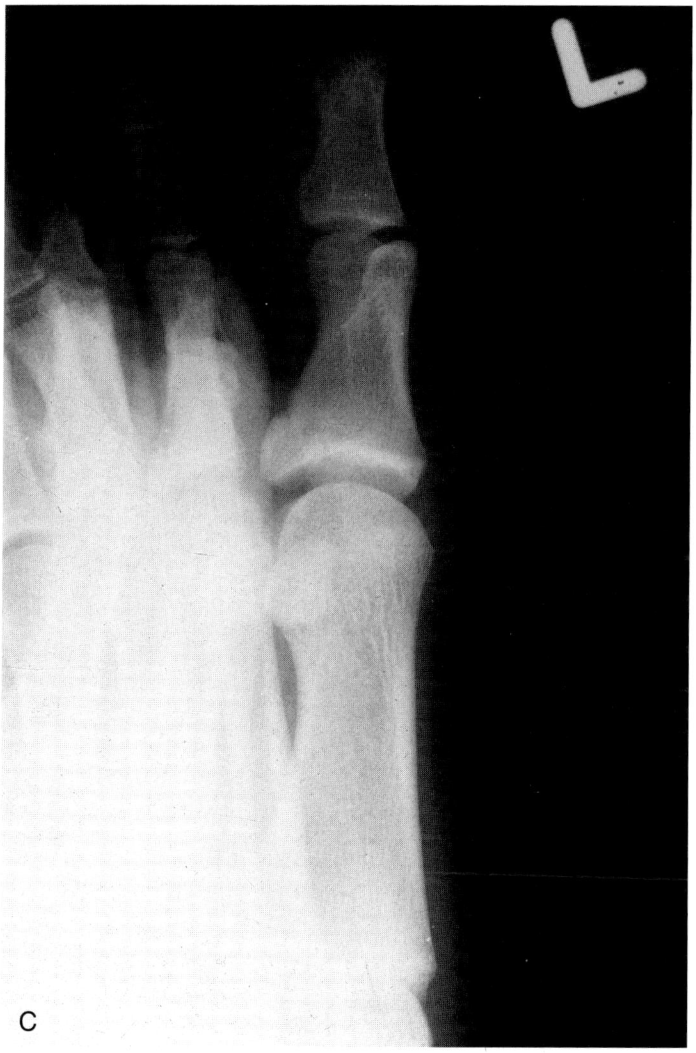

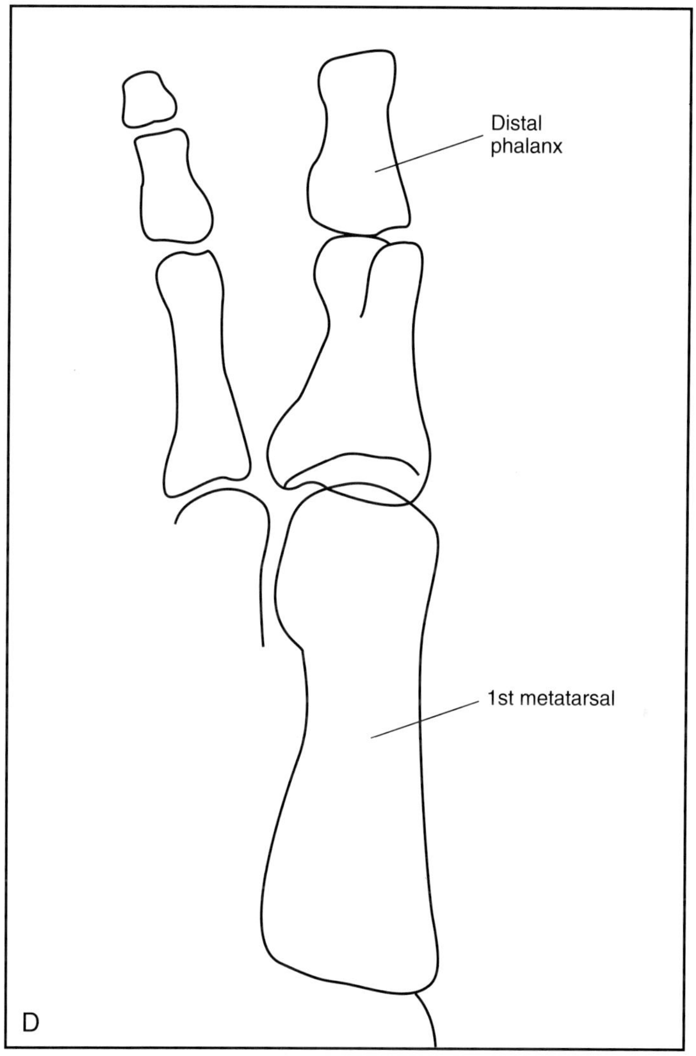

Figure 10.15 *(Continued)* C and D, AP oblique 1st toe.

Toes

Position/Projection

Plantodorsal oblique (PA) projection

Film Size:
8 × 10 inches (20 × 24 cm)
crosswise or lengthwise
tabletop
Divide cassette in halves or thirds

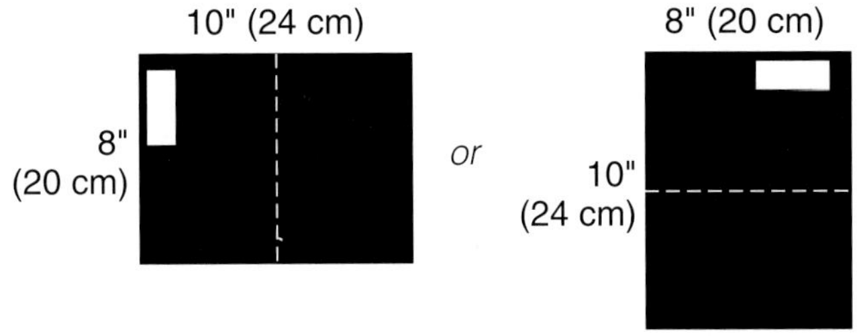

Patient Position

Prone, rotate laterally toward affected foot (Fig. 10.16).

Part Position

Align cassette with long axis of foot. Rotate patient laterally to place plantar surface of foot 30° to plane of cassette.

Central Ray

Perpendicular to 3rd metatarsophalangeal joint or to metatarsophalangeal joint of affected toe.

Structures Demonstrated

PA oblique projection of phalanges, interphalangeal joints, metatarsophalangeal joints, and distal end of metatarsals (Fig. 10.17).

Evaluation Criteria

1. Phalanx or phalanges should be seen with no overlapping.
2. Distal end of metatarsals should be oblique.
3. Joint spaces of 2nd through 5th metatarsophalangeals should be open (sometimes not completely open).

NOTE: Some departments require all toes to be included on the radiograph—center at the 3rd metatarsophalangeal joint. Some departments require just the affected toe on the radiograph—center at the metatarsophalangeal joint of the affected toe. This projection is seldom performed owing to patient discomfort.

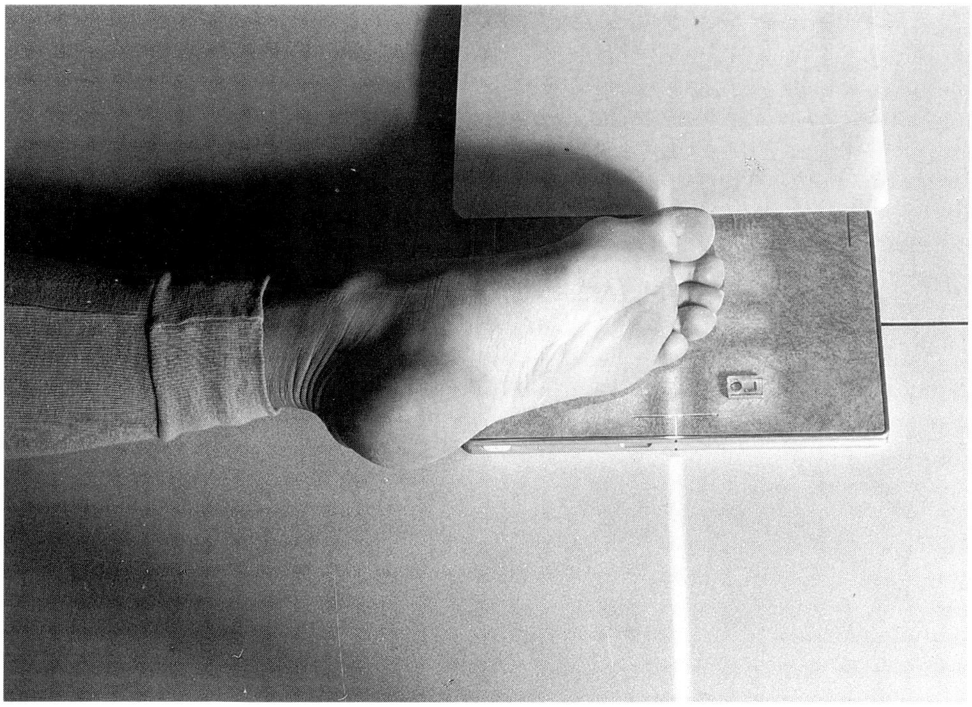

Figure 10.16. PA oblique toes.

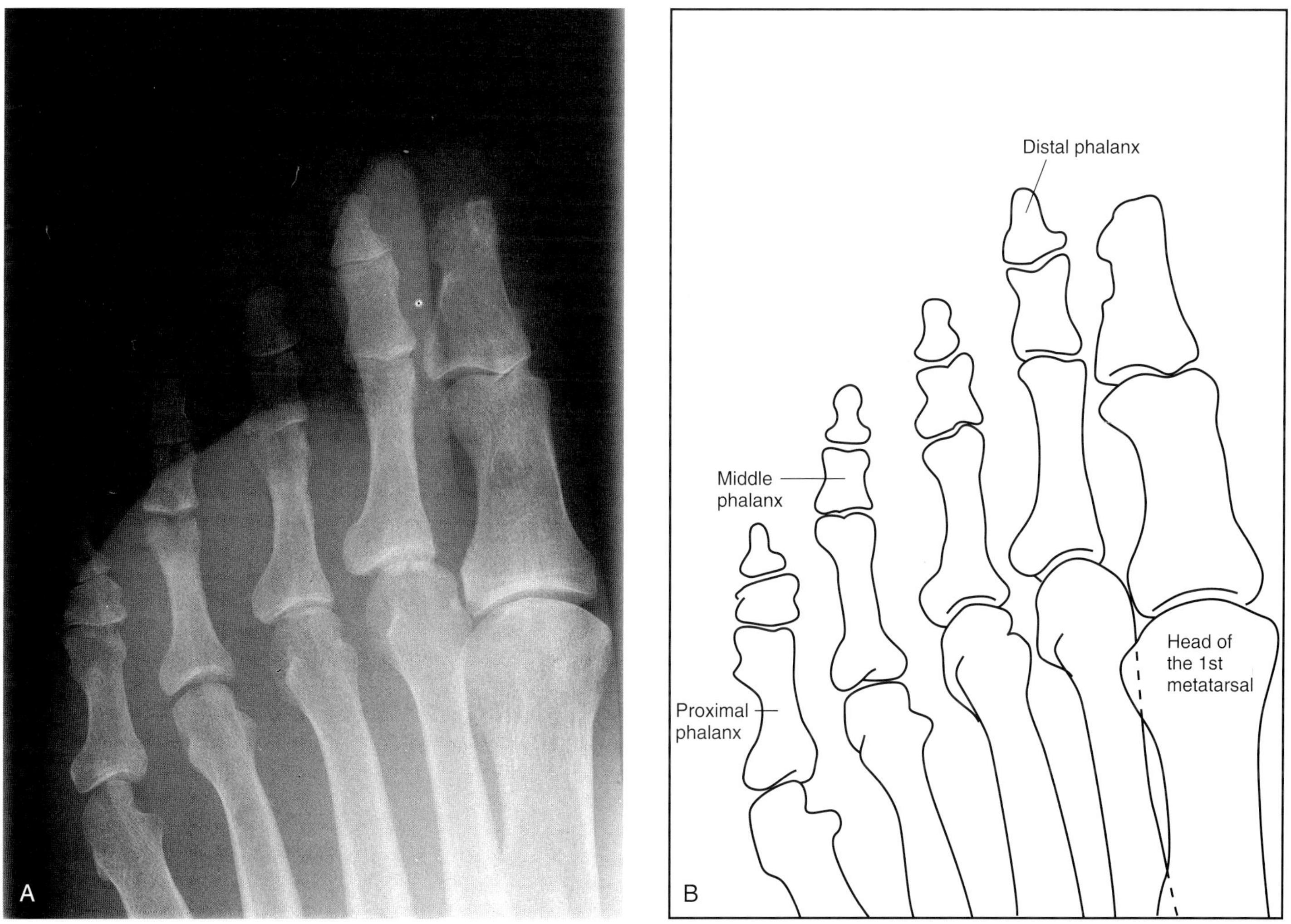

Figure 10.17. A and B, PA oblique toes.

Toes

Position/Projection

Lateral projection

Film Size:
8 × 10 inches (20 × 24 cm)
crosswise or lengthwise
tabletop
Divide cassette in halves or
thirds

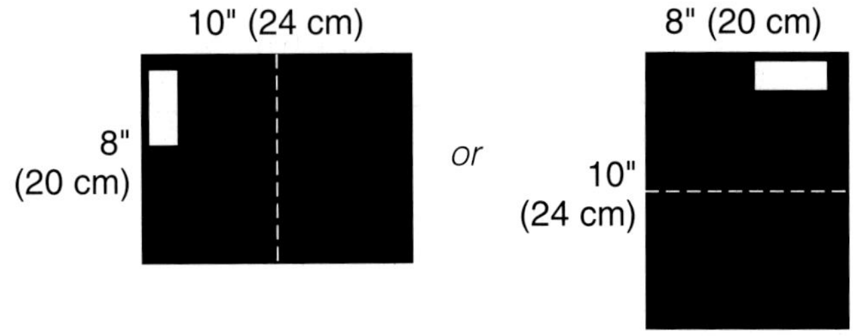

Patient Position

Lateral recumbent position, either lateral can be done, but if possible, place affected toe closest to cassette.

Part Position

Align long axis of toes to unmasked portion of cassette. Place plantar surface perpendicular to plane of cassette.

For Great Toe
Place toe in true lateral position and center interphalangeal joint to midpoint of unmasked portion of cassette (Figs. 10.18 and 10.19).

For 2nd Through 5th Toes
Place toe in true lateral position and center proximal interphalangeal joint to midpoint of unmasked portion of cassette (Figs. 10.20 to 10.23).

Use tape or gauze to place toes above and below toe in question in flexed position to prevent superimposition.

Central Ray

Perpendicular to interphalangeal joint of great toe or perpendicular to proximal interphalangeal joint of 2nd through 5th toes.

Structures Demonstrated

Presents lateral projection of phalanges and interphalangeal joints (see Fig. 10.19).

Evaluation Criteria

1. Affected phalanx should be free of superimposition.
2. Phalanx should be in true lateral position.
3. Interphalangeal joint spaces should be open.
4. Metatarsophalangeal joint spaces should be open.

NOTE: Some departments require all toes to be included on the radiograph—center at the 3rd metatarsophalangeal joint. Some departments require just the affected toe on the radiograph—center at the metatarsophalangeal joint of the affected toe.

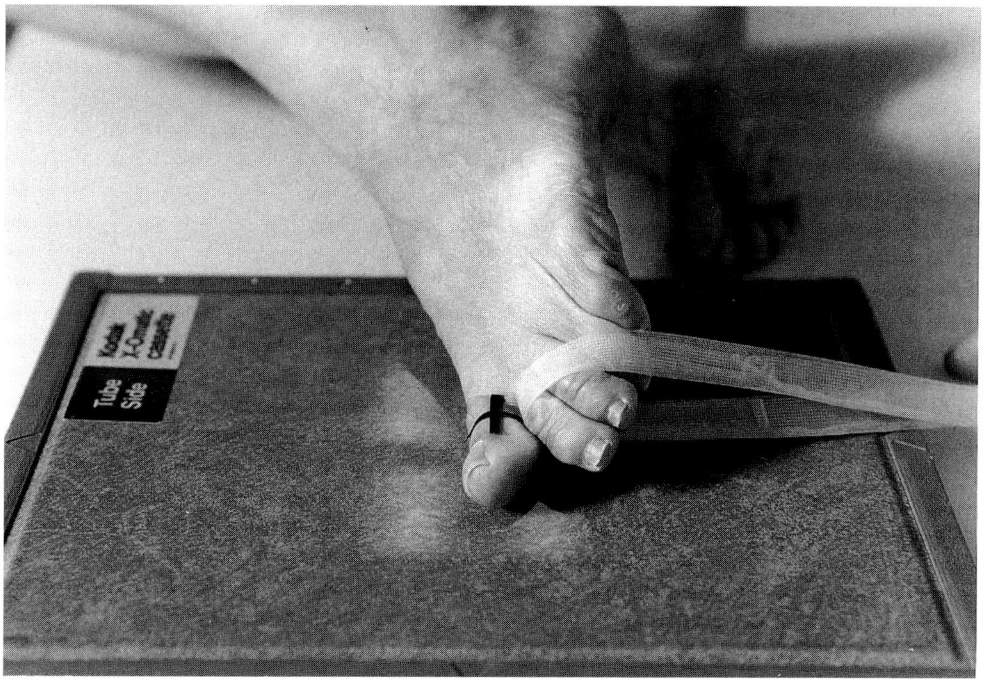

Figure 10.18. Lateral 1st toe.

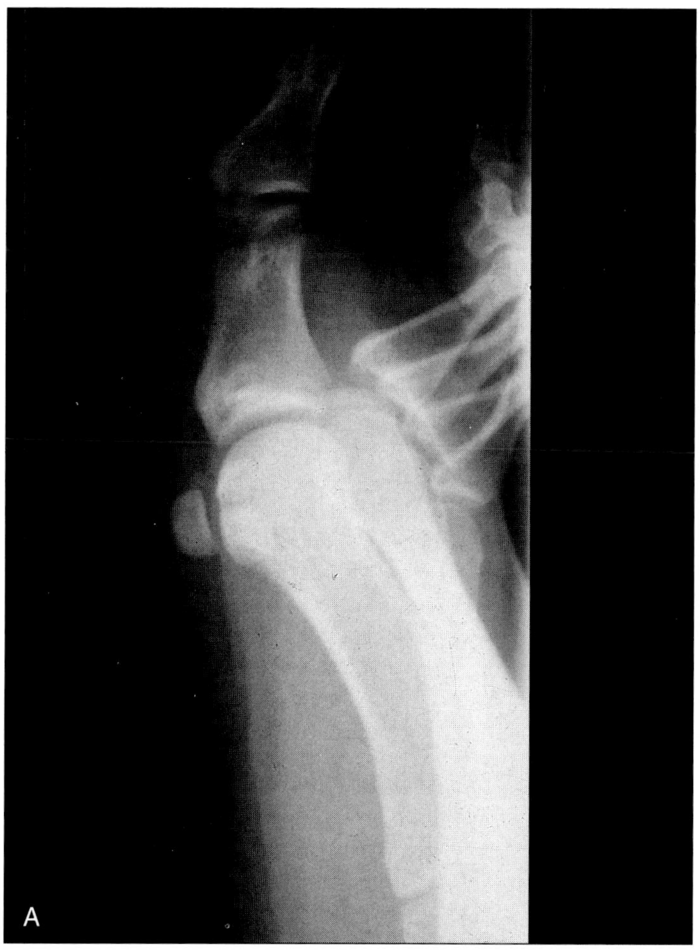

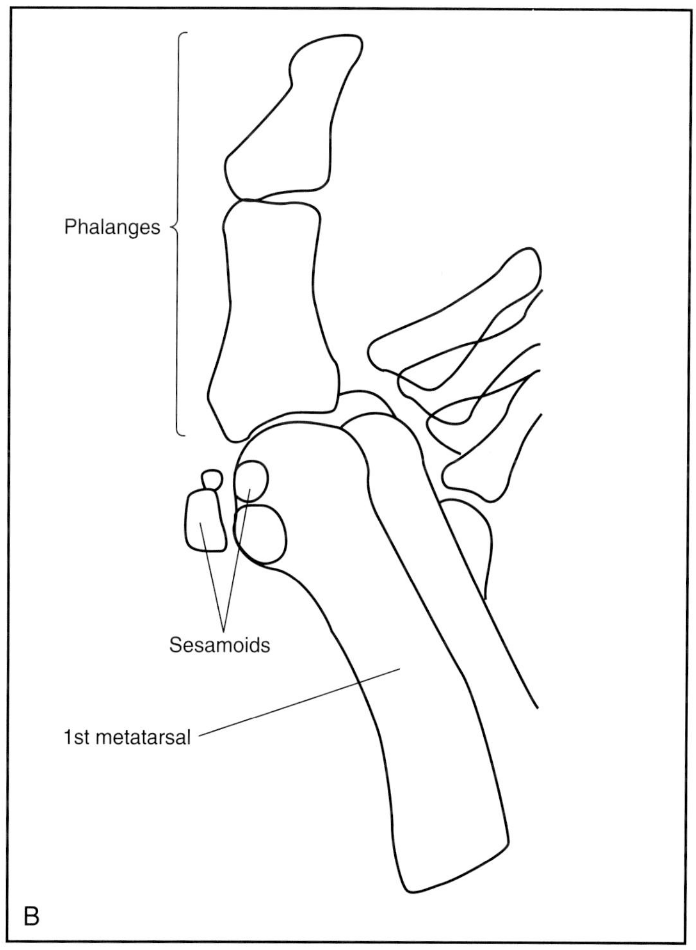

Figure 10.19. A and B, Lateral 1st toe.

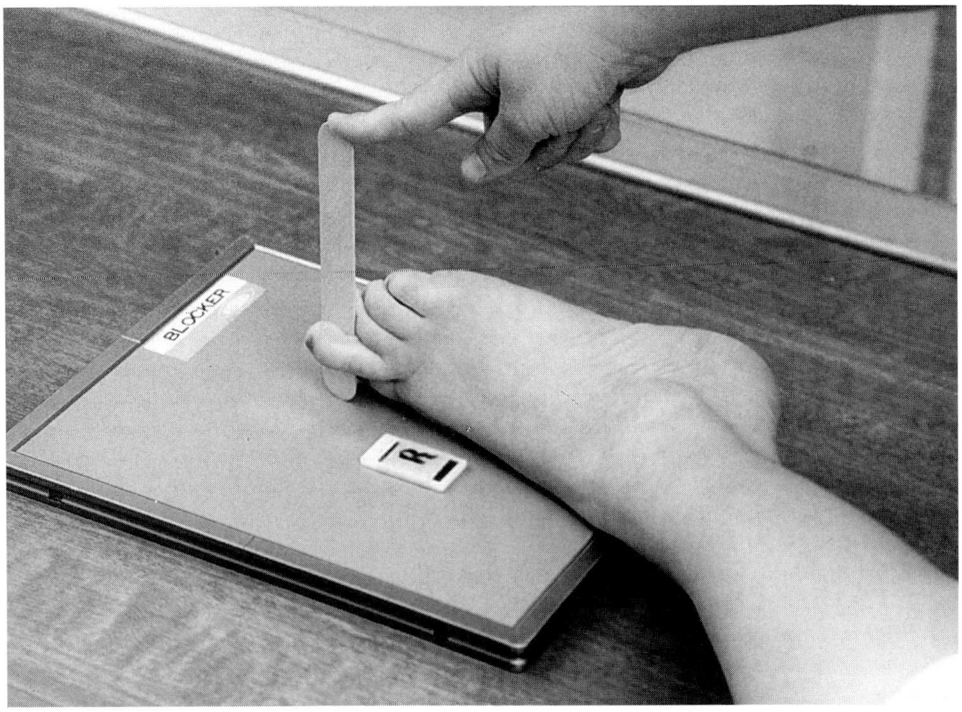

Figure 10.20. Lateral 2nd toe.

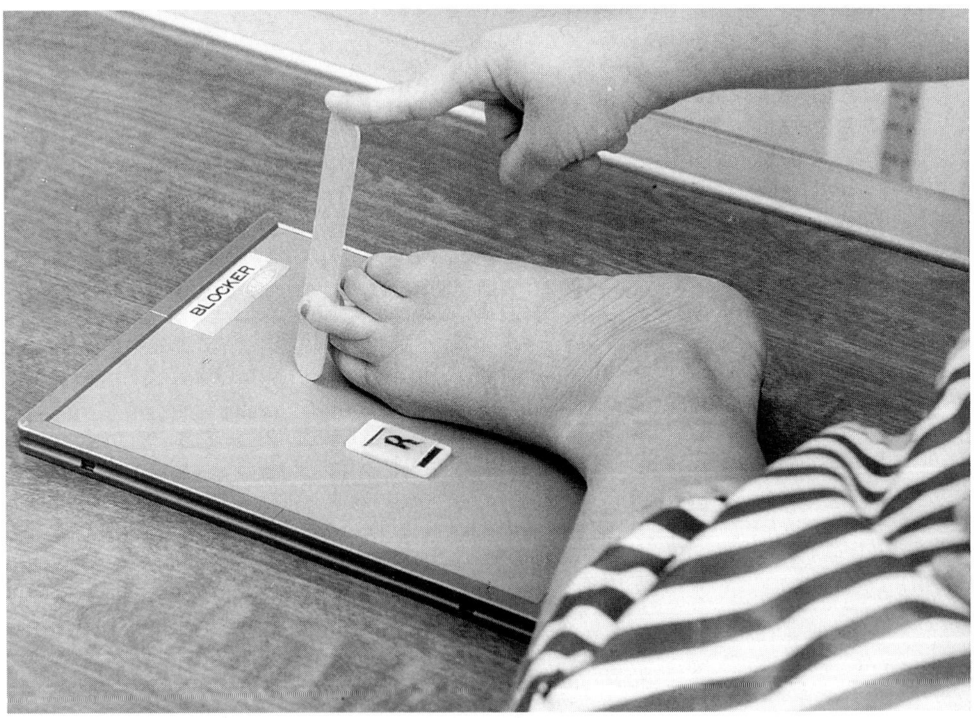

Figure 10.21. Lateral 3rd toe.

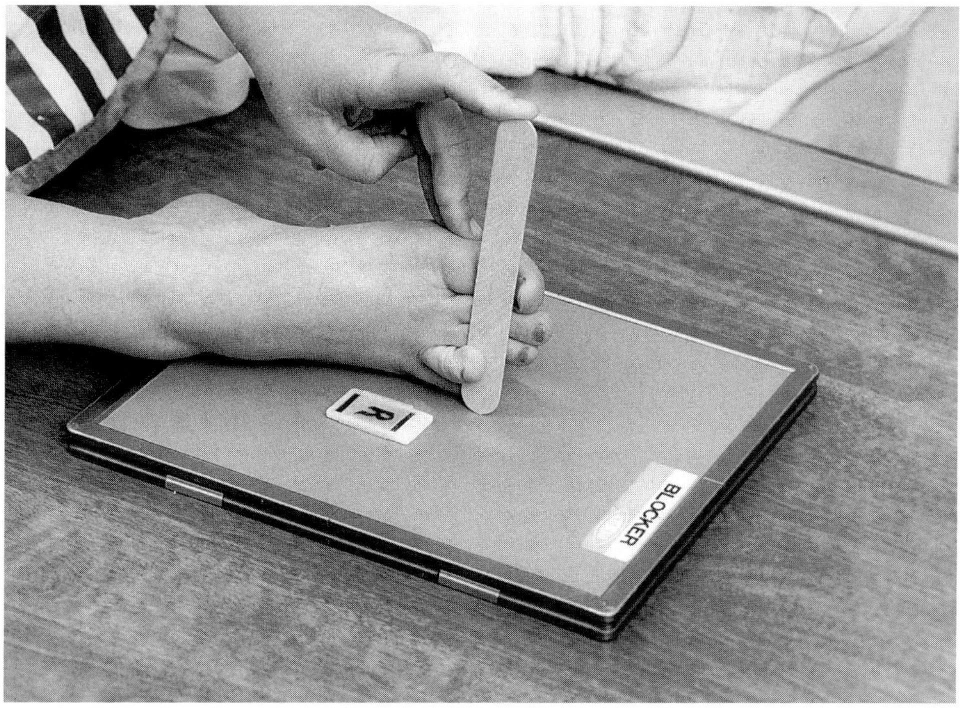

Figure 10.22. Lateral 4th toe.

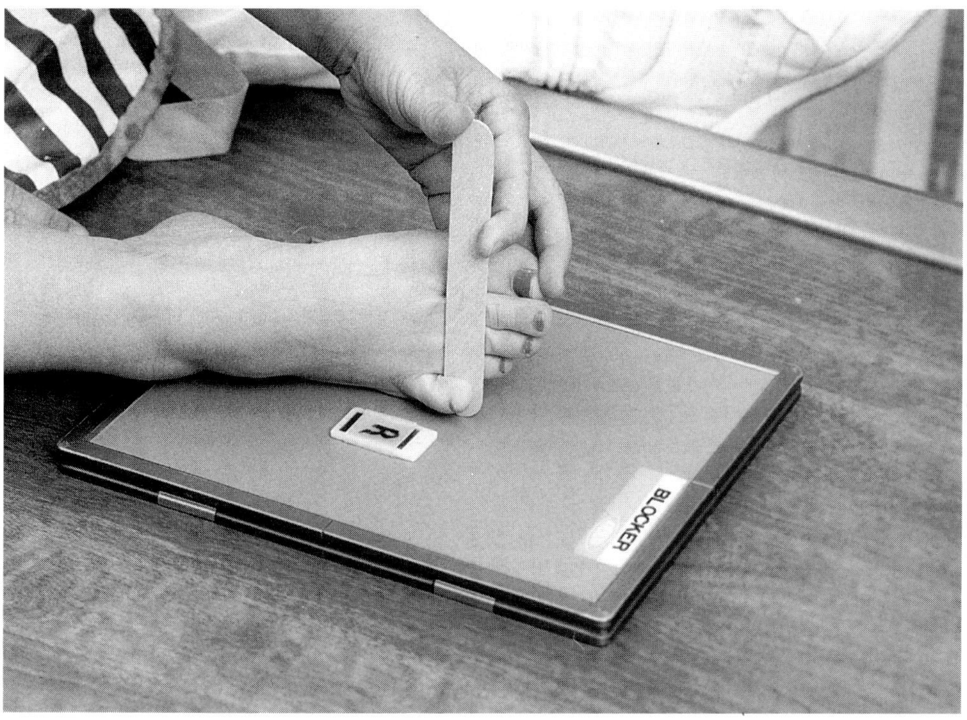

Figure 10.23. Lateral 5th toe.

Sesamoids (Metatarsophalangeal)

Position/Projection

Tangential projection—Lewis' method

Film Size:
8 × 10 inches (20 × 24 cm)
lengthwise or crosswise
tabletop

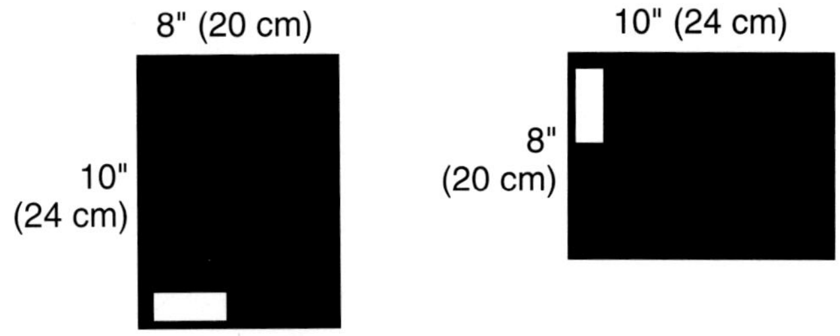

Patient Position

Prone (Fig. 10.24).

Part Position

Align long axis of leg to cassette. Extend leg of affected foot. Rest foot on dorsiflexed 1st toe to place ball of foot perpendicular to plane of cassette. Center distal end of 2nd metatarsal to midpoint of cassette.

NOTE: This position is very uncomfortable and difficult to maintain.

Central Ray

Perpendicular to distal end (head) of 2nd metatarsal.

Structures Demonstrated

Tangential projection of metatarsal heads and sesamoids (Fig. 10.25).

Evaluation Criteria

1. Sesamoid projected free of superimposition of any portion of 1st metatarsal.
2. All five metatarsal heads (distal end) should be seen.

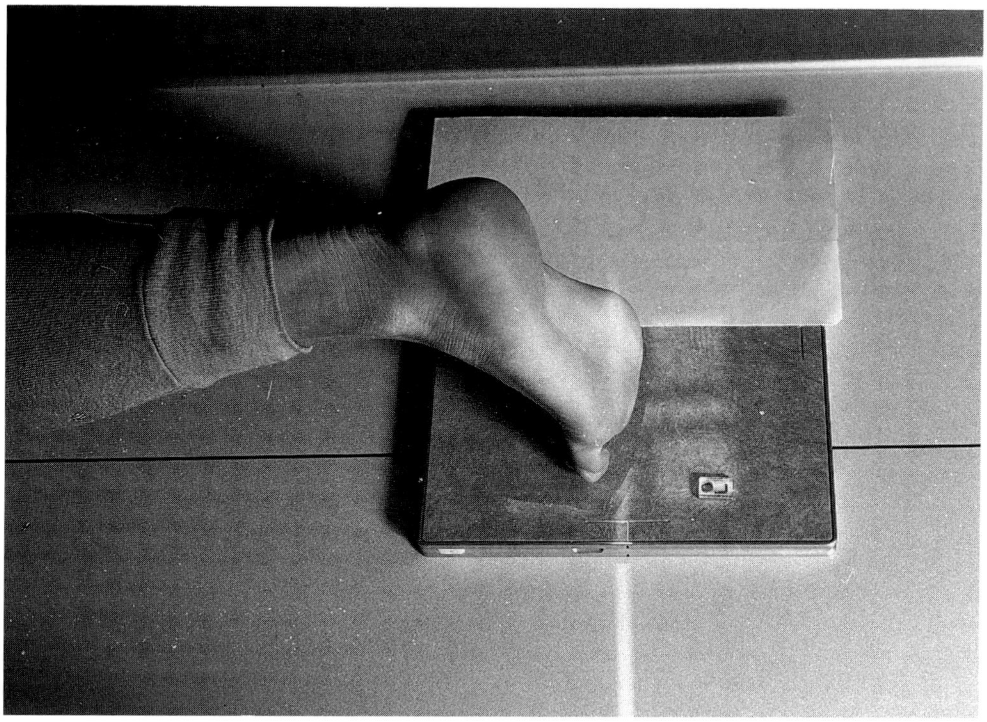

Figure 10.24. Sesamoids, tangential projection.

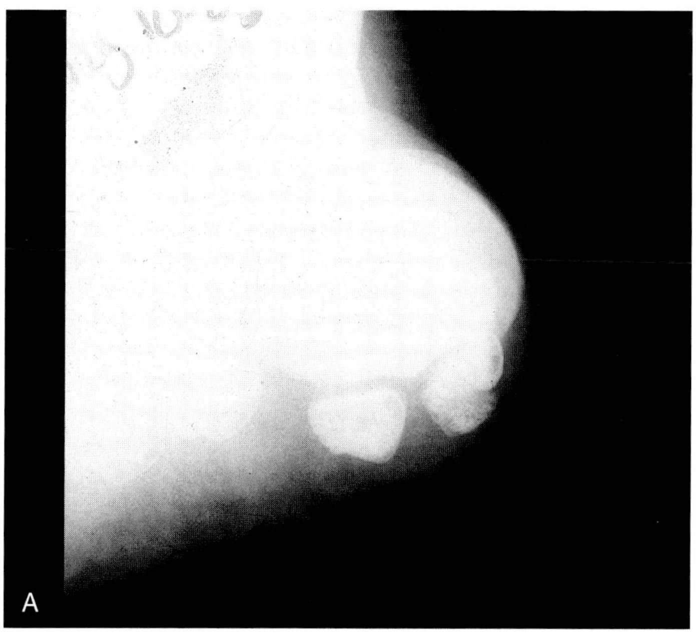

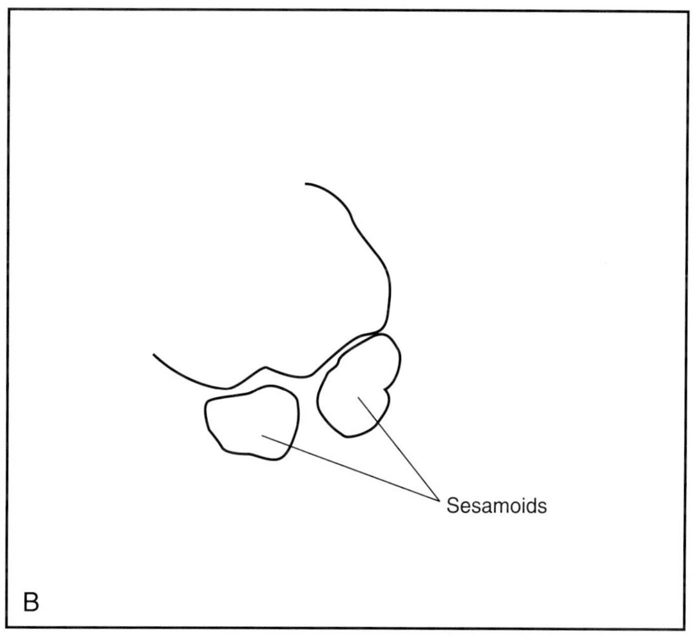

Figure 10.25. A and B, Sesamoids, tangential projection.

Sesamoids (Metatarsophalangeal)

Position/Projection

Lateromedial tangential projection—Causton's method

Film Size:
8 × 10 inches (20 × 24 cm)
crosswise or lengthwise
tabletop

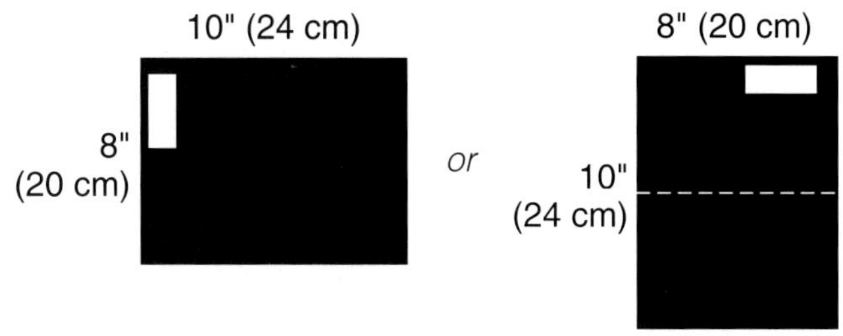

Patient Position

Lateral recumbent turned toward unaffected side with knee flexed (Fig. 10.26).

Part Position

Affected foot in lateral position. Center lower metatarsal region to midpoint of unmasked portion of cassette.

Central Ray

40° cephalic angle toward heel to enter 1st metatarsophalangeal joint.

Structures Demonstrated

Tangential projection of 1st metatarsophalangeal sesamoids (Fig. 10.27).

Evaluation Criteria

Sesamoids projected with no overlapping.

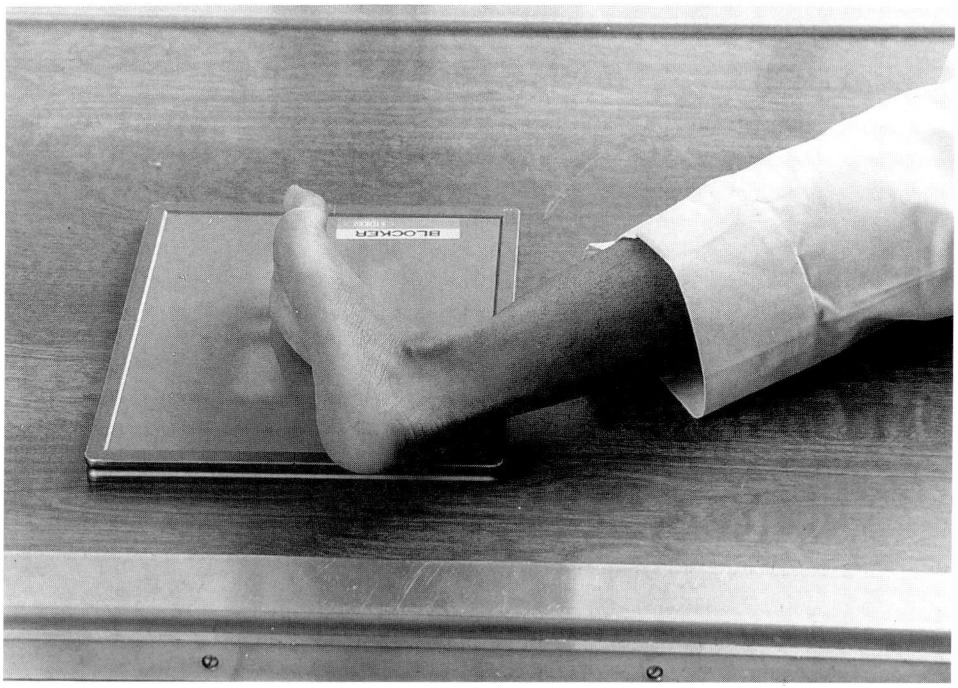

Figure 10.26. Sesamoids, lateromedial tangential projection.

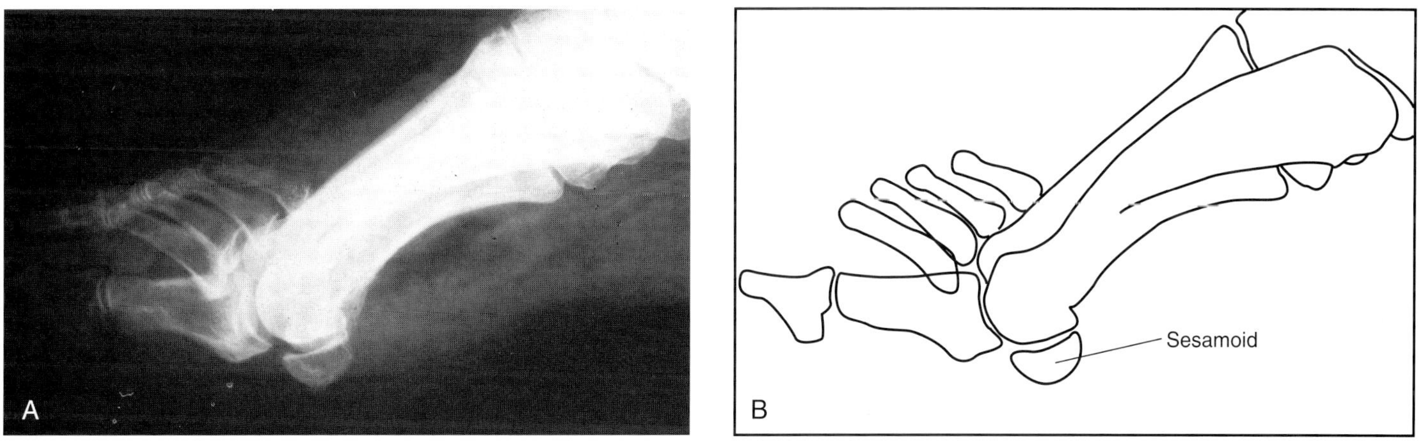

Figure 10.27. A and B, Sesamoids, lateromedial projection.

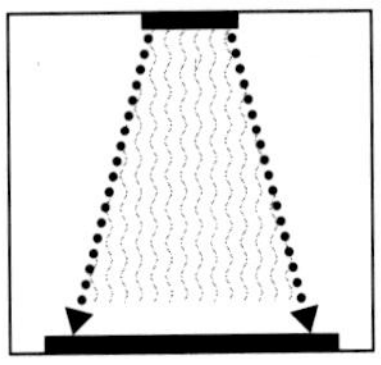

Foot

Position/Projection

Dorsoplantar (AP) projection

Film Size:
10 × 12 inches (24 × 30 cm) lengthwise tabletop
Divide cassette in half
Cassette needs to be at least 2 inches (5 cm) longer than foot

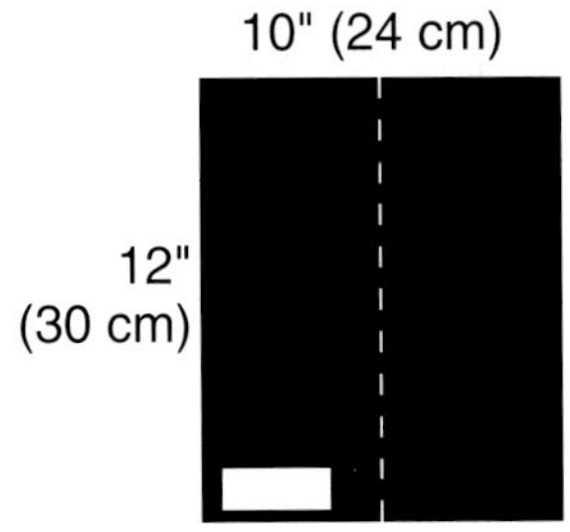

Patient Position

Supine or sitting with knee of affected foot flexed and plantar surface of foot resting flat on cassette (Fig. 10.28).

Part Position

Adjust position of foot so that its longitudinal plane coincides with long axis of unmasked half of cassette. Center base of 3rd metatarsal to midpoint of unmasked half of cassette.

Central Ray

Perpendicular to midpoint of cassette through base of 3rd metatarsal.

Structures Demonstrated

Tarsal anterior to talus, metatarsals, and phalanges (Fig. 10.29).

Evaluation Criteria

1. Foot should be seen without rotation (indicated by equal distance between adjacent midshafts of 2nd through 5th metatarsals) from distal phalanges of toes through tarsal.
2. Visualization of phalanges, tarsal distal to talus, metatarsals, cuneiforms, cuboid, and navicular.

NOTE: If the metatarsals are of primary interest, angle the central ray 10° cephalad (may vary 5° to 15°) to place it perpendicular to their plane rather than to the plane of the cassette. Remember to demonstrate the same anatomic parts at the same end of the film.

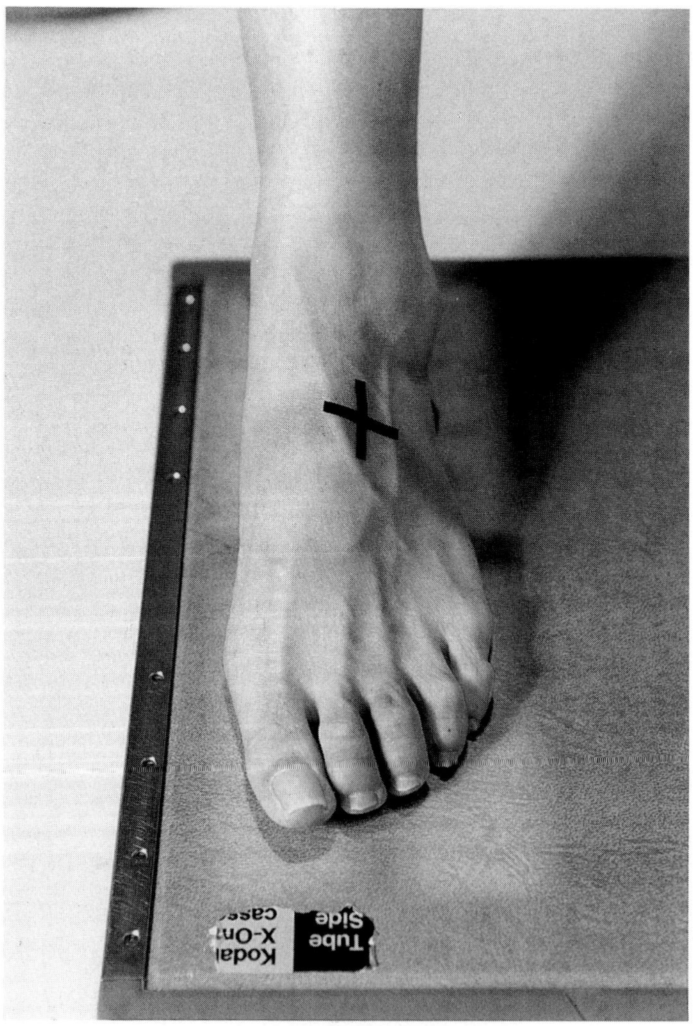

Figure 10.28. AP foot, dorsoplantar projection.

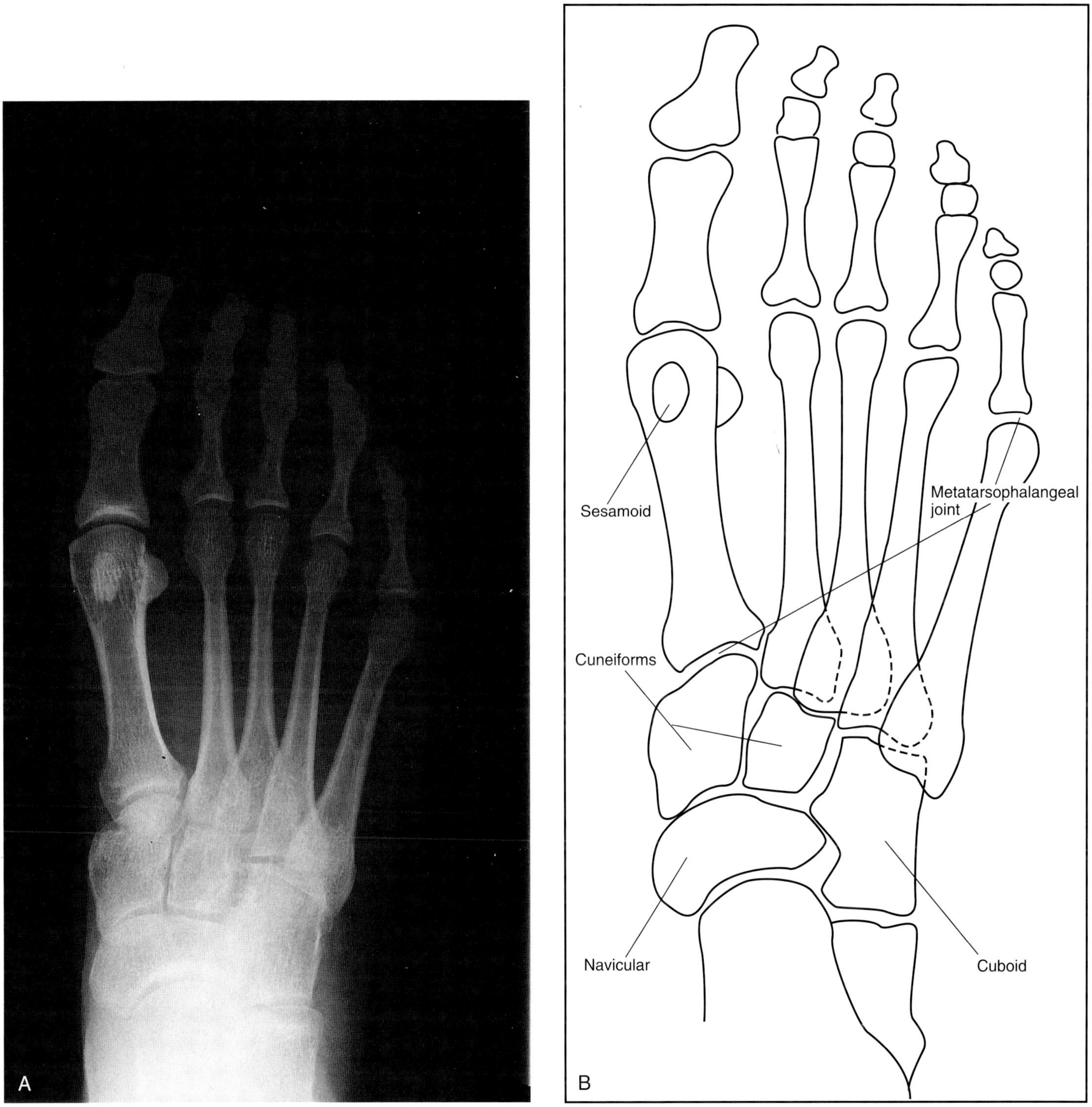

Figure 10.29. A and B, AP foot.

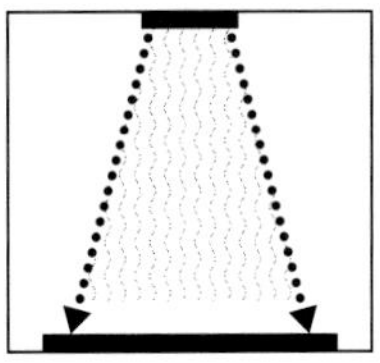

Foot

Position/Projection

Medial oblique projection

Film Size:
10 × 12 inches (24 × 30 cm) lengthwise tabletop
Divide cassette in half
Cassette needs to be at least 2 inches (5 cm) longer than foot

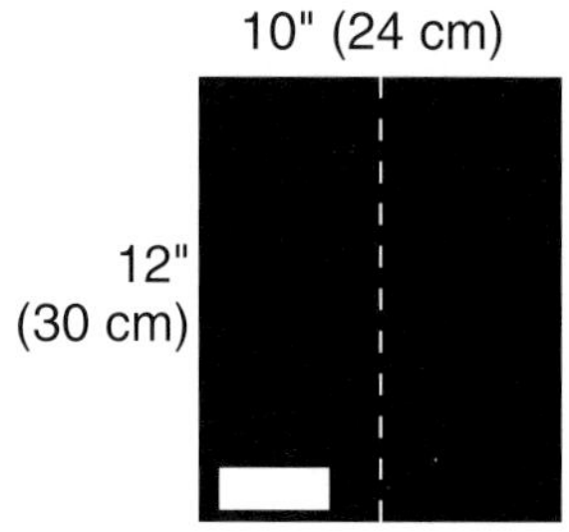

Patient Position

Supine or sitting; rotate affected leg medially until sole of foot forms 30° angle to cassette (Fig. 10.30).

Part Position

Align long axis of cassette with long axis of foot. Center midpoint of foot at level of base of 5th metatarsal to midpoint of cassette.

Central Ray

Perpendicular to base of 3rd metatarsal.

Structures Demonstrated

Interspaces between cuboid and calcaneus, between cuboid and 4th and 5th metatarsals, between cuboid and 3rd cuneiform, and between talus and navicular (Fig. 10.31).

Evaluation Criteria

1. Distal phalanges of toes through tarsal should be visualized.
2. 3rd through 5th metatarsal bases should be free of superimposition.
3. 1st and 2nd metatarsals partially superimposed.
4. Equal space between shafts of 2nd through 5th metatarsals.
5. Sinus tarsi should be seen.
6. Tarsometatarsal and intertarsal joints should be seen.

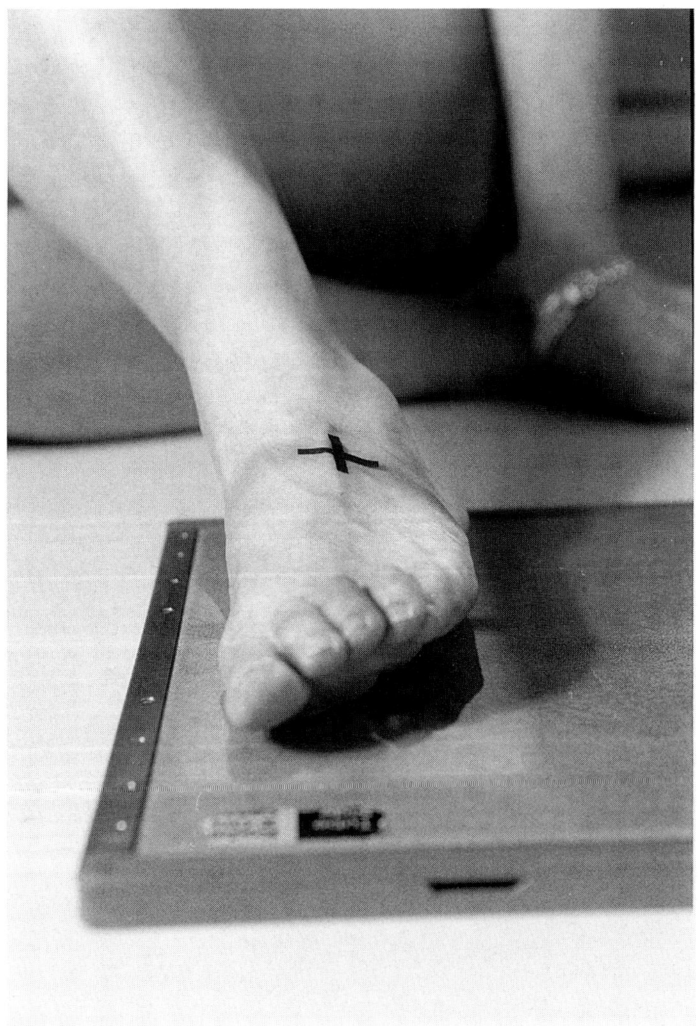

Figure 10.30. Medial oblique foot.

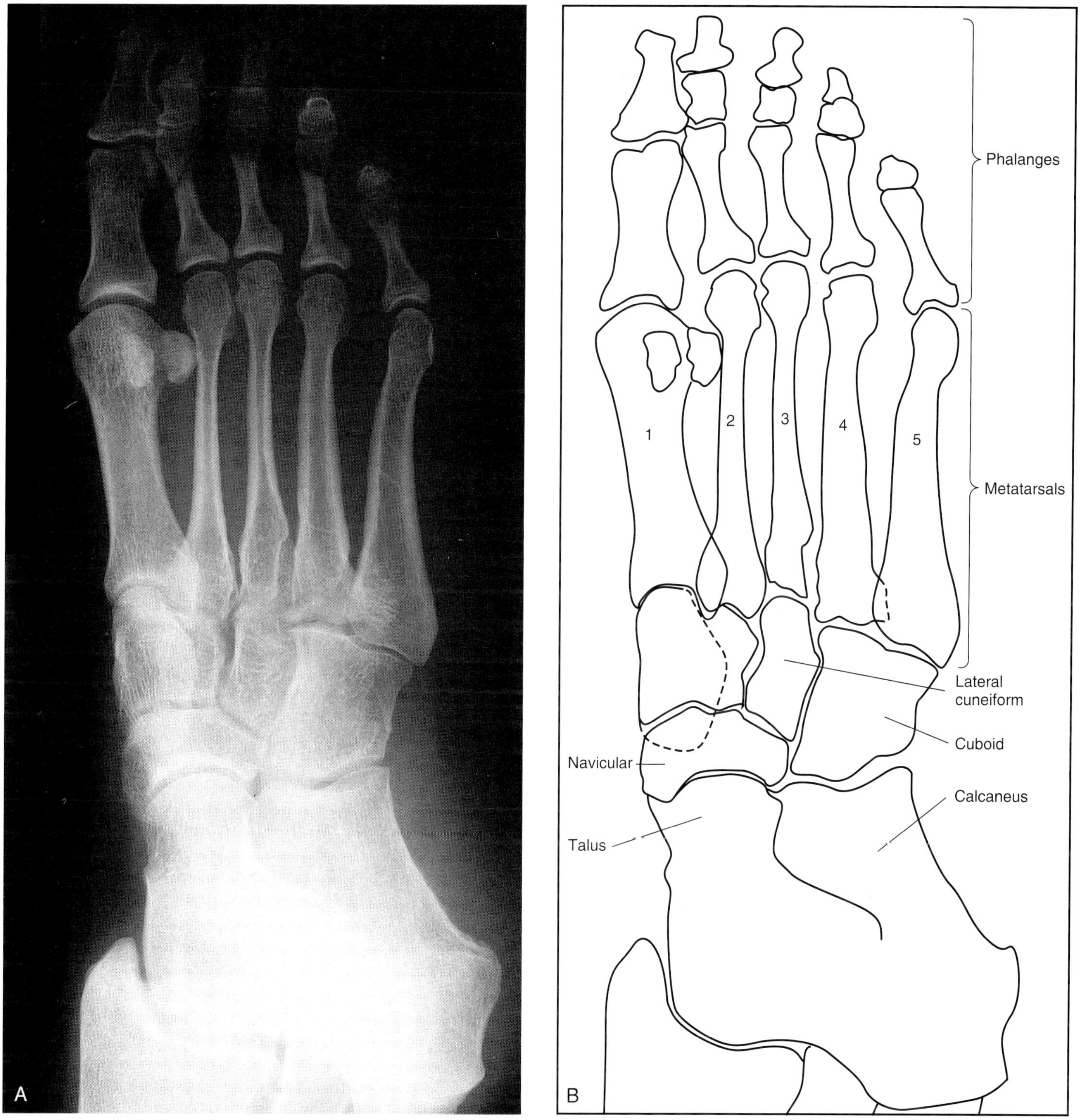

Figure 10.31. A and B, Medial oblique foot.

Foot

Position/Projection

Lateral oblique projection

Film Size:
10 × 12 inches (24 × 30 cm)
lengthwise tabletop
Divide cassette in half
Cassette needs to be at least 2 inches (5 cm) longer than foot

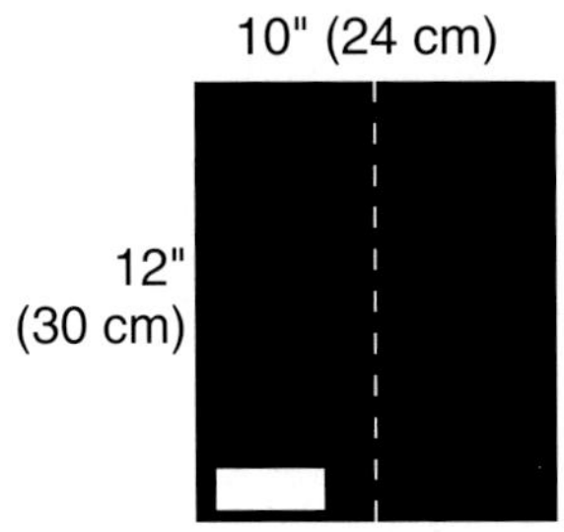

Patient Position

Supine or sitting; rotate affected leg laterally until foot is rotated 30° laterally (Fig. 10.32).

Part Position

Align long axis of cassette with long axis of foot. Center midpoint of foot at level of base of 5th metatarsal to midpoint of cassette. Rotate foot and leg laterally until plantar surface of foot forms an angle of 30° with film plane.

Central Ray

Perpendicular to base of 3rd metatarsal.

Structures Demonstrated

Interspaces between 1st and 2nd metatarsals. Interspaces between 1st and 2nd cuneiforms (Fig. 10.33).

Evaluation Criteria

1. 1st and 2nd cuneiforms not superimposed.
2. No overlapping of 1st and 2nd metatarsal bases.
3. Navicular demonstrated more clearly in this projection.
4. Demonstration of phalanges, metatarsals, and tarsal.

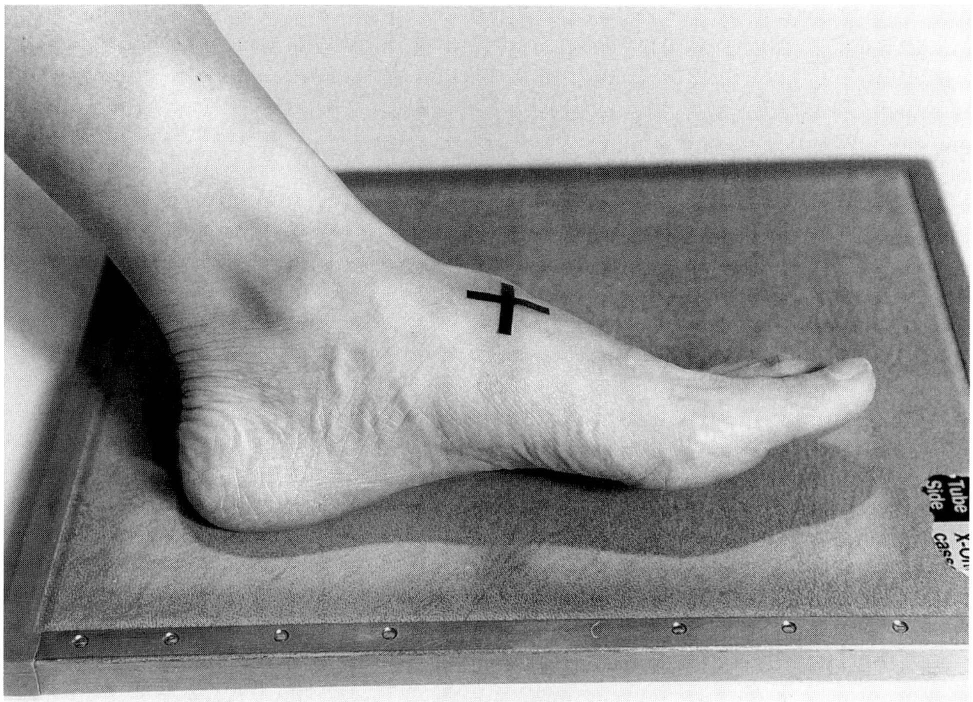

Figure 10.32. Lateral oblique foot.

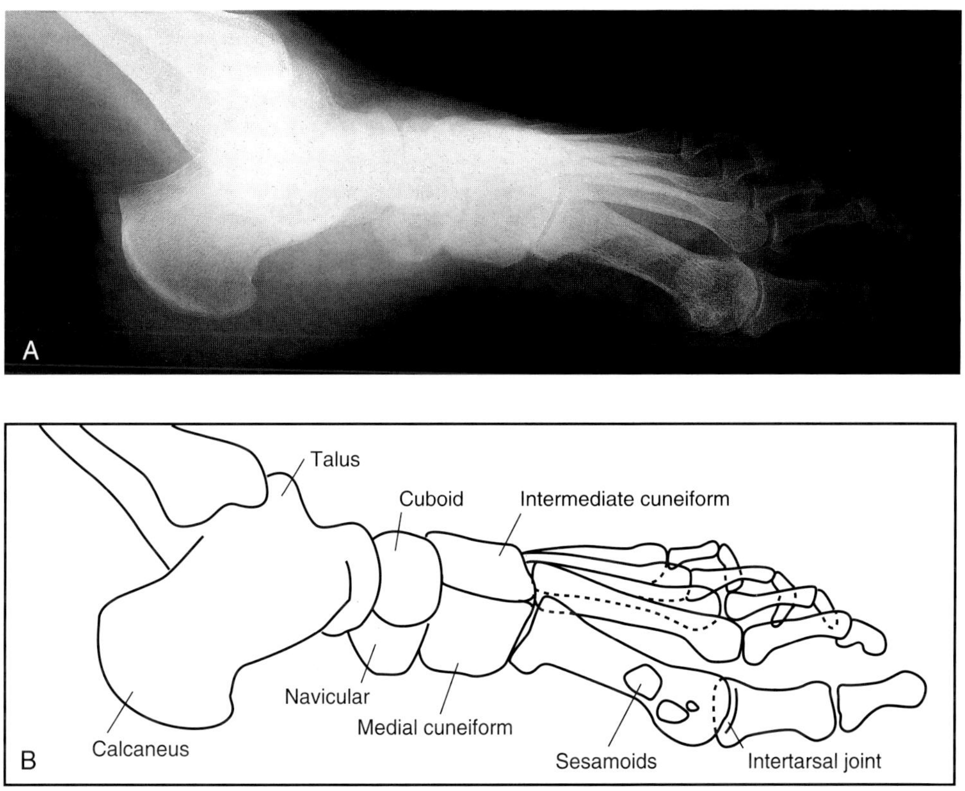

Figure 10.33. A and B, Lateral oblique foot.

Foot

Position/Projection

Lateromedial projection

Film Size:
10 × 12 inches (24 × 30 cm) lengthwise tabletop
Divide cassette in half
Cassette needs to be at least 2 inches (5 cm) longer than foot

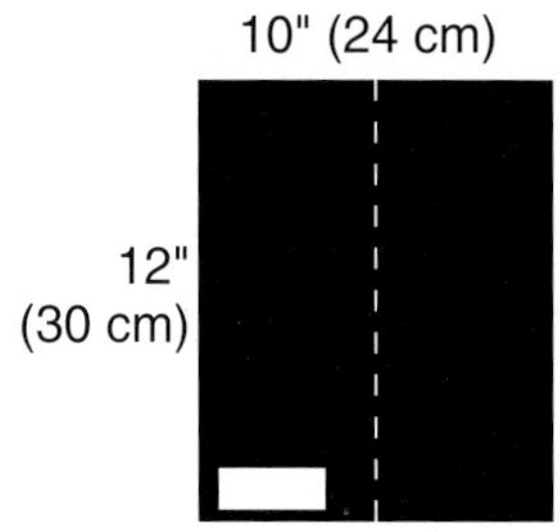

Patient Position

Supine; turn patient away from affected side until leg and foot are laterally placed (Fig. 10.34).

Part Position

Place plantar surface of foot perpendicular to cassette. Adjust foot to place its longitudinal plane parallel with plane of cassette. Place support under knee to position patella perpendicular to table.

Central Ray

Perpendicular to midpoint of cassette through bases of metatarsals (approximate center of foot).

Structures Demonstrated

True lateral projection of foot, ankle joint, and distal ends of tibia and fibula (Fig. 10.35).

Evaluation Critera

1. Distal phalanges of toes to calcaneus and distal tibia and fibula should be seen.
2. Phalanges superimposed.
3. Metatarsals superimposed.
4. Tibia superimposed over fibula.

NOTE: This projection is seldom performed owing to patient discomfort. To include the entire foot, the cassette may have to be turned diagonally to place the long axis of the foot across the diagonal length of the cassette.

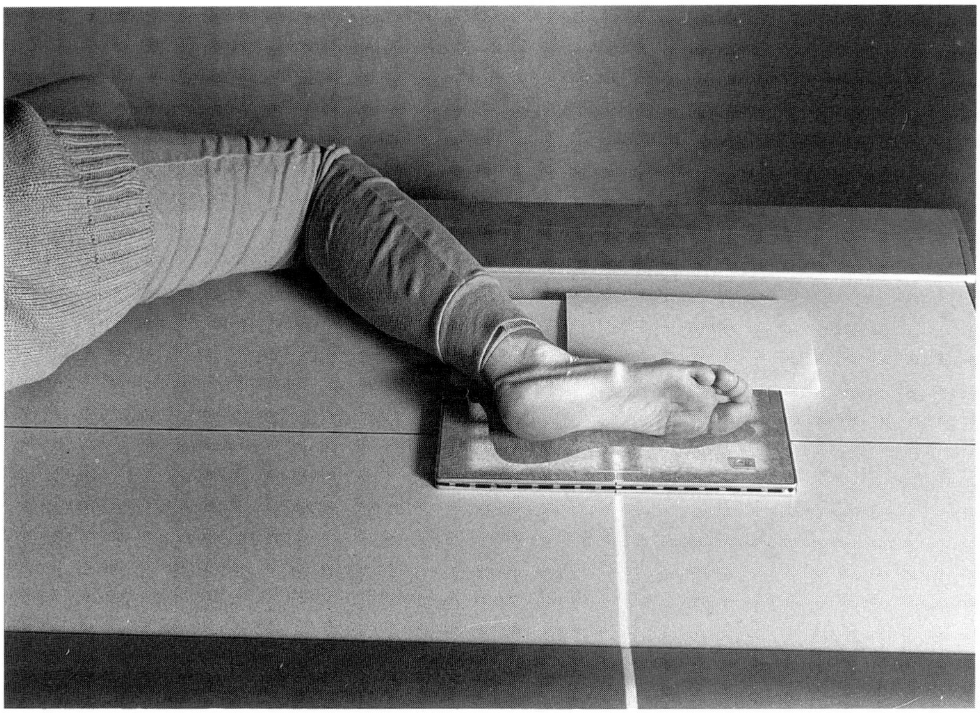

Figure 10.34. Lateromedial foot.

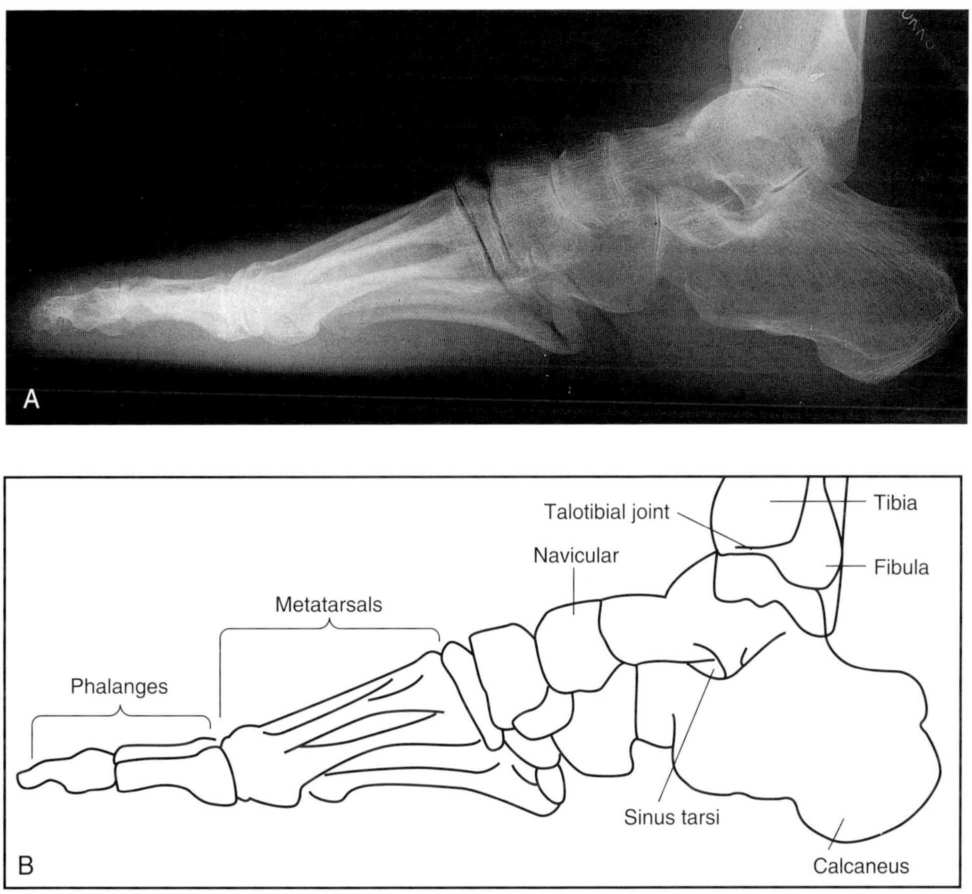

Figure 10.35. A and B, Lateromedial foot.

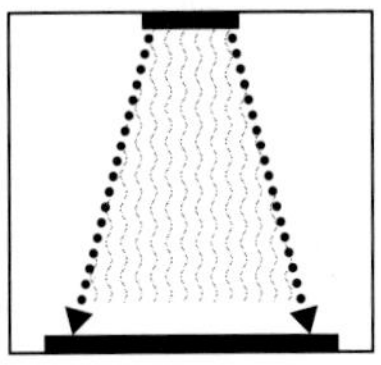

Foot

Position/Projection

Mediolateral projection

Film Size:
10 × 12 inches (24 × 30 cm) lengthwise tabletop
Divide cassette in half
Cassette needs to be at least 2 inches (5 cm) longer than foot

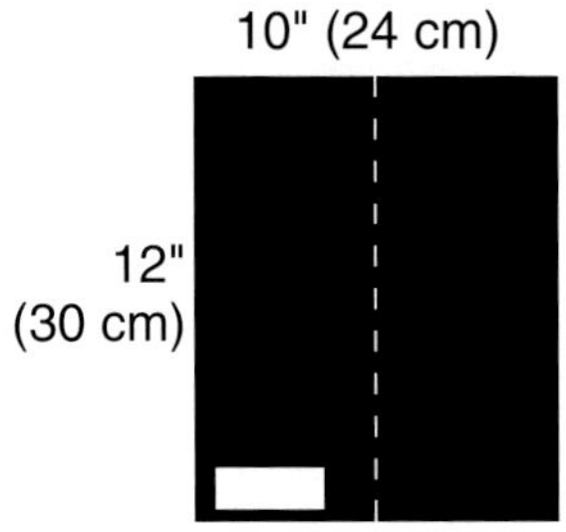

Patient Position

Supine; turn patient toward affected side and rotate body until foot is in lateral profile position (Fig. 10.36).

Part Position

Place plantar surface of foot perpendicular to cassette. Adjust foot to place its longitudinal plane parallel with plane of cassette. Place support under knee to place patella perpendicular to table.

Central Ray

Perpendicular to midpoint of cassette through bases of metatarsals (approximately center of foot).

Structures Demonstrated

Lateral projection of foot, ankle joint, and distal ends of tibia and fibula (Fig. 10.37).

Evaluation Criteria

1. Distal phalanges of toes to calcaneus and distal tibia and fibula should be seen.
2. Phalanges superimposed.
3. Metatarsals superimposed.
4. Tibia superimposed over fibula.

NOTE: This projection is normally performed for patient comfort. To include the entire foot, the cassette may have to be turned diagonally to place the long axis of the foot across the diagonal length of the cassette.

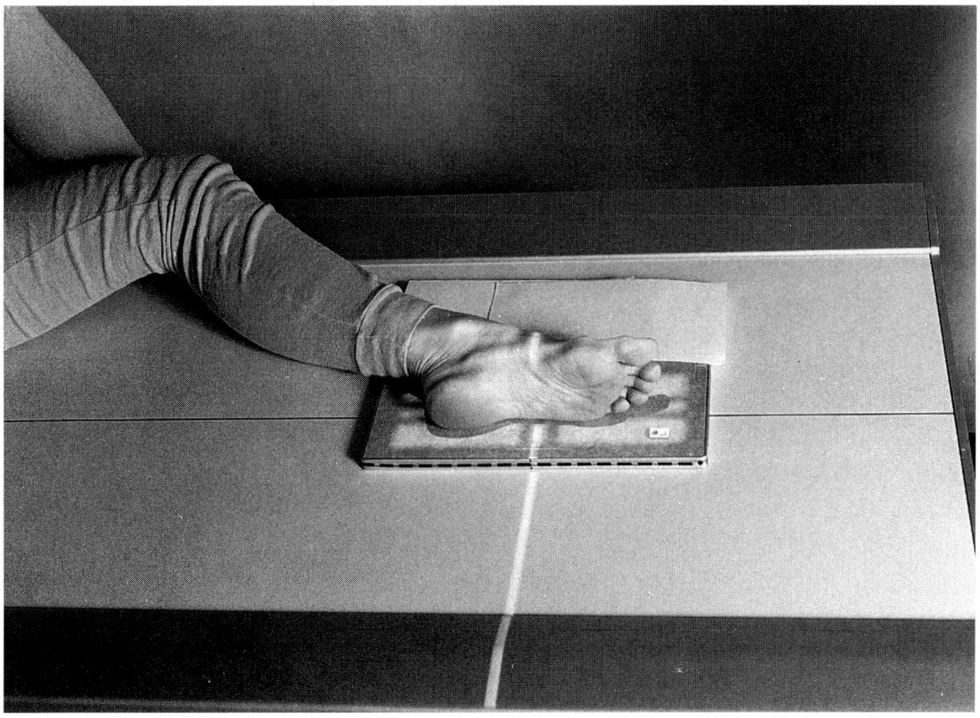

Figure 10.36. Mediolateral foot.

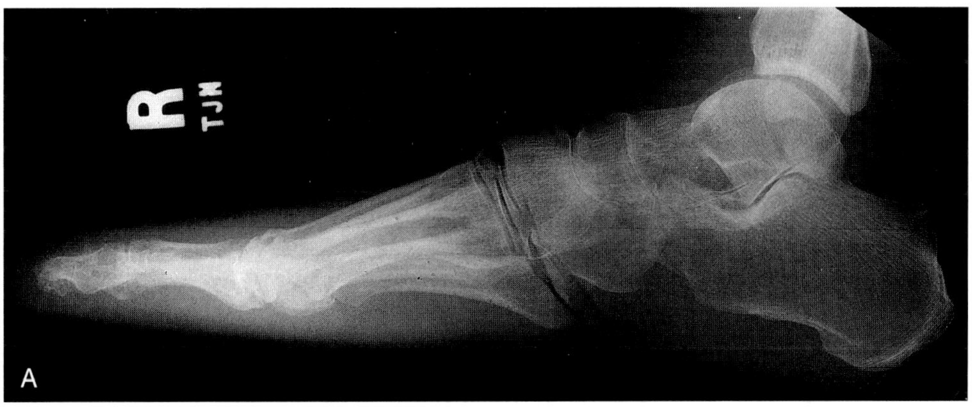

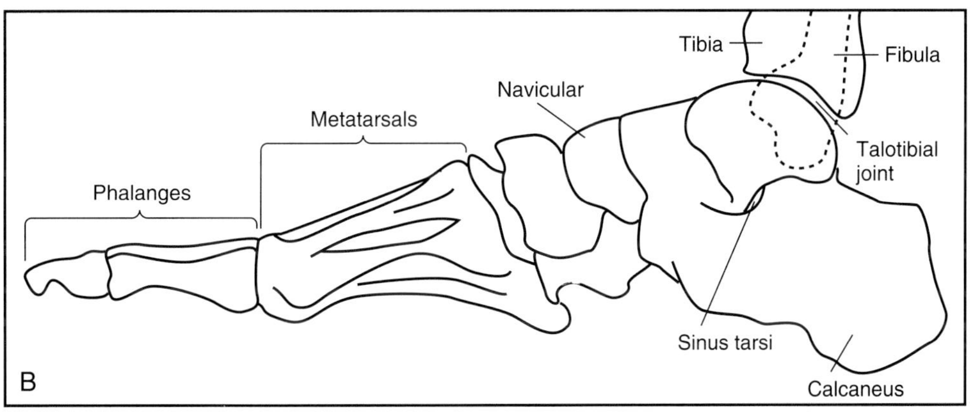

Figure 10.37. A and B, Mediolateral foot.

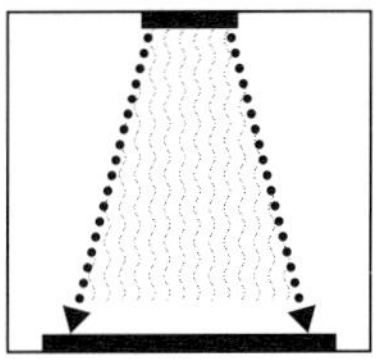

Foot

Position/Projection

Longitudinal arch lateral projection (weight-bearing position)

Film Size:
10 × 12 inches (24 × 30 cm) crosswise tabletop

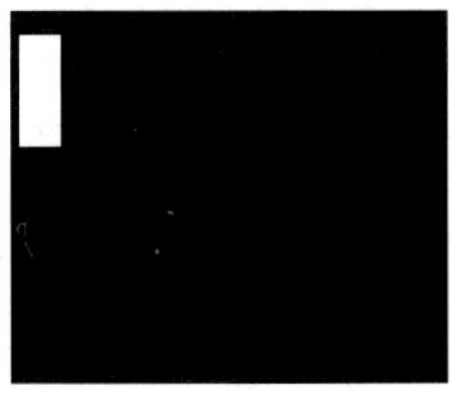

Patient Position

Erect, with weight distributed equally on both feet (Fig. 10.38).

Part Position

Place cassette between feet. Align long axis of foot to long axis of cassette. Cassette should be placed low enough to include plantar surface of foot. Base of metatarsals centered to cassette.

Central Ray

Horizontal beam perpendicular to bases of metatarsals.

Structures Demonstrated

Phalanges, metatarsals, tarsals, calcaneus, and distal ends of tibia and fibula (Fig. 10.39).

Evaluation Criteria

1. Entire foot should be seen. Phalanges should be superimposed. Metatarsals should be superimposed.
2. Distal tibia should be superimposed by distal fibula.
3. Longitudinal arch should be seen.

NOTE: This projection demonstrates the longitudinal arch or "fallen arches." It is usually necessary to stand the patient on blocks, a platform, or a footstool to demonstrate the entire foot, since most radiographic units do not go to the floor.

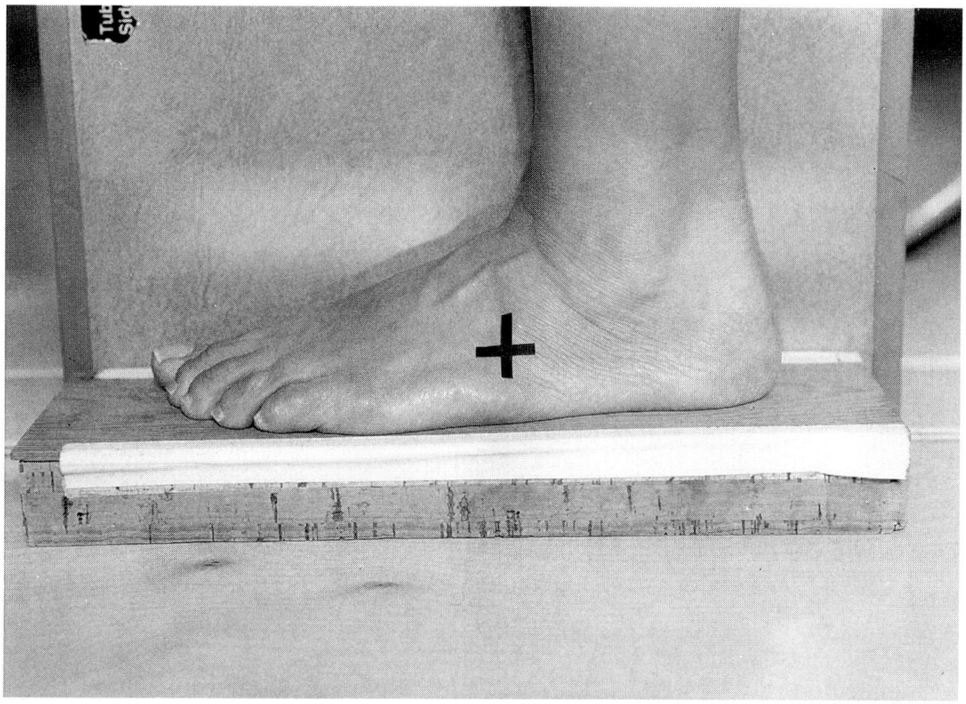

Figure 10.38. Longitudinal arch, weight-bearing.

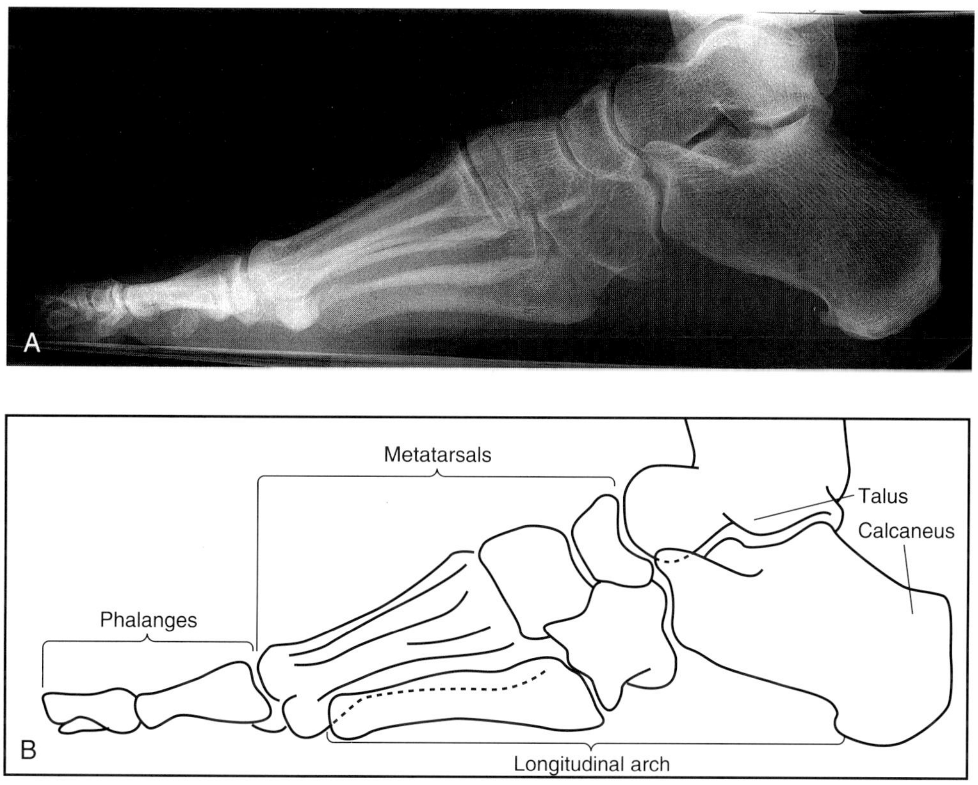

Figure 10.39. A and B, Longitudinal arch, lateral weight-bearing.

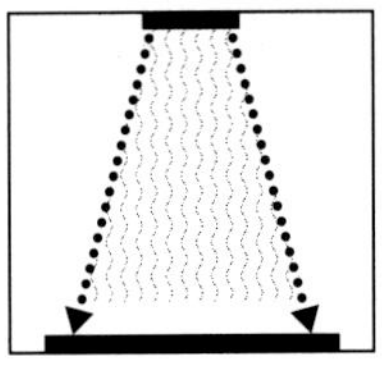

Foot

Position/Projection

Composite dorsoplantar projection (weight-bearing, axial projection)

Film Size:
10 × 12 inches (24 × 30 cm) lengthwise

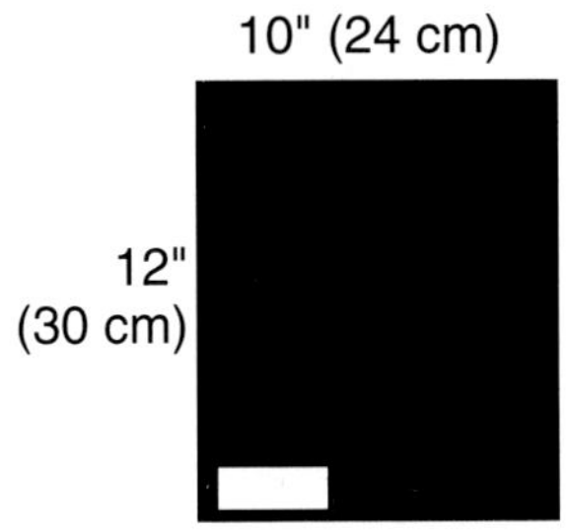

Patient Position

Erect, standing on cassette (Fig. 10.40).

Part Position

Align long axis of foot to long axis of cassette. When forefoot is point of interest, place unaffected foot one step backward. When calcaneus is point of interest, place unaffected foot one step forward.

Central Ray

Make two projections on same cassette. Stress to patient to maintain same position of foot for both projections.

Projection #1
Place tube in front of patient, angle 15° toward heel entering scaphoid and exiting midpoint of cassette. Place unaffected foot one step backward. Be sure patient and cassette do not move.

Projection #2
Place tube behind patient, angle 25° toward toes entering posterior surface of heel and exiting plantar surface at level of lateral malleolus. Place unaffected foot one step forward.

Structures Demonstrated

Weight-bearing, axial projection of foot. Foot is projected free of shadow of leg (Fig. 10.41).

Evaluation Criteria

Phalanges, metatarsals, tarsals, and calcaneus should be seen free of shadow of leg.

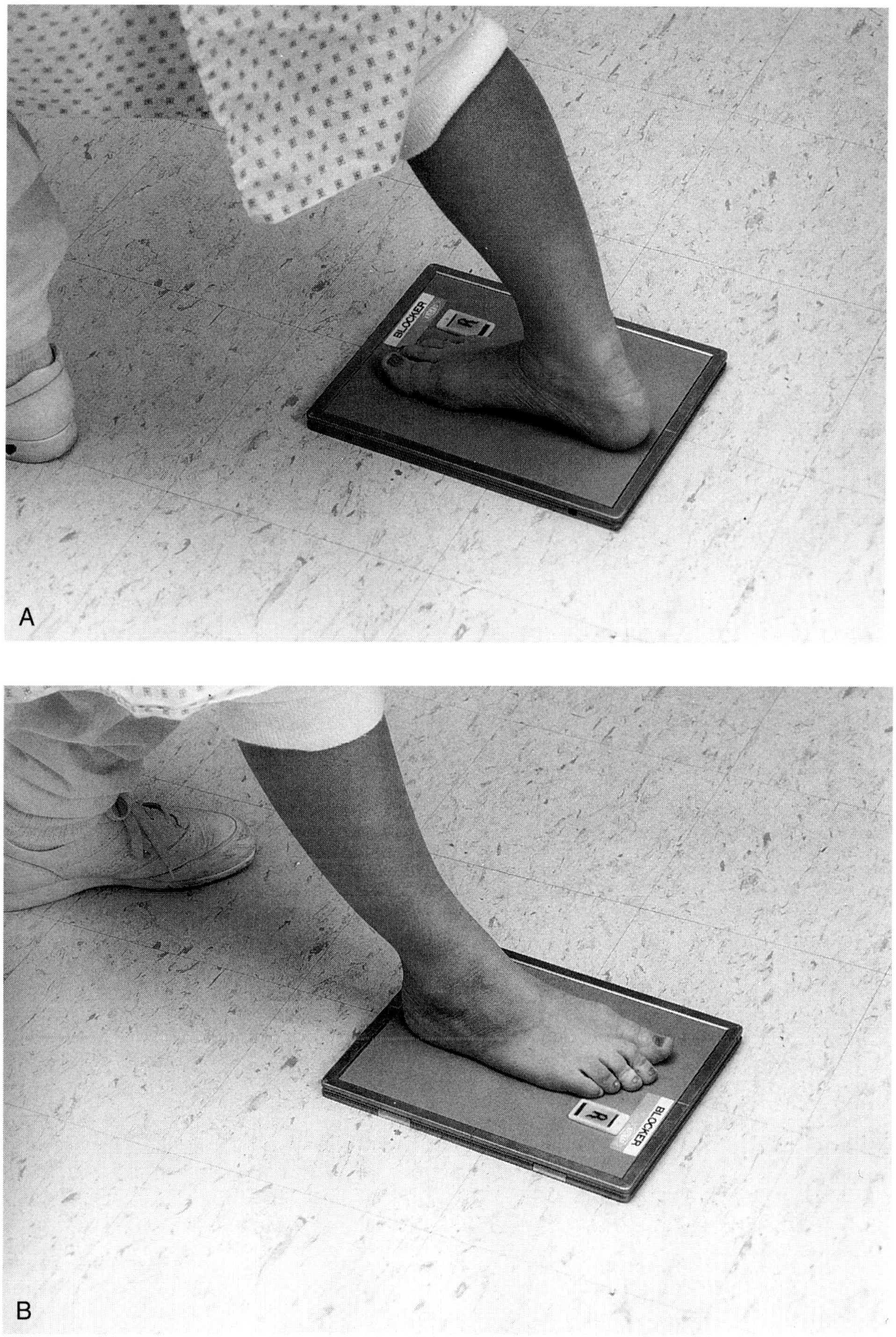

Figure 10.40. A, Composite dorsoplantar posterior angular. B, Composite dorsoplantar anterior angular.

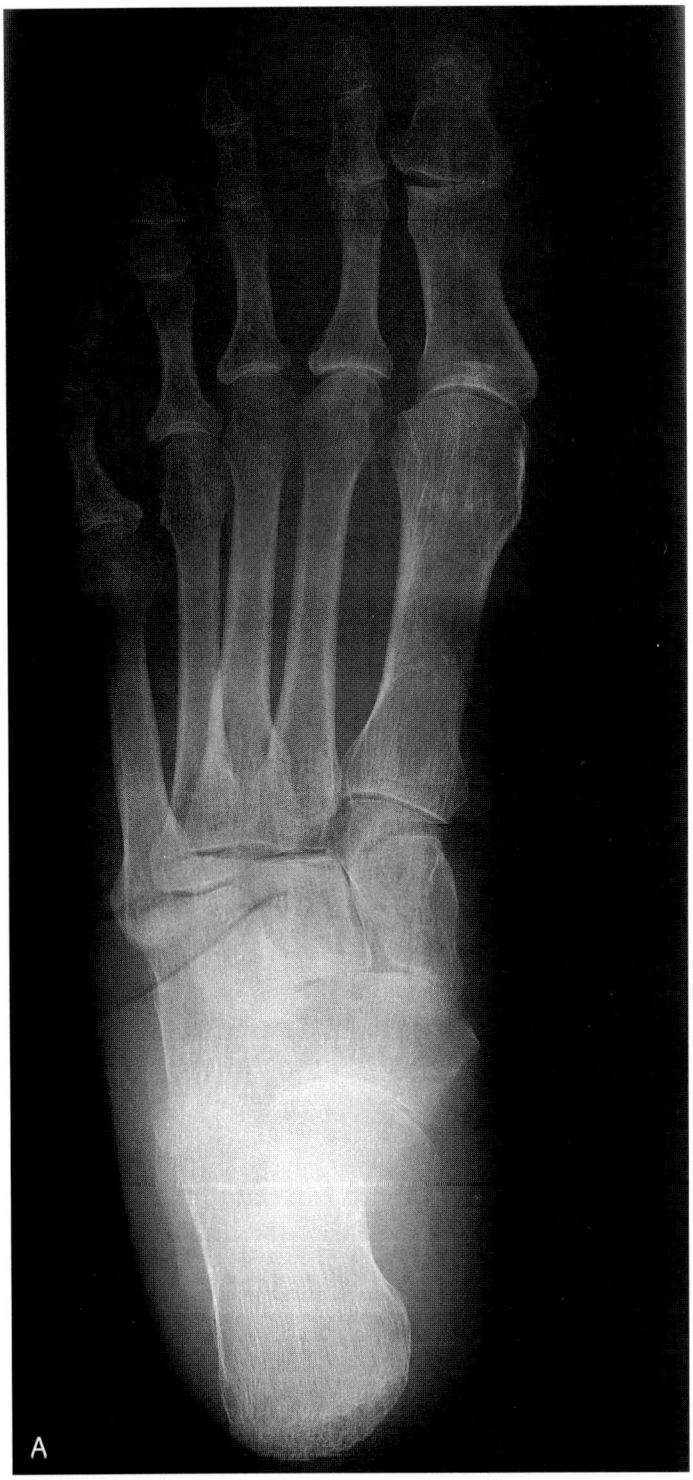

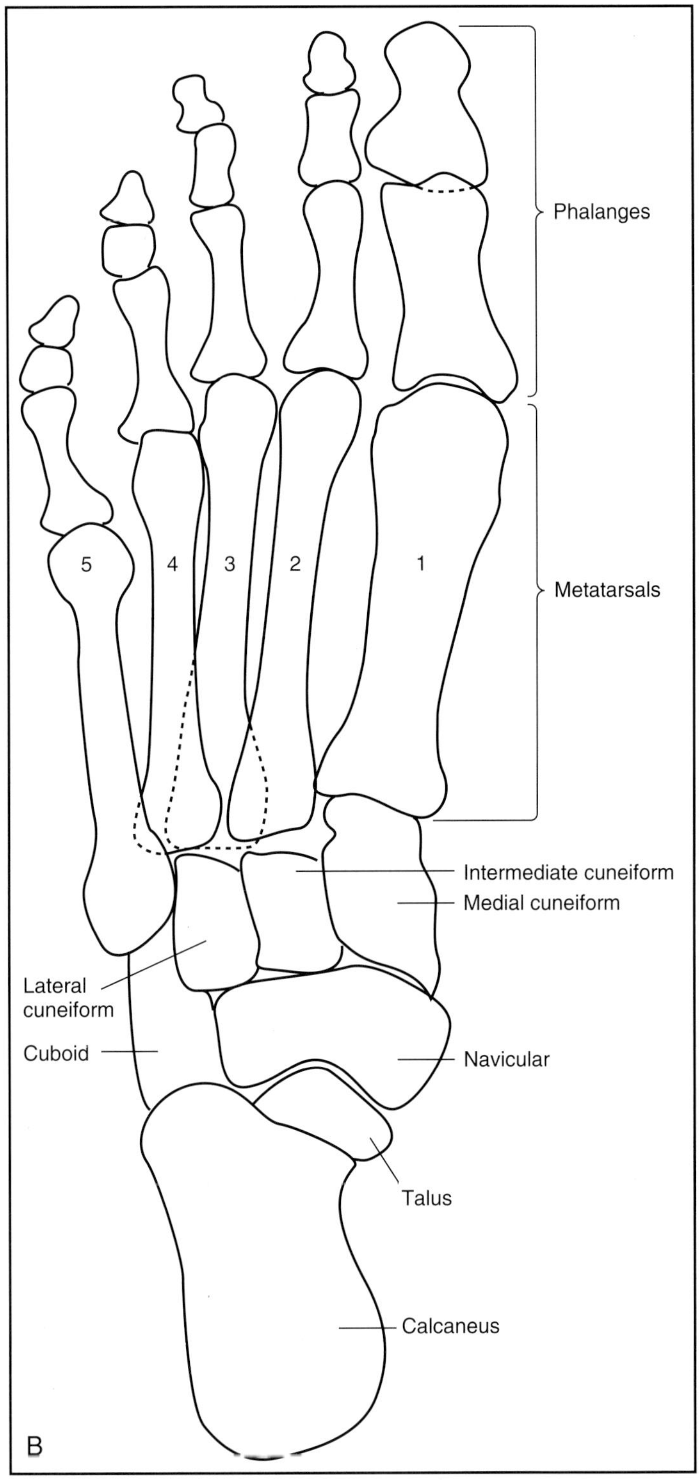

Figure 10.41. A and B, Composite dorsoplantar.

Congenital Clubfoot

Position/Projection

Dorsoplantar projection—Kite's method

Film Size:
8 × 10 inches (20 × 24 cm)
lengthwise or crosswise
tabletop

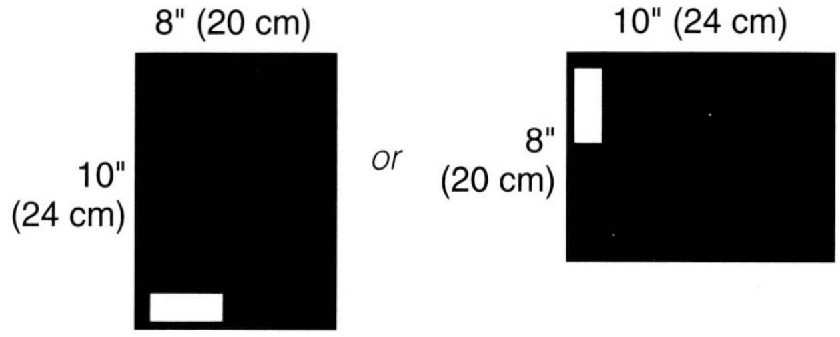

Patient Position

Supine with knee flexed (Fig. 10.42).

Part Position

Align long axis of foot to cassette. No attempt should be made to change abnormal alignment of foot. Center tarsal area to cassette. Generally, a bilateral study of feet is performed unless overlapping of feet occurs when adduction deformity is great.

Central Ray

15° angle toward heel to exit midpoint of cassette.

Structures Demonstrated

Degree of adduction of forefoot and degree of inversion of calcaneus (Fig. 10.43).

Evaluation Criteria

1. No medial or lateral rotation of leg.
2. Entire foot should be seen with no overlapping of other foot.

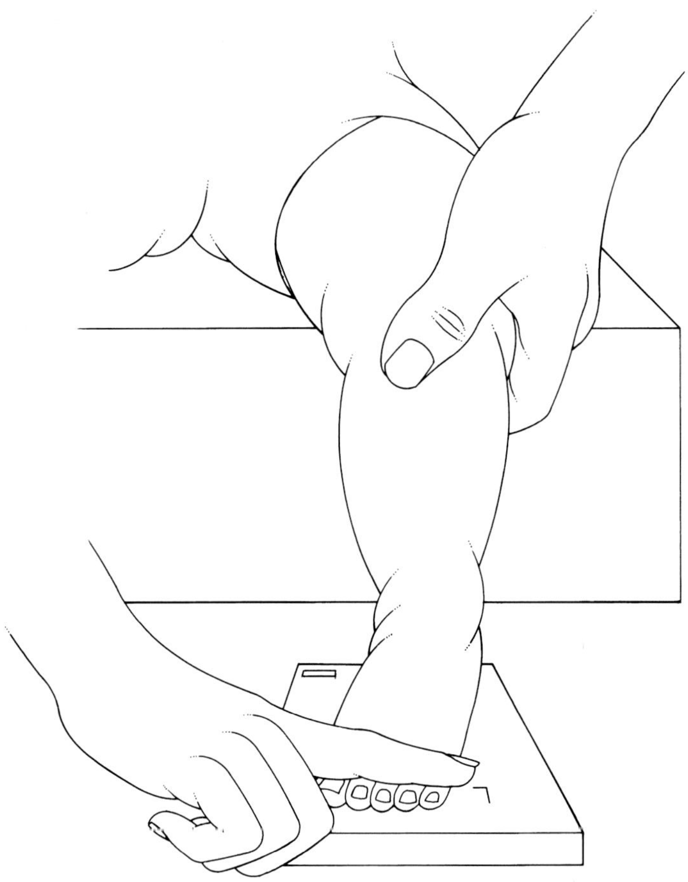

Figure 10.42. Congenital clubfoot, dorsoplantar.
(From Ballinger PW: Merrill's Atlas of Radiographic Positions and Radiologic Projections. 7th ed. Vol. 1. St. Louis: Mosby–Year Book, 1991.)

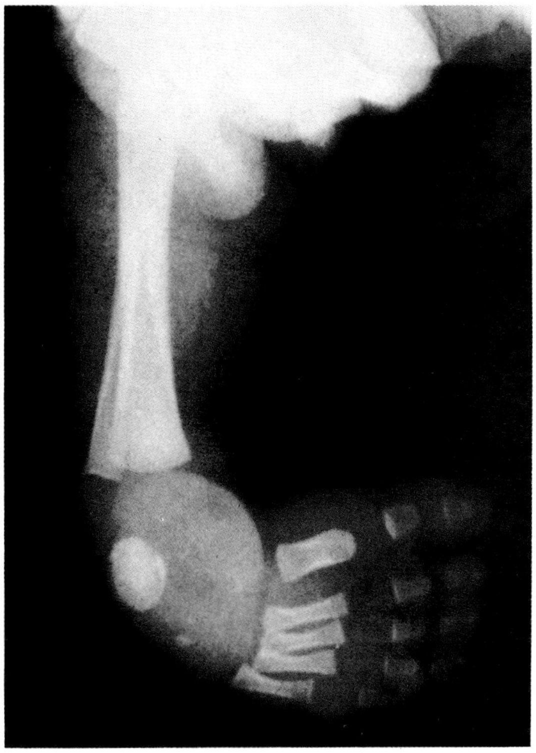

Figure 10.43. Kite's projection, dorsoplantar position for congenital clubfoot.

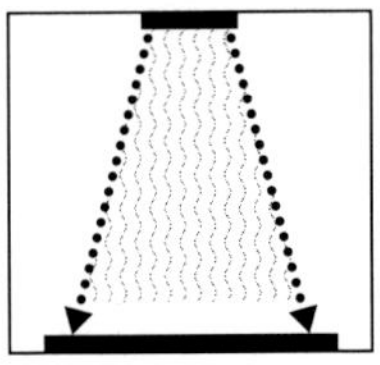

Congenital Clubfoot

Position/Projection

Lateral projection—Kite's method

Film Size:
8 × 10 inches (20 × 24 cm)
crosswise tabletop

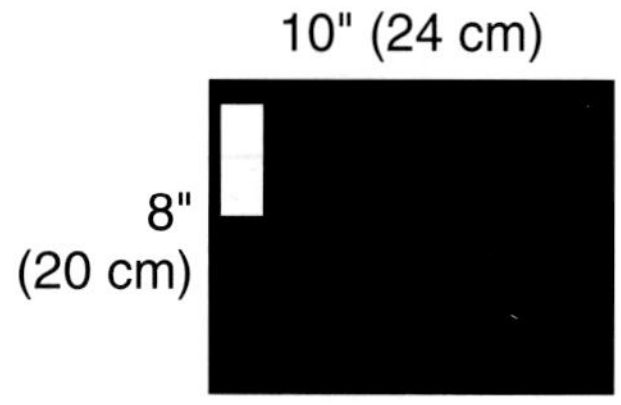

Patient Position

Infant turned laterally on affected side, unaffected leg flexed and placed in front of affected leg (Fig. 10.44).

Part Position

Align long axis of foot to long axis of cassette (cassette can be turned diagonally if needed). No attempt should be made to change abnormal alignment of foot. Center midtarsal area to cassette.

Central Ray

Perpendicular to midtarsal area to exit midpoint of cassette.

Structures Demonstrated

Anterior talar subluxation and degree of plantar flexion (Fig. 10.45).

Evaluation Criteria

1. Fibula should overlap posterior half of tibia.
2. Entire foot should be seen.

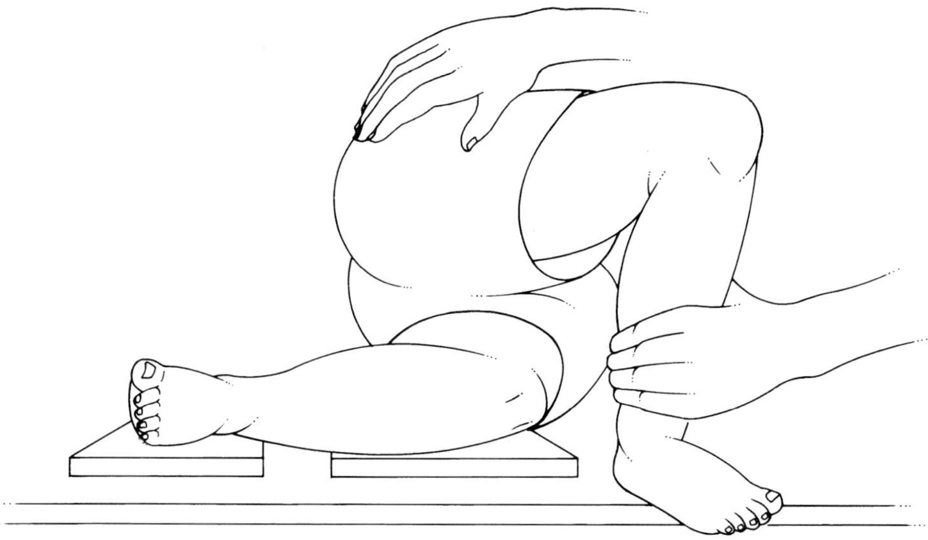

Figure 10.44. Lateral projection, Kite's method. (From Ballinger PW: Merrill's Atlas of Radiographic Positions and Radiologic Procedures. 7th ed. Vol. 1. St. Louis: Mosby–Year Book, 1991.)

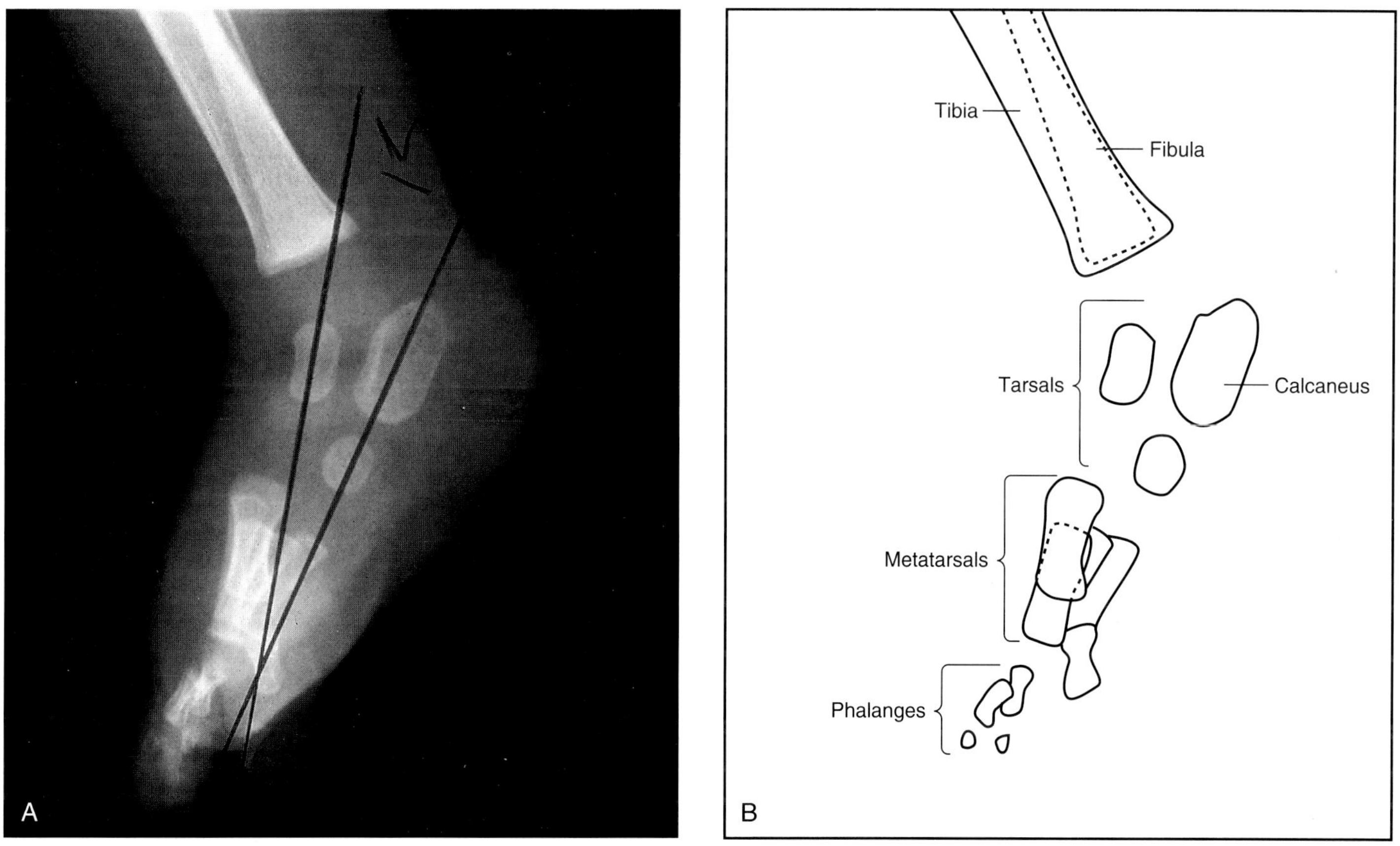

Figure 10.45. A and B, Lateral projection, Kite's method.

Congenital Clubfoot

Position/Projection

Dorsoplantar projection—Kandel's method

Film Size:
8 × 10 inches (20 × 24 cm)
crosswise tabletop

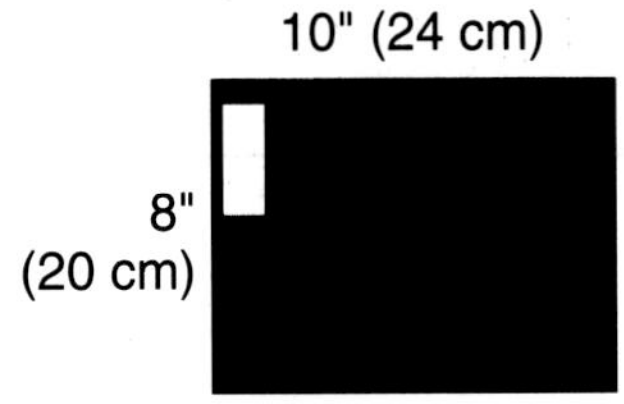

Patient Position

Infant held in standing or bending forward position (Fig. 10.46).

Part Position

Sole of foot should touch cassette. Center tarsals to midpoint of cassette.

Central Ray

Place tube behind patient; 40° angle toward toes to enter posterior of heel and exit level of base of 3rd metatarsal.

Structures Demonstrated

Sustentaculum talar joint and calcaneus.

Evaluation Criteria

No medial or lateral angulation of leg.

NOTE: It is recommended that four radiographs be made with varying angles (35°, 40°, 45°, and 55°).

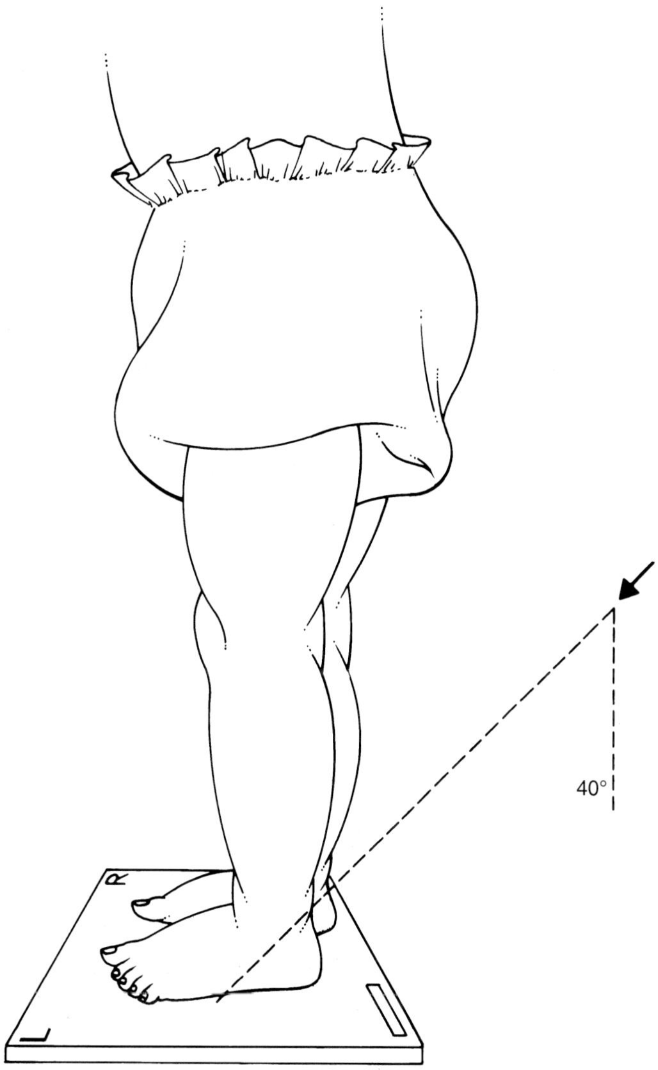

Figure 10.46. Kandel's method, dorsoplantar. (From Ballinger PW: Merrill's Atlas of Radiographic Positions and Radiologic Procedures. 7th ed. Vol. 1. St. Louis: Mosby–Year Book, 1991.)

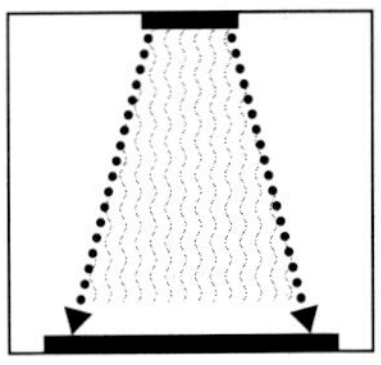

Tarsus: Calcaneus (Os Calcis)—Heel

Position/Projection

Axial plantodorsal projection

Film Size:
8 × 10 inches (20 × 24 cm)
crosswise or lengthwise
tabletop (2 projections)
Divide cassette in half

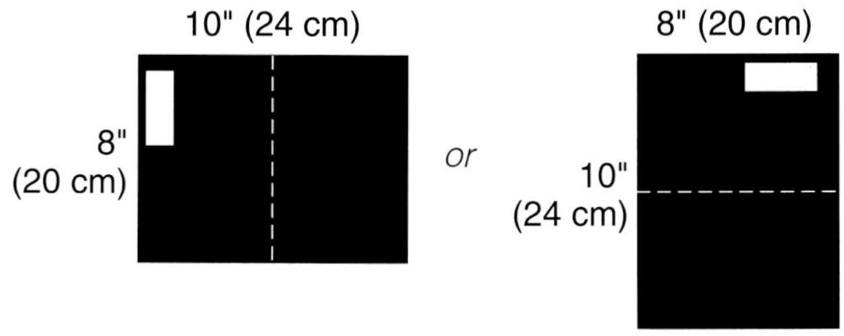

Patient Position

Supine or seated with legs extended (Fig. 10.47).

Part Position

Center cassette to midpoint between tips of lateral malleolus. Immobilize part by having patient hold gauze bandage around ball of foot. Flex ankle in right-angle dorsiflexion (plantar surface of foot perpendicular to cassette).

NOTE: This position is very uncomfortable and difficult to maintain.

Central Ray

Directed to midpoint of cassette at 40° cephalic angle to long axis of foot. Central ray to enter plantar surface of foot at base of 3rd metatarsal and exit midpoint of cassette.

Structures Demonstrated

Semiaxial projection of calcaneus (Fig. 10.48).

Evaluation Criteria

1. Entire calcaneus seen without rotation.
2. Talocalcaneal joint should be seen.
3. Calcaneus should be visualized from tuberosity to sustentaculum tali and trochlear process.
4. Bases of 1st and 5th metatarsals should be superimposed by calcaneus.

NOTE: The calcaneus is a dense area of bone that requires an exposure greater than that needed to radiograph a foot.

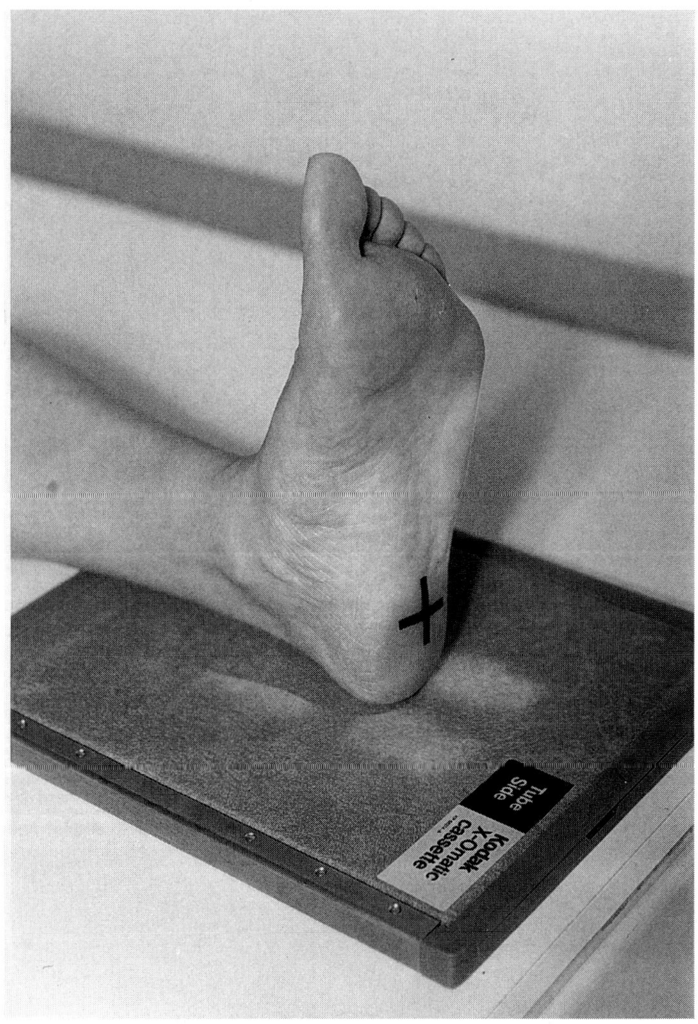

Figure 10.47. Axial plantodorsal calcaneus.

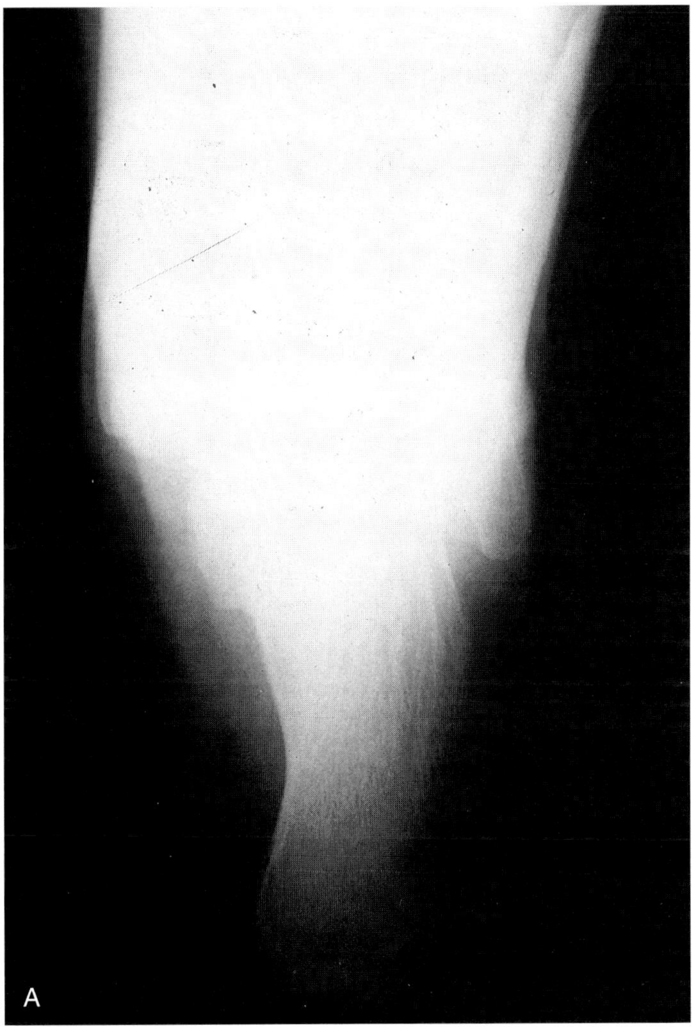

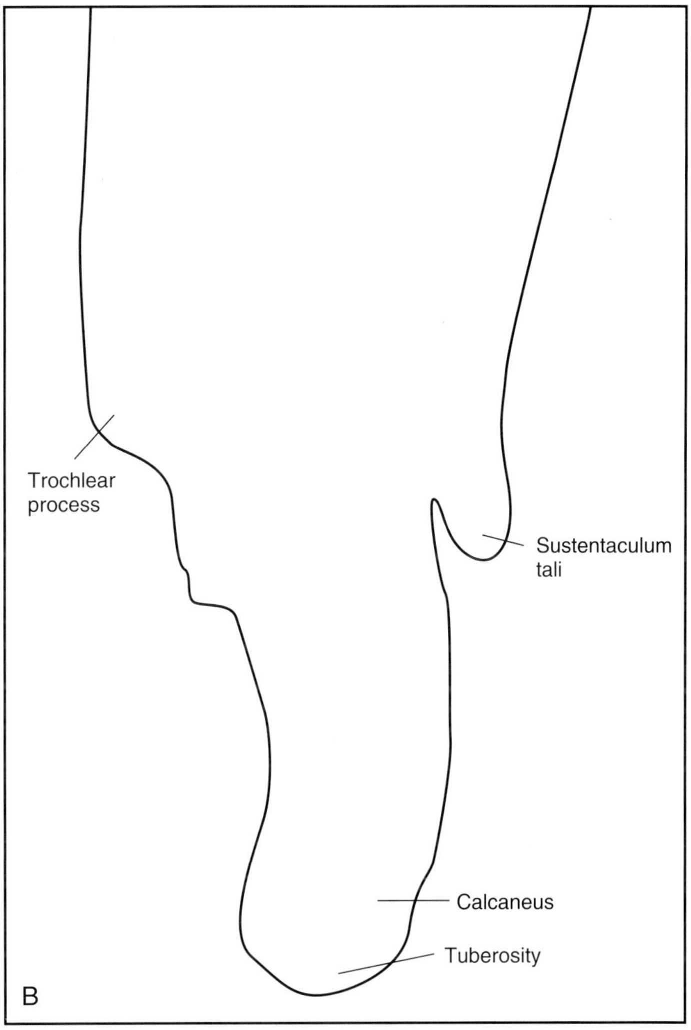

Figure 10.48. A and B, Plantodorsal calcaneus.

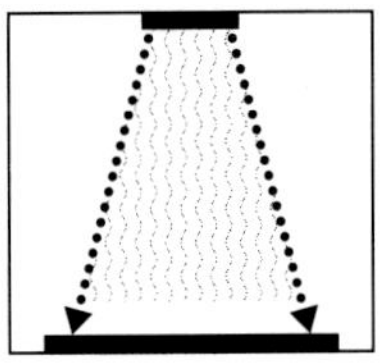

Tarsus: Calcaneus (Os Calcis)—Heel

Position/Projection

Axial dorsoplantar projection

Film Size:
8 × 10 inches (20 × 24 cm) crosswise tabletop (2 projections)
Divide cassette in half

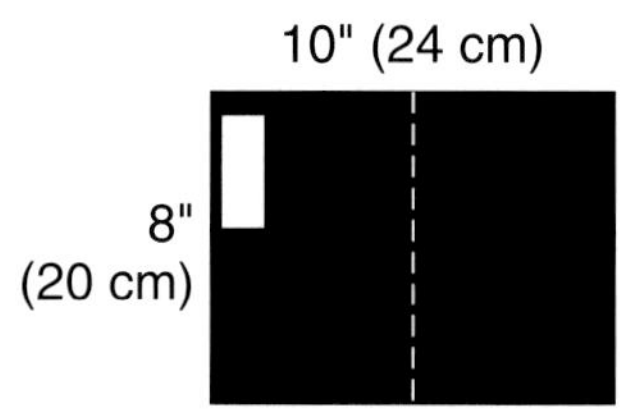

Patient Position

Prone with leg extended (Fig. 10.49).

Part Position

Elevate ankle to a position that allows foot to be dorsiflexed so plantar surface is perpendicular to plane of table. Support ankle with sandbags. Cassette is placed perpendicular to table against plantar surface of foot with long axis of foot aligned with long axis of cassette. Support cassette with vertical holder or sandbags. Superior edge of cassette placed 2 inches (5 cm) above level of posterior surface of calcaneus.

NOTE: This position is very uncomfortable and difficult to maintain.

Central Ray

Directed to midpoint of cassette at 40° caudal angle to long axis of foot. Central ray to enter dorsal surface of ankle joint to exit plantar surface at level of base of 5th metatarsal.

Structures Demonstrated

Axial projection of calcaneus (Fig. 10.50).

Evaluation Criteria

1. Entire calcaneus seen without rotation.
2. Talocalcaneal joint should be seen.
3. Calcaneus should be visualized from tuberosity to sustentaculum tali and trochlear process.
4. Base of 1st and 5th metatarsals should be superimposed by calcaneus.

NOTE: The calcaneus is a dense area of bone that requires an exposure greater than that needed to radiograph a foot. This projection is not normally done as part of the routine procedure of the calcaneus.

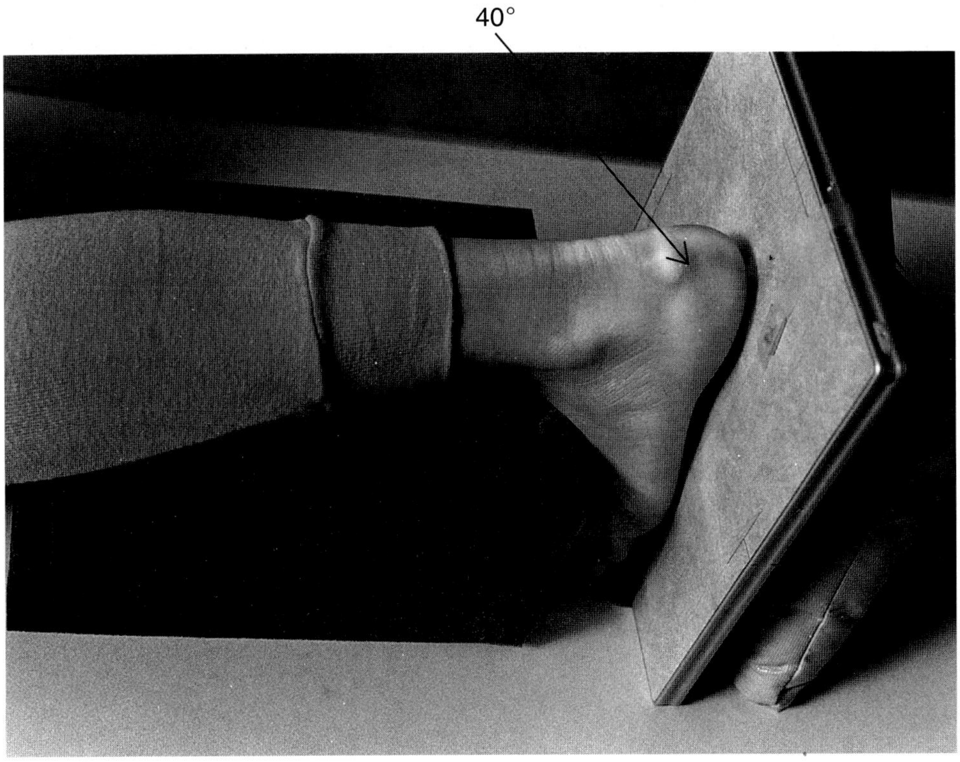

Figure 10.49. Axial dorsoplantar calcaneus.

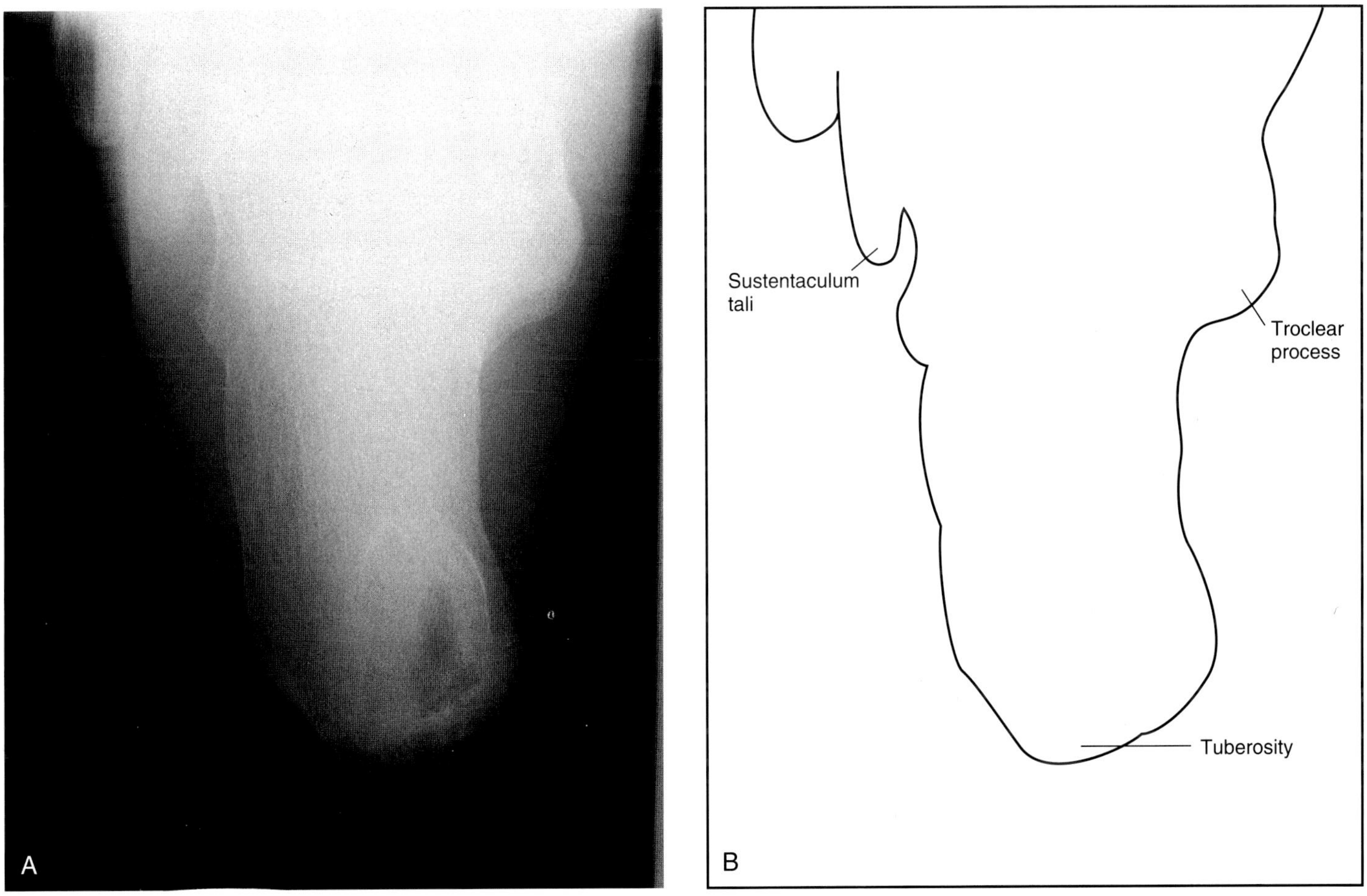

Figure 10.50. A and B, Dorsoplantar calcaneus.

Tarsus: Calcaneus (Os Calcis)—Heel

Position/Projection

Weight-bearing "coalition" projection

Film Size:
8 × 10 inches (20 × 24 cm)
lengthwise

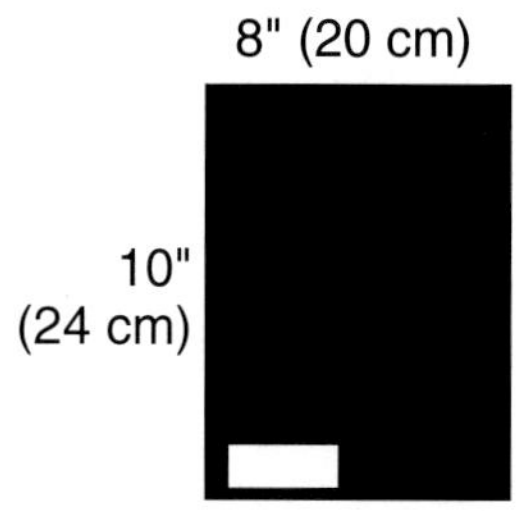

Patient Position

Standing erect position with unaffected foot one step forward (Fig. 10.51).

Part Position

Posterior surface of affected heel at edge of cassette. Cassette centered to long axis of calcaneus at level of base of 5th metatarsal.

Central Ray

Anterior angle of 45° through posterior surface of ankle to exit plantar surface at level of base of 5th metatarsal.

Structures Demonstrated

Calcaneotalar coalition; tarsal coalition (Fig. 10.52).

Evaluation Criteria

Calcaneus seen without rotation.

NOTE: This project is important in diagnosing flatfoot.

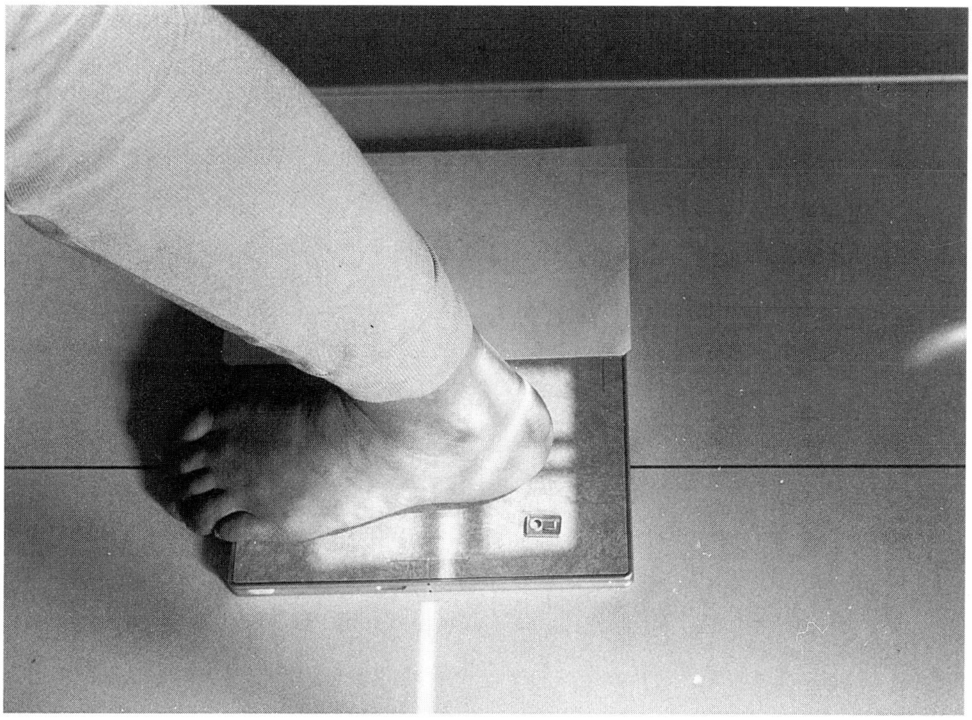

Figure 10.51. Weight-bearing "coalition."

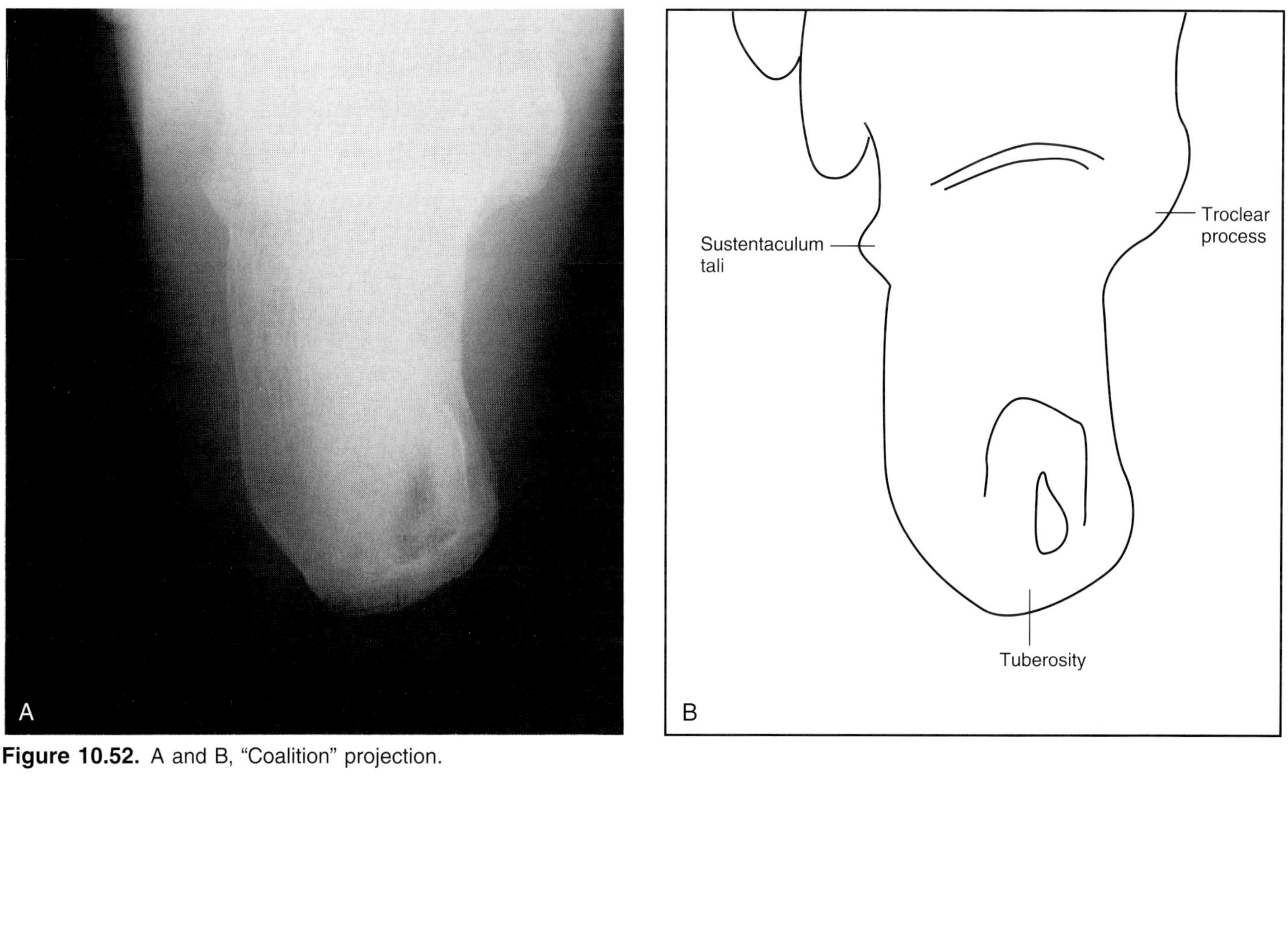

Figure 10.52. A and B, "Coalition" projection.

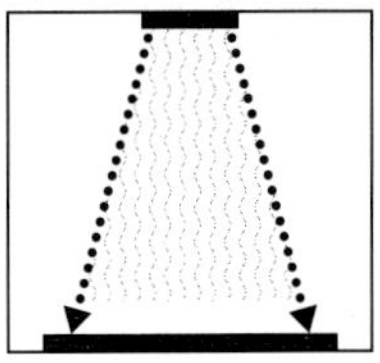

Tarsus: Calcaneus (Os Calcis)—Heel

Position/Projection

Lateral projection

Film Size:
8 × 10 inches (20 × 24 cm) crosswise tabletop (2 projections)
Divide cassette in half

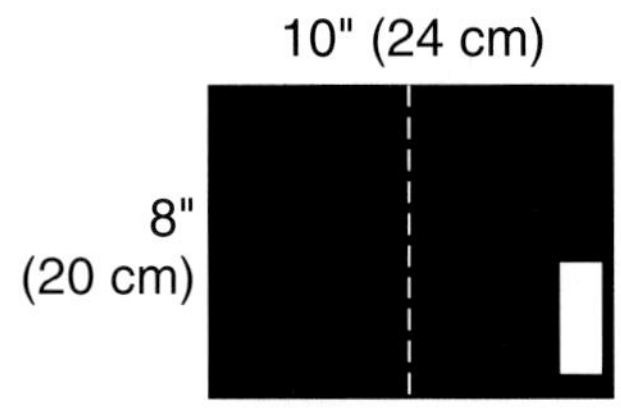

Patient Position

Supine or seated with legs extended (Fig. 10.53).

Part Position

Place affected foot in true lateral position on its lateral surface. Center midportion of heel (1 to 1½ inches [2.5 to 4 cm] distal to medial malleolus) to midpoint of unmasked half of cassette. Place long axis of plantar surface of heel parallel to long axis of unmasked half of cassette. Plantar surface of foot perpendicular to plane of cassette.

Central Ray

Perpendicular to midpoint of cassette.

Structures Demonstrated

Lateral projection of calcaneus and ankle joint (Fig. 10.54).

Evaluation Criteria

1. Sinus tarsi should be seen.
2. Ankle joint and adjacent tarsals should be seen.
3. Calcaneus should be in lateral profile without rotation.

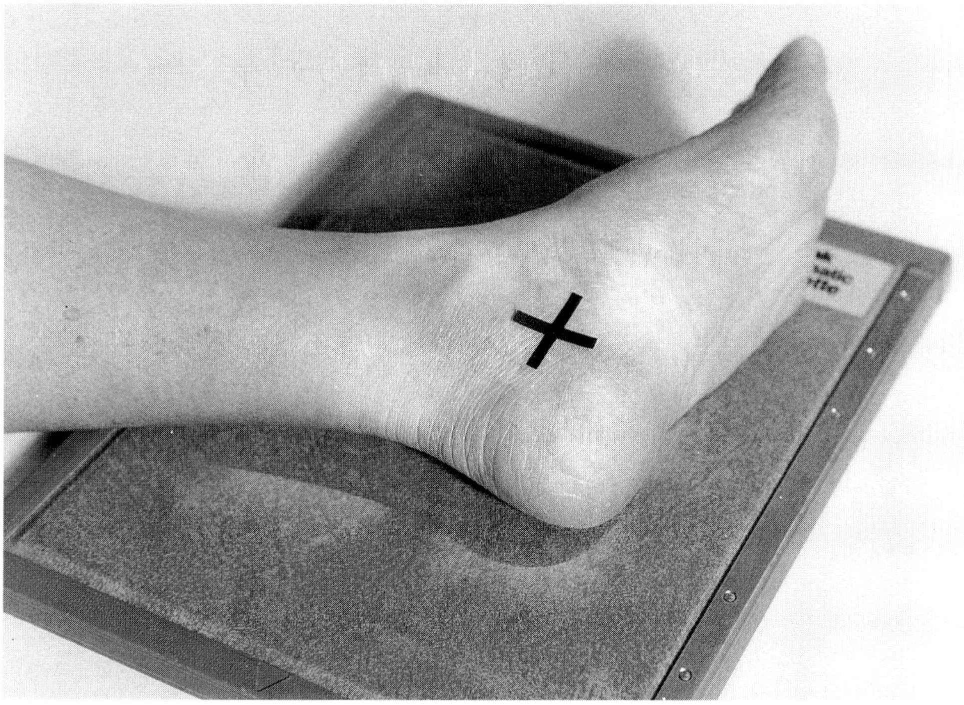

Figure 10.53. Lateral calcaneus.

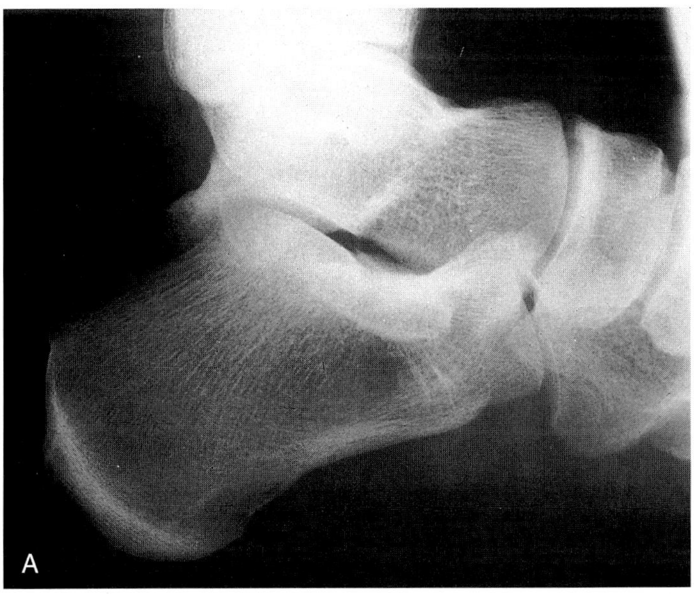

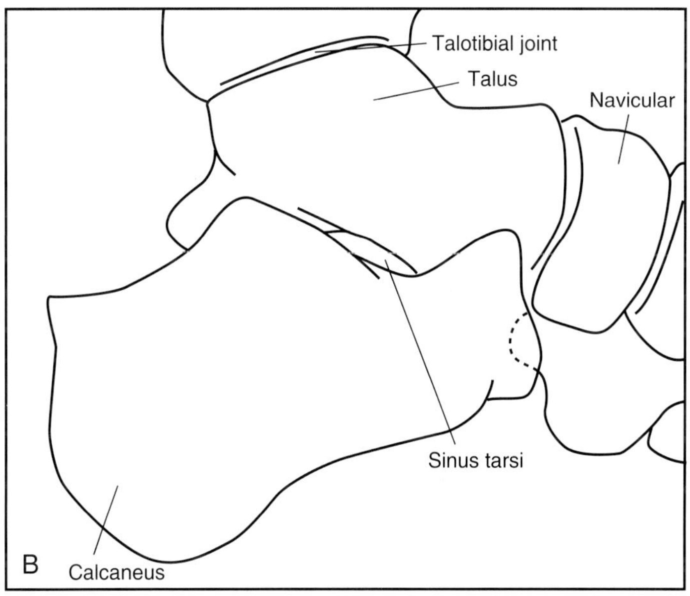

Figure 10.54. A and B, Lateral calcaneus.

Tarsus: Calcaneus (Os Calcis)—Heel

Position/Projection

Oblique projection

Film Size:
8 × 10 inches (20 × 24 cm)
lengthwise tabletop

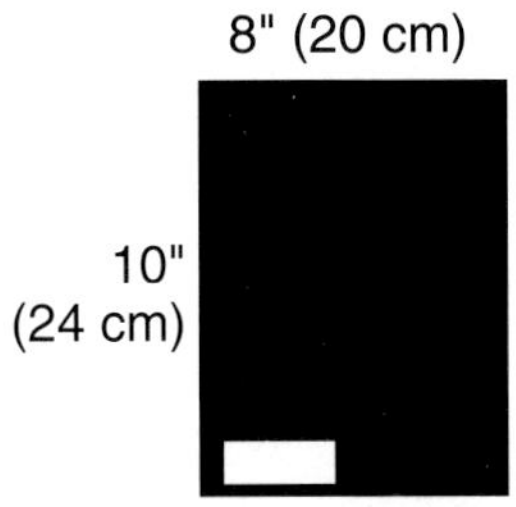

Patient Position

Standing erect position with affected heel placed toward lateral border of cassette (Fig. 10.55).

Part Position

Affected leg perpendicular to cassette. Center affected heel close to lateral border of cassette.

Central Ray

Directed medially to lateral malleolus with 45° caudal angle.

Structures Demonstrated

Oblique weight-bearing to demonstrate calcaneal tubercle (Fig. 10.56).

Evaluation Criteria

Sinus tarsi, cuboid, and calcaneal tubercle should be seen.

NOTE: This projection is important in diagnosing stress fractures of the calcaneus or tubercle.

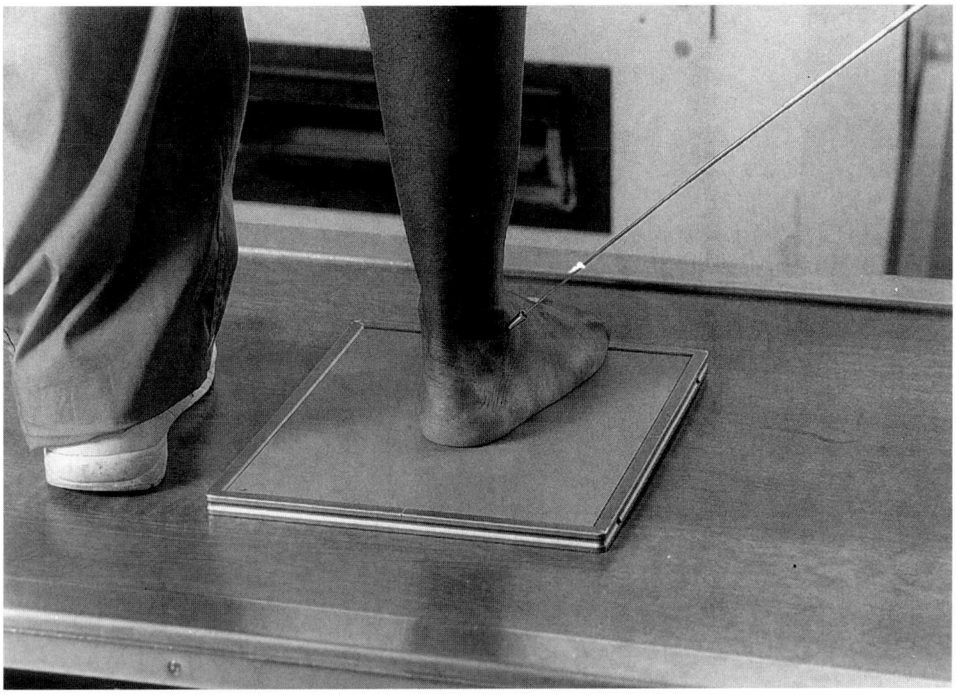

Figure 10.55. Oblique weight-bearing calcaneus.

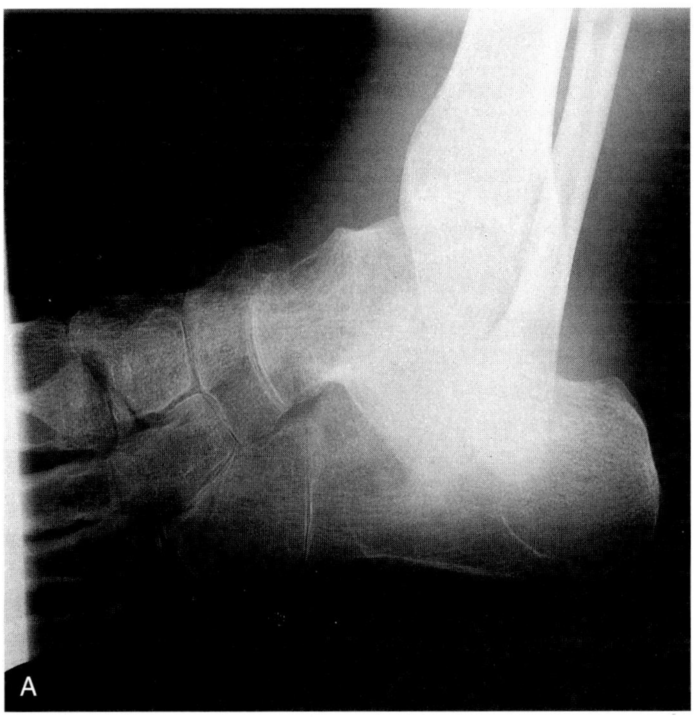

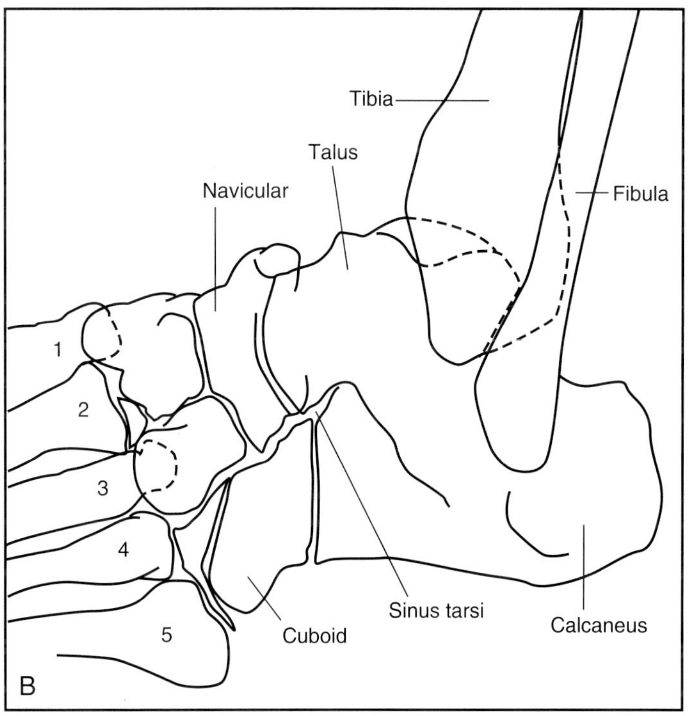

Figure 10.56. A and B, Oblique weight-bearing calcaneus.

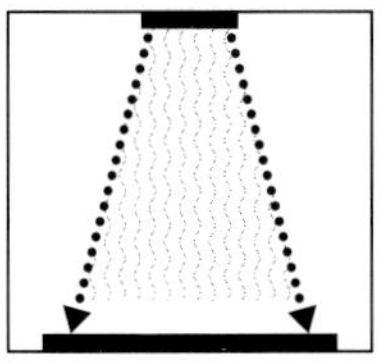

Subtalar Joint

Position/Projection

Anterior articulation; superoinferior oblique projection

Film Size:
8 × 10 inches (20 × 24 cm)
crosswise tabletop

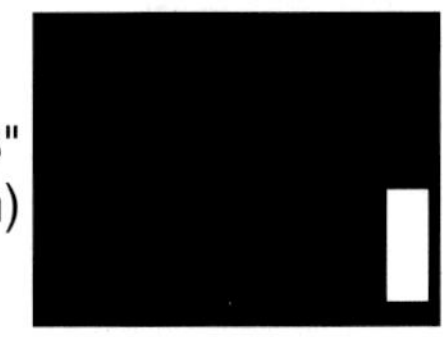

Patient Position

Lateral recumbent on affected side with affected extremity extended (Fig. 10.57).

Part Position

Roll affected extremity slightly forward. Oblique foot to elevate heel $1\frac{1}{2}$ inches (4 cm) from lateral position. Angle ball of foot forward 25°. Midpoint of cassette should be centered 1 to $1\frac{1}{2}$ inches (2.5 to 4 cm) distal to ankle joint.

Central Ray

23° caudal angle and 5° anterior angle to ankle joint.

Structures Demonstrated

Anterior and posterior articulations of subtalar joint. Lateral malleolus, talus, talocalcaneal articulation, sinus tarsi, navicular, talonavicular joint, and calcaneus should be demonstrated (Fig. 10.58).

Evaluation Criteria

1. Subtalar joint articulations and sinus tarsi should be open.
2. Lateral malleolus should be in profile.

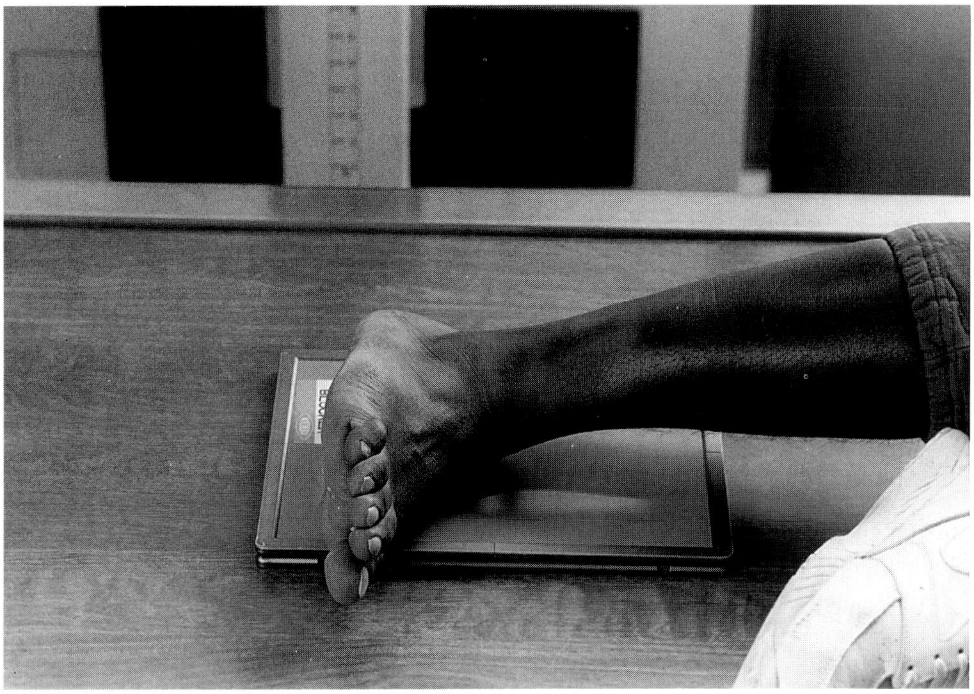

Figure 10.57. Subtalar joint, superoinferior oblique.

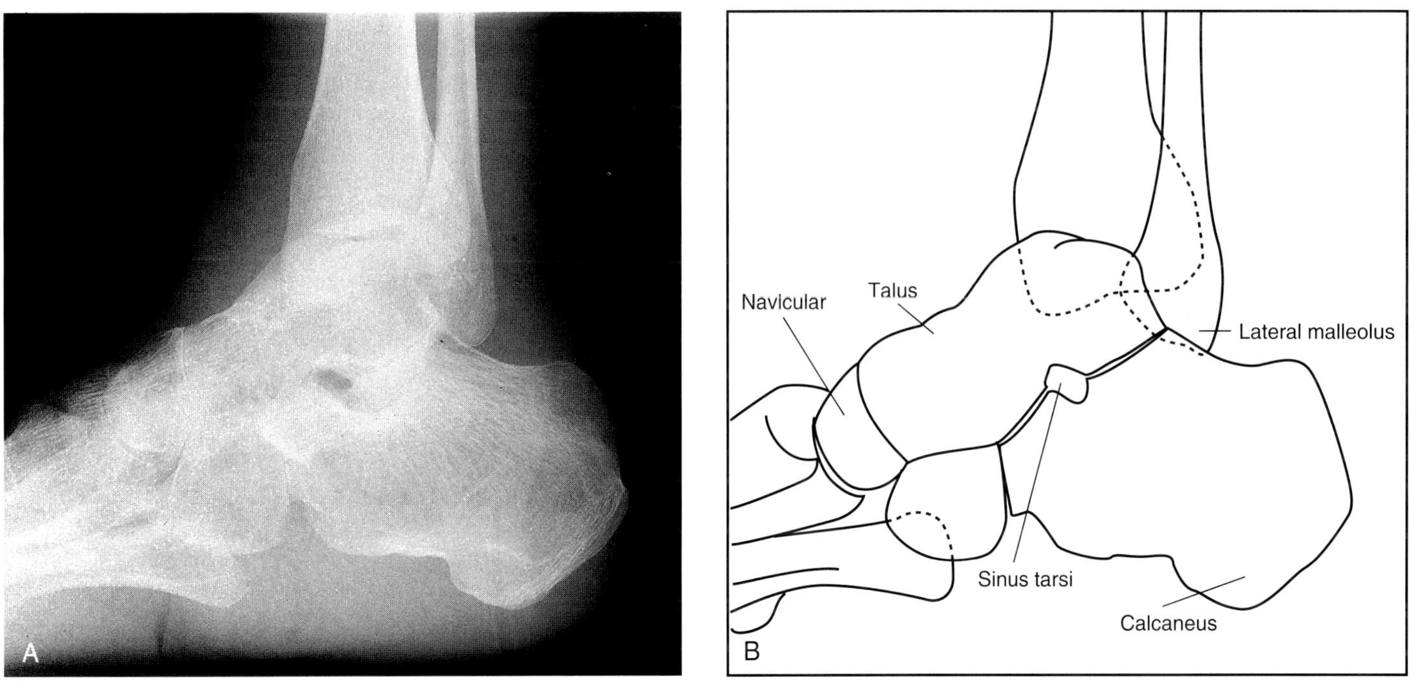

Figure 10.58. A and B, Subtalar joint.

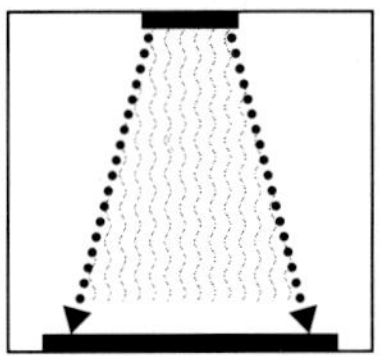

Subtalar Joint

Position/Projection

Lateromedial oblique projection

Film Size:
8 × 10 inches (20 × 24 cm)
crosswise tabletop

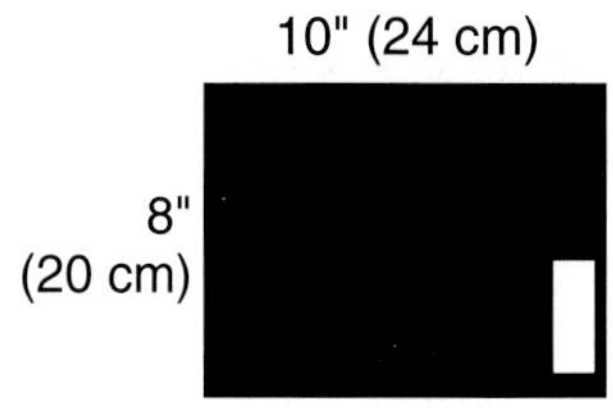

Patient Position

Supine with leg extended (Fig. 10.59).

Part Position

Place ankle joint in right-angle flexion. Rotate leg and foot 45° medially. Place lower edge of cassette at least 1 inch (2.5 cm) distal to plantar surface of heel.

Central Ray

Four projections should be taken at 40°, 30°, 20°, and 10°. Cephalic angle directed ¾ inch (2 cm) caudoanteriorly to lateral malleolus at midpoint of imaginary line from most prominent point of lateral malleous to base of 5th metatarsal and to exit at midpoint of cassette.

Structures Demonstrated

10° angle demonstrates posterior portion of subtalar joint. 40° angle demonstrates anterior portion of posterior facet. 20° and 30° angles demonstrate articulation between talus and sustentaculum tali (Fig. 10.60).

Evaluation Criteria

Anterior and posterior portions of subtalar joint should be seen.

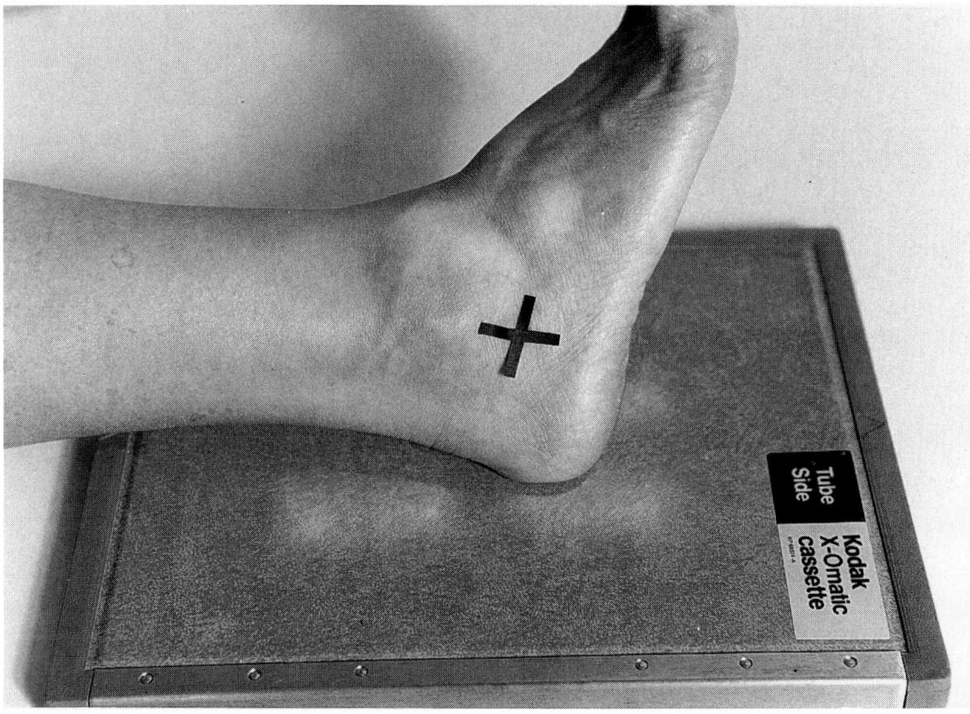

Figure 10.59. Lateromedial subtalar joint.

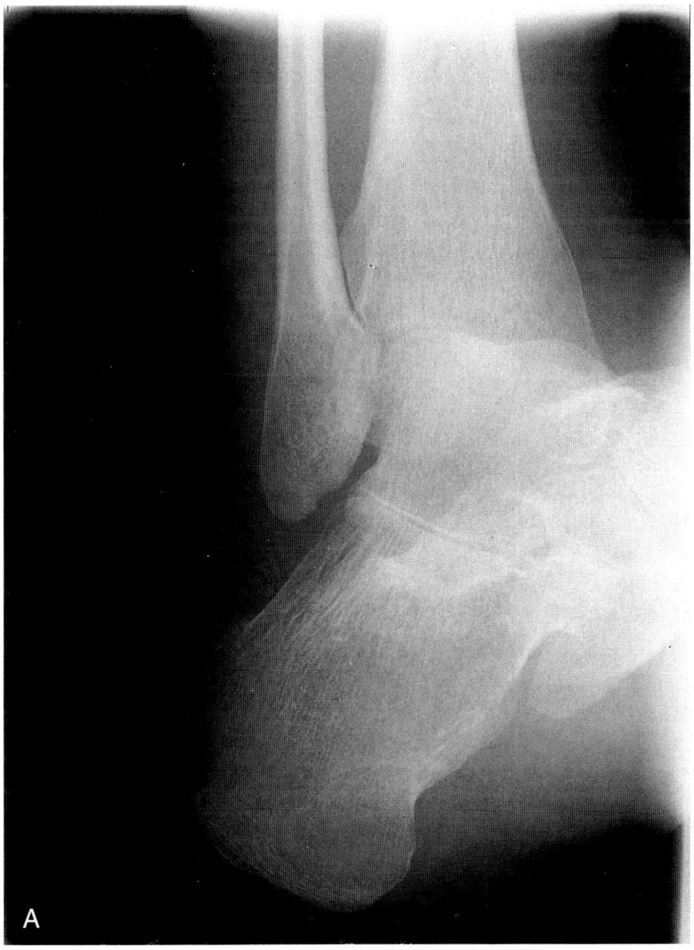

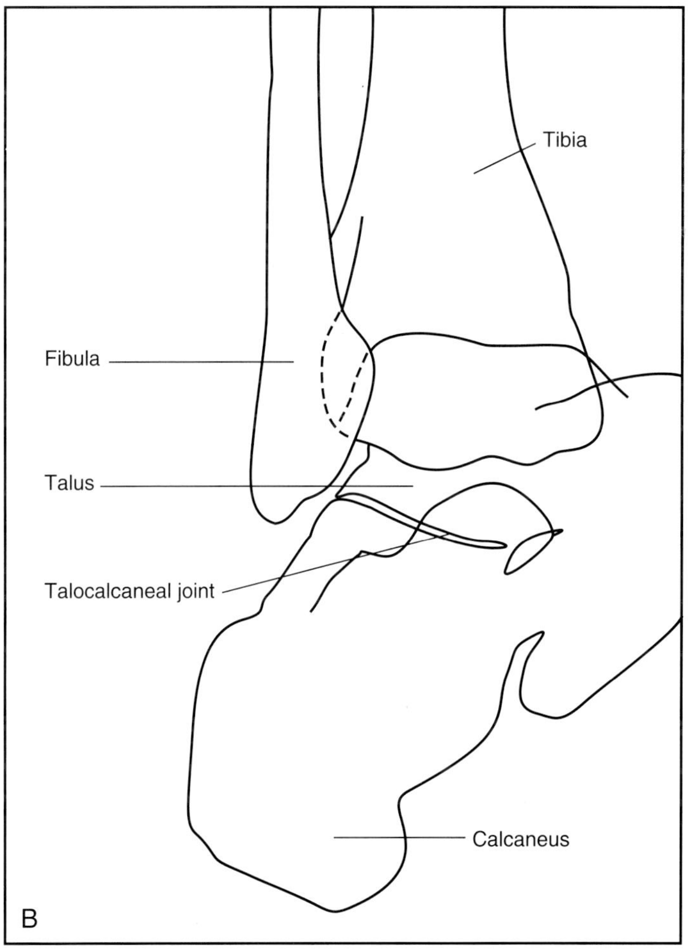

Figure 10.60. A and B, Lateromedial subtalar joint.

Subtalar Joint

Position/Projection

Mediolateral oblique projection

Film Size:
8 × 10 inches (20 × 24 cm)
crosswise tabletop

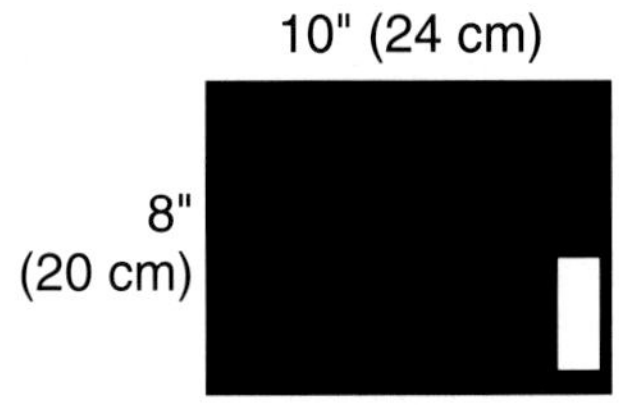

Patient Position

Supine with leg extended (Fig. 10.61).

Part Position

Place ankle joint in right-angle flexion. Rotate leg and foot 45° laterally. Place lower edge of cassette at least 1 inch (2.5 cm) distal to plantar surface of heel.

Central Ray

15° cephalic angle to enter ¾ inch (2 cm) distal and ¾ inch (2 cm) anterior to medial malleolus. Do two or three projections with 3° to 4° difference in angulation. Central ray should exit midpoint of cassette.

Structures Demonstrated

Posterior facet of calcaneous in profile. Articulation between talus and sustentaculum tali should be seen. Posterior talocalcaneal joint should be seen (Fig. 10.62).

Evaluation Criteria

Posterior portion of subtalar joint should be seen.

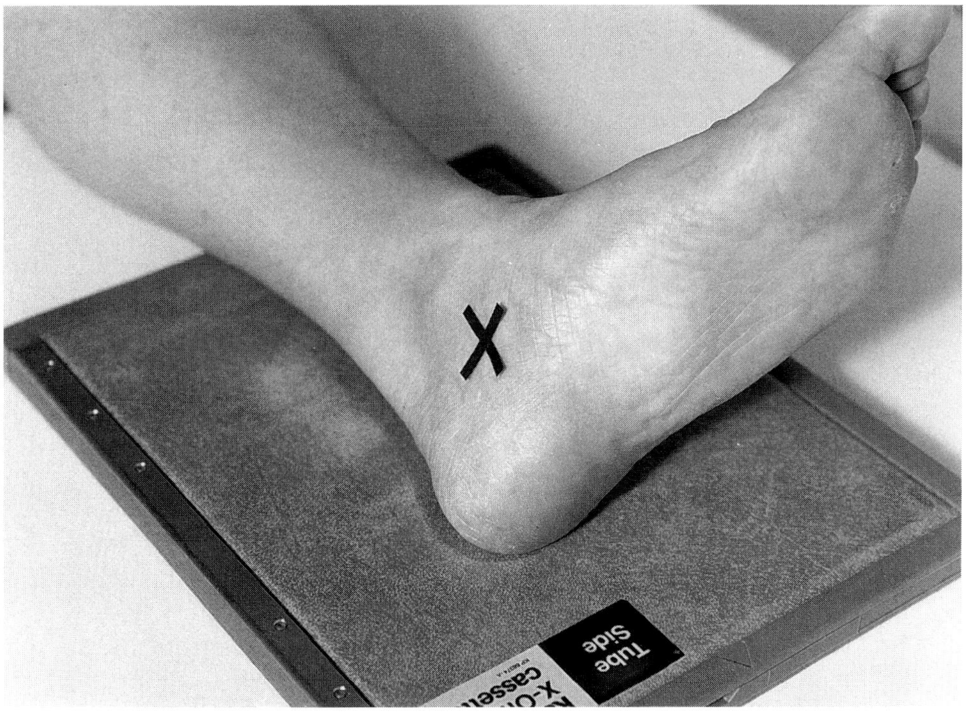

Figure 10.61. Mediolateral subtalar joint.

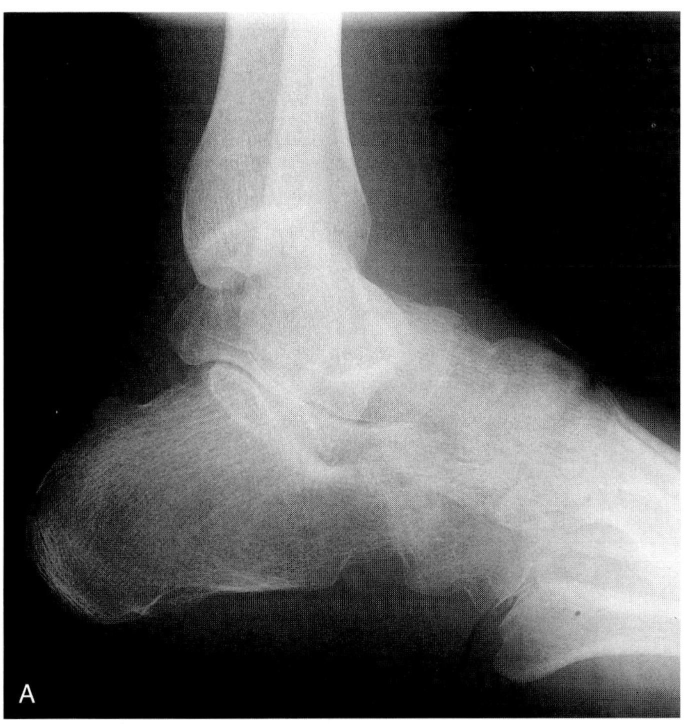

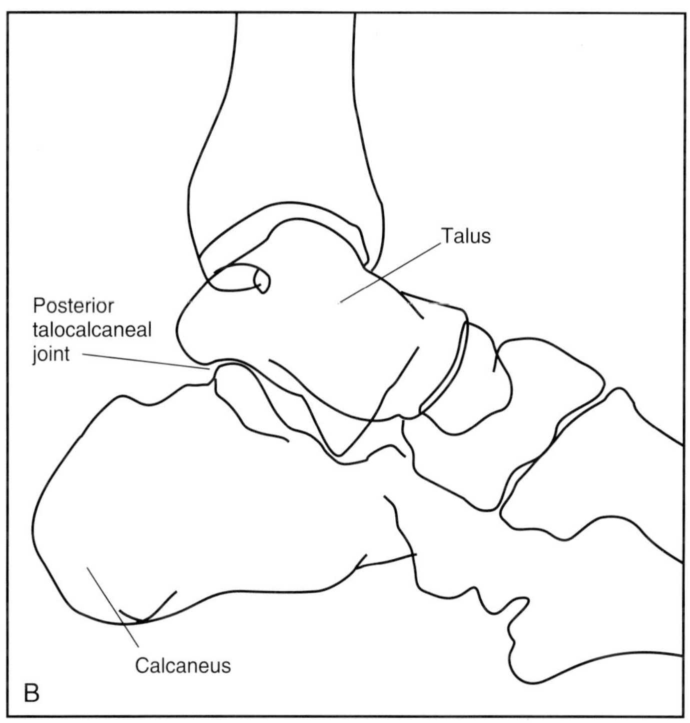

Figure 10.62. A and B, Mediolateral subtalar joint.

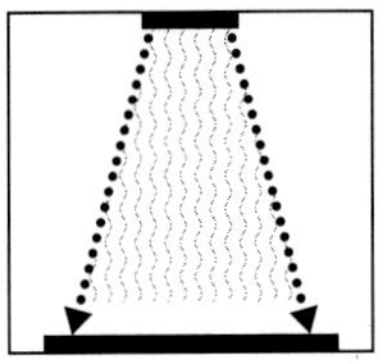

Ankle

Position/Projection

AP projection

Film Size:
8 × 10 inches (20 × 24 cm) lengthwise tabletop (1 projection)

or

10 × 12 inches (24 × 30 cm) crosswise tabletop (2 projections)
Divide cassette in half

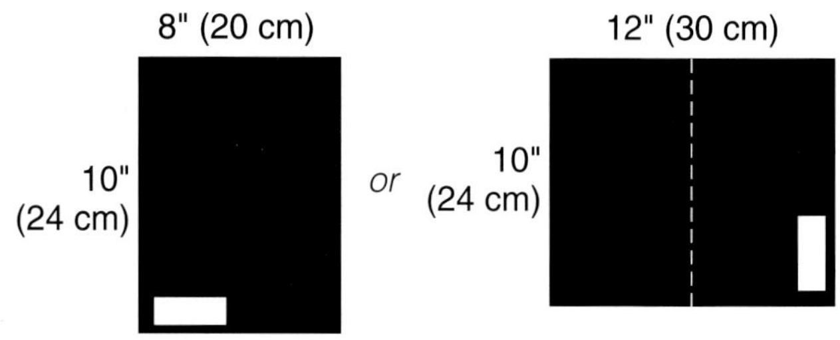

Patient Position

Supine or seated with legs extended (Fig. 10.63).

Part Position

Align long axis of leg to unmasked half of cassette. Center a point midway between lateral malleolus and medial malleolus to midpoint of unmasked half of cassette. Dorsiflex foot with 5° medial rotation to place intermalleolar line parallel to cassette and to place plantar surface of foot perpendicular to cassette.

Central Ray

Perpendicular to midpoint of unmasked portion of cassette through ankle joint at point midway between malleoli.

Structures Demonstrated

AP projection of ankle joint, distal tibia, distal fibula, and proximal talus (Fig. 10.64).

Evaluation Criteria

1. Distal tibia and fibula to talus should be seen with slight overlapping of distal tibiofibular articulation.
2. Talotibial joint space should be seen.
3. Ankle joint should be centered to film.
4. Medial and lateral malleoli should be seen with medial malleolus free of superimposition and lateral malleolus slightly superimposed by talus.

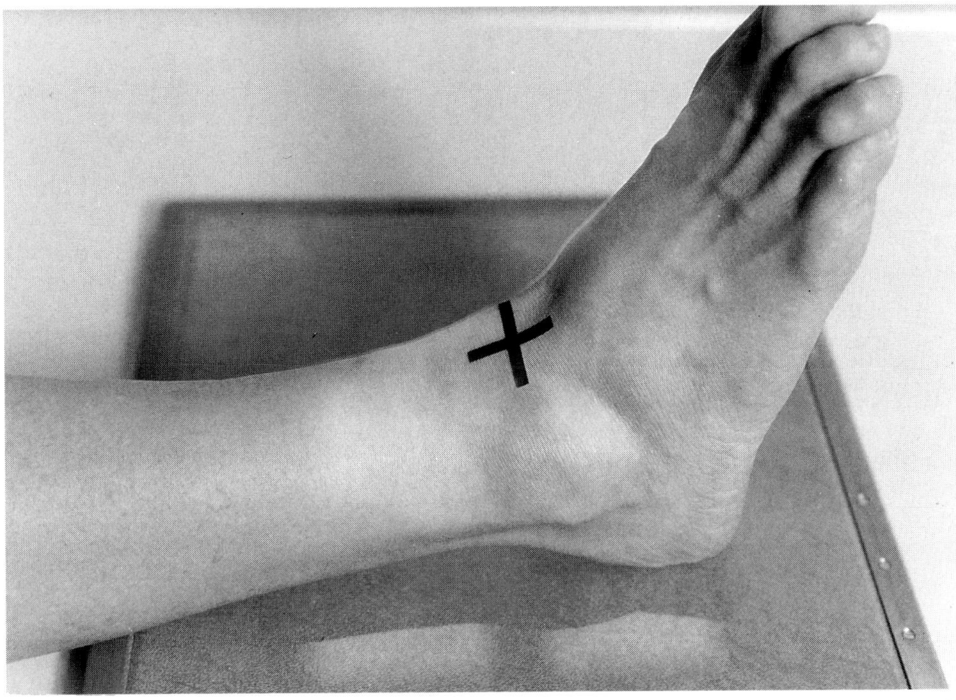

Figure 10.63. AP ankle.

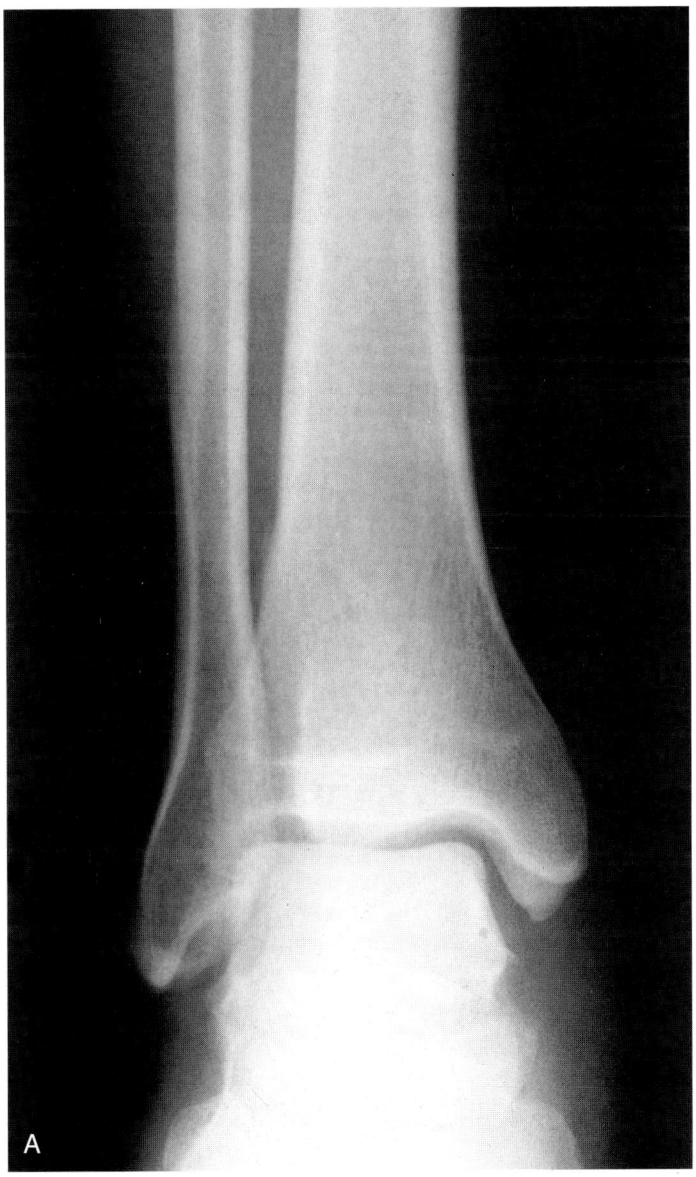

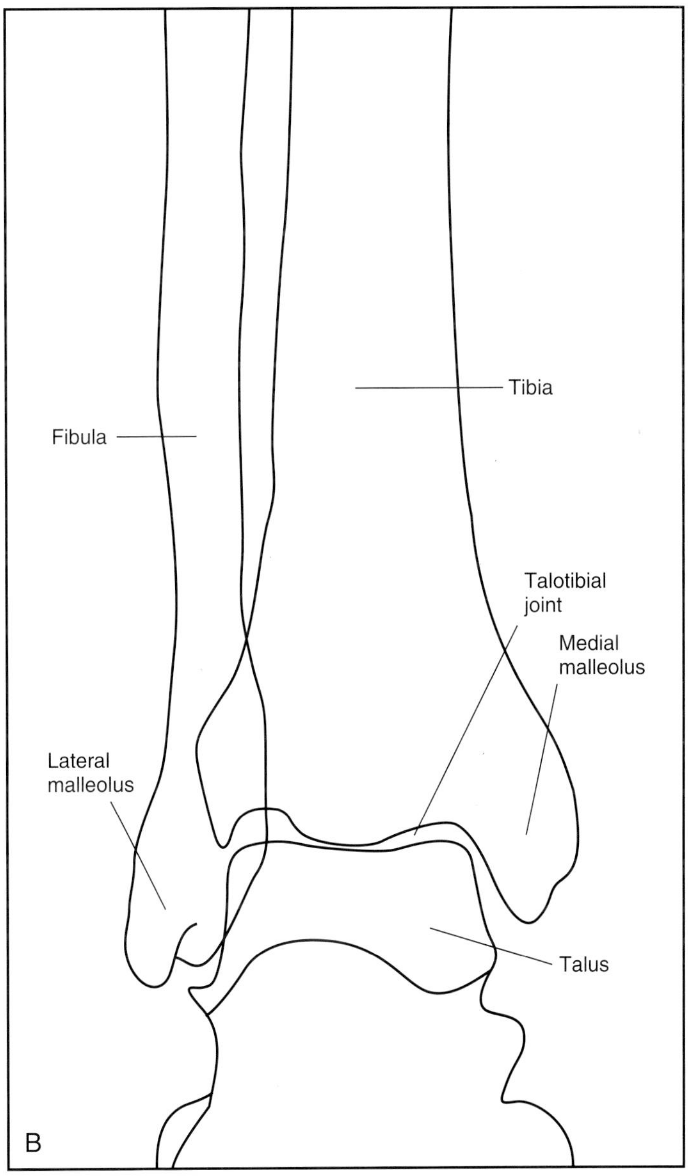

Figure 10.64. A and B, AP ankle.

Ankle

Position/Projection

Lateral projection (lateromedial projection)

Film Size:
8 × 10 inches (20 × 24 cm) lengthwise (1 projection)
or
10 × 12 inches (24 × 30 cm) crosswise (2 projections)
Divide cassette in half

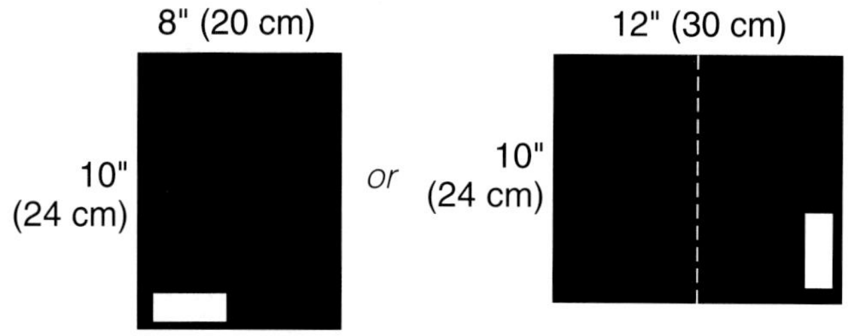

Patient Position

Supine or seated; turn patient away from affected side (Fig. 10.65).

Part Position

Center cassette to ankle joint (about ½ inch [1 cm] above distal tip of medial malleolus or ¾ inch [2 cm] above distal tip of lateral malleolus). Adjust foot in lateral position and place plane of patella perpendicular to table. Dorsiflex foot to place plantar surface parallel to cassette. Support foot and body in this position.

Central Ray

Perpendicular to midpoint of cassette or unmasked portion through ankle joint midway between anterior and posterior surfaces.

Structures Demonstrated

Lateral projection of distal tibia and fibula, ankle joint, and tarsus (Fig. 10.66).

Evaluation Criteria

1. Distal tibia and fibula, talus, and adjacent tarsals should be seen.
2. Talotibial joint should be seen.
3. Ankle joint should be centered to film.
4. Fibula should superimpose posterior half of tibia.

NOTE: This projection places the ankle joint closer to the cassette for "better image detail," but because of patient discomfort, the mediolateral projection is normally performed.

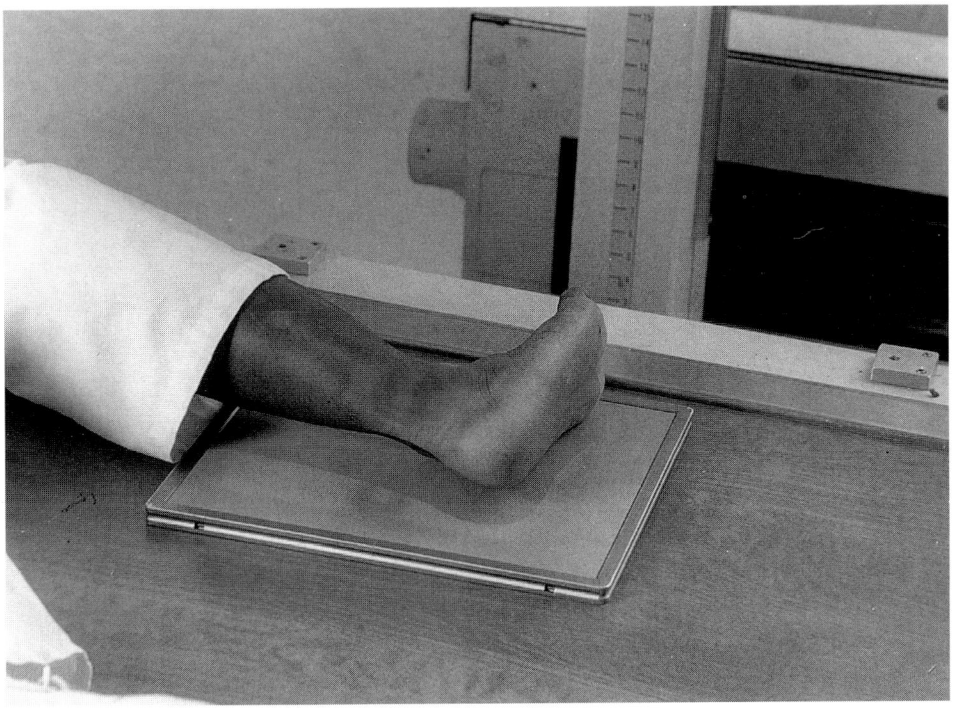

Figure 10.65. Lateromedial ankle.

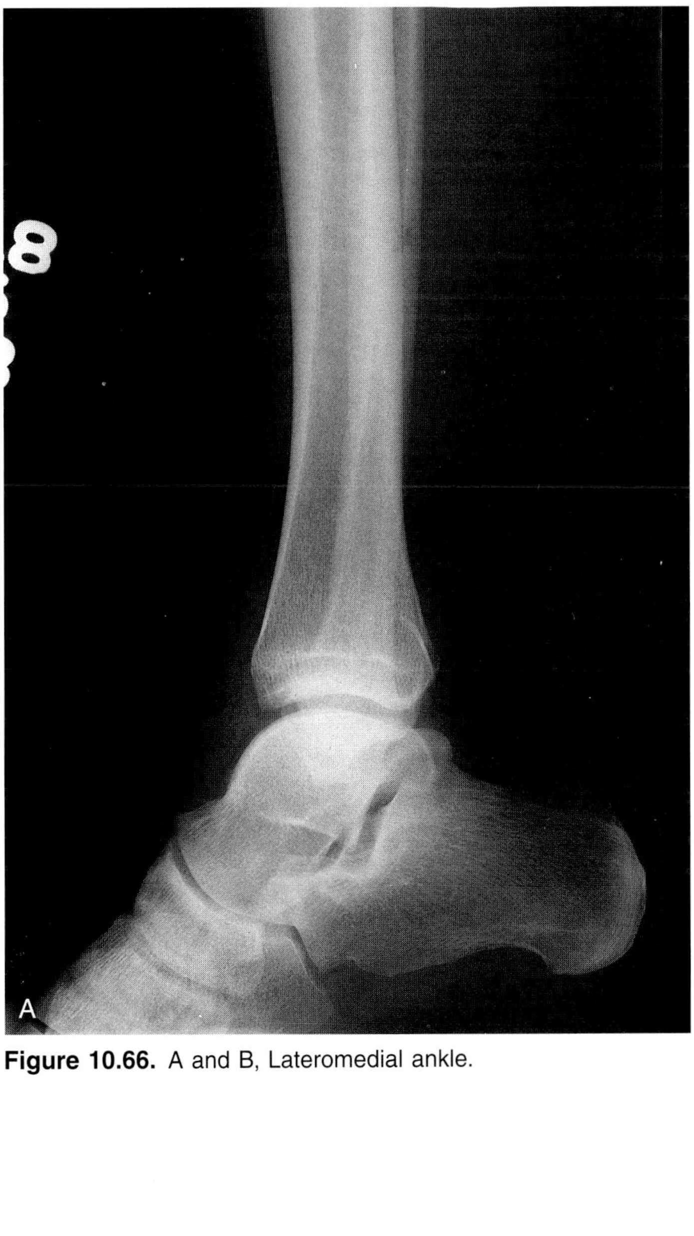

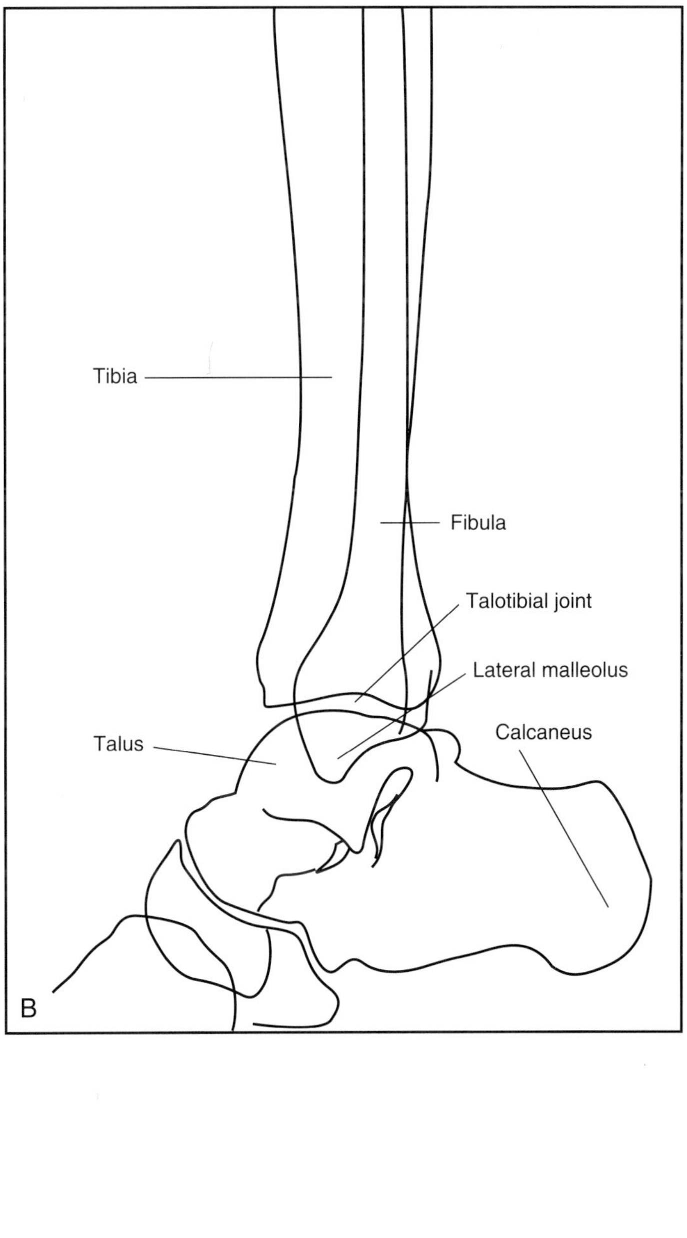

Figure 10.66. A and B, Lateromedial ankle.

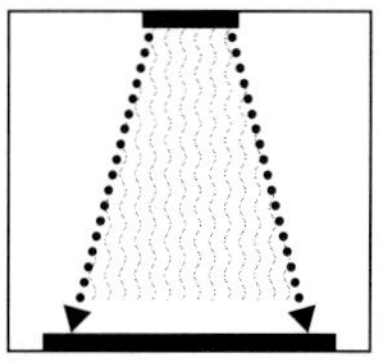

Ankle

Position/Projection

Lateral projection (mediolateral projection)

Film Size:
8 × 10 inches (20 × 24 cm) lengthwise tabletop (1 projection)

or

10 × 12 inches (24 × 30 cm) crosswise tabletop (2 projections)
Divide cassette in half

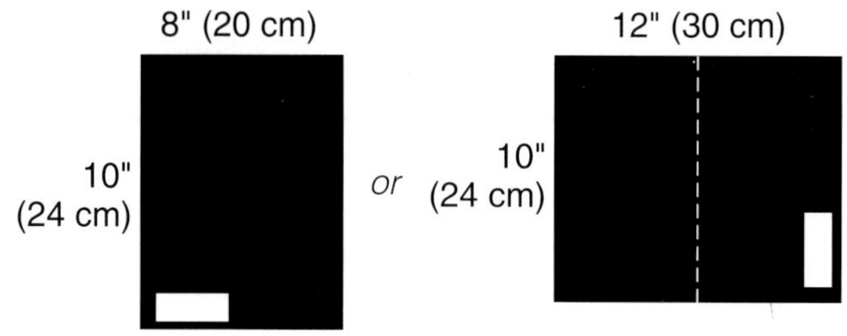

Patient Position

Supine or seated; turn patient toward affected side (Fig. 10.67).

Part Position

Center cassette to ankle joint about ½ inch (1 cm) above distal top of medial malleolus or ¾ inch (2 cm) above distal tip of lateral malleolus. Adjust foot in lateral position and place plane of patella perpendicular to table. Dorsiflex foot to place plantar surface parallel to cassette. Support foot and body in this position.

Central Ray

Perpendicular to midpoint of cassette or unmasked portion through ankle joint midway between anterior and posterior surfaces.

Structures Demonstrated

Lateral projection of distal tibia and fibula, ankle joint, and tarsal (Fig. 10.68).

Evaluation Criteria

1. Distal tibia and fibula, talus, and adjacent tarsals should be seen.
2. Talotibial joint space should be seen.
3. Ankle joint should be centered to film.
4. Fibula should superimpose posterior half of tibia.

NOTE: This projection is preferred for patient comfort.

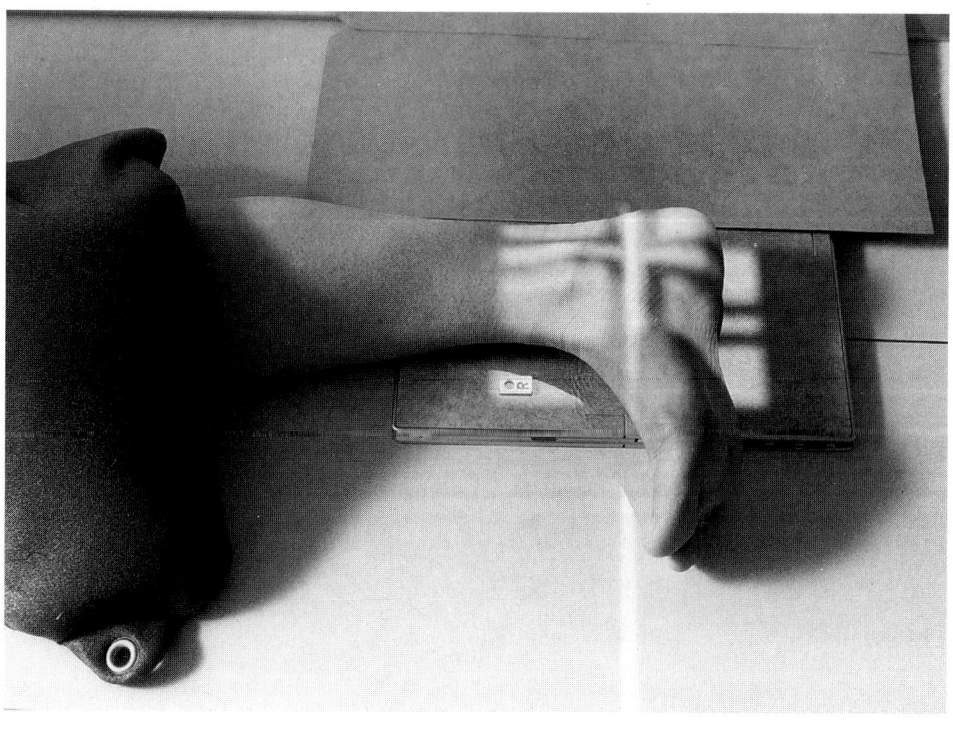

Figure 10.67. Mediolateral ankle.

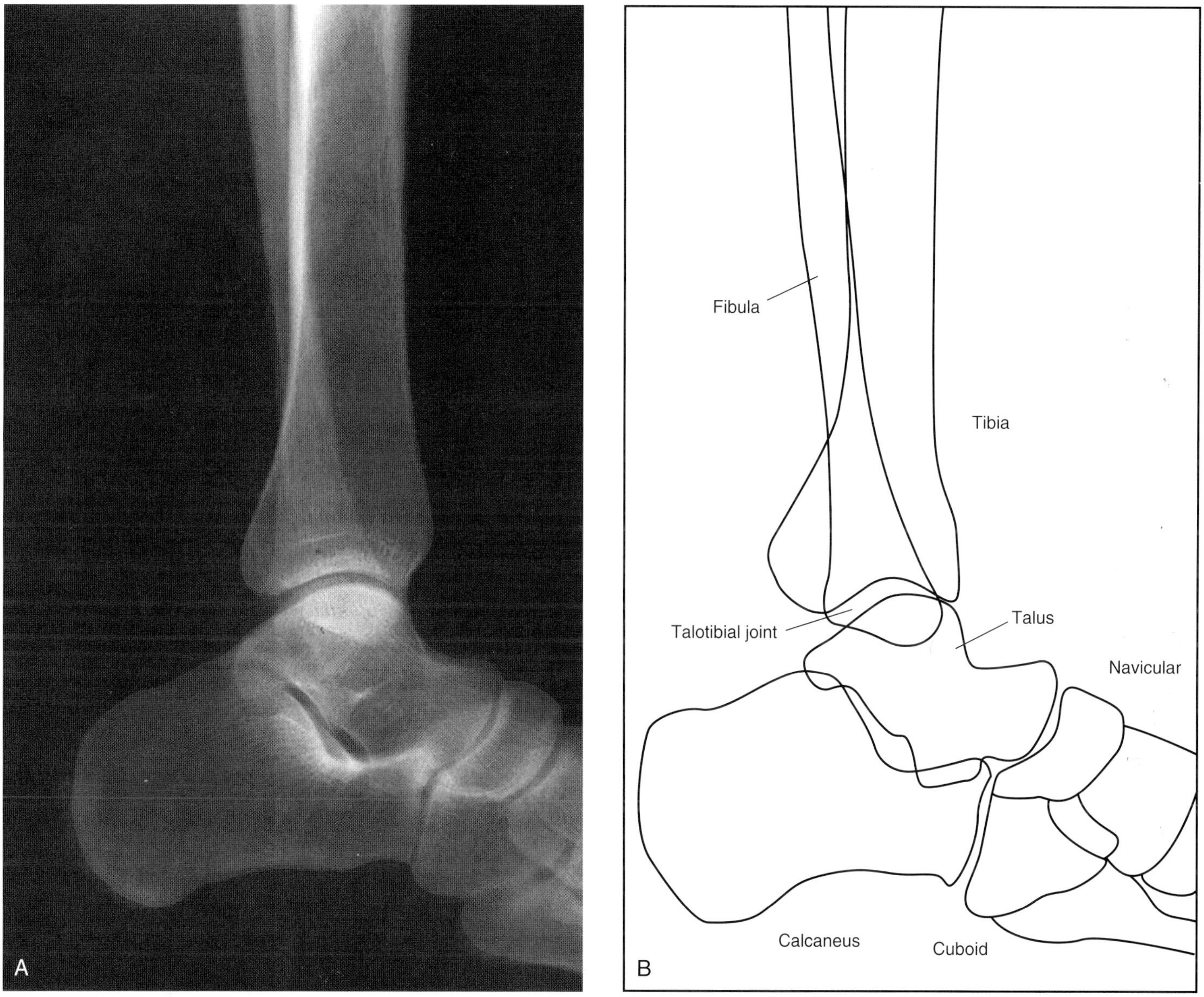

Figure 10.68. A and B, Mediolateral ankle.

Ankle

Position/Projection

Medial oblique projection

Film Size:
8 × 10 inches (20 × 24 cm) lengthwise tabletop (1 projection)

or

10 × 12 inches (24 × 30 cm) crosswise tabletop (2 projections)
Divide cassette in half

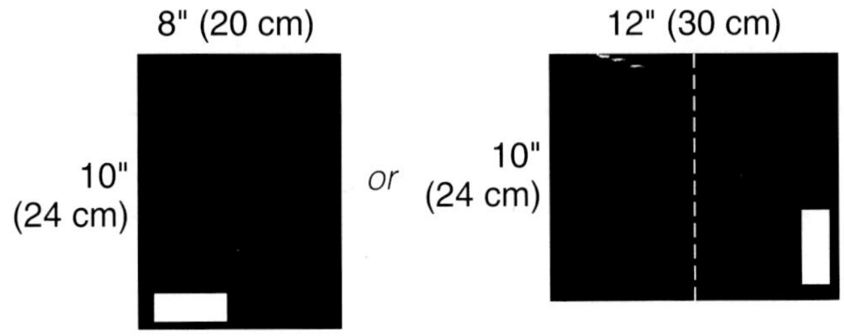

Patient Position

Supine or seated with legs extended (Fig. 10.69).

Part Position

Align long axis of leg to long axis of unmasked half of cassette. Entire lower extremity must be rotated (since knee is a hinge joint, rotation of extremity can come only from hip joint). Rotate affected ankle medially until imaginary line between malleoli is 45° to plane of cassette. Center unmasked half of cassette to ankle joint midway between malleoli. Adjust support under hip so medial side of ankle and foot rest against 45° foam wedge. Place sandbag support under knee. Dorsiflex foot enough to prevent superimposition of lateral malleolus and calcaneus. Dorsiflexion should place ankle at nearly right-angle flexion.

Central Ray

Perpendicular to unmasked portion of cassette through ankle joint midway between malleoli.

Structures Demonstrated

Oblique projection of distal tibia and fibula. Lateral malleolus is well demonstrated in medial oblique projection (Fig. 10.70).

Evaluation Criteria

1. Distal tibia and fibula, talus, and adjacent tarsals should be seen.
2. Talofibular articulation with lateral and medial malleolus should be seen without superimposition over calcaneus.

NOTE: This projection is best for evaluating the ankle mortise. It separates the joint space between distal tibia and fibula (tibiofibular articulation).

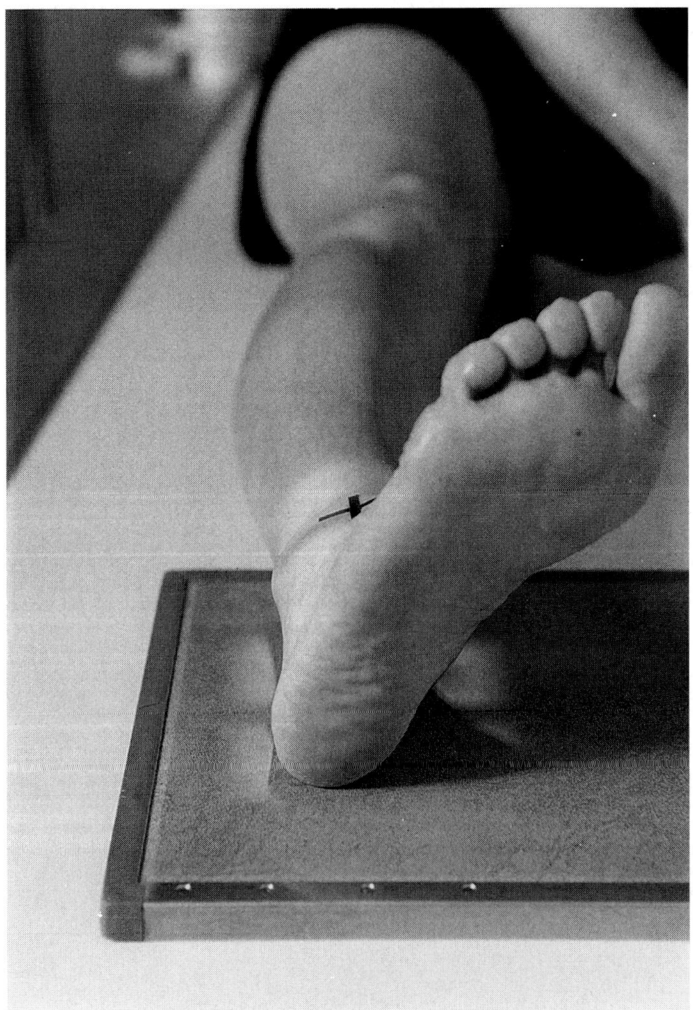

Figure 10.69. Medial oblique ankle.

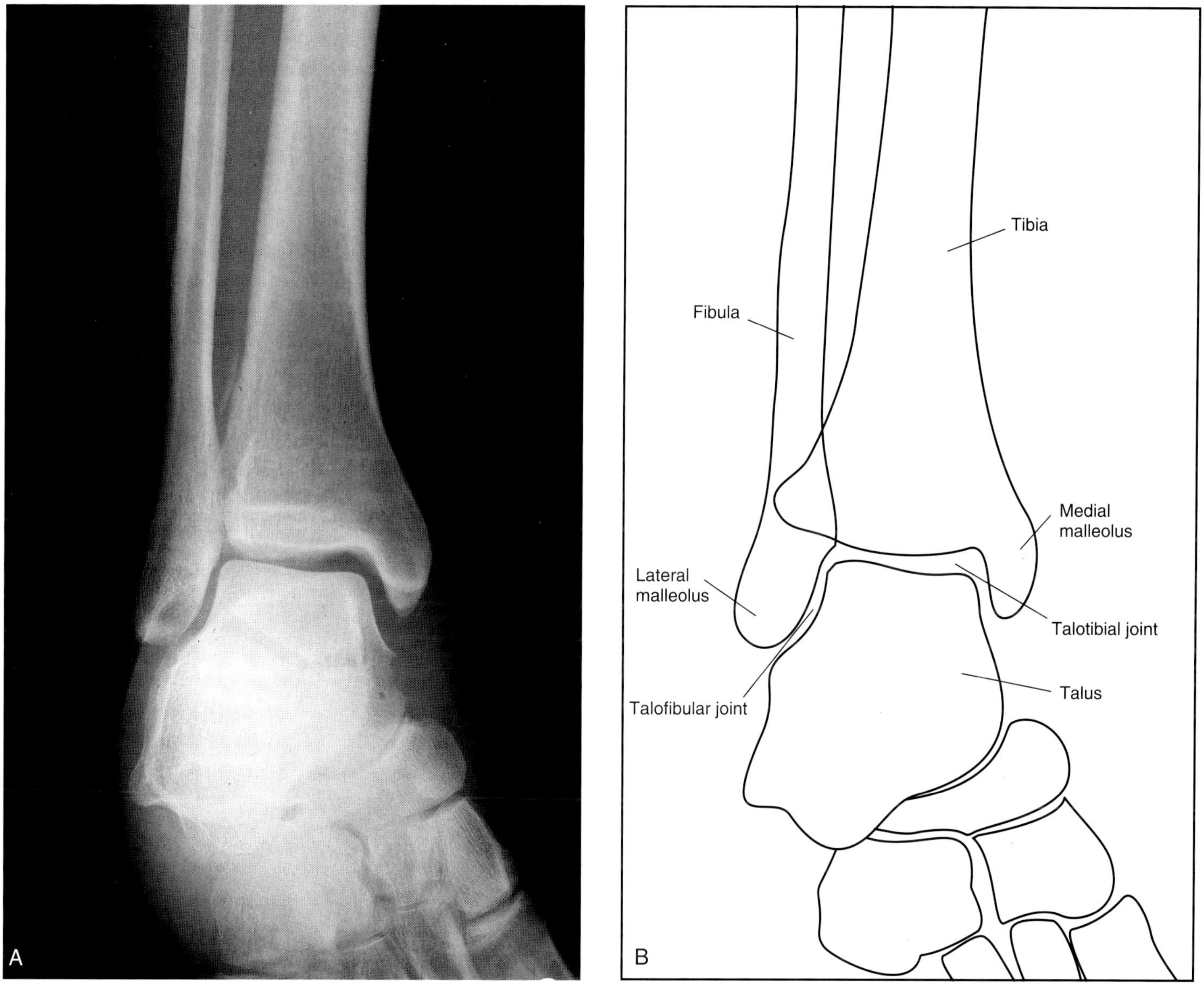

Figure 10.70. A and B, Medial oblique ankle.

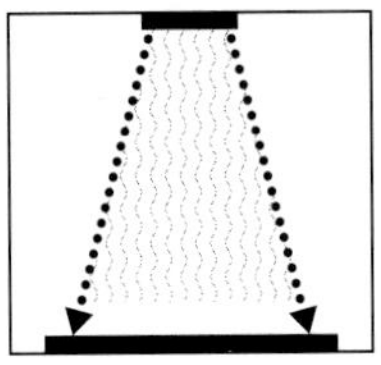

Ankle

Position/Projection

Lateral oblique projection

Film Size:
8 × 10 inches (20 × 24 cm) lengthwise tabletop (1 projection)

or

10 × 12 inches (24 × 30 cm) crosswise tabletop (2 projections)
Divide cassette in half

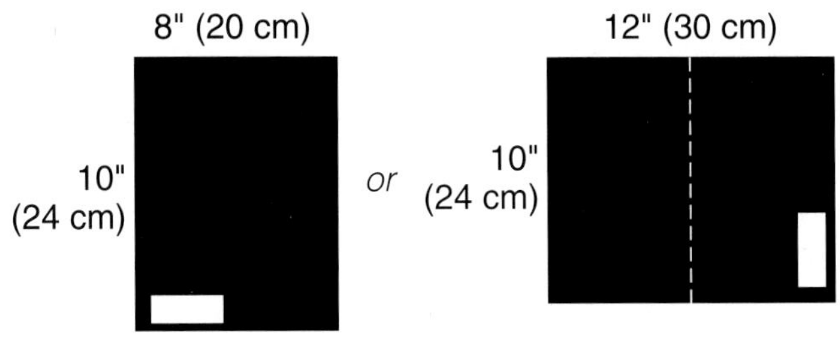

Patient Position

Supine or seated with legs extended (Fig. 10.71).

Part Position

Align long axis of leg to unmasked half of cassette. Entire lower extremity must be rotated (since knee is a hinge joint, rotation can come only from hip joint). Rotate affected ankle laterally until imaginary line between malleoli is 45° to plane of cassette. Center unmasked half of cassette to ankle joint midway between malleoli. Adjust support under hip so lateral side of ankle and foot rest against 45° foam wedge.

Central Ray

Perpendicular to unmasked portion of cassette through ankle joint midway between malleoli.

Structures Demonstrated

Oblique projection of distal tibia and fibula. Calcaneal sulcus is demonstrated (Fig. 10.72).

Evaluation Criteria

1. Distal tibia, fibula, talus, and adjacent tarsals should be seen.
2. Talocalcaneal joint should be demonstrated along with calcaneal sulcus.

NOTE: This projection is useful to determine subtle fractures.

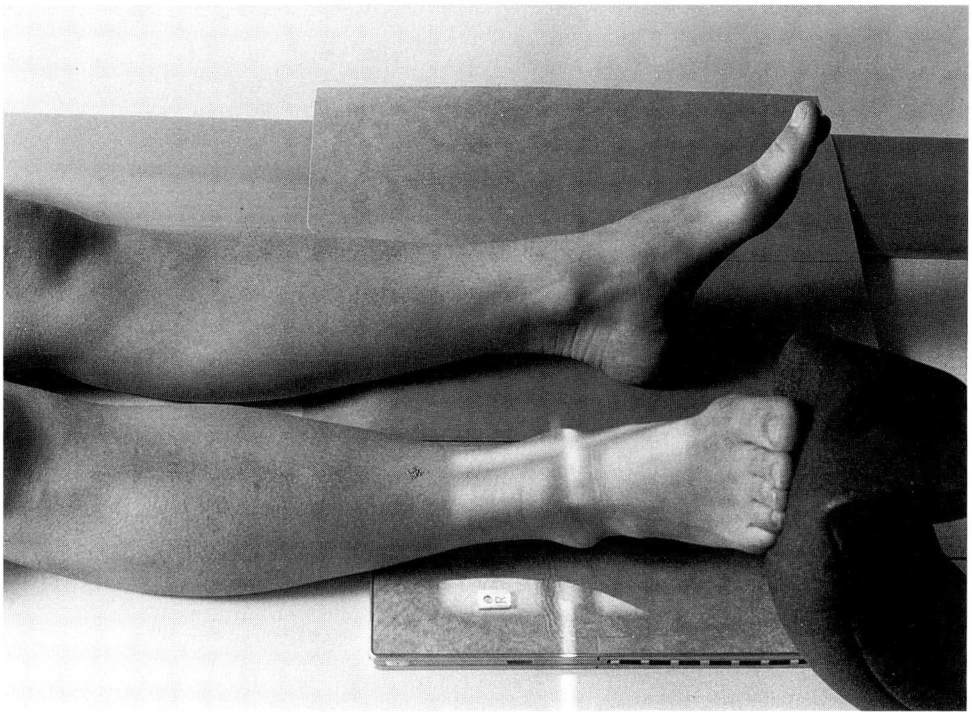

Figure 10.71. Lateral oblique ankle.

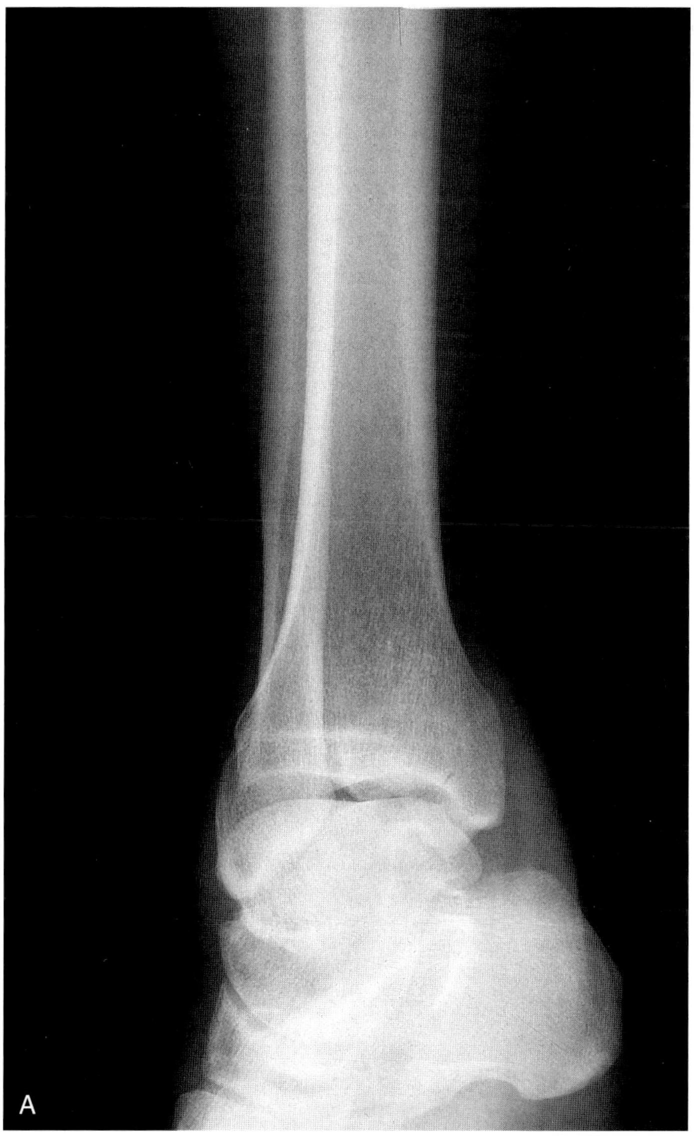

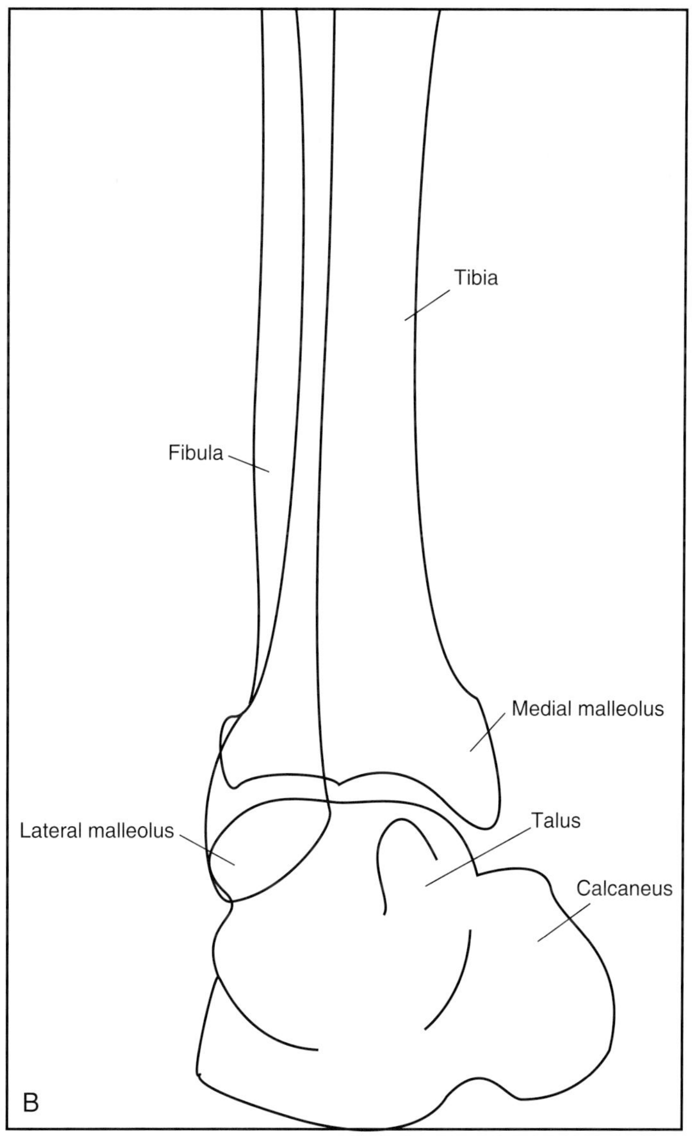

Figure 10.72. A and B, Lateral oblique ankle.

Ankle

Position/Projection

AP stress studies

Film Size:
8 × 10 inches (20 × 24 cm) lengthwise tabletop (1 projection)

or

10 × 12 inches (24 × 30 cm) crosswise tabletop (2 projections)
Divide cassette in half

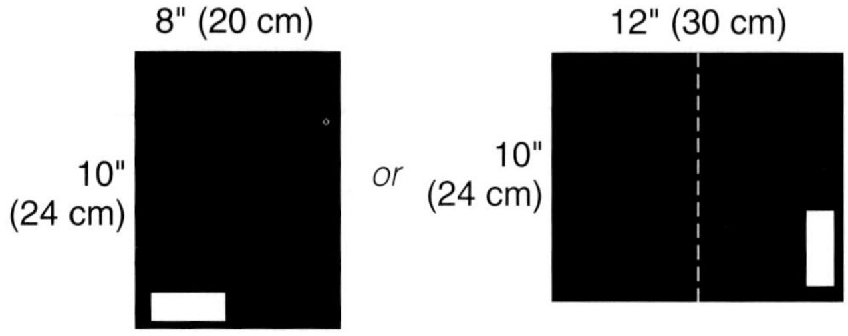

Patient Position

Supine or seated with legs extended (Fig. 10.73).

Part Position

Stress studies are usually positioned by physician. Align long axis of leg to unmasked portion of cassette. Center point midway between lateral and medial malleoli to midpoint of unmasked half of cassette. Dorsiflex foot with 5° medial rotation to place intermalleolar line parallel to cassette and to place plantar surface of foot perpendicular to cassette. Dorsiflex foot with 5° medial rotation to place intermalleolar line parallel to cassette and to place plantar surface of foot perpendicular to cassette. For first projection, place foot in extreme inversion. For second projection, place foot in extreme eversion.

Central Ray

Perpendicular to midpoint of unmasked portion of cassette midway between malleoli.

Structures Demonstrated

AP stress projection of ankle joint, distal tibia and fibula, and proximal talus (Fig. 10.74). Demonstrates ligament tears.

Evaluation Criteria

1. Distal tibia and fibula to talus should be seen with slight overlapping of distal tibiofibular articulation.
2. Talotibial joint space should be seen.
3. Ankle joint should be centered to film.
4. Medial and lateral malleoli should be seen with medial malleolus free of superimposition and lateral malleolus slightly superimposed by talus.

NOTE: Stress studies are usually done to rule out a ligamentous tear after an inversion or supination injury. To see the tear, the joint space needs to be widened on the injured side so the foot is forced toward the opposite side. A short exposure technique is used, since this projection is very uncomfortable and painful for the patient.

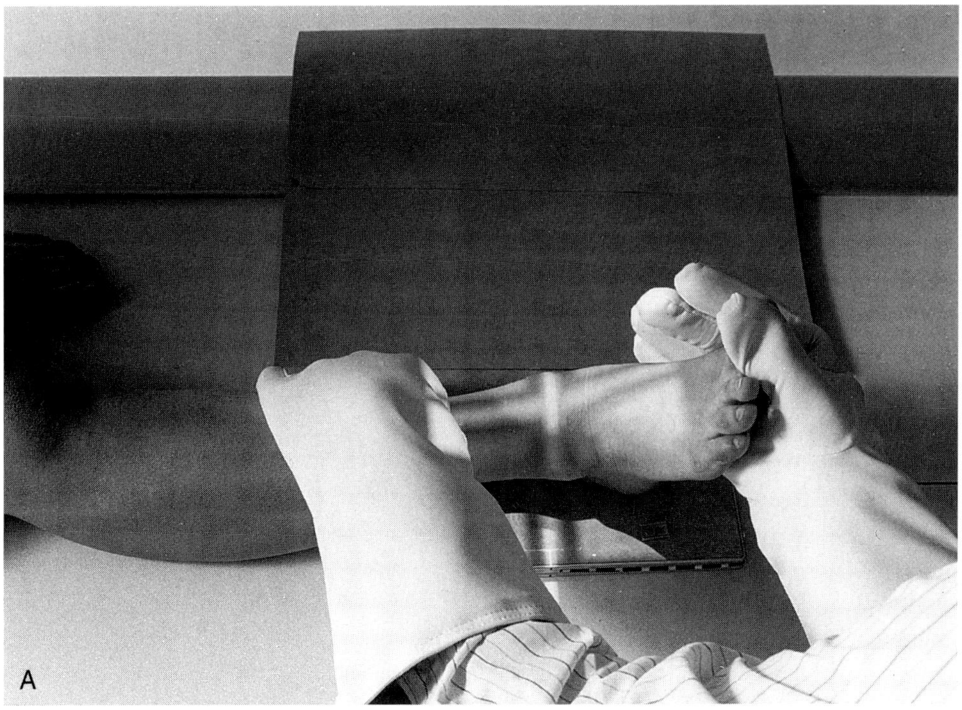
A

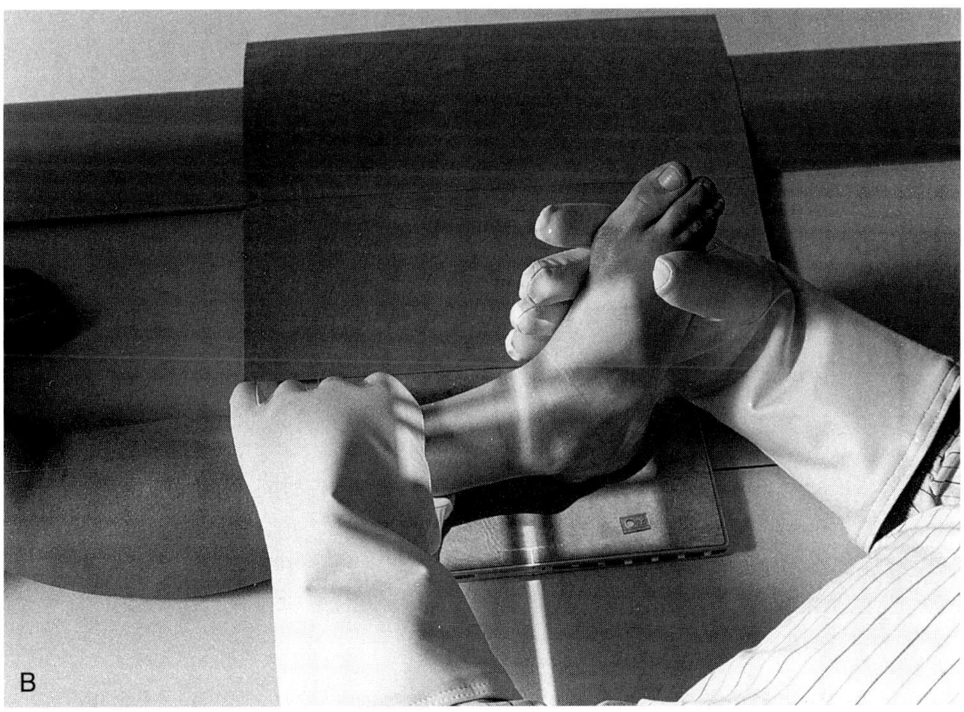
B

Figure 10.73. A and B, AP stress studies.

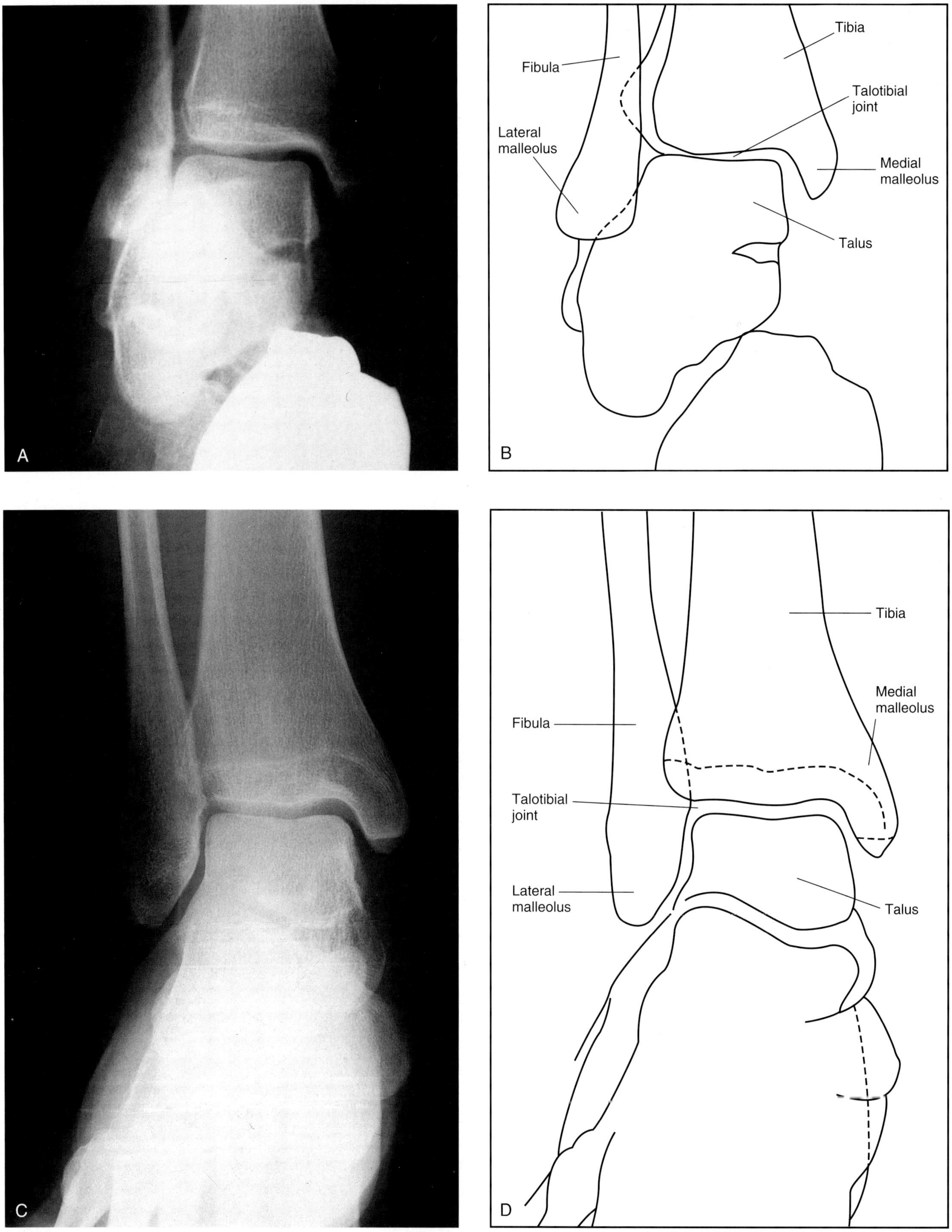

Figure 10.74. A–D, AP stress studies.

Leg

Position/Projection

AP projection

Film Size:
14 × 17 inches (35 × 43 cm) lengthwise tabletop (for adults)
Divide cassette in half
Cassette needs to be long enough to include all of knee joint and all of ankle joint
Cassette needs to extend 1 to 1½ inches (2.5 to 4 cm) beyond joints
Cassette can be lengthwise or diagonal

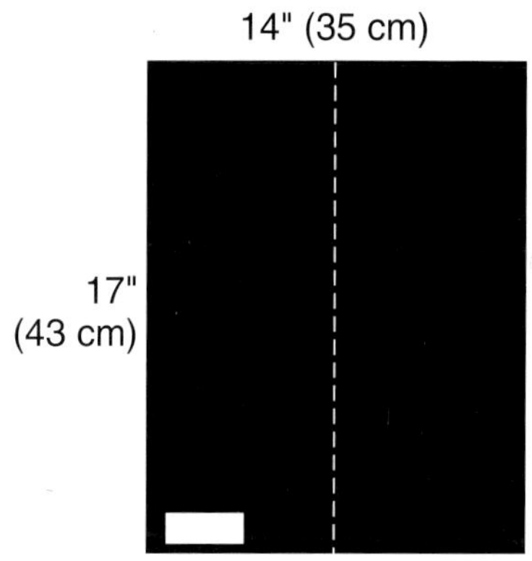

Patient Position
Supine or seated with knee extended (Fig. 10.75).

Part Position
Align long axis of leg to long axis of cassette. Adjust leg in AP position with foot slightly inverted (do not rotate leg). Center leg to midline of cassette. Check positioning to make sure both joints included on cassette.

Central Ray
Perpendicular to midpoint of cassette through midshaft of tibia.

Structures Demonstrated
AP projection of entire tibia, fibula, knee joint, and ankle joint (Fig. 10.76).

Evaluation Criteria
1. Entire leg, including knee joint and ankle joint, should be seen.
2. Entire leg should be seen without rotation (should see equal spaces on both sides of knee joint).
3. Talotibial joint space should be seen.
4. Technique should provide density to visualize trabecular markings and soft tissue of entire leg.

NOTE: Before exposure is made of the lower leg, check position of part and cassette to assure both joints will be included in their entirety in the image. If the entire extremity is not included, then have a longer film to include one joint and direct the central ray perpendicular to the midpoint of the cassette. With the patient and part in the same position, choose a smaller cassette and center the extremity to include the other joint and overlap the first image by about 2 inches (5 cm); direct central ray perpendicular to the midpoint of the cassette.

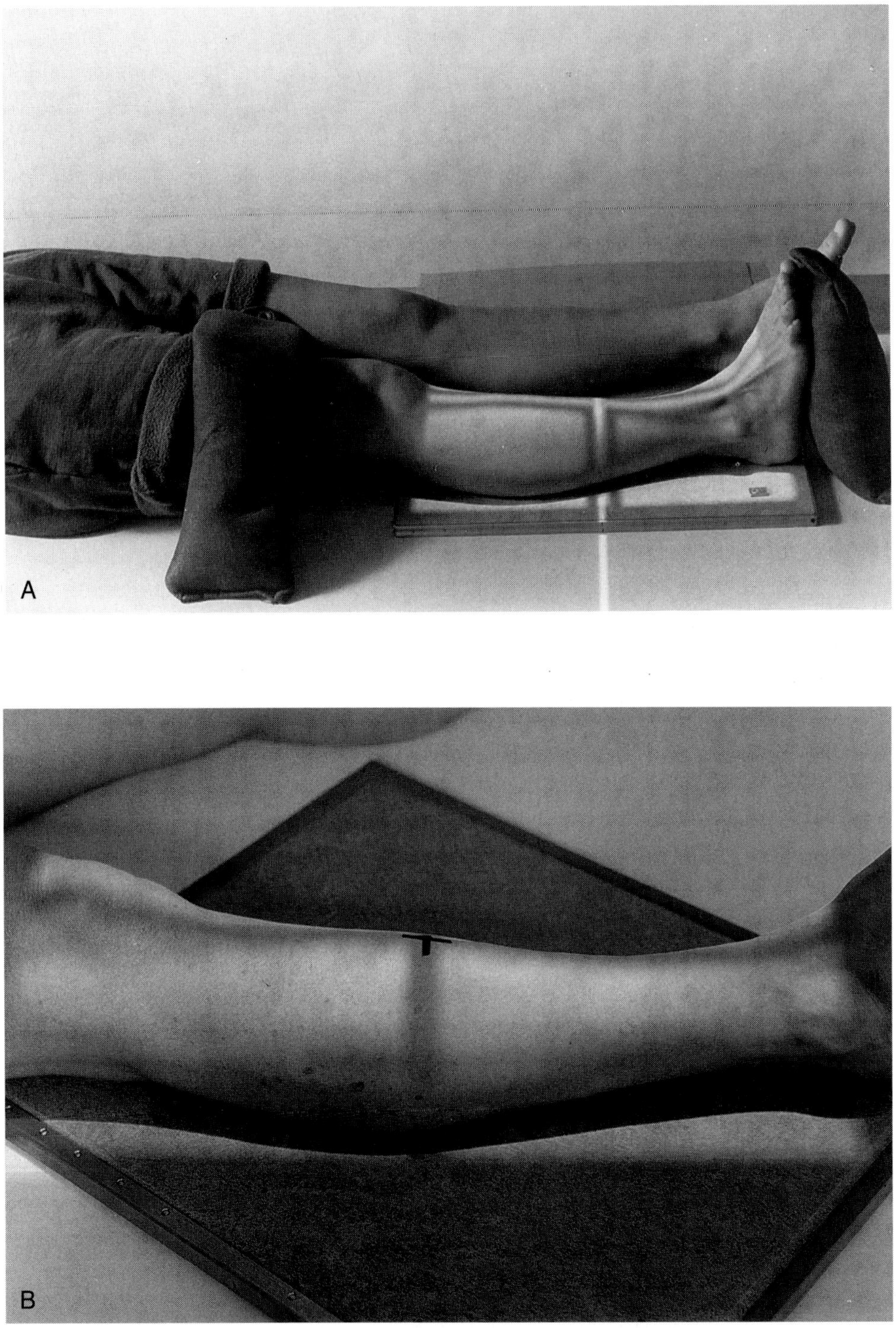

Figure 10.75. A, AP tibia and fibula. B, AP tibia and fibula, placed diagonally.

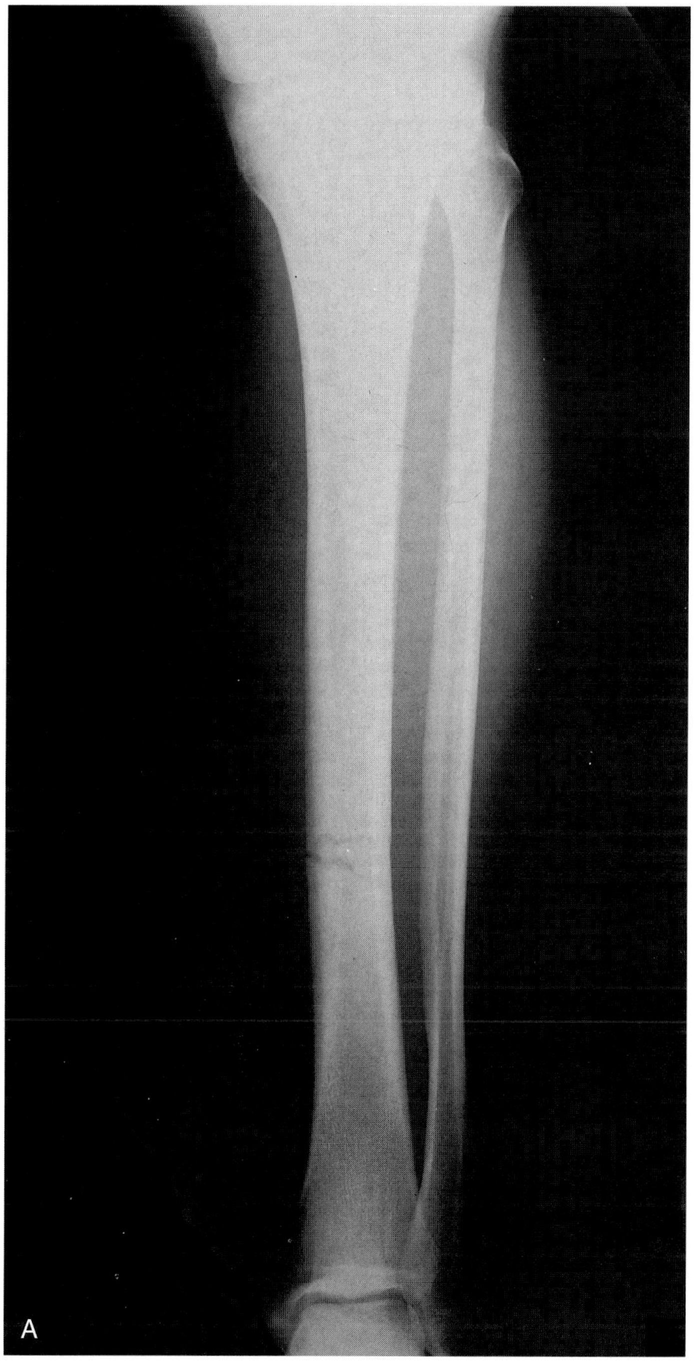

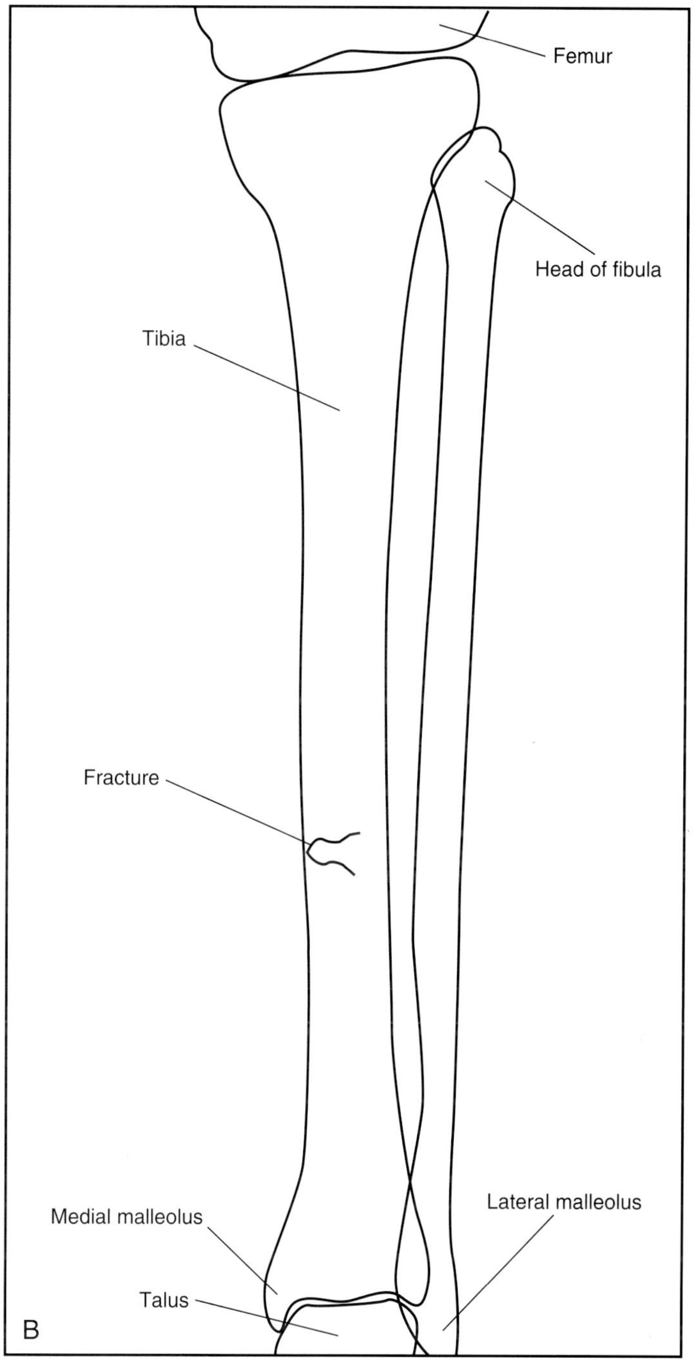

Figure 10.76. A and B, AP tibia and fibula.

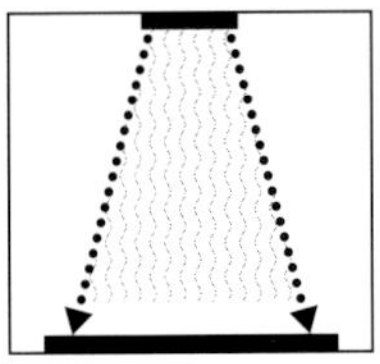

Leg

Position/Projection

Lateral projection

Film Size:
14 × 17 inches (35 × 43 cm) lengthwise tabletop (for adults)
Divide cassette in half
Cassette needs to be long enough to include all of knee joint and all of ankle joint
Cassette needs to extend 1 to 1½ inches (2.5 to 4 cm) beyond joints
Cassette can be lengthwise or diagonal

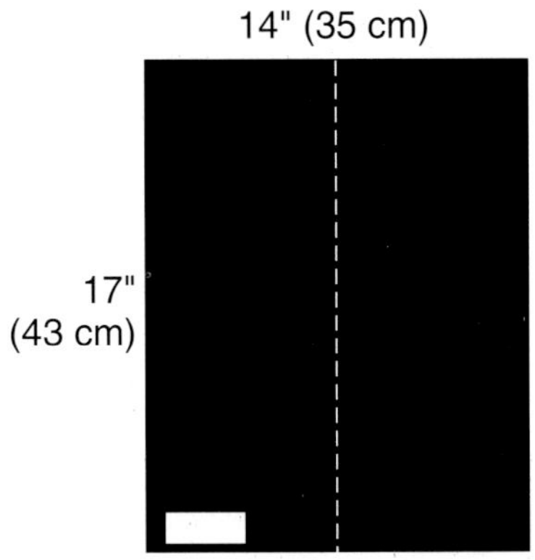

Patient Position

Supine or seated, patient turned laterally toward affected extremity (Fig. 10.77).

Part Position

Align long axis of leg to long axis of cassette. Turn patient laterally toward affected side. Position leg to place plane of patella perpendicular to cassette. Center midpoint of leg to unmasked half of cassette. Dorsiflex foot to place plantar surface parallel to plane of cassette. Check positioning to make sure both joints are included on cassette.

Central Ray

Perpendicular to midpoint of cassette through midshaft of tibia.

Structures Demonstrated

Lateral projection of entire tibia, fibula, knee joint, and ankle joint (Fig. 10.78).

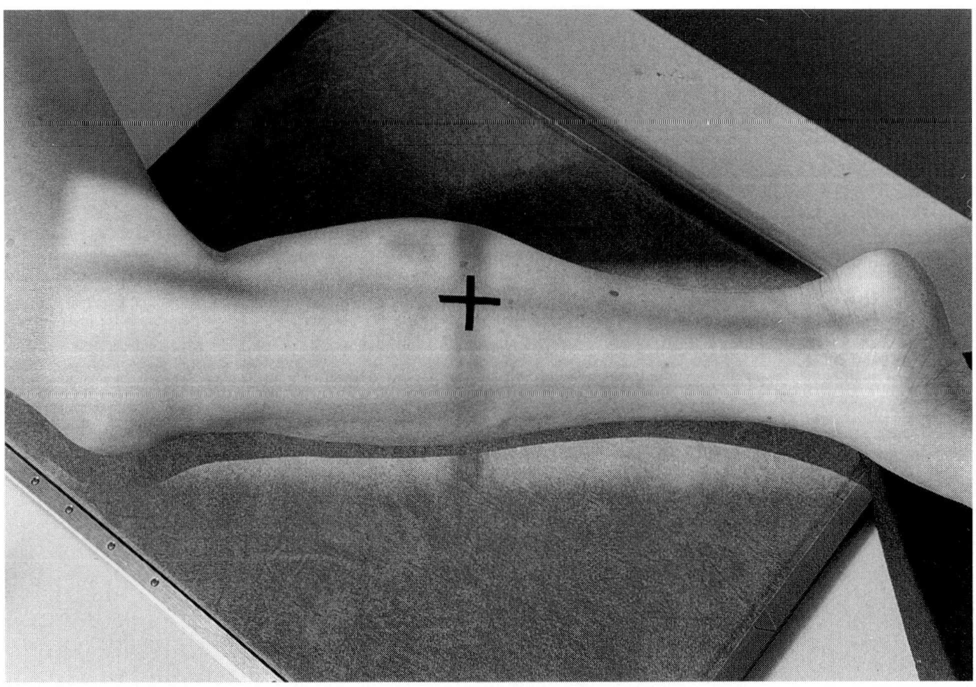

Figure 10.77. Lateral tibia and fibula.

Evaluation Criteria

1. Entire leg, including knee joint and ankle joint, should be seen.
2. Distal fibula should superimpose posterior half of tibia.
3. Tibia should completely superimpose lateral malleolus of distal fibula.
4. Technique should provide density to visualize trabecular markings and soft tissue of entire leg.

NOTE: The lateral projection of the lower leg is normally performed using the mediolateral projection. If the patient cannot turn in the lateral position, a cross-table lateral can be performed. This can be done with the lower leg in an AP position with the film in a vertical position on its side between the extremities. The central ray is directed horizontally and perpendicular to midpoint of cassette through the lateral side of affected leg.

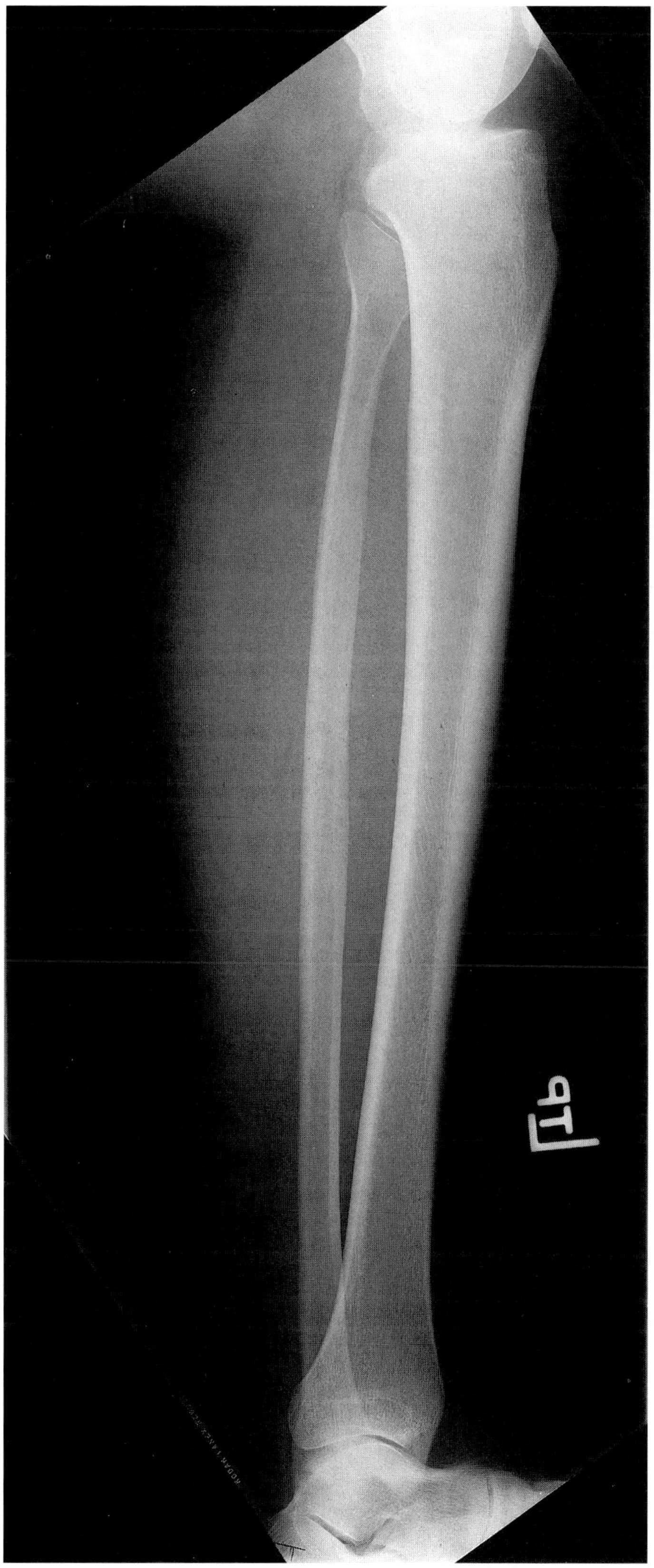

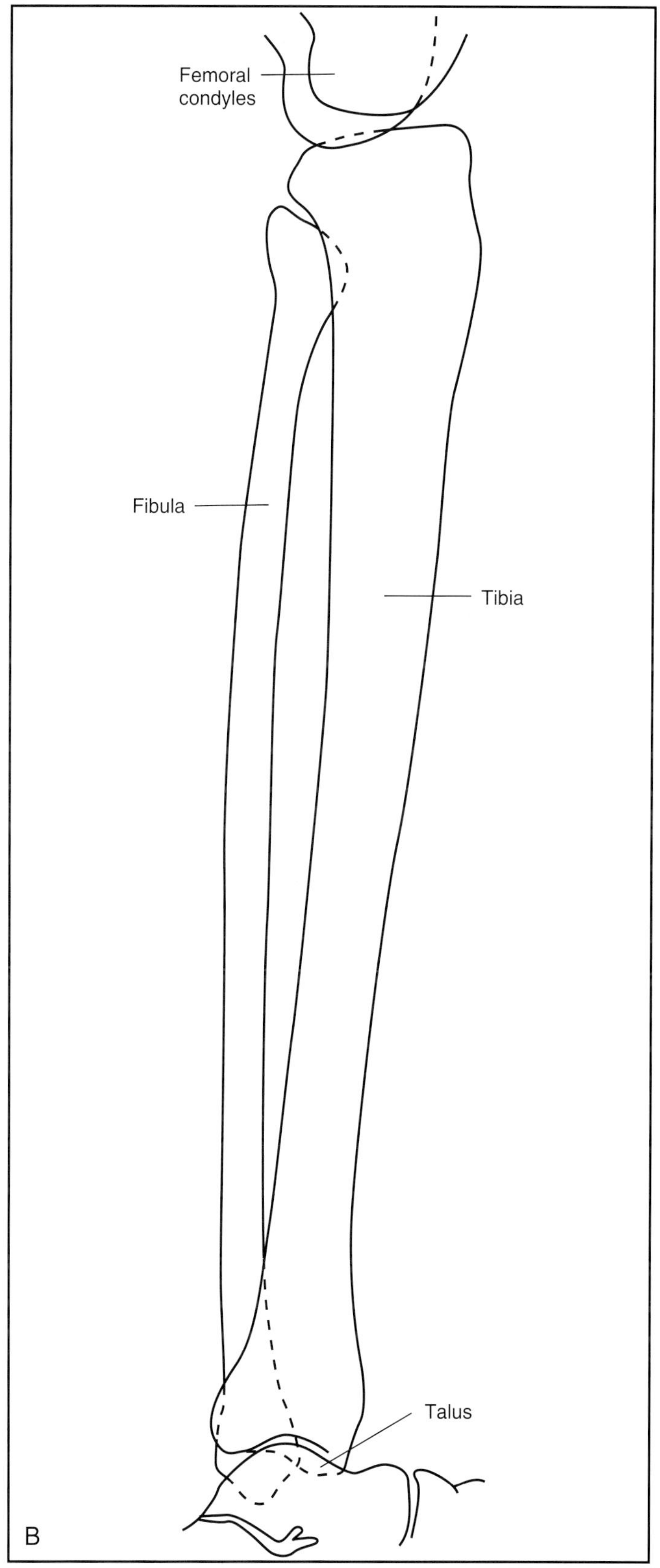

Figure 10.78. A and B, Lateral tibia and fibula.

Lower Leg

Position/Projection

Oblique projections

Film Size:
14 × 17 inches (35 × 43 cm) lengthwise tabletop (for adults)
Divide cassette in half
Cassette needs to be long enough to include all of knee joint and all of ankle joint
Cassette needs to extend 1 to 1½ inches (2.5 to 4 cm) beyond joints
Cassette can be lengthwise or diagonal

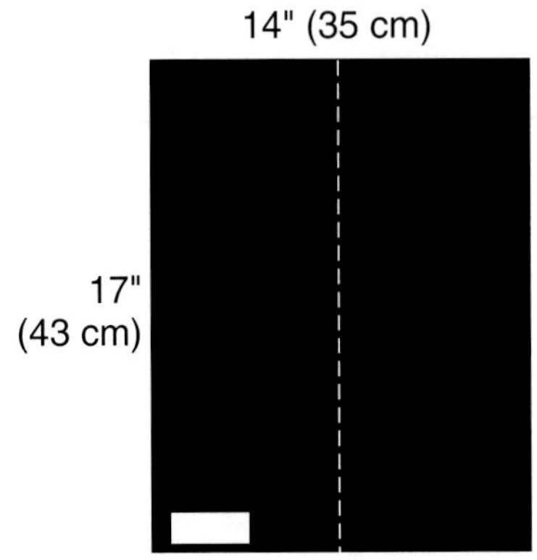

Patient Position

Supine or seated with leg extended (Fig. 10.79).

Part Position

Align long axis of leg to long axis of cassette. Center midpoint of leg to unmasked half of cassette. For medial oblique (internal rotation), rotate extremity 45° medially. For lateral oblique (external rotation), rotate extremity 45° laterally.

Central Ray

Perpendicular to midpoint of cassette.

Structures Demonstrated

45° oblique projections of lower leg with adjacent joints included (Fig. 10.80).

Evaluation Criteria

Medial Oblique

1. Entire leg, including knee joint and ankle joint, should be seen.
2. Fibula superimposed by lateral portion of tibia.

Lateral Oblique

1. Entire leg, including knee joint and ankle joint, should be seen.
2. Distal and proximal tibiofibular articulations should be seen.

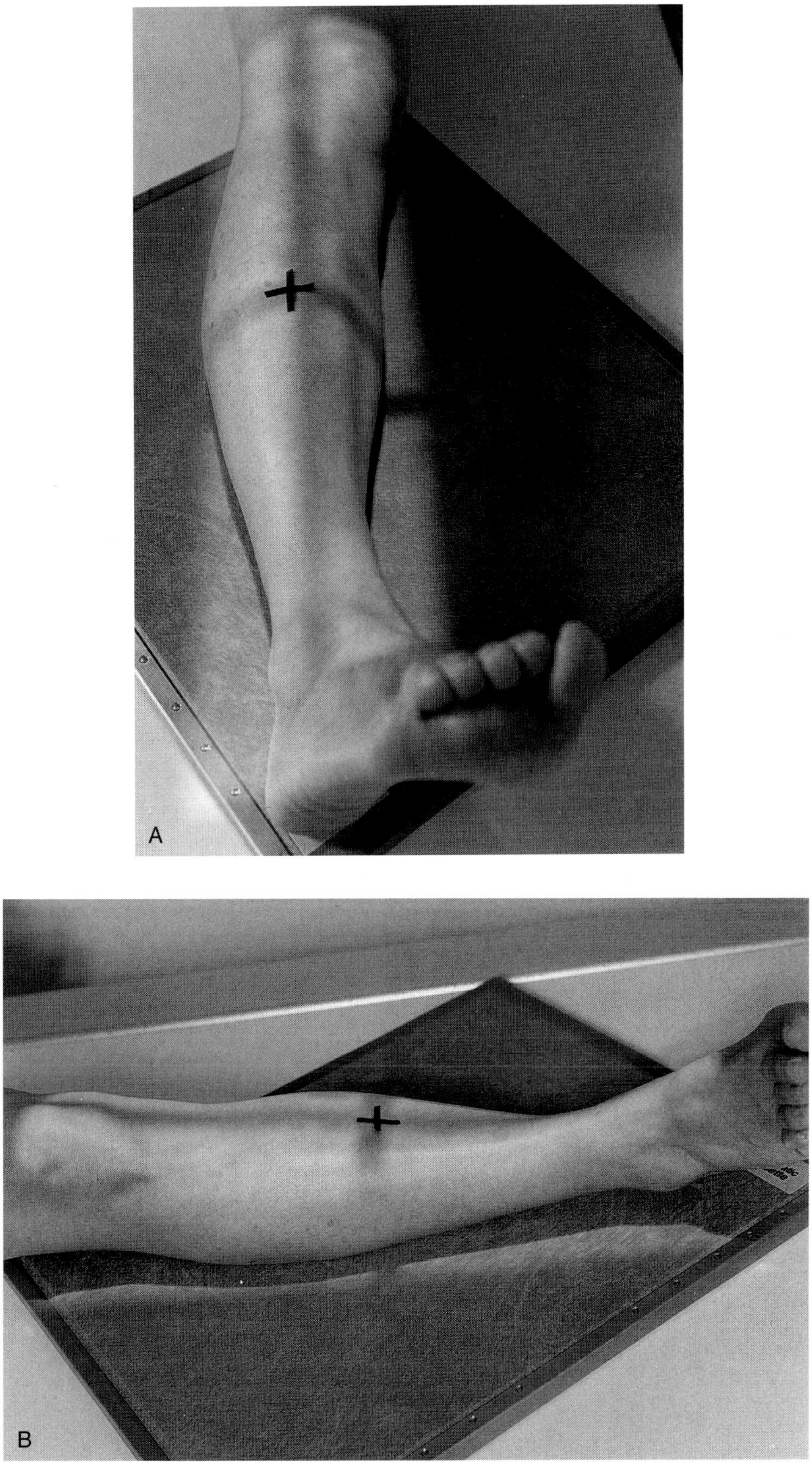

Figure 10.79. A, Medial oblique. B, Lateral oblique.

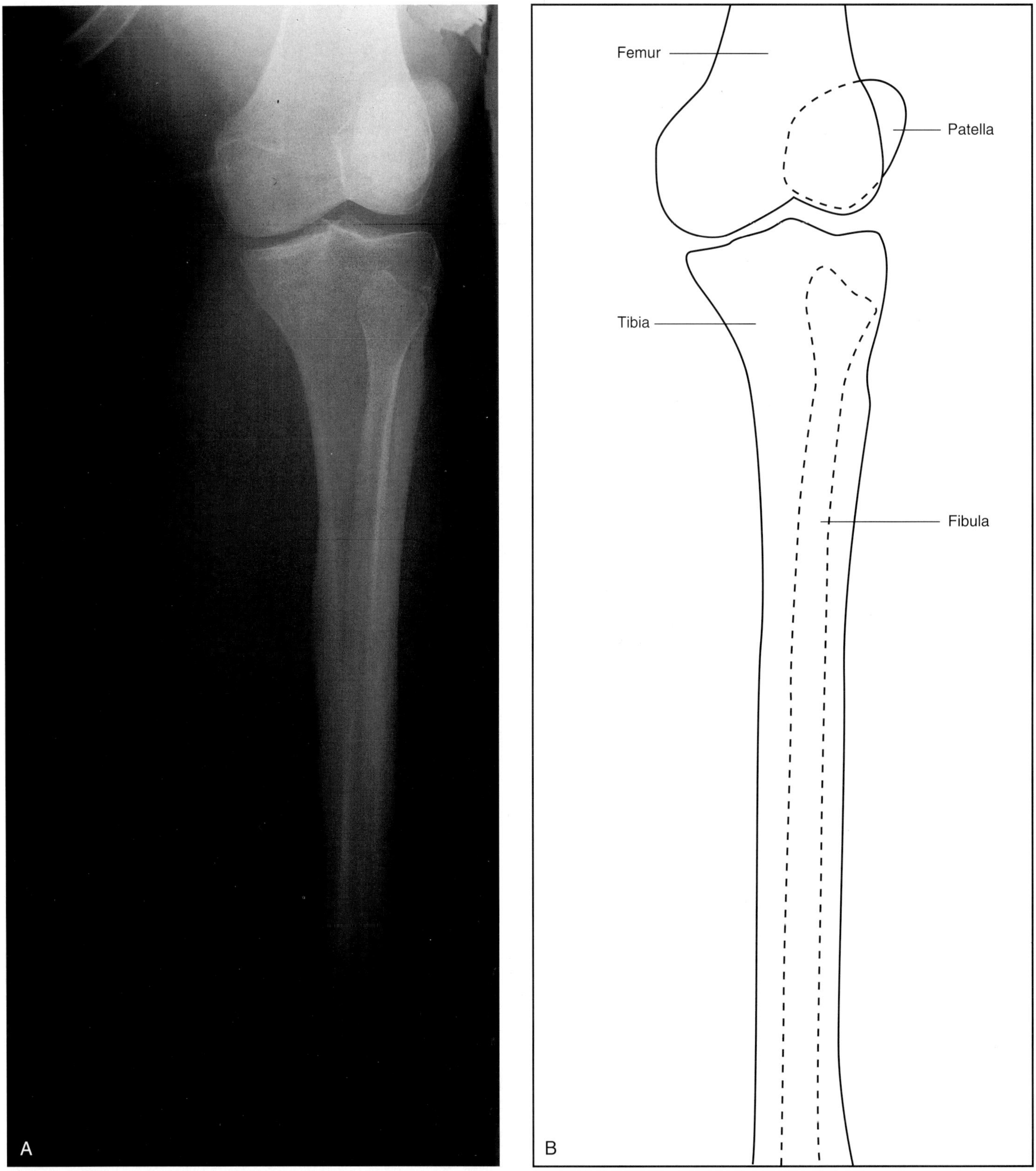

Figure 10.80. A–D, Medial oblique tibia and fibula.

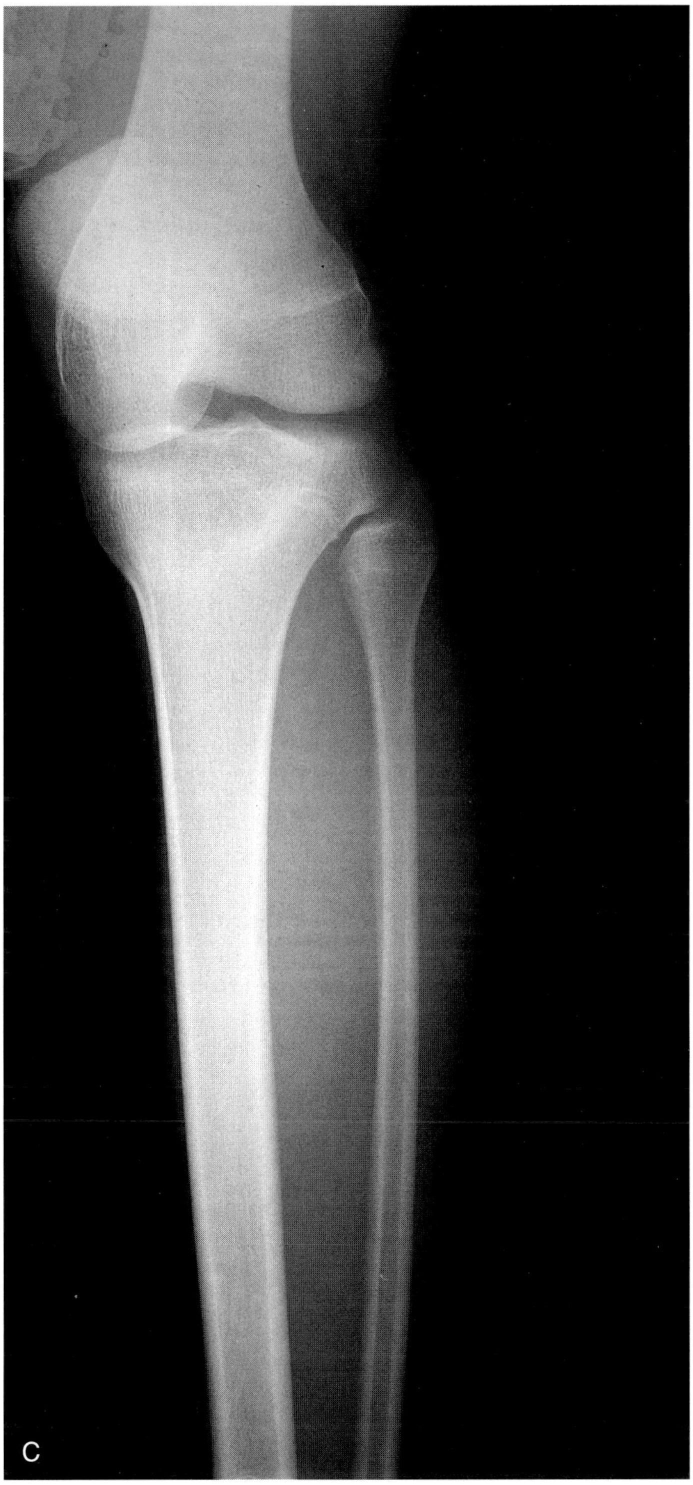

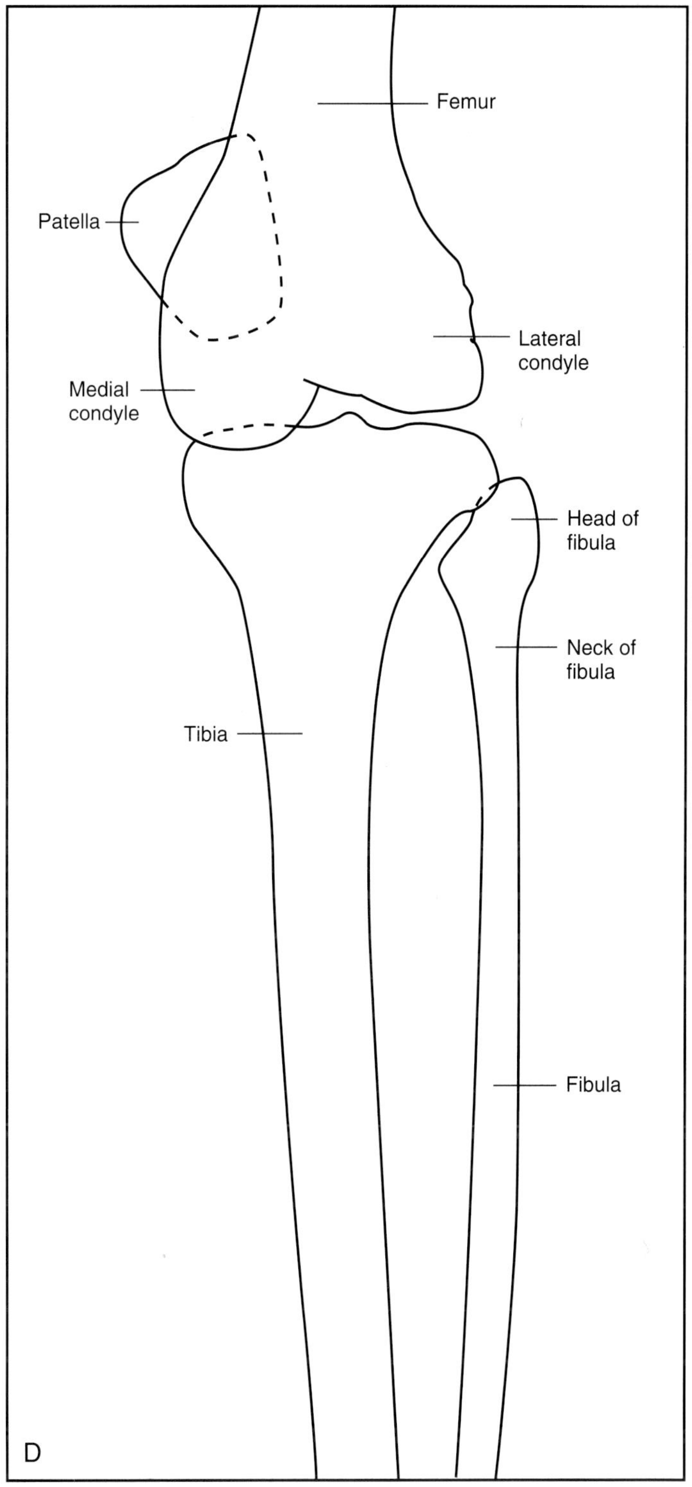

Figure 10.80 *(Continued)*

Knee

Position/Projection

PA projection

Film Size:
8 × 10 inches (20 × 24 cm) lengthwise (small to normal) Bucky

or

10 × 12 inches (24 × 30 cm) lengthwise (large) Bucky

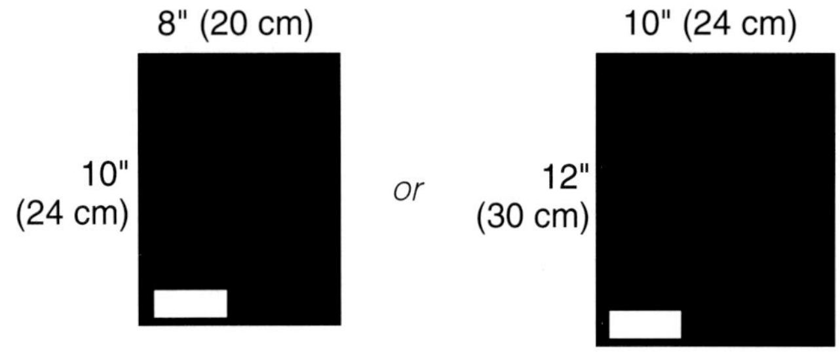

Patient Position

Prone, with legs extended (Fig. 10.81).

Part Position

Align long axis of affected leg with midline of table. Rotate entire leg of affected knee 5° internally (places imaginary line between femoral condyles parallel with plane of table). Support ankle to prevent pressure on toes.

Central Ray

Perpendicular ½ inch (1 cm) below apex of patella (with the lower leg elevated, there is no need for angulation because central ray enters perpendicular to the tibia plateau so the joint space is open). Center cassette to central ray.

Structures Demonstrated

PA projection of distal femur, proximal tibia and fibula, and patella. Open joint space (Fig. 10.82).

Evaluation Criteria

1. Lateral and medial portions of joint space should be equal.
2. Joint space should be seen without superimposition by patella.

NOTE: If there is deterioration of the joint space caused by trauma or pathology, the medial and lateral portions may not be equal.

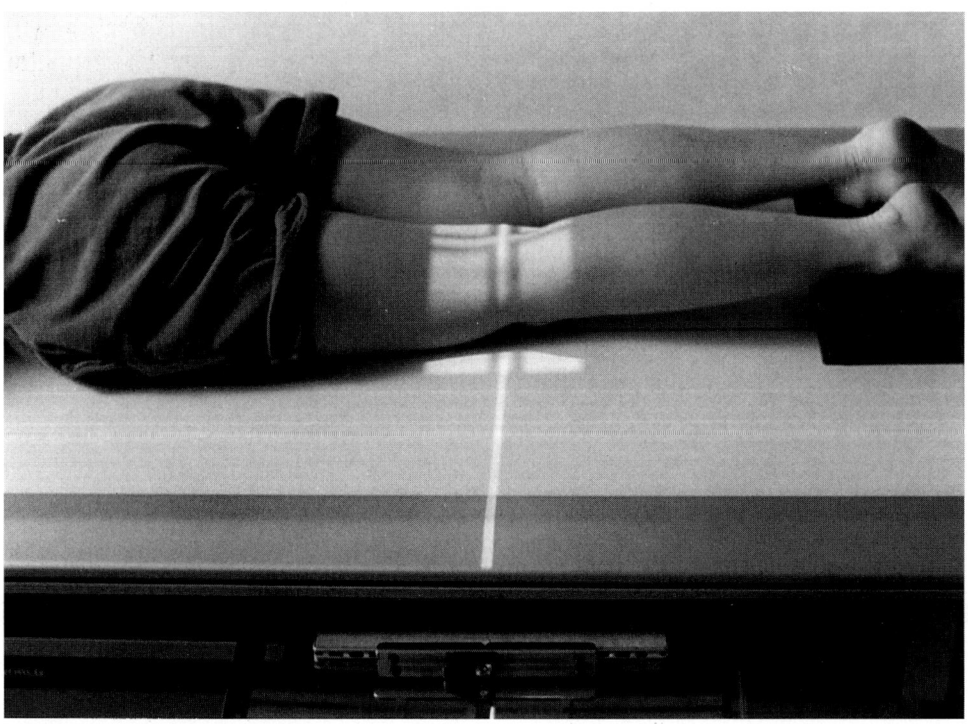

Figure 10.81. PA knee.

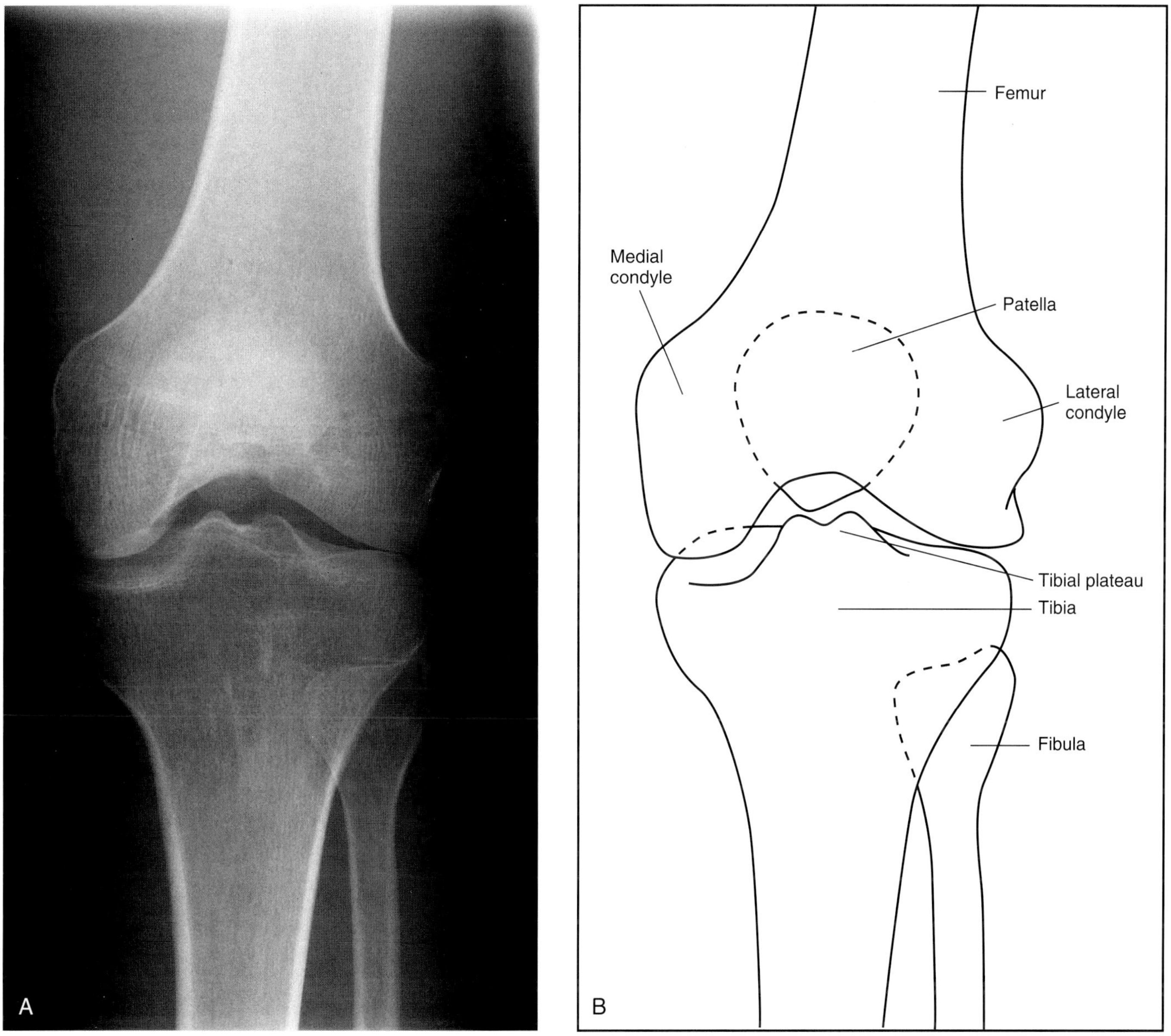

Figure 10.82. A and B, PA knee.

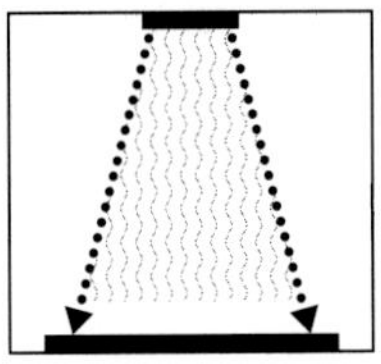

Knee

Position/Projection

AP projection

Film Size:
8 × 10 inches (20 × 24 cm) lengthwise (small to normal) Bucky

or

10 × 12 inches (24 × 30 cm) lengthwise (large) Bucky

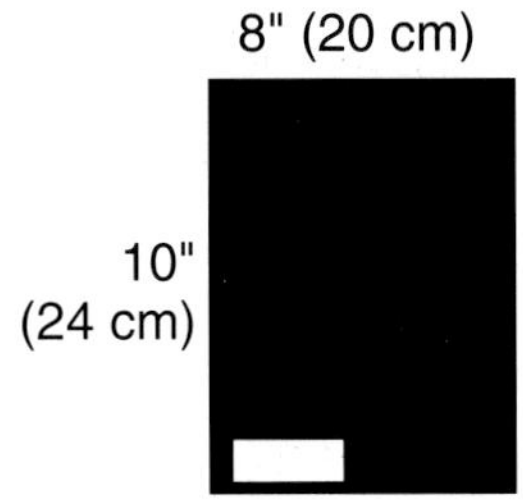

or

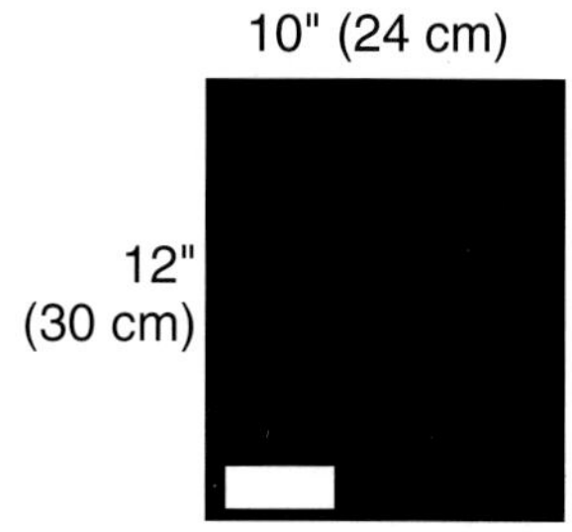

Patient Position

Supine or seated with legs extended (Fig. 10.83).

Part Position

Align long axis of affected leg with midline of table. Adjust leg in true AP position; plane of patella parallel with plane of cassette. Rotate entire leg of affected knee 5° internally (places imaginary line between femoral condyles parallel with plane of table). Central ray enters knee about ½ inch (1 cm) below apex of patella (knee joint space lies, with lower extremity extended, approximately ½ inch (1 cm) below level of apex of patella).

Central Ray

5° cephalic angle through knee joint to demonstrate joint space. Direct central ray perpendicular to knee joint to demonstrate distal end of femur or proximal ends of tibia and fibula.

Structures Demonstrated

AP projection of distal femur, proximal tibia and fibula, and patella. Central ray angled demonstrates joint space without superimposition by patella. Central ray perpendicular demonstrates joint space superimposed by patella (Fig. 10.84).

Evaluation Criteria

1. Lateral and medial portions of joint space should be equal.
2. If central ray angled, joint space should be seen without superimposition by patella; patella should superimpose femur.
3. If central ray perpendicular, patella should superimpose joint space.

NOTE: If there is deterioration of the joint space caused by trauma or pathology, the medial and lateral portions may not be equal.

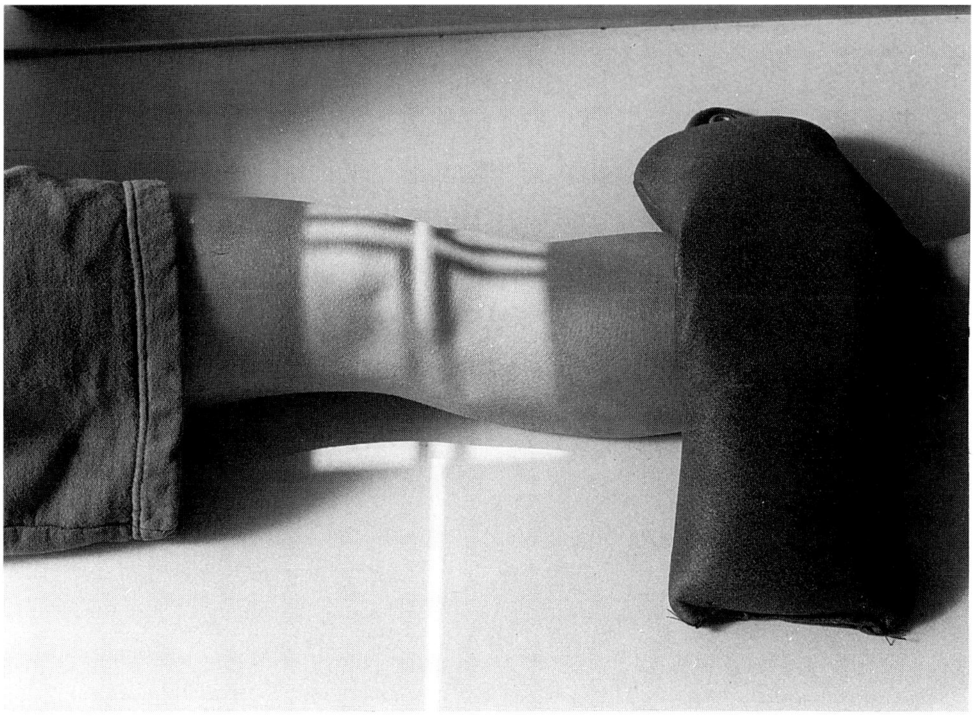

Figure 10.83. AP knee.

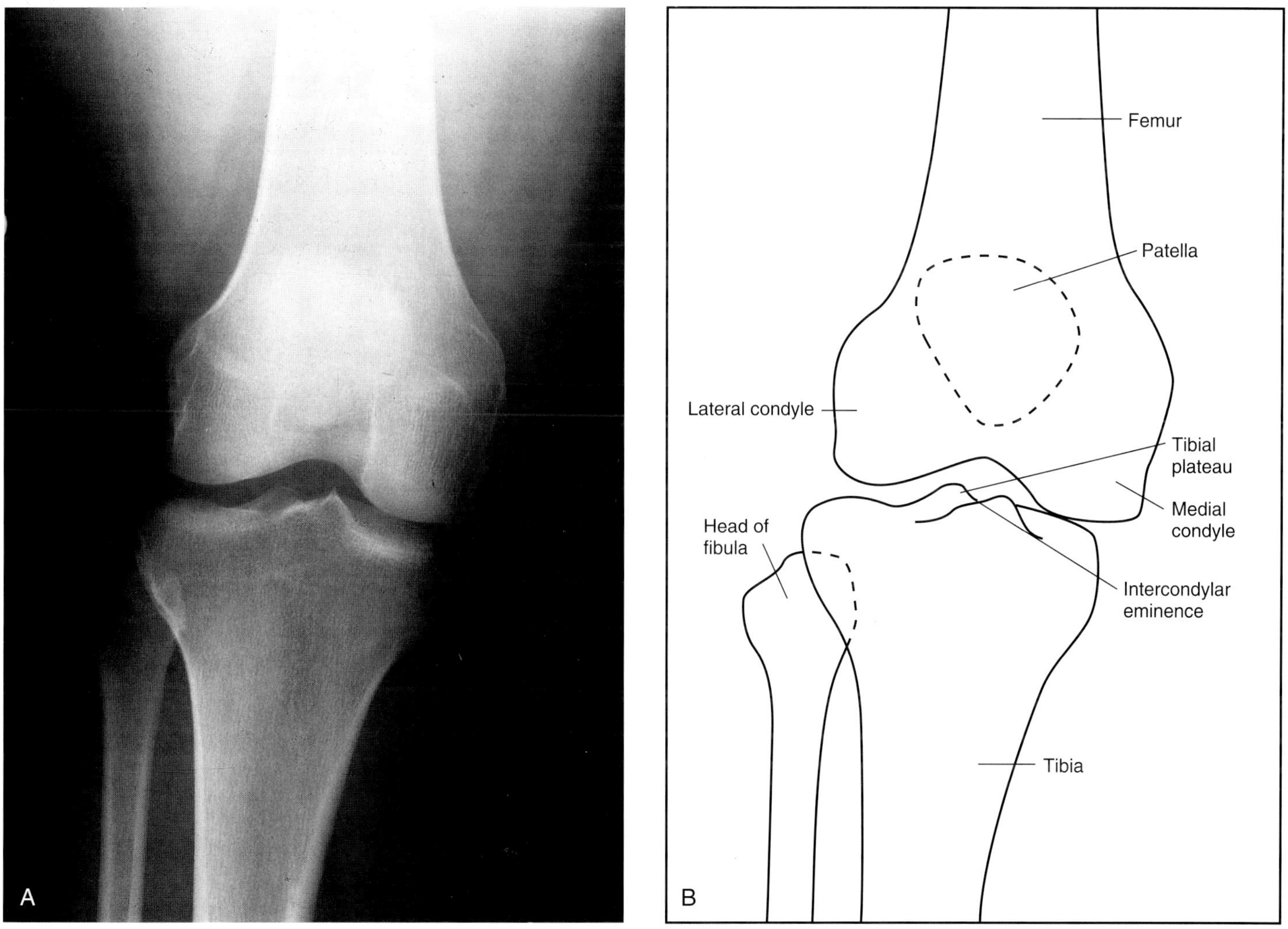

Figure 10.84. A and B, AP knee.

Knee

Position/Projection

Lateral projection

Film Size:
8 × 10 inches (20 × 24 cm) lengthwise (small to normal) Bucky

or

10 × 12 inches (24 × 30 cm) lengthwise (large) Bucky

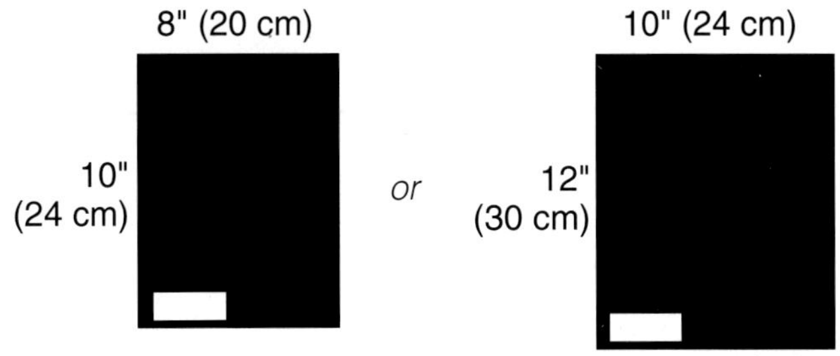

Patient Position

Laterally recumbent on affected side (Fig. 10.85).

Part Position

Align long axis of femur of affected leg to midline of table. Flex knee 45°; patella perpendicular to plane of table.

Central Ray

5° cephalic angle through knee joint (depression between medial femoral and tibial condyles). Center cassette to central ray.

Structures Demonstrated

Lateral projection of distal femur, proximal tibia and fibula, patella, and joint space (Fig. 10.86).

Evaluation Criteria

1. Femoral condyles should be superimposed.
2. Patella in profile.
3. Slight superimposition of head of fibula by proximal tibia.

NOTE: If a fracture of the patella is suspected or known, do not flex the knee. If a patient has very large hips, the central ray will need to be angled more than 5° so it will be perpendicular to the joint space.

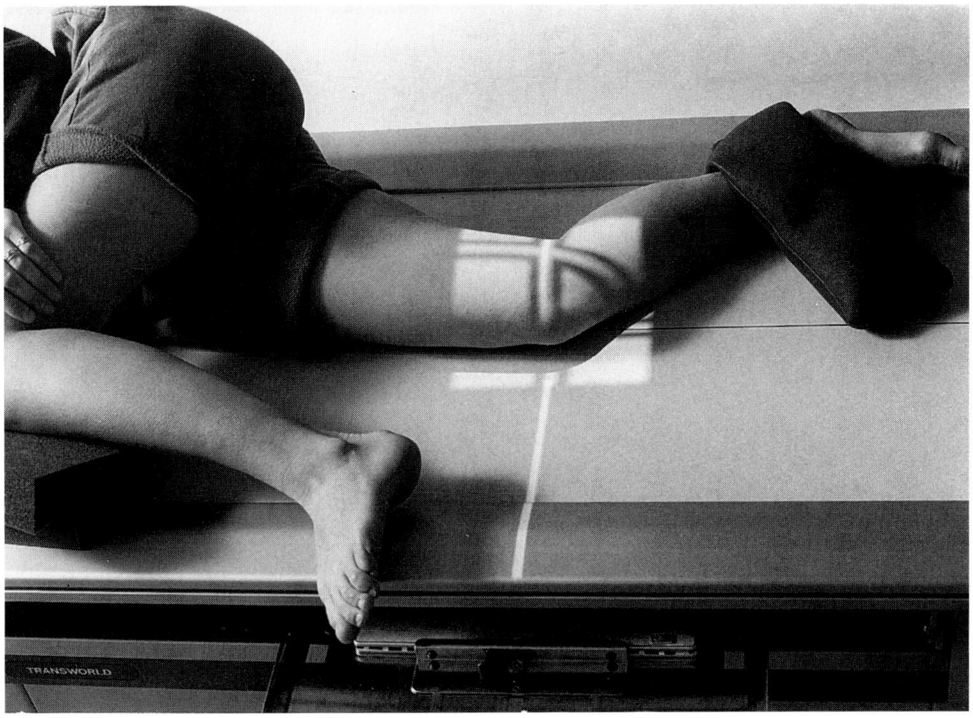

Figure 10.85. Lateral knee.

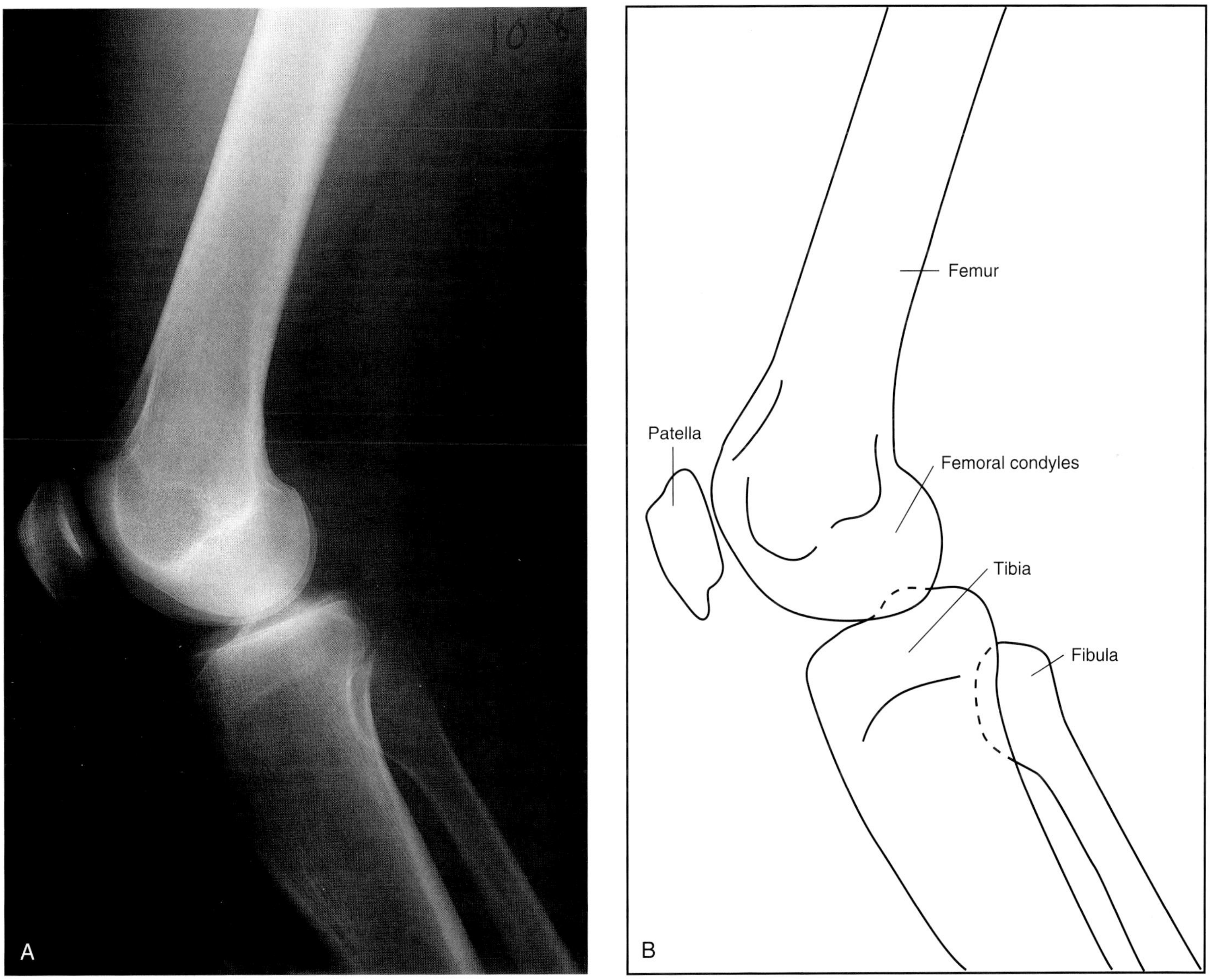

Figure 10.86. A and B, Lateral knee.

Knee

Position/Projection

PA oblique projections

Film Size:
8 × 10 inches (20 × 24 cm)
lengthwise Bucky

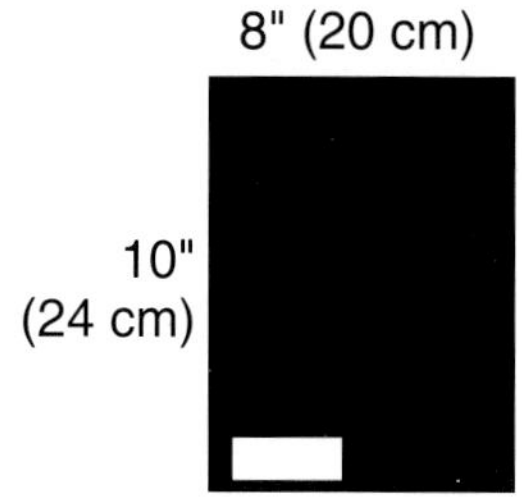

Patient Position

Prone (Fig. 10.87).

Part Position

Posteromedial Oblique Projection

Align long axis of affected leg to midline of table. Elevate affected side and rotate affected extremity externally until knee forms 45° angle.

Posterolateral Oblique Projection

Align long axis of affected leg to midline of table. Elevate unaffected extremity internally until knee forms 45° angle.

Central Ray

Perpendicular entering posterior surface of knee and exiting either medial or lateral surface of knee through knee joint.

Structures Demonstrated

PA oblique projections of knee demonstrating femoral condyles, tibial plateaus, and patella (Fig. 10.88).

Evaluation Criteria

Posteromedial Oblique Projection

1. Knee joint should be open.
2. Medial, femoral, tibial condyles, and tibial plateaus should be seen.
3. Lateral portion of tibia should be superimposed by fibula.
4. Portion of patella will project slightly in front of femoral condyle.

Posterolateral Oblique Projection

1. Knee joint should be open.
2. Lateral femoral condyles and lateral tibial condyles should be demonstrated.
3. Tibial plateaus should be visualized.
4. Portion of patella will project slightly in front of femoral condyle.
5. Knee can be flexed slightly for patient comfort.

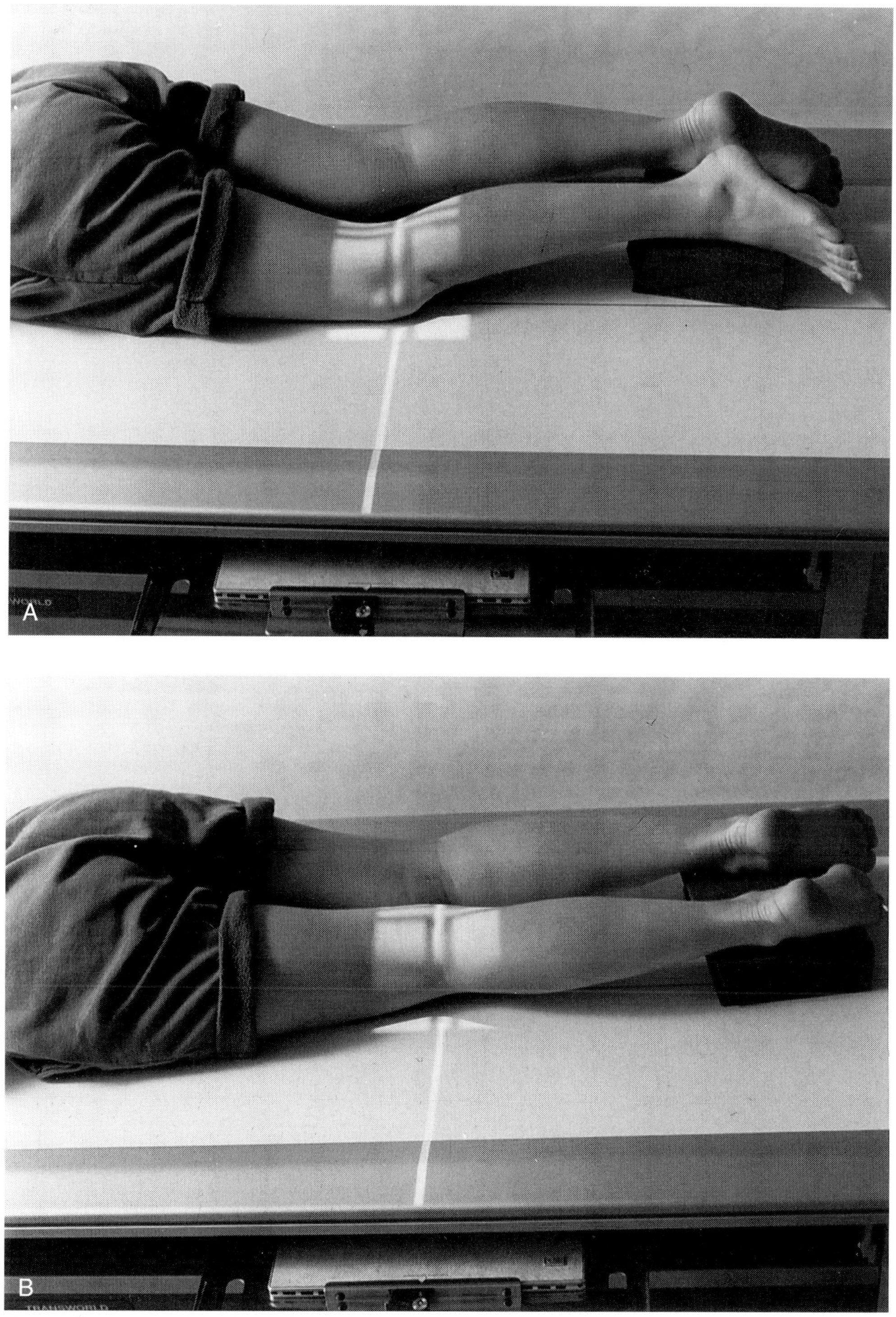

Figure 10.87. A, Posteromedial oblique. B, Posterolateral oblique.

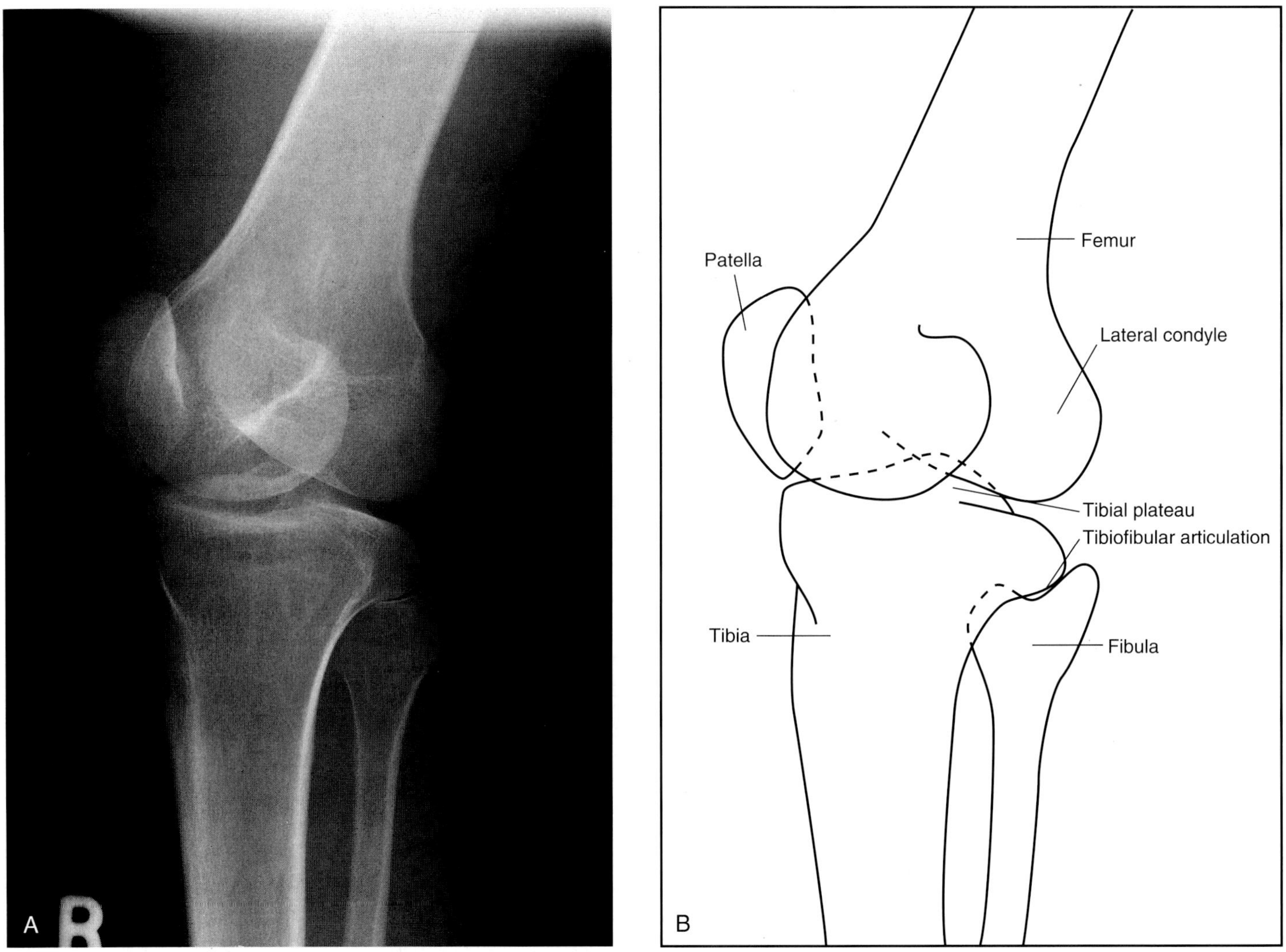

Figure 10.88. A and B, Posteromedial oblique.

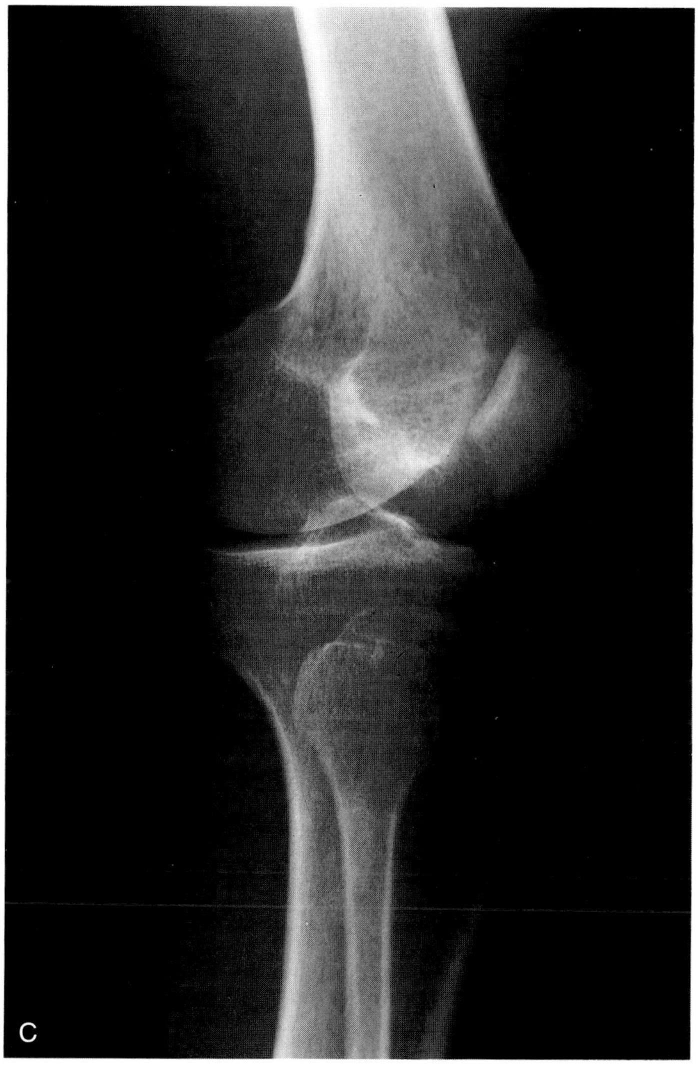

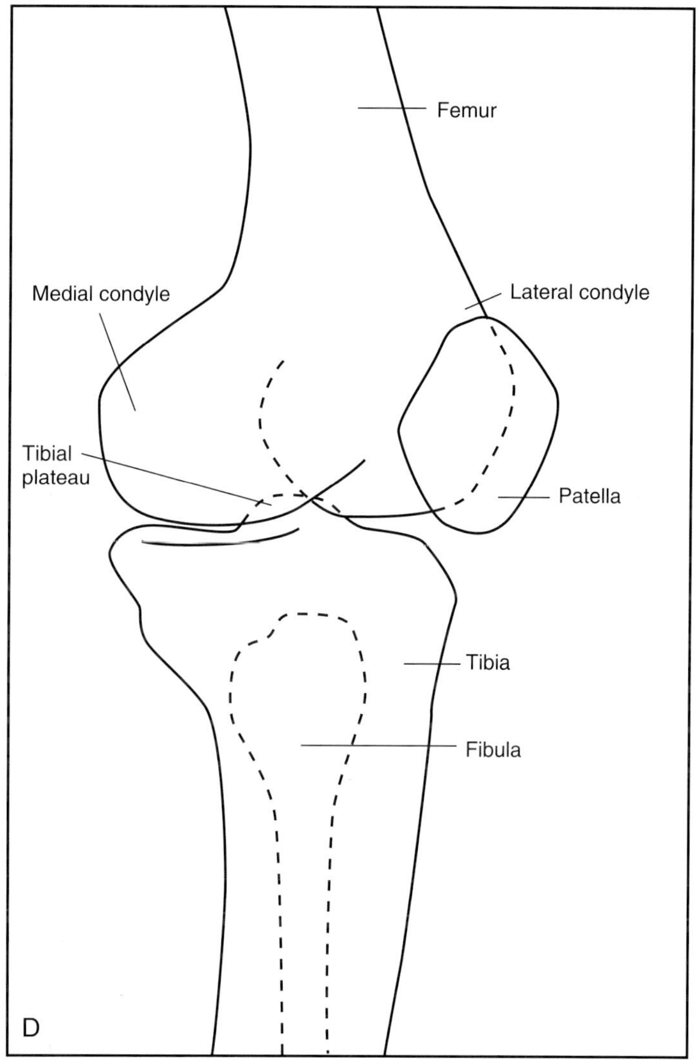

Figure 10.88 *(Continued)* C and D, Posterolateral oblique.

Knee

Position/Projection

Medial oblique projection

Film Size:
8 × 10 lengthwise (small to normal) Bucky
or
10 × 12 lengthwise (large) Bucky

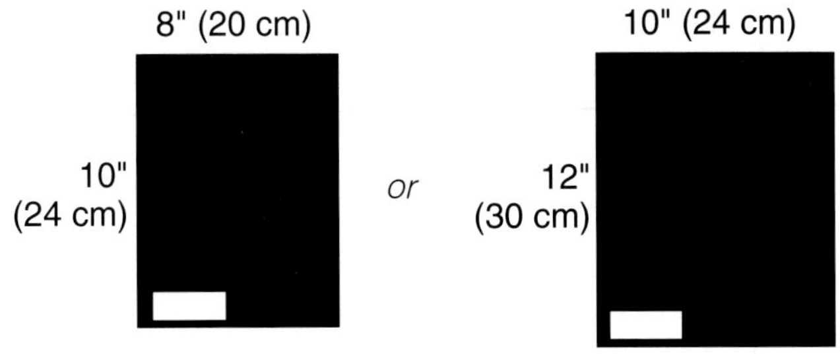

Patient Position

Supine or seated with legs extended (Fig. 10.89).

Part Position

Align long axis of affected leg with midline of table. Rotate affected extremity 45° medially by inverting hip of affected side. Support elevated hip.

Central Ray

Perpendicular to level approximately ½ inch (1 cm) below apex of patella. Center cassette to central ray.

Structures Demonstrated

Medial anterior oblique projection of femoral condyles, patella, tibial condyles, and head of fibula. Proximal tibiofibular articulation is well demonstrated in anteromedial oblique (internal) projection (Fig. 10.90).

Evaluation Criteria

1. Fibula should be free of superimposition by tibia.
2. Lateral condyles of femur and tibia should be demonstrated.
3. Tibial plateau should be well demonstrated.
4. Part of medial portion of patella should be seen free of superimposition by medial condyle of femur.

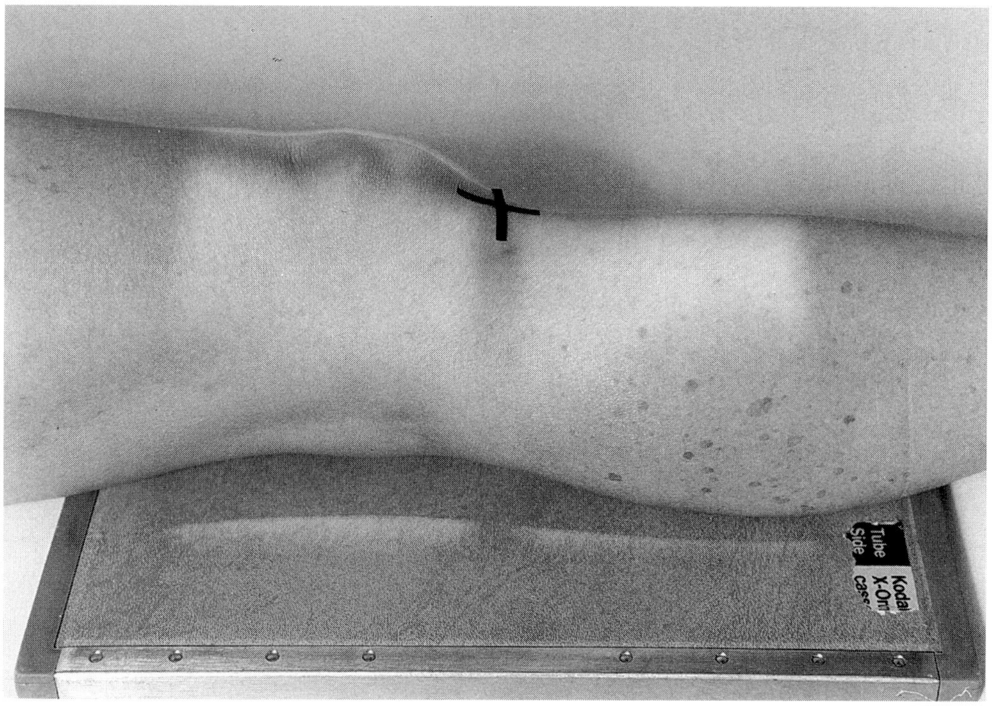

Figure 10.89. Medial oblique knee.

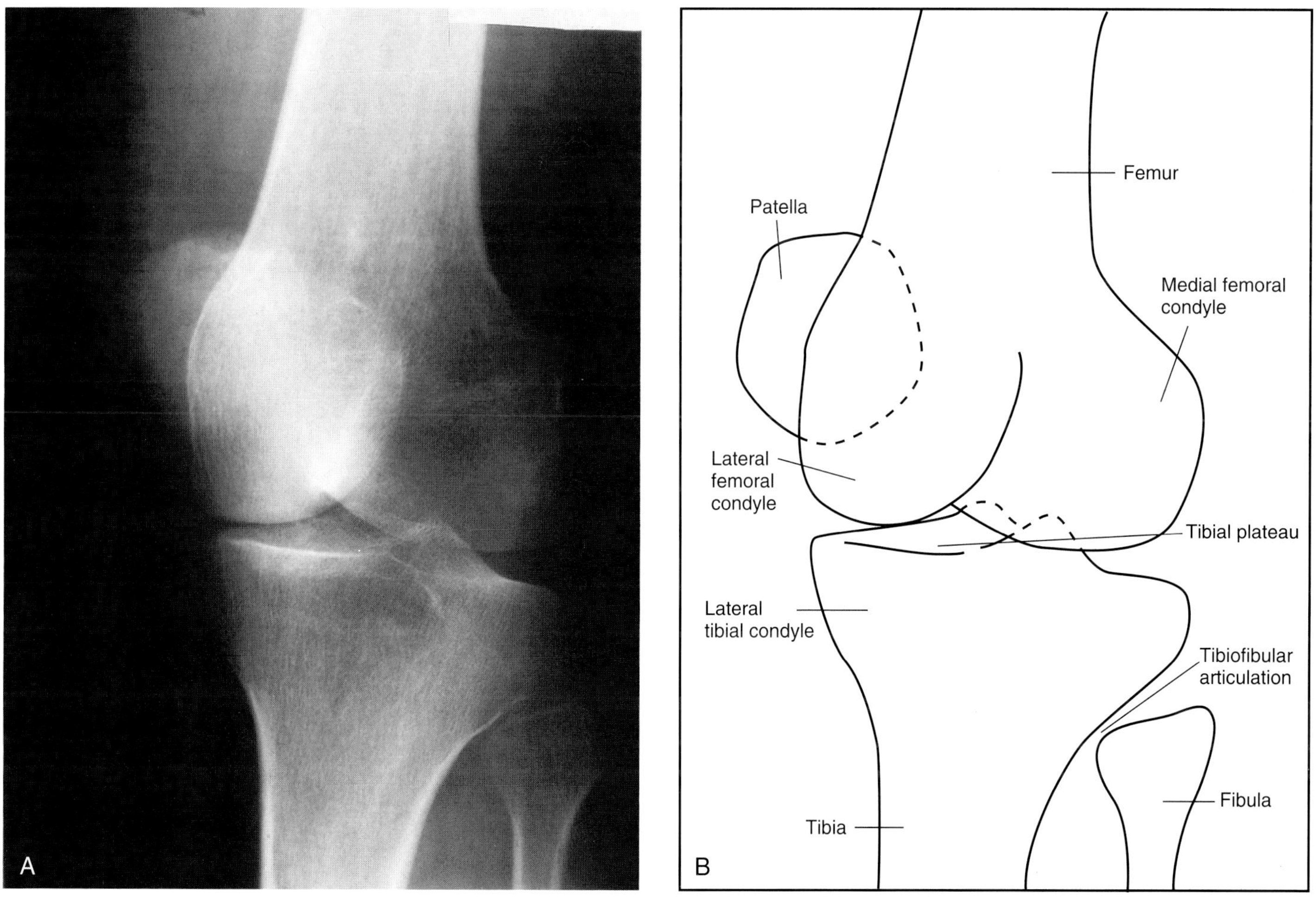

Figure 10.90. A and B, Medial oblique.

Knee

Position/Projection

Lateral oblique projection

Film Size:
8 × 10 inches (20 × 24 cm) lengthwise (small to normal) Bucky

or

10 × 12 inches (24 × 30 cm) lengthwise (large) Bucky

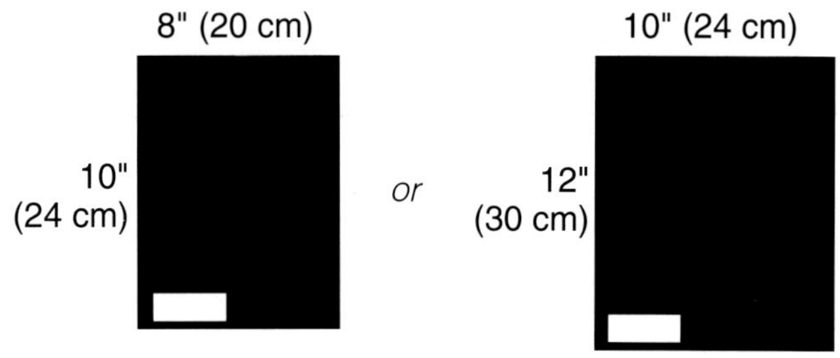

Patient Position

Supine or seated with legs extended (Fig. 10.91).

Part Position

Align long axis of affected leg with midline of table. Rotate affected extremity 45° laterally. If necessary, elevate hip of unaffected side. Support or elevate hip and knee.

Central Ray

Perpendicular to level approximately ½ inch (1 cm) below apex of patella. Center cassette to central ray.

Structures Demonstrated

Lateral anterior oblique projection of femoral condyles, patella, tibial condyles, and head of fibula (Fig. 10.92).

Evaluation Criteria

1. Fibula is superimposed by tibia.
2. Medial condyles of femur and tibia should be demonstrated.
3. Part of lateral portion of patella should be seen free of superimposition by lateral condyle of femur.

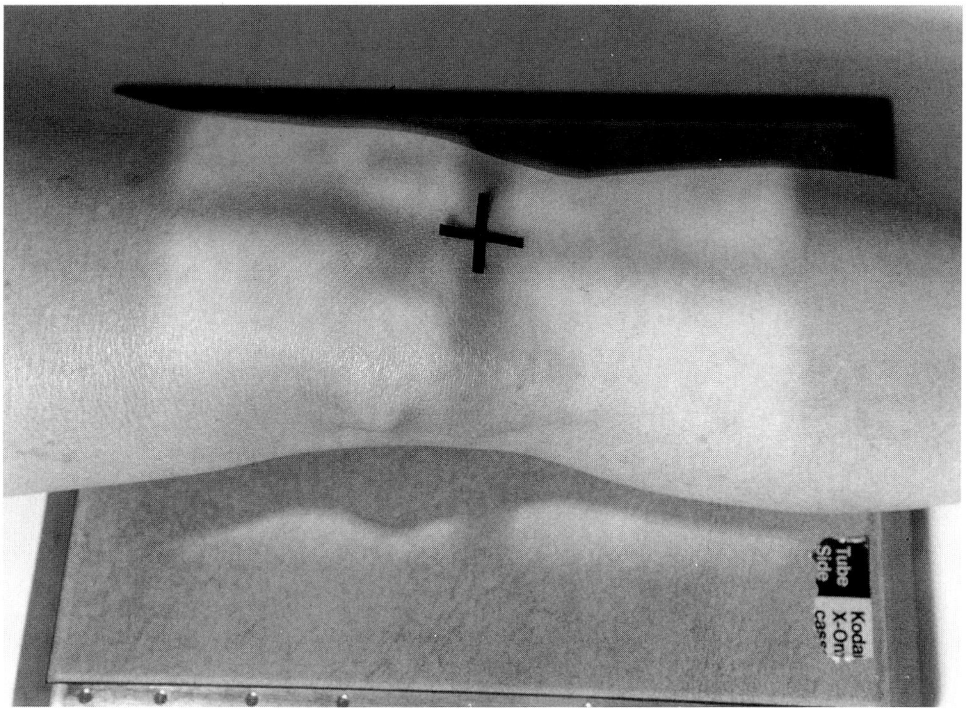

Figure 10.91. Lateral oblique knee.

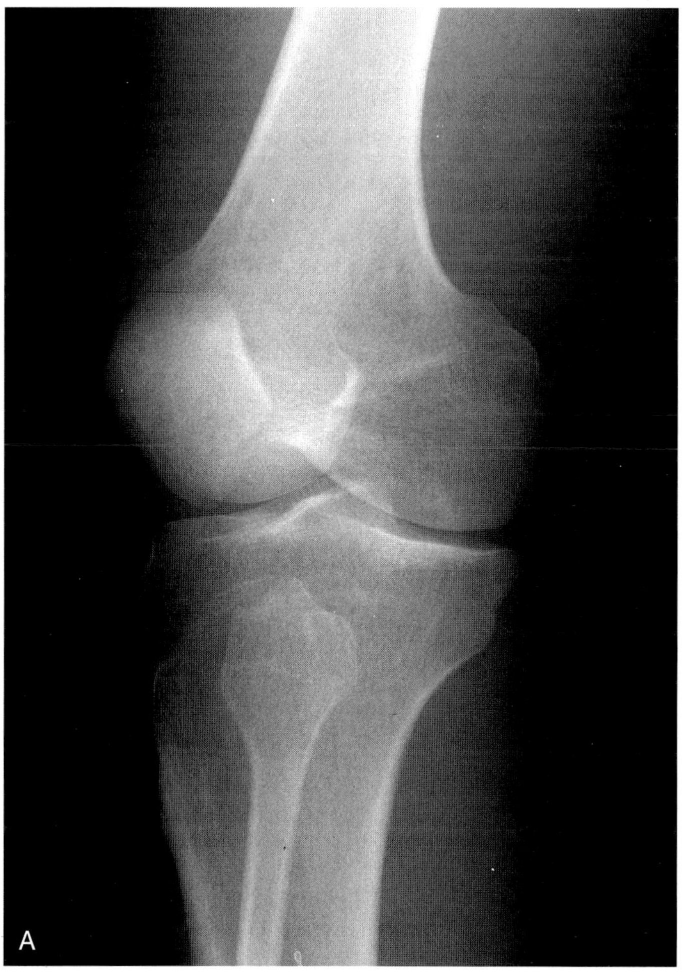

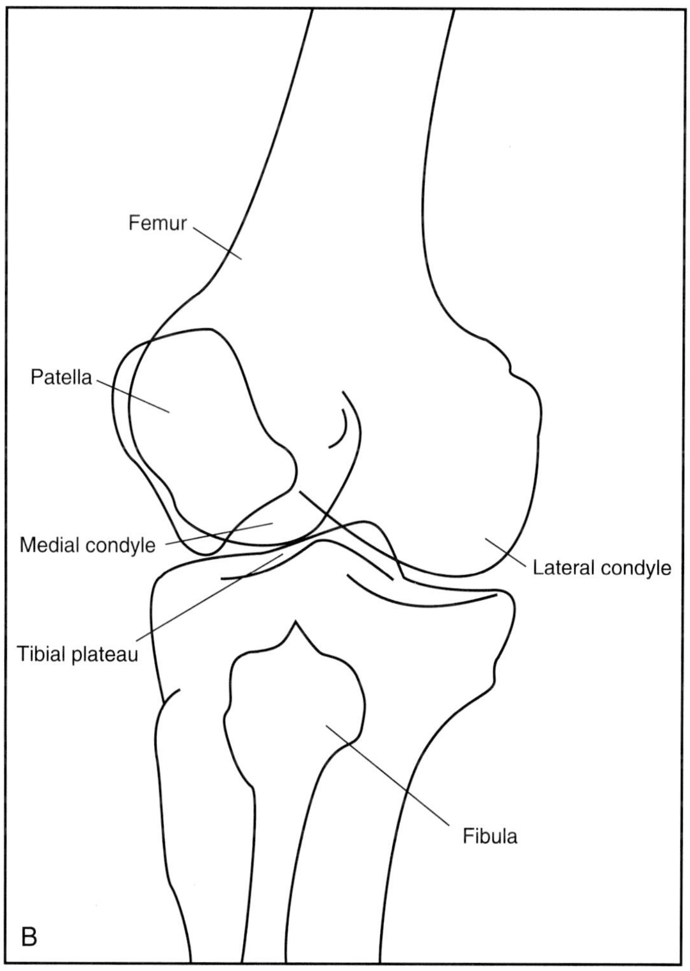

Figure 10.92. A and B, Lateral oblique.

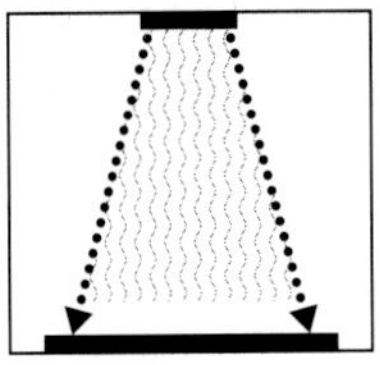

Weight-Bearing Knee

Position/Projection

AP projection

Film Size:
10 × 12 inches (24 × 30 cm) lengthwise (unilateral projection)

or

11 × 14 inches (28 × 35 cm) crosswise (bilateral projection)
Cassette in vertical grid device

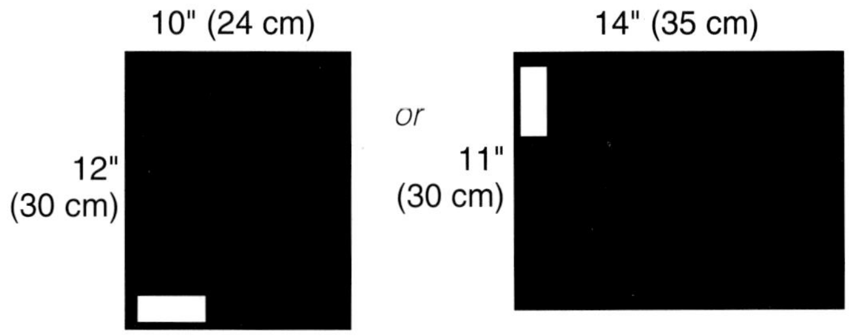

Patient Position

Erect (Fig. 10.93).

Part Position

Bilateral
Separate feet for good balance, fully extend knees, and distribute weight equally on feet.

Unilateral
Separate knees for good balance, fully extend knees, and put all weight on affected knee.

Central Ray

Center midpoint of cassette to central ray.

Bilateral
Horizontal midway between knees at level of apex of patella.

Unilateral
Horizontal at level of apex of patella.

Structures Demonstrated

Narrowing of joint space. Degree of lower extremity varus or valgus deformity (Fig. 10.94).

Evaluation Criteria

1. No medial or lateral rotation of knee.
2. Knee joint should be in center of film.
3. Longitudinal axis of femoral and tibial shafts should be seen.

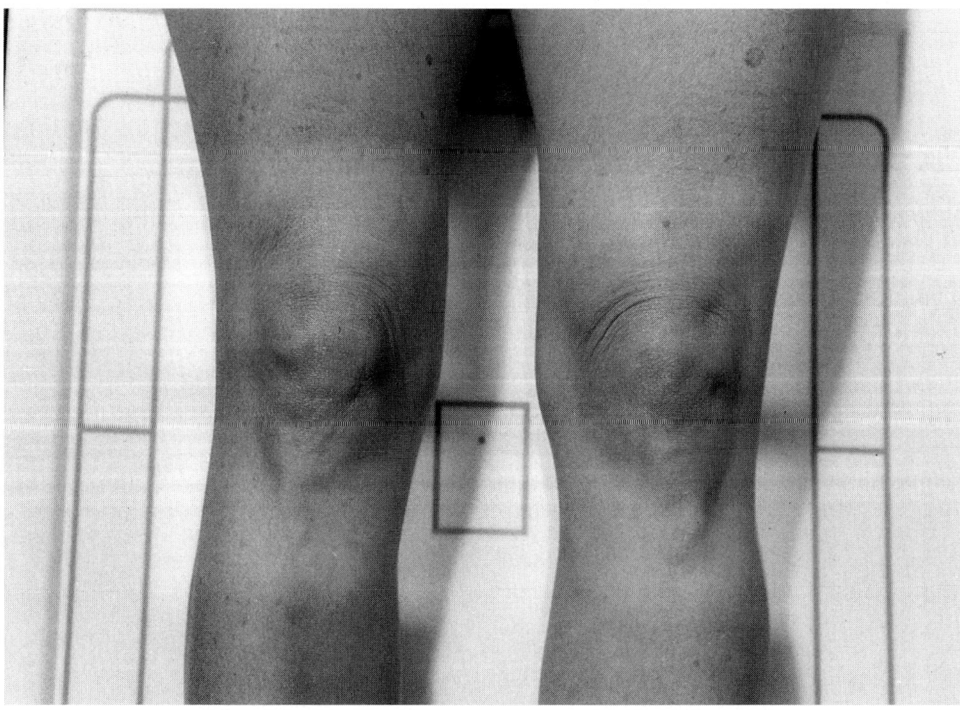

Figure 10.93. AP weight-bearing knee.

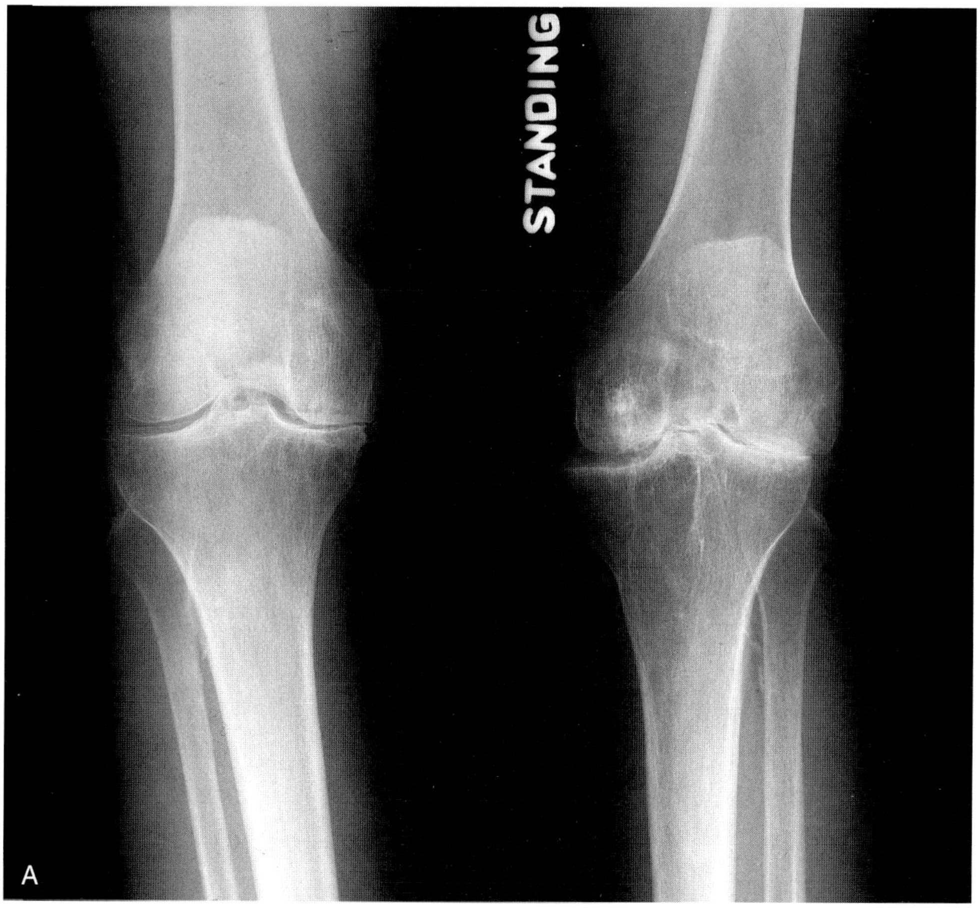

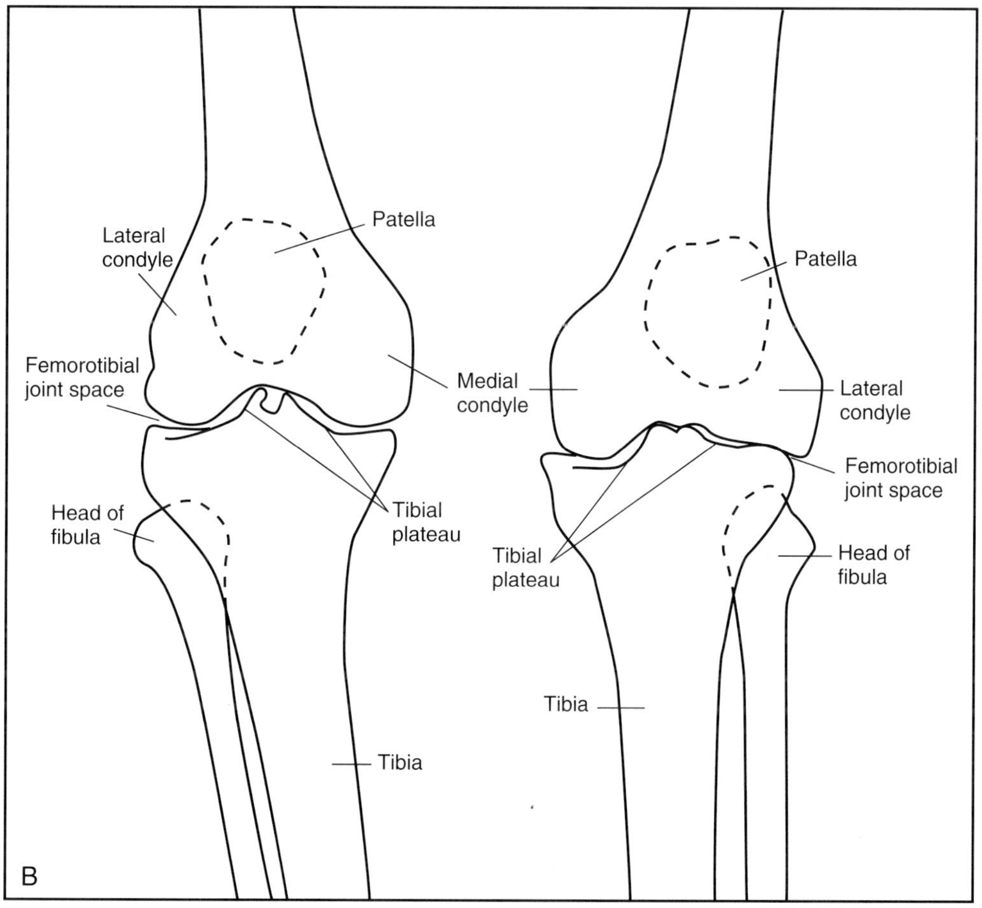

Figure 10.94. A and B, AP weight-bearing knee.

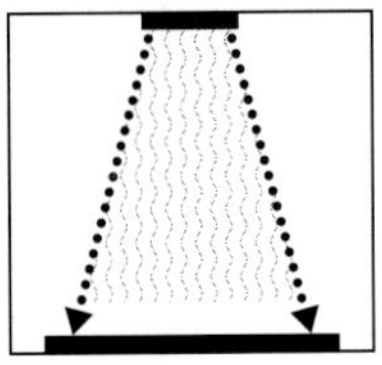

Intercondylar Fossa

Position/Projection

PA axial projection—Camp-Coventry method

Film Size:
8 × 10 inches (20 × 24 cm)
lengthwise tabletop

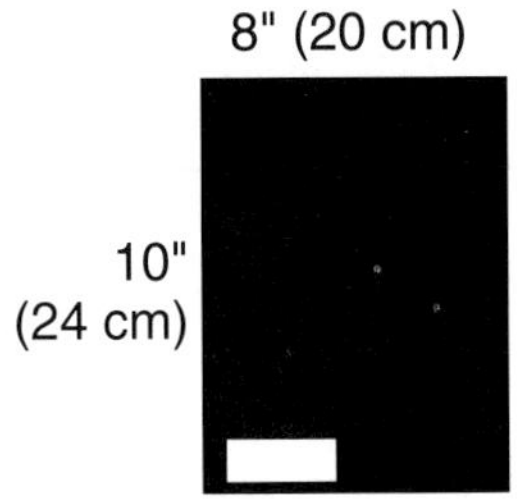

Patient Position

Prone with legs extended (Fig. 10.95).

Part Position

Affected knee flexed at 40° angle to cassette. Center knee joint to proximal half of cassette.

Central Ray

40° caudal angle to enter knee joint over popliteal depression. Central ray should exit midpoint of cassette.

Structures Demonstrated

Open image of intercondylar fossa (Fig. 10.96).

Evaluation Criteria

1. Intercondylar fossa should be open.
2. No medial or lateral rotation of knee.
3. Joint space and tibial eminences should be demonstrated.
4. Fossa should not be superimposed by patella.
5. Posteroinferior surface of femoral condyles should be seen.

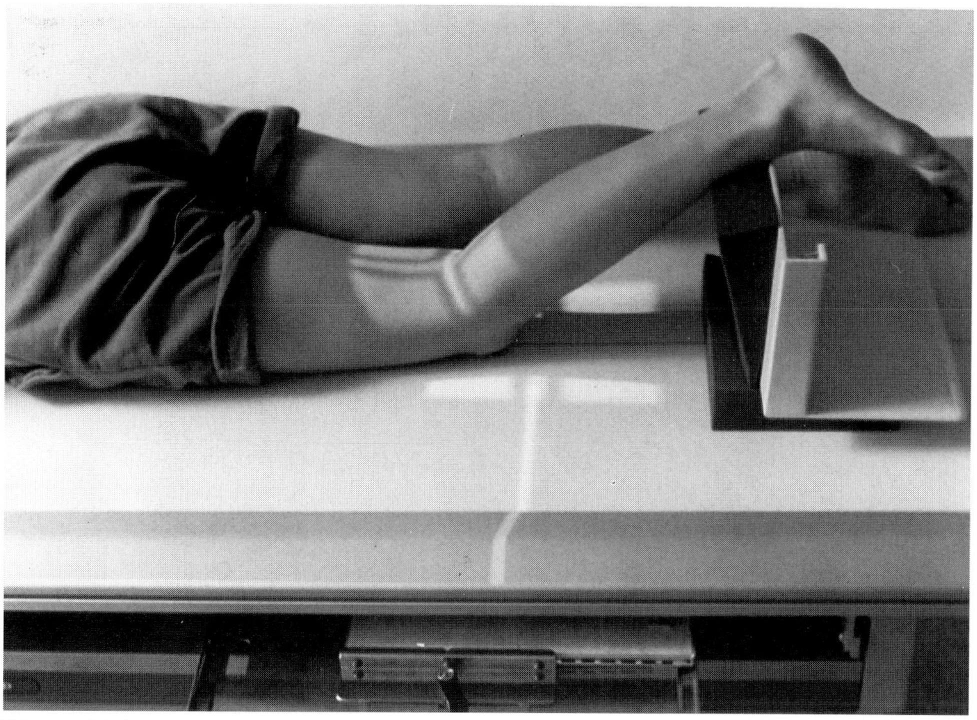

Figure 10.95. Camp-Coventry method, intercondylar fossa.

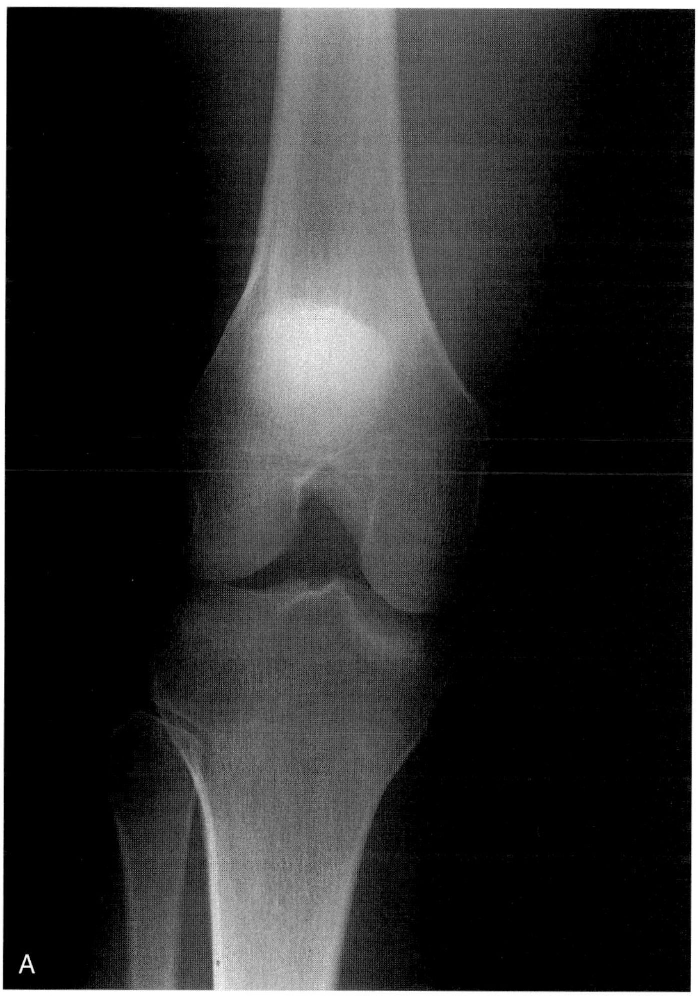

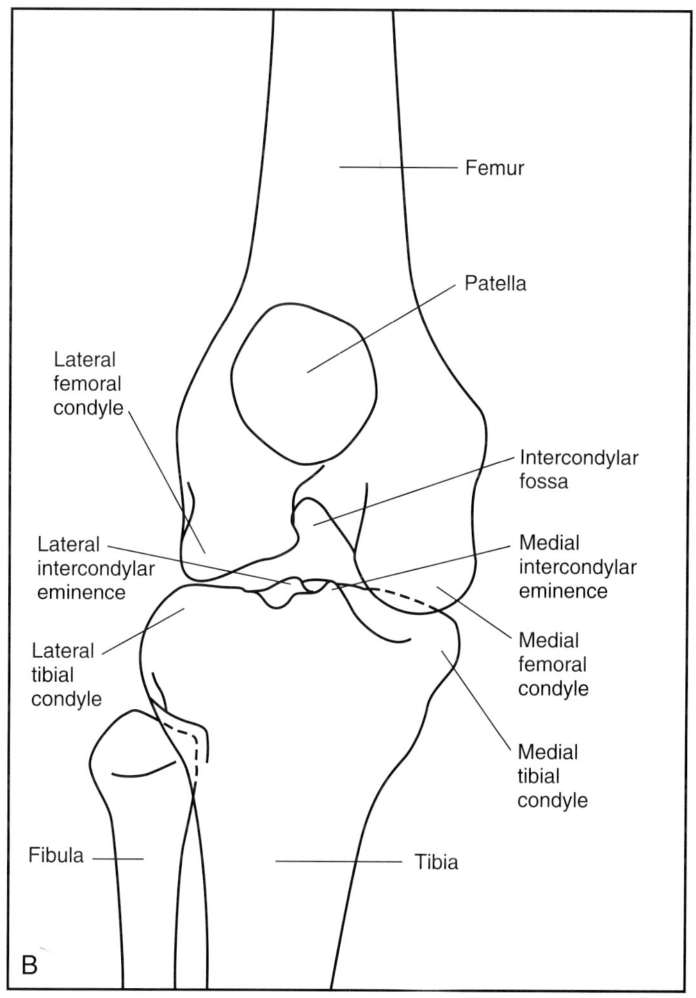

Figure 10.96. A and B, Camp-Coventry method, intercondylar fossa. (A and B [redrawn], From Meschan I: Radiographic Positioning and Related Anatomy. 2nd ed. Philadelphia: WB Saunders, 1978, p 109.)

Intercondylar Fossa

Position/Projection

Semiaxial PA projection—Holmblad's method

Film Size:
8 × 10 inches (20 × 24 cm)
lengthwise tabletop

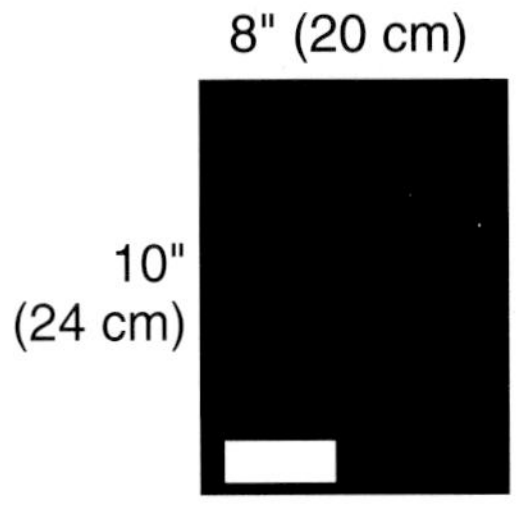

Patient Position

Kneeling (Fig. 10.97).

Part Position

Place patient in "all-fours" position. Have patient lean forward to move femur and buttocks out of central ray and away from affected knee. Be sure most of patient's weight is supported on unaffected leg.

Central Ray

Perpendicular entering knee joint over popliteal depression. Central ray should exit midpoint of cassette.

Structures Demonstrated

Open image of intercondylar fossa, tibial spine, tibial plateau, knee joint, and distal femur (Fig. 10.98).

Evaluation Criteria

1. Intercondylar fossa should be open.
2. No medial or lateral rotation of knee.
3. Joint space and tibial eminences should be demonstrated.
4. Fossa should not be superimposed by patella.
5. Posteroinferior surface of femoral condyles should be seen.

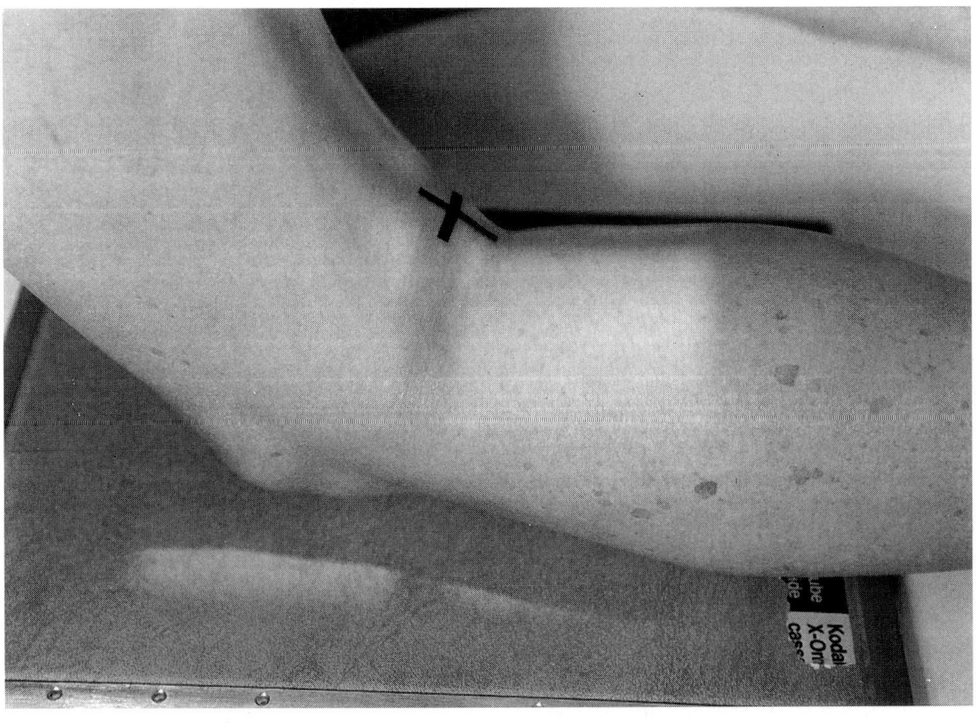

Figure 10.97. Semiaxial PA, Holmblad's method.

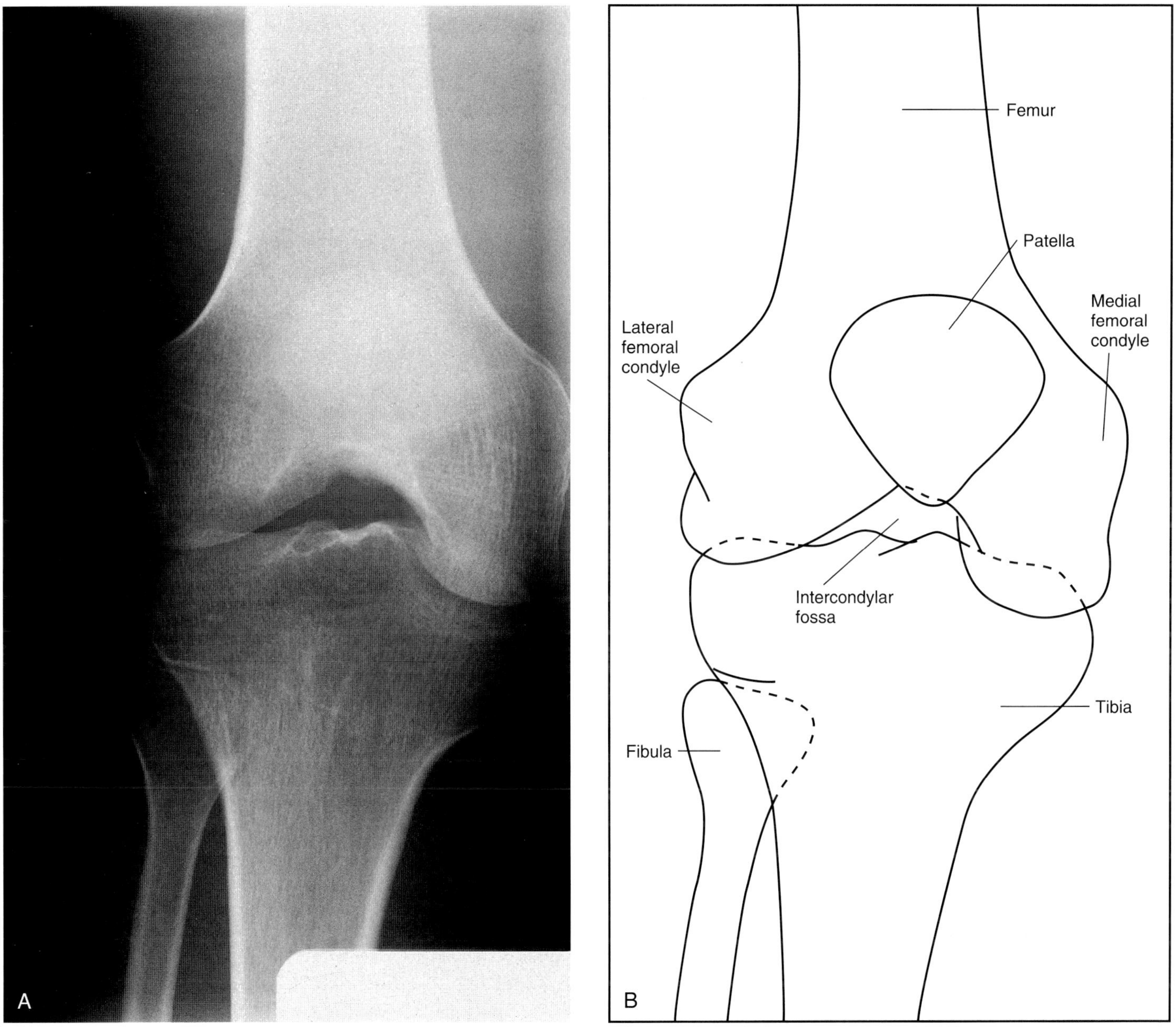

Figure 10.98. A and B, Holmblad's method.

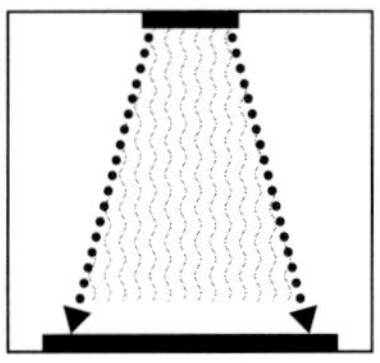

Patella

Position/Projection

PA projection

Film Size:
8 × 10 inches (20 × 24 cm)
lengthwise Bucky

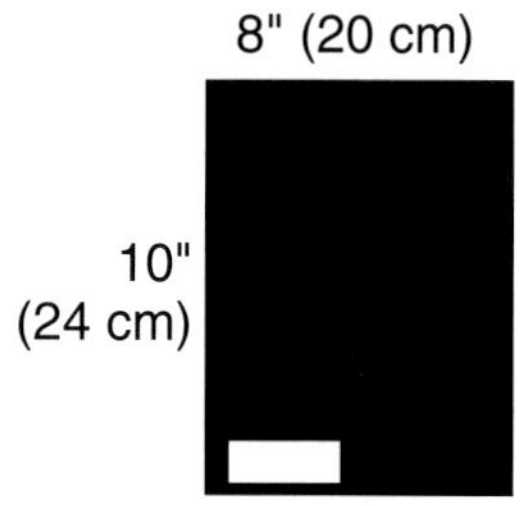

Patient Position

Prone with legs extended (Fig. 10.99)

Part Position

Align long axis of affected leg to midline of table. Place patella parallel to plane of table.

Central Ray

Perpendicular entering posterior leg to exit midpoint of patella. Center midpoint of cassette to central ray.

Structures Demonstrated

PA projection of patella and knee joint (Fig. 10.100).

Evaluation Criteria

1. Patella superimposed by femur.
2. Outline of patella clearly visible without rotation.
3. Knee joint should be seen.

NOTE: The PA projection will demonstrate the patella in more detail, but is usually contraindicated in cases of trauma owing to patient discomfort.

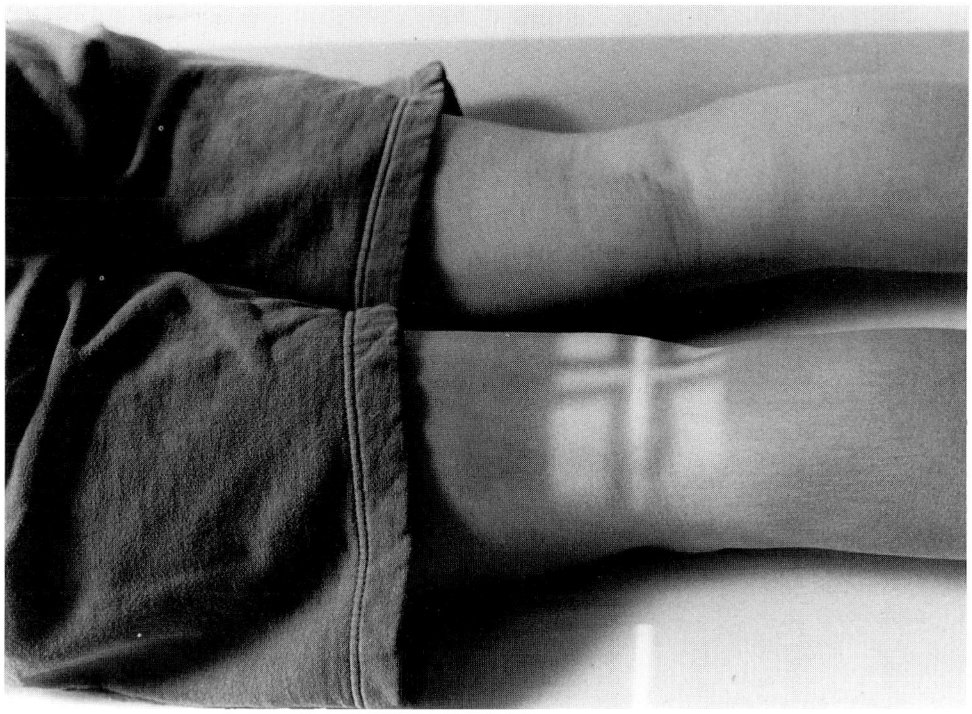

Figure 10.99. PA patella.

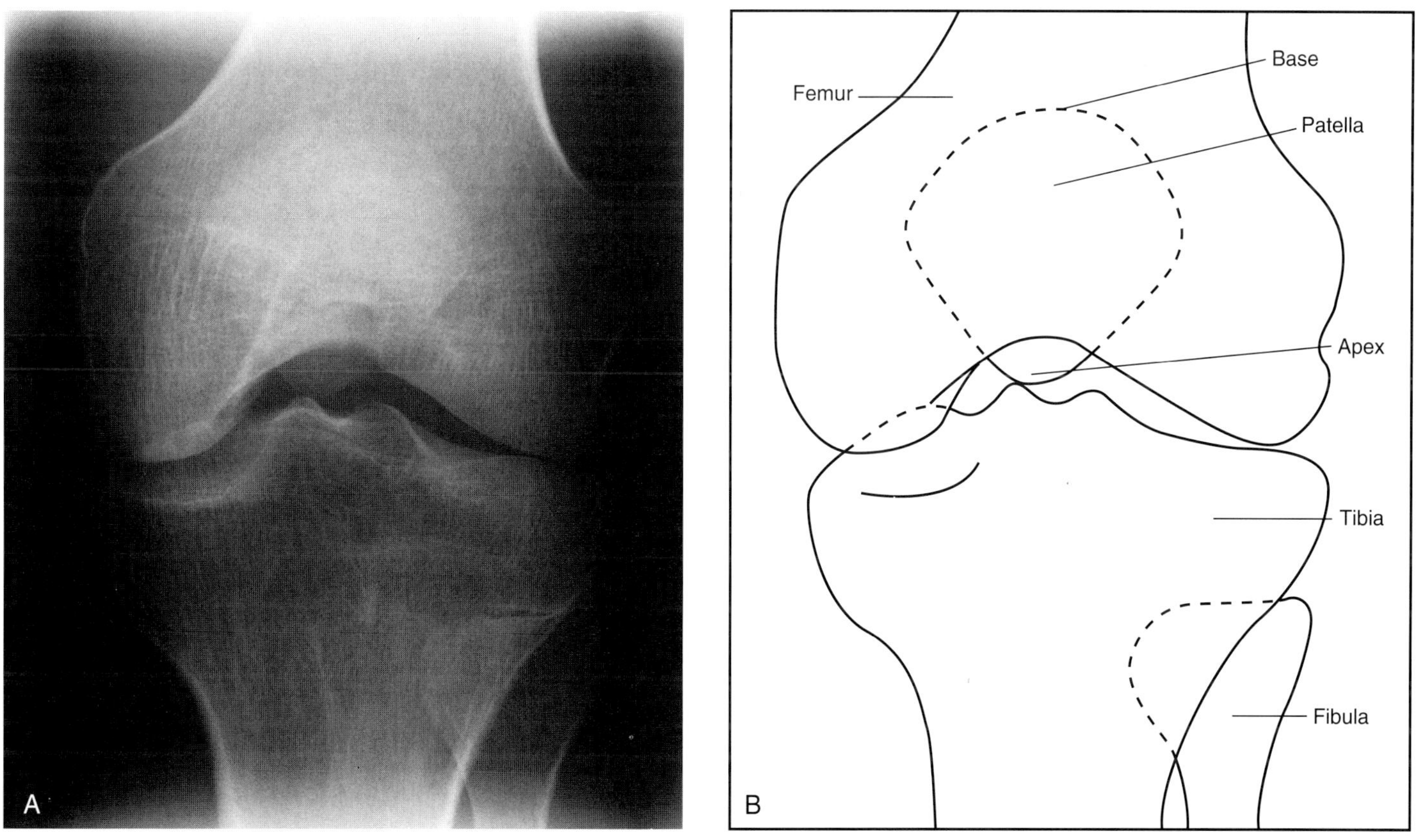

Figure 10.100. A and B, PA patella.

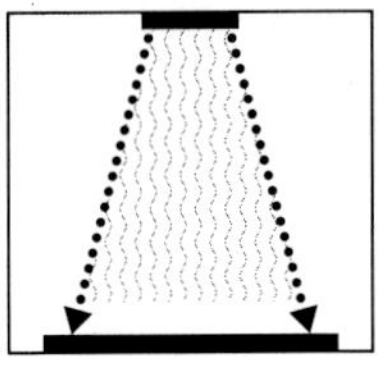

Patella

Position/Projection

Medial oblique projection

Film Size:
8 × 10 inches (20 × 24 cm)
lengthwise Bucky

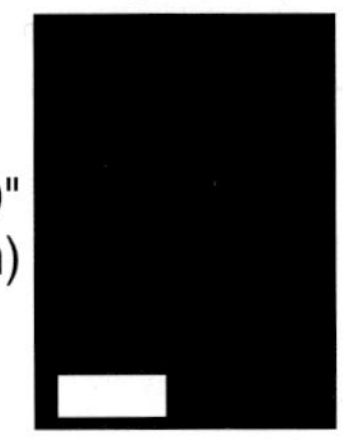

Patient Position

Prone with legs extended (Fig. 10.101).

Part Position

Align long axis of affected leg with long axis of table. Patella centered to midline of table. Flex knee slightly and turn knee slightly lateral from PA position. Anteromedial portion of knee will rest against table.

Central Ray

25° to 30° caudal angle to enter posterior surface of patella through joint space that lies between patella and femoral condyles.

Structures Demonstrated

Slight PA oblique projection of the patella (Fig. 10.102).

Evaluation Criteria

1. Patella free of most superimposition.
2. Most of patella projected out from femur.
3. Outline of patella superimposed by portion of patella.

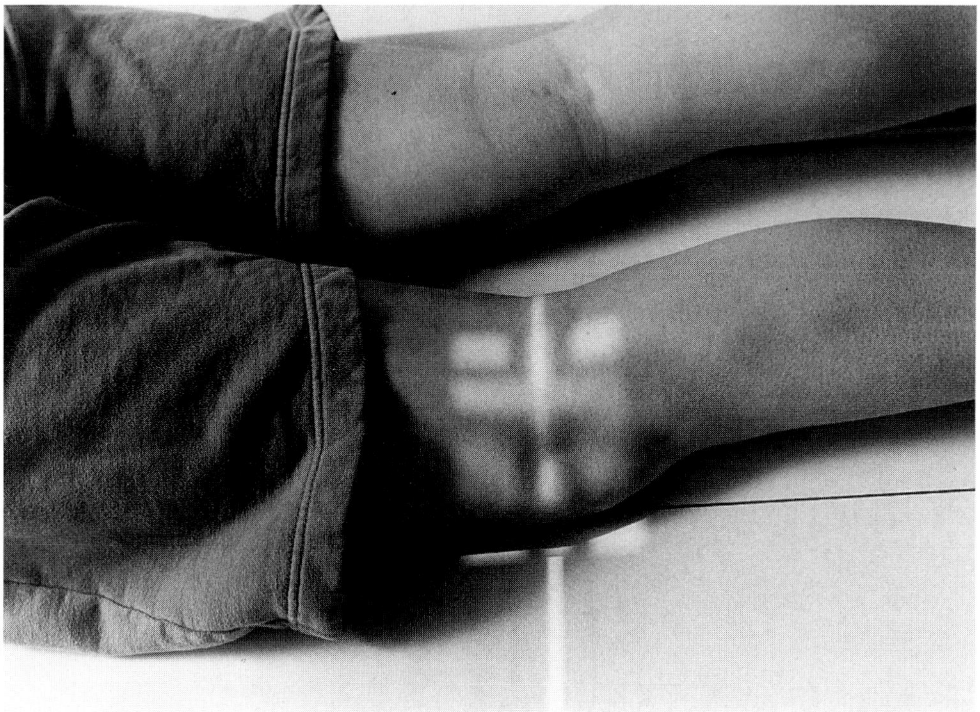

Figure 10.101. Medial oblique patella.

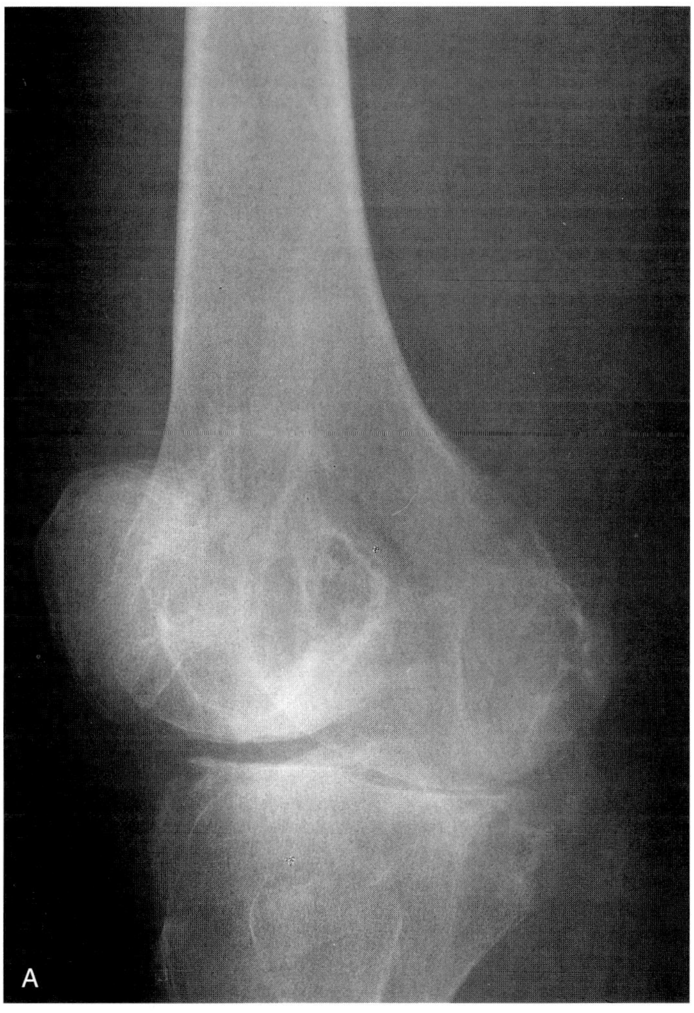

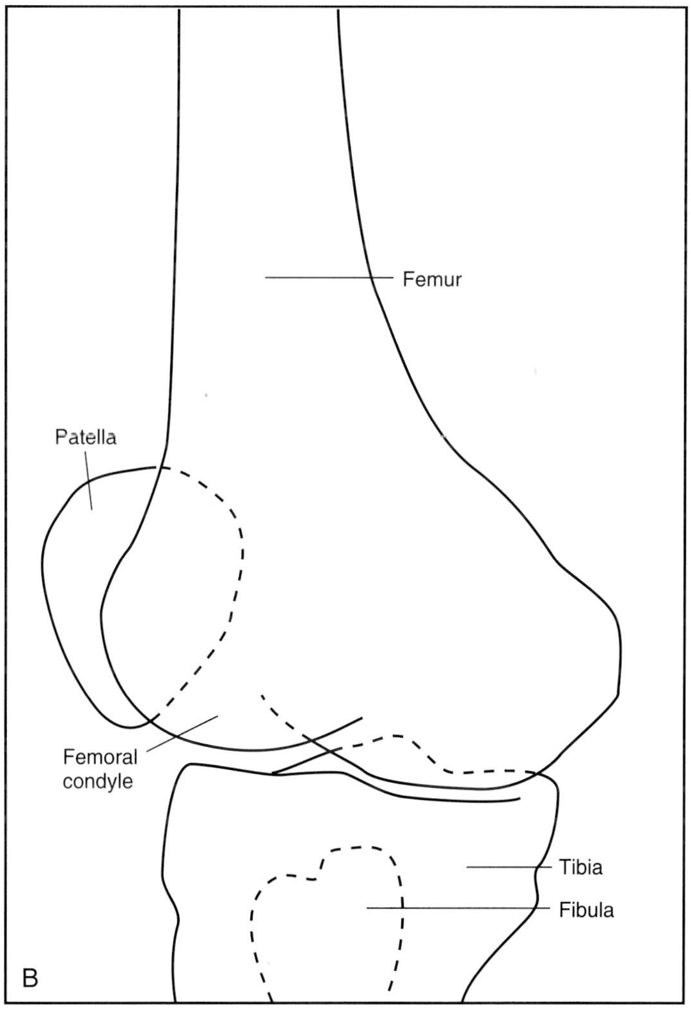

Figure 10.102. Medial oblique patella.

Patella

Position/Projection

Lateral projection

Film Size:
8 × 10 inches (20 × 24 cm)
lengthwise Bucky or tabletop

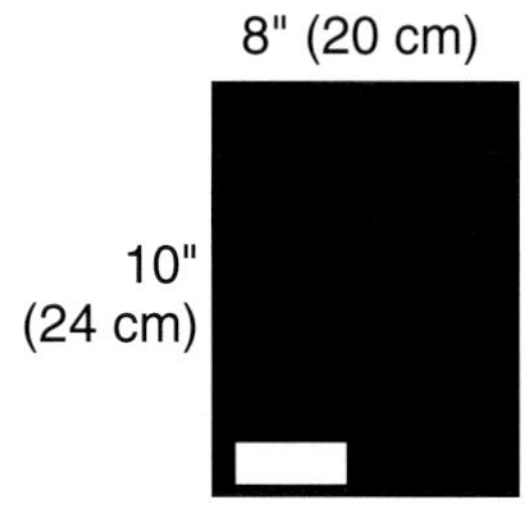

Patient Position

Laterally recumbent on affected side (Fig. 10.103).

Part Position

Patella centered to middle of table. Patella perpendicular to plane of table.

Central Ray

Perpendicular to midpoint of patella. Center midpoint of cassette to central ray.

Structures Demonstrated

Lateral projection of patella, femoropatellar joint space, distal femur, and proximal tibia and fibula (Fig. 10.104).

Evaluation Criteria

1. Patella demonstrated in profile.
2. Femoropatellar joint space demonstrated well.
3. Femoral condyles should be superimposed.

NOTE: Do not flex the knee if there is a known or suspected fracture of the patella. Utilize close collimation, but be sure to include the knee joint.

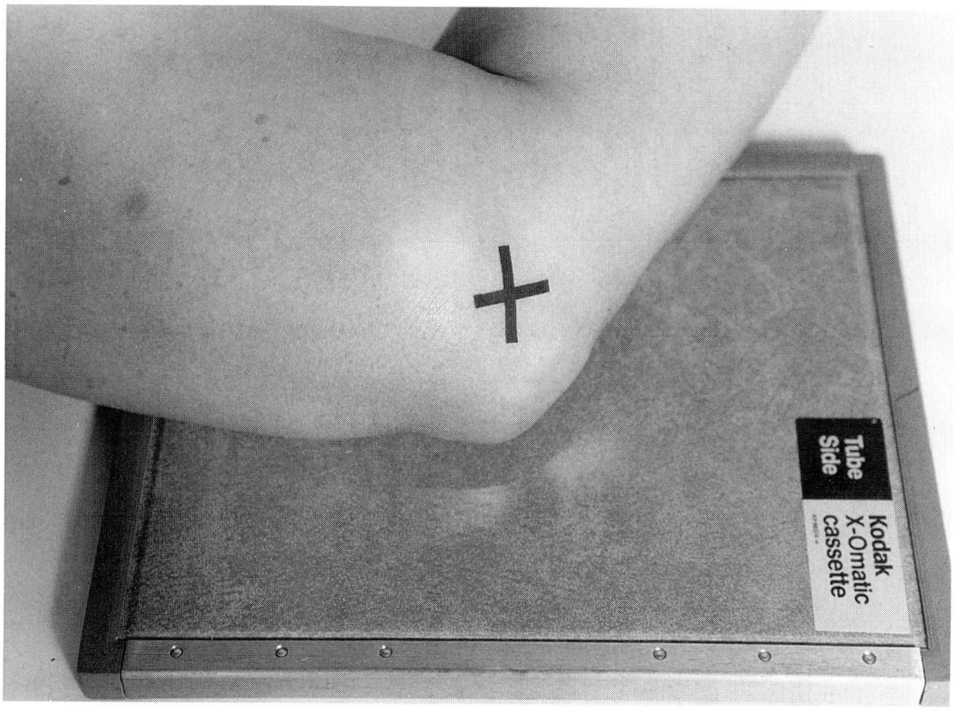

Figure 10.103. Lateral patella.

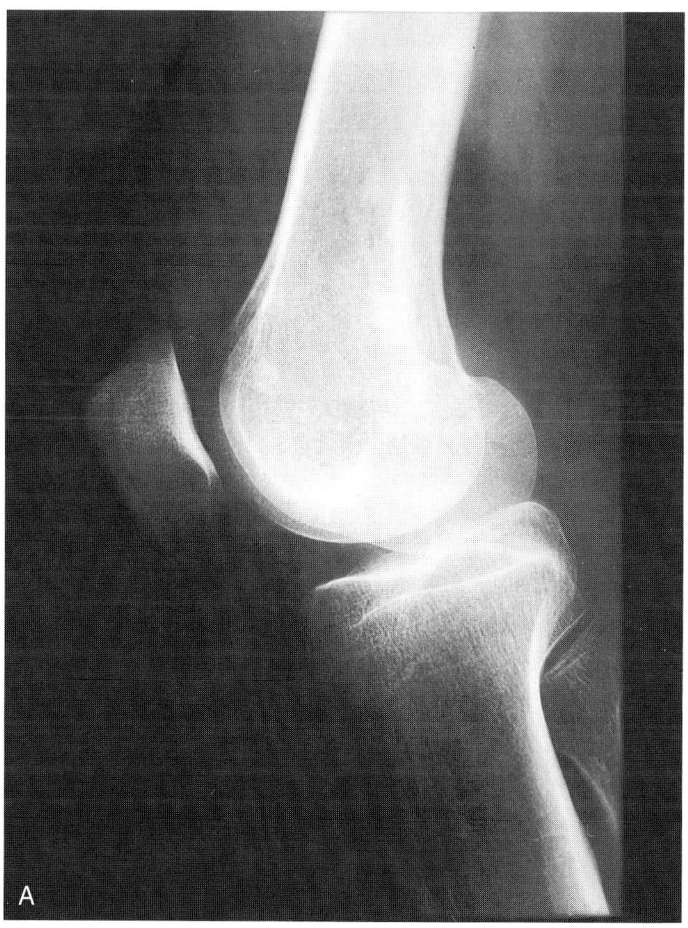

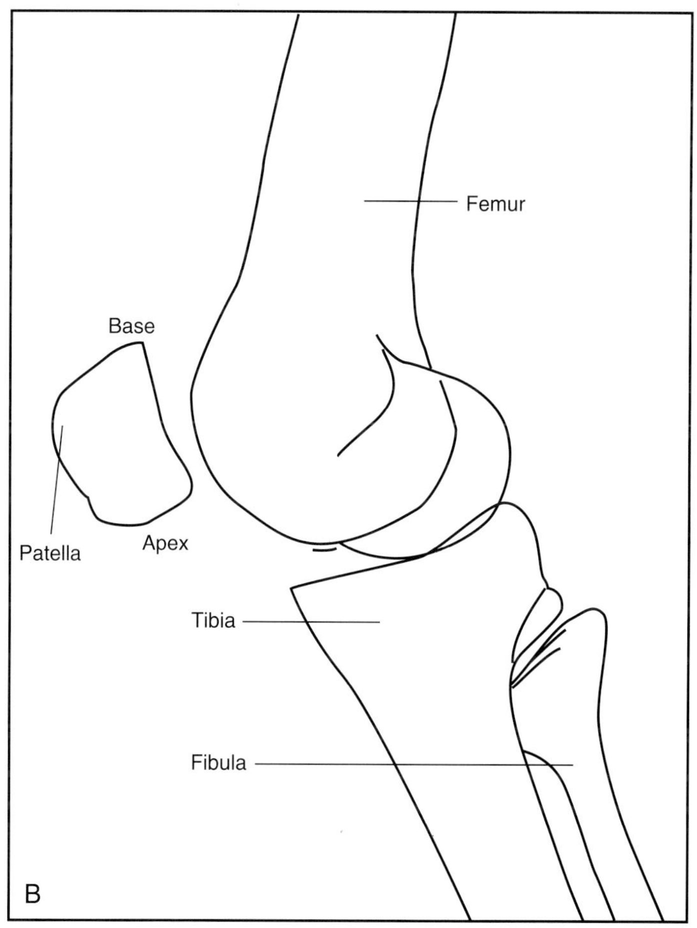

Figure 10.104. A and B, Lateral patella.

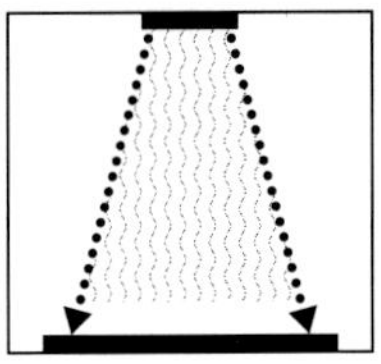

Patella

Position/Projection

Settegast's method, sunrise/skyline

Film Size:
8 × 10 inches (20 × 24 cm)
lengthwise

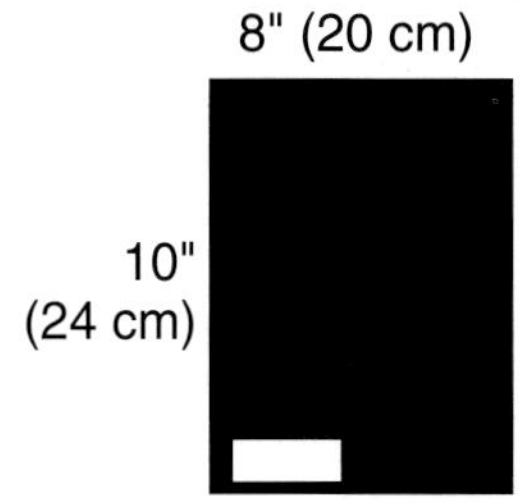

Patient Position

Prone, seated or supine (Figs. 10.105 and 10.106).

Part Position

Align affected knee to midline of cassette or to midline of table. Have patient flex affected knee in acute flexion until patellar surface is perpendicular to plane of table. Long strip of gauze can be placed around ankle or foot with patient grasping ends over shoulder to immobilize leg. Do not attempt this projection until a transverse fracture has been ruled out. If projection is done tabletop, center joint space between patella and femoral condyles to midpoint of cassette.

Central Ray

Perpendicular through femoropatellar space. If there is inadequate flexion of knee, angle central ray cephalic until it passes through femoropatellar space. Use close collimation. Center midpoint of cassette to central ray if done Bucky.

Structures Demonstrated

Vertical fractures of patella. Femoropatellar articulation (Figs. 10.107 and 10.108).

Evaluation Criteria

1. Femoropatellar space should be open.
2. Patella should be in profile.

NOTE: This projection can also be obtained with the patient sitting or in the supine position if the same part-film and tube-film relationships are maintained with the knee flexed and the central ray directed through the femoropatellar space. Bilateral examination can also be obtained.

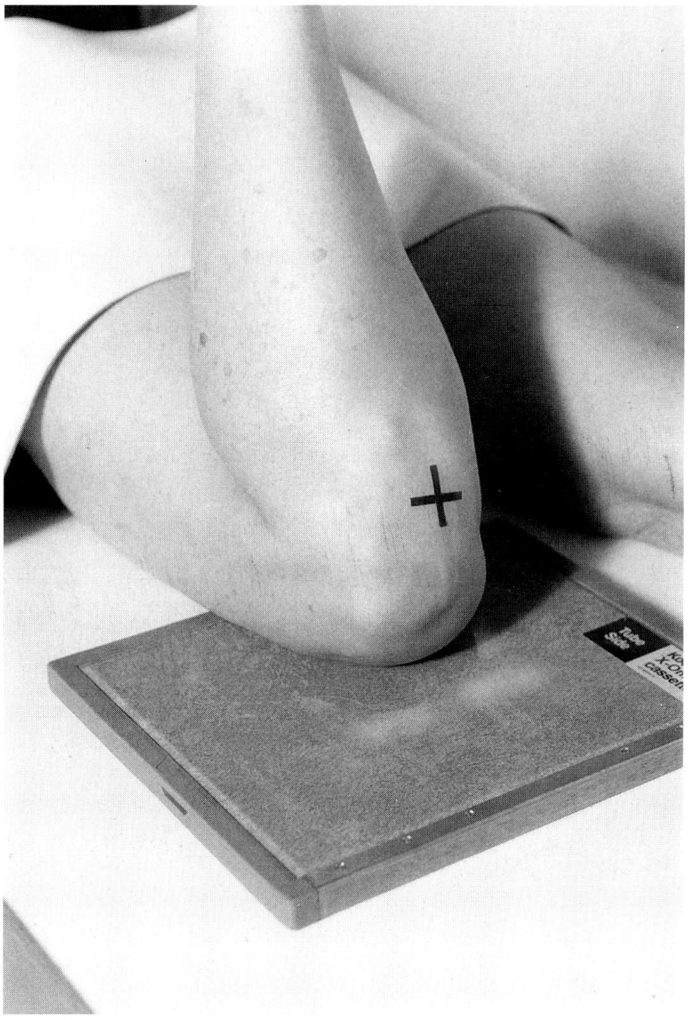

Figure 10.105. Settegast's method.

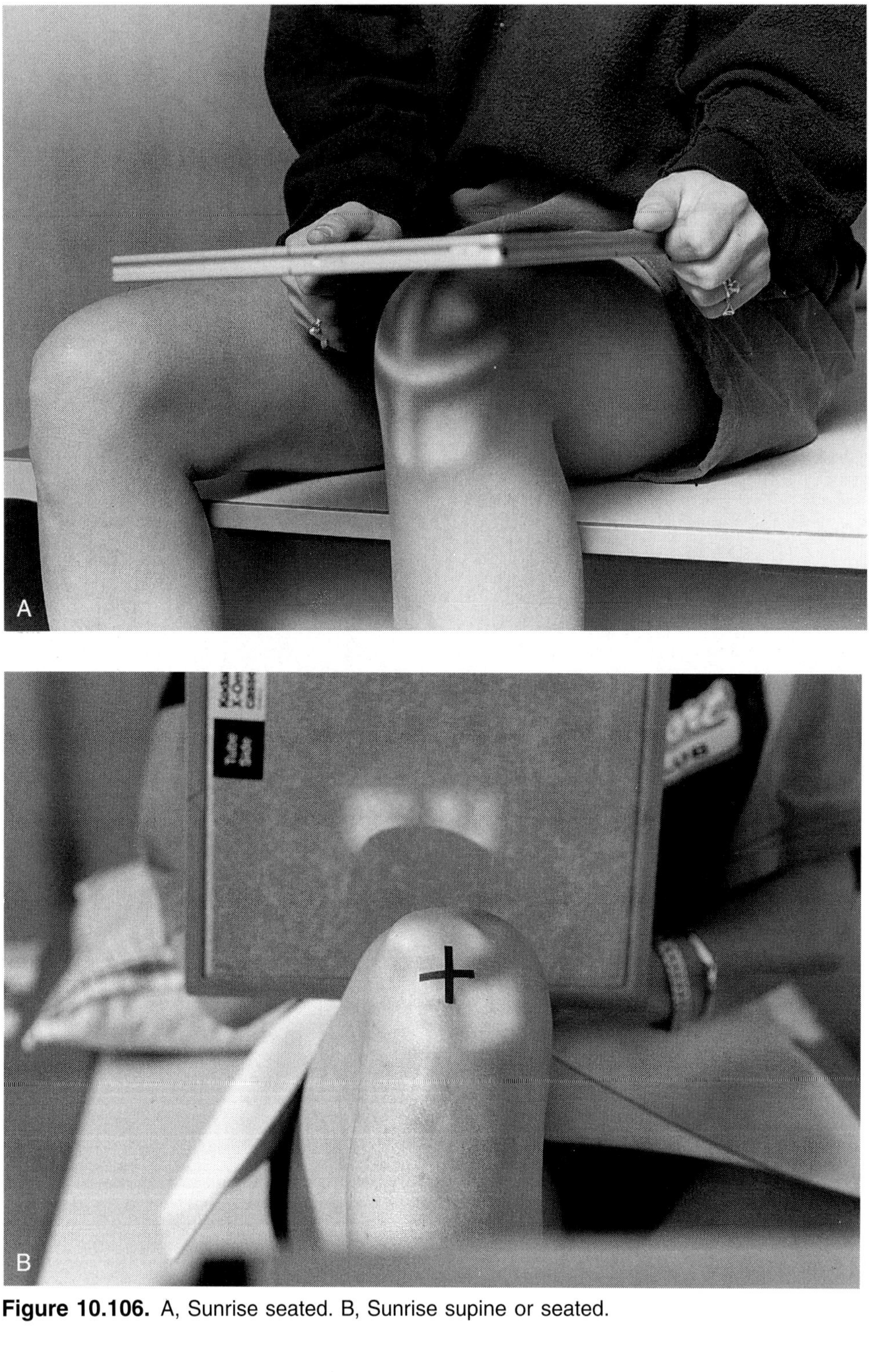

Figure 10.106. A, Sunrise seated. B, Sunrise supine or seated.

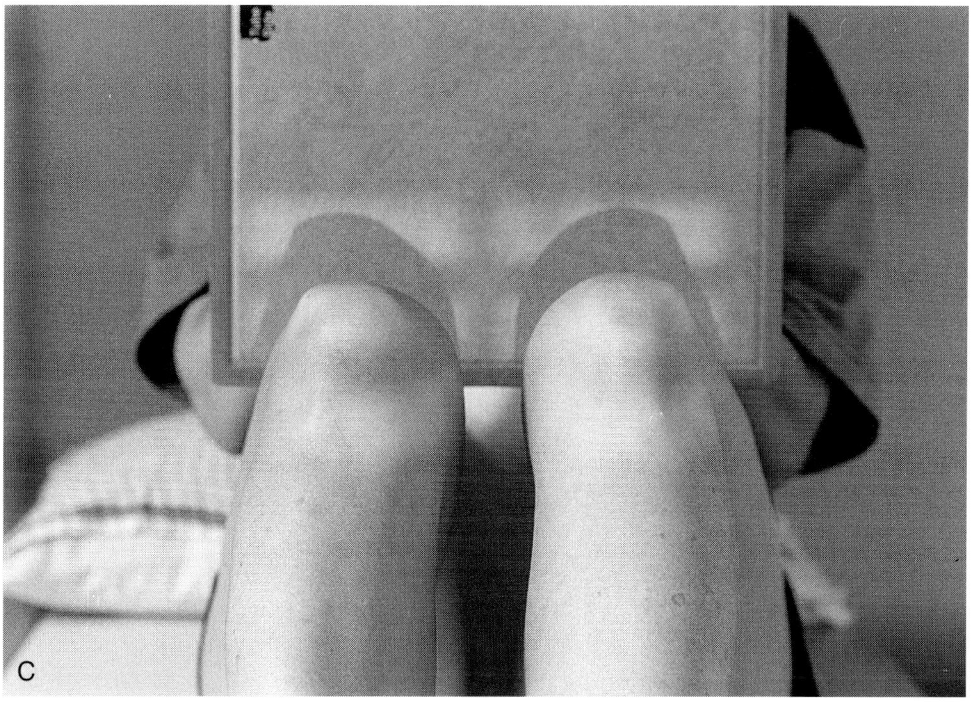

Figure 10.106 *(Continued)* C, Sunrise bilateral.

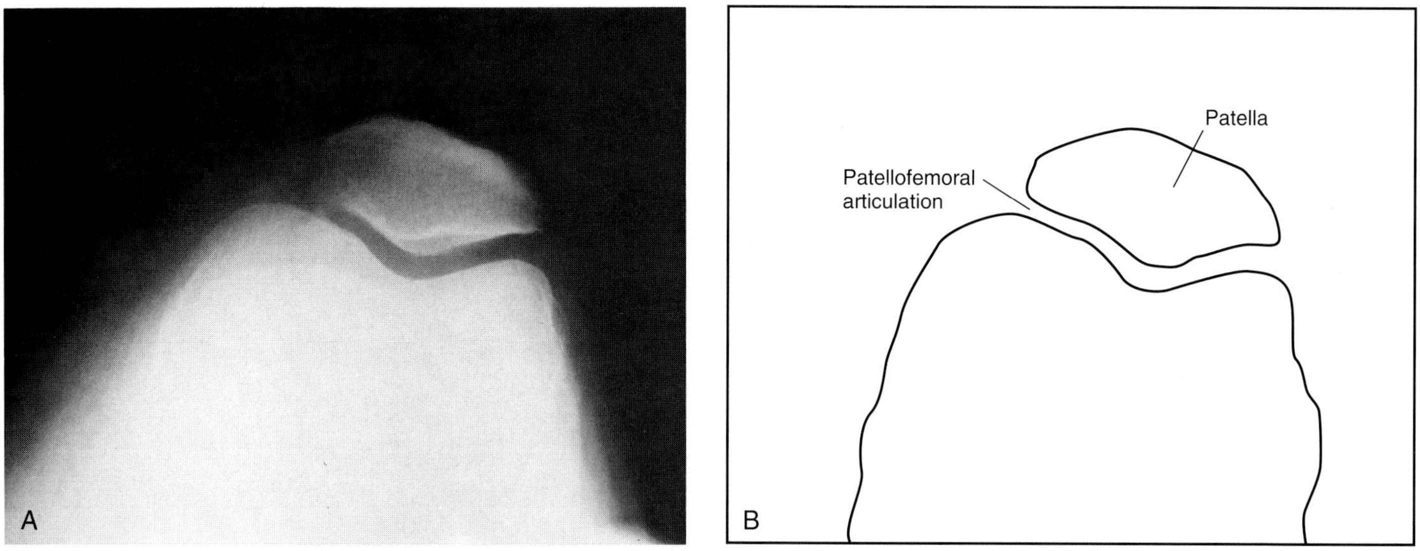

Figure 10.107. A and B, Settegast's method.

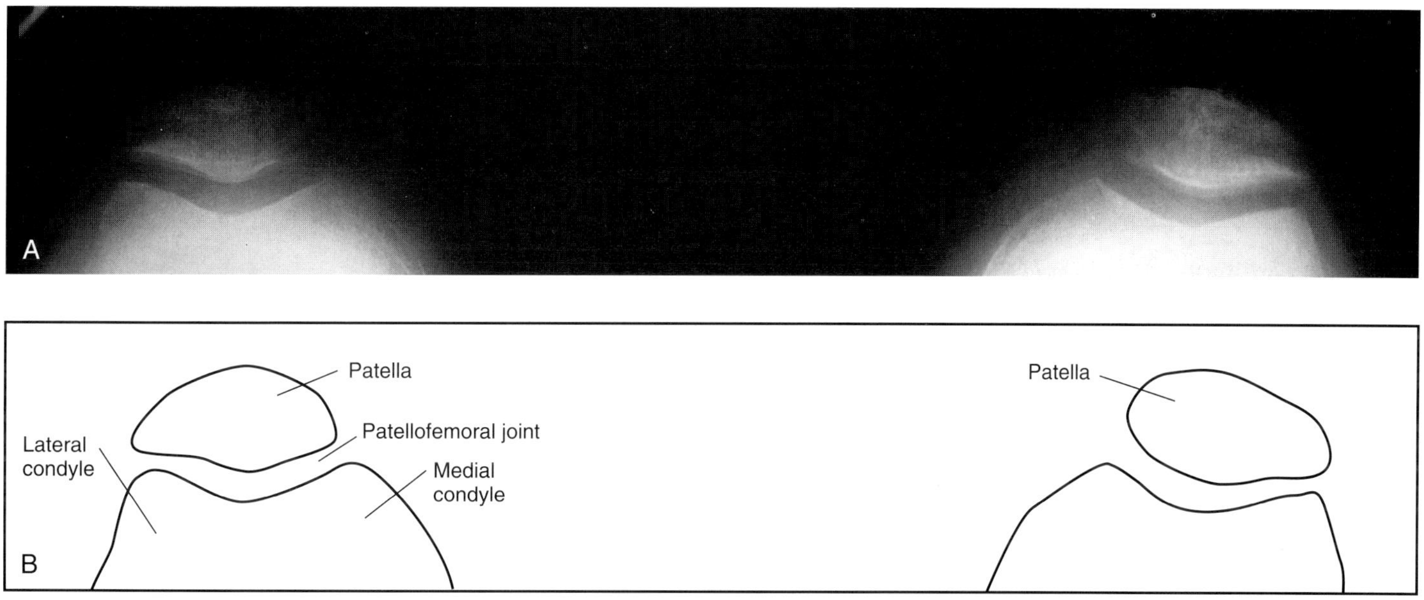

Figure 10.108. A and B, Sunrise.

Femur

Position/Projection

AP projection

Film Size:
14 × 17 inches (35 × 43 cm) (1 projection) Bucky
or
14 × 17 inches (35 × 43 cm) and 8 × 10 inches (20 × 24 cm) lengthwise (2 projections)

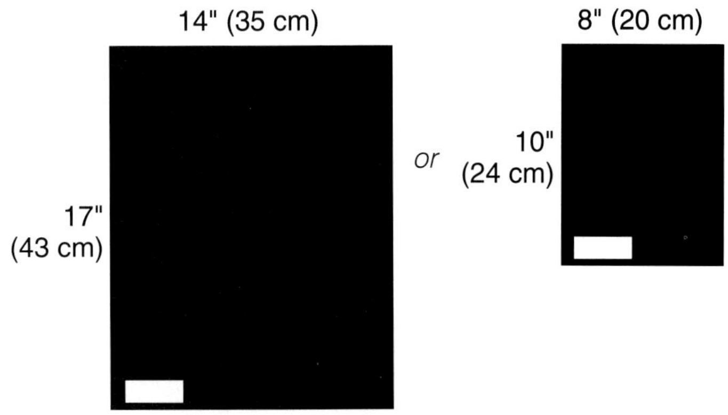

Patient Position
Supine, lower extremities extended (Fig. 10.109).

Part Position
Legs extended, pelvis not rotated. Align long axis of affected femur to midline of table. Invert foot 15° to overcome anteversion of femoral necks. Center cassette to midshaft of femur to include hip joint or knee joint, or both.

Central Ray
Perpendicular to midpoint of cassette through midshaft of femur.

Structures Demonstrated
AP femur, AP hip joint, or AP knee joint (Fig. 10.110).

Evaluation Criteria
1. Entire femur should be seen, to include joint closest to site of interest.
2. If hip joint is seen, neck of femur should be visualized without foreshortening.
3. Lesser trochanter should not be seen.
4. If lesser trochanter is not superimposed, leg has not been rotated enough internally.
5. If knee joint is seen, patella and femur should be superimposed.
6. Proximal tibia should slightly superimpose head of fibula.
7. No rotation of knees.

NOTE: The entire length of the femur, including both joints, should be visualized on one film. If this is not possible, an additional AP projection can be done on a smaller cassette to include the joint that was not included on the first film. Usually after the initial set of radiographs, it is necessary to include only the joint closest to the injury site or the portion of the femur in question. If an orthopedic appliance is present, it needs to be visualized in its entirety in one radiograph.

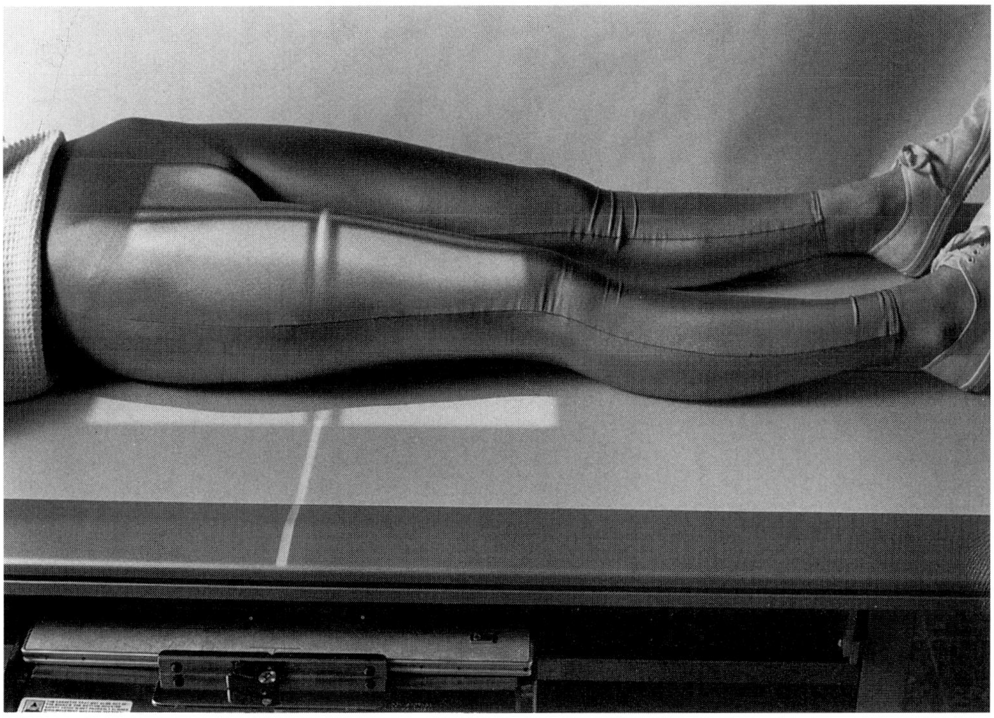

Figure 10.109. AP femur.

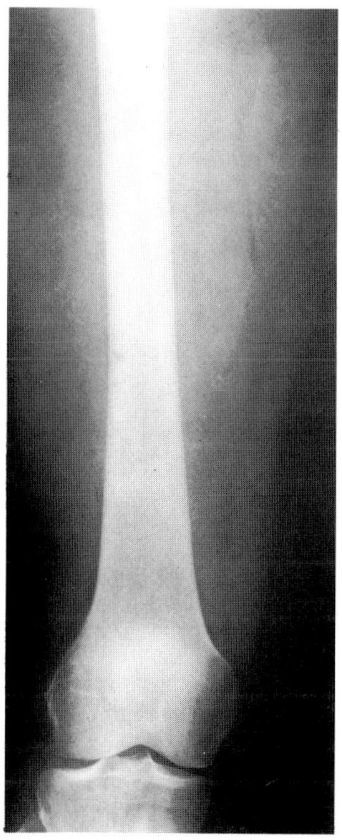

A

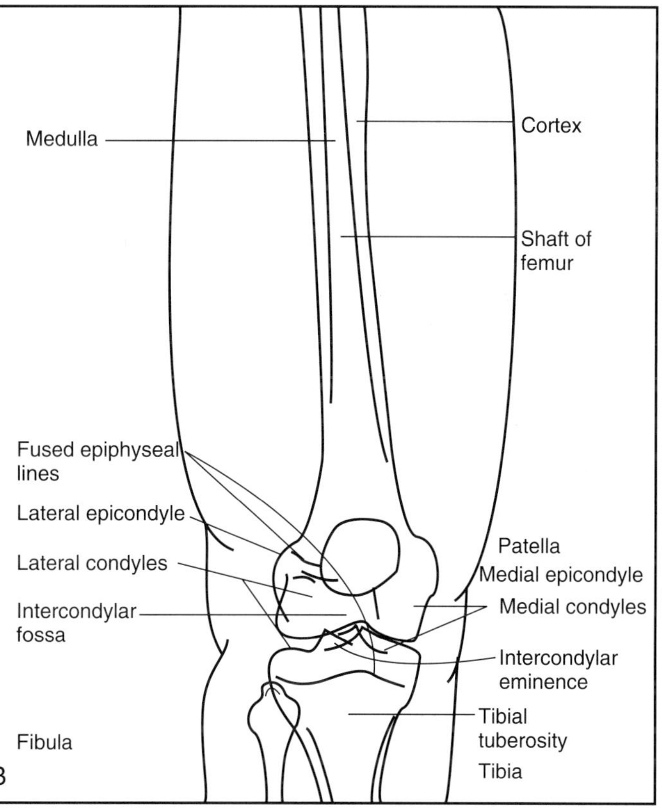

B

Figure 10.110. A and B, AP femur. (A and B [redrawn], From Meschan I: Radiographic Positioning and Related Anatomy. 2nd ed. Philadelphia: WB Saunders, 1978, p 116.)

Femur

Position/Projection

Lateral projection

Film Size:
14 × 17 inches (35 × 43 cm) lengthwise (1 projection) Bucky

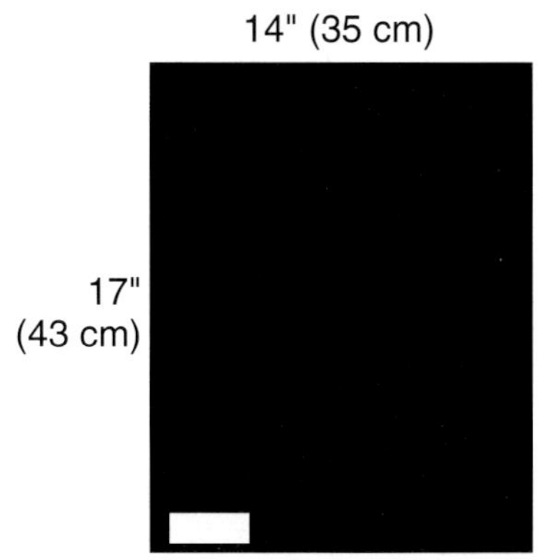

Patient Position

Laterally recumbent on affected side; knee flexed (Fig. 10.111).

Part Position

Center thigh to midline of table. Adjust lower extremity so patella is perpendicular to plane of table. Place unaffected extremity behind affected extremity.

To Include Hip Joint
Have unaffected leg behind dependent leg. Roll pelvis backward enough to prevent its superimposition on affected femur (go out 15° from lateral).

To Include Knee Joint
Bring unaffected leg forward. Adjust pelvis to true lateral position.

Central Ray

Perpendicular to midpoint of cassette through midshaft of femur.

Structures Demonstrated

Lateral projection of three fourths of femur and adjacent joint (Fig. 10.112).

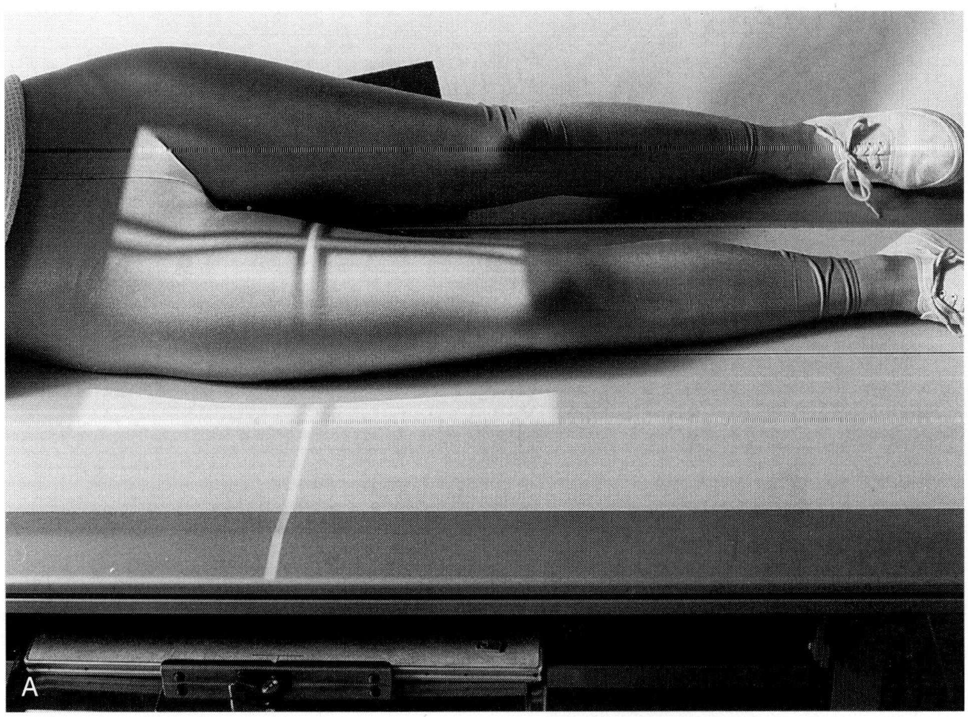

Figure 10.111. A and B, Lateral femur.

Evaluation Criteria

1. Entire lateral femur should be seen, to include joint closest to site of interest.
2. If hip joint is seen, there should be no superimposition of pelvis and affected femur.
3. Femur should superimpose lesser and greater trochanters.
4. If knee joint is to be seen, unaffected extremity should not be over affected thigh.
5. Femoropatellar space should be open and femoral condyles should be slightly superimposed.

NOTE: This projection should not be done on patients with a new or recent femoral fracture. This projection could cause more fracture fragment displacement. If the patient has a new or recent fracture, a cross-table lateral should be performed instead of the lateral projection. Patient is supine with affected extremity extended. The cassette is placed on either the lateral or the medial side of the affected leg (normally placed on the lateral side). To include the hip joint, the cassette has to be placed on the lateral side. Raise the unaffected leg so the horizontal beam will enter the midshaft of the affected femur. Place the cassette to include the posterior surface of the affected femur. The cassette should have a grid if the patient's thigh measures 4 inches (10 cm) or more.

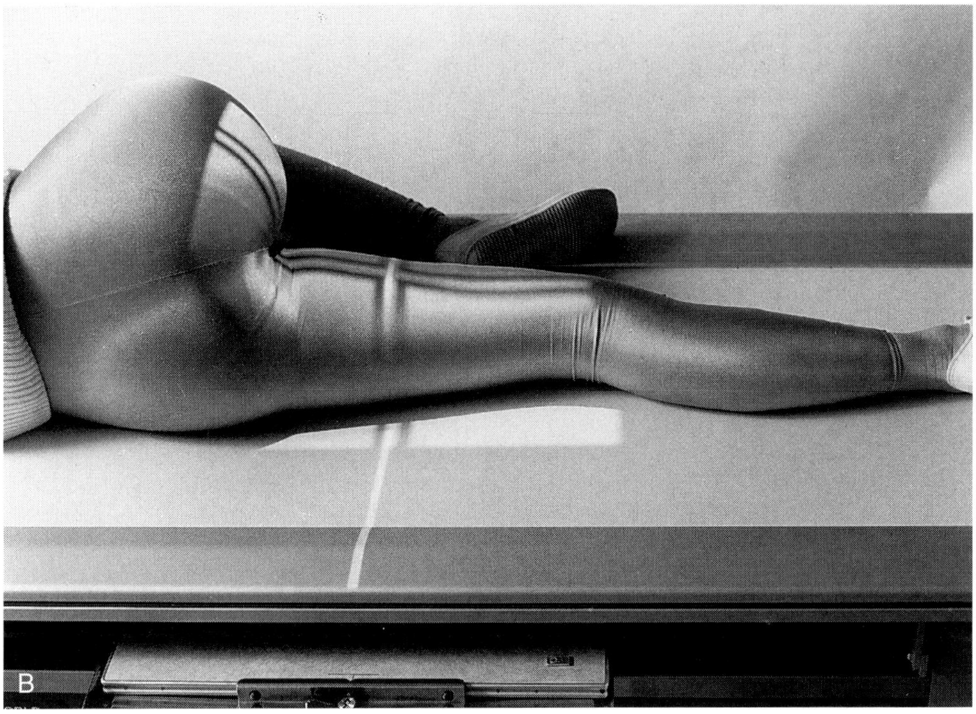

Figure 10.111 *(Continued)*

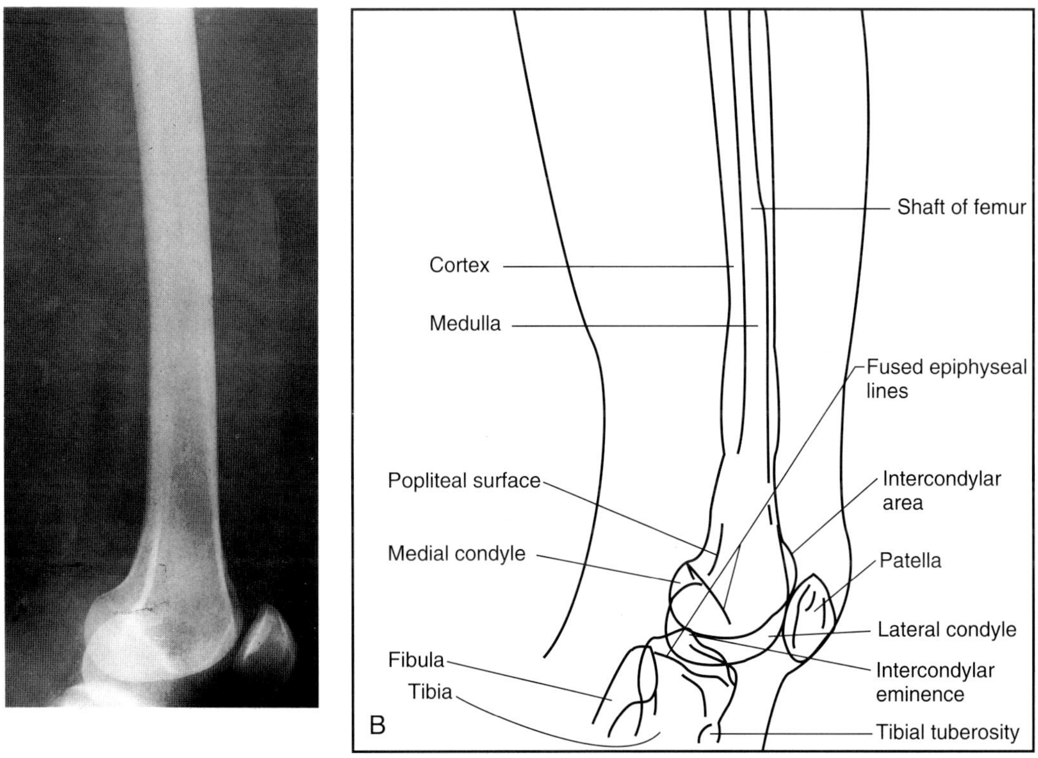

Figure 10.112. A and B, Lateral femur. (A and B [redrawn], From Meschan I: Radiographic Positioning and Related Anatomy. 2nd ed. Philadelphia: WB Saunders, 1978, p 116.)

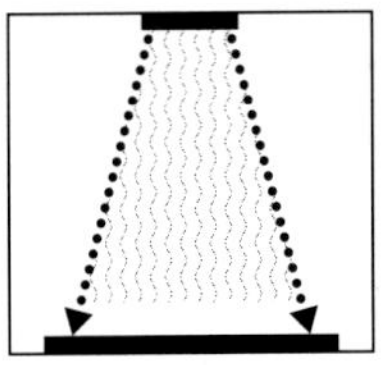

Pelvis

Position/Projection

AP projection

Film Size:
14 × 17 inches (35 × 43 cm) crosswise Bucky

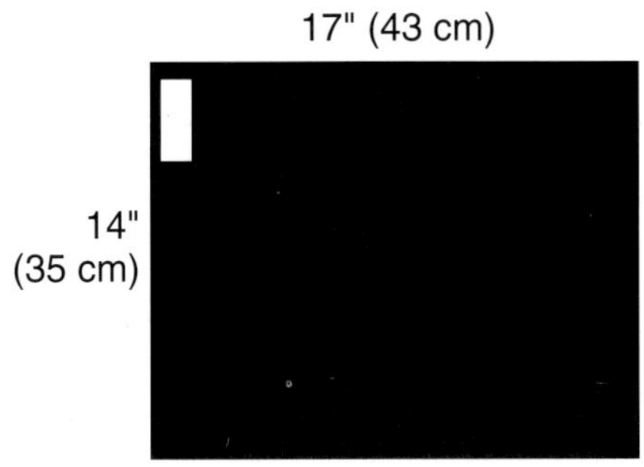

Patient Position

Recumbent (supine) with lower extremities extended. Center midsagittal plane of body to midline of table (Fig. 10.113).

Part Position

Adjust body in true AP position, making sure both anterior superior iliac spines (ASISs) are equidistant from table. Invert toes of both extremities medially 15° to overcome anteversion of femoral necks and place their long axis parallel with film. Center cassette at level of soft tissue depression just above greater trochanter. Top of cassette should be 1½ inches (4 cm) above level of iliac crest.

Central Ray

Perpendicular to midpoint of cassette.

Structures Demonstrated

AP projection of pelvic girdle, hip joint, and proximal femora (Fig. 10.114).

Evaluation Criteria

1. Entire pelvis should be seen including proximal portions of femurs.
2. Femoral heads should be seen.
3. No evidence of rotation of pelvis (greater trochanters should be of equal size and free of superimposition).
4. Lesser trochanters should not be seen.
5. No foreshortening of femoral necks.

NOTE: If the radiograph is being done for internal hip fixation or for a prosthesis, center lower to demonstrate more of the femur including the complete fixation or prosthesis. Generally, the head of the femur (acetabulum) to the tip of the length of the pin must be included on the radiograph. If more than the tip of the lesser trochanter is seen, the legs have not been rotated internally enough.

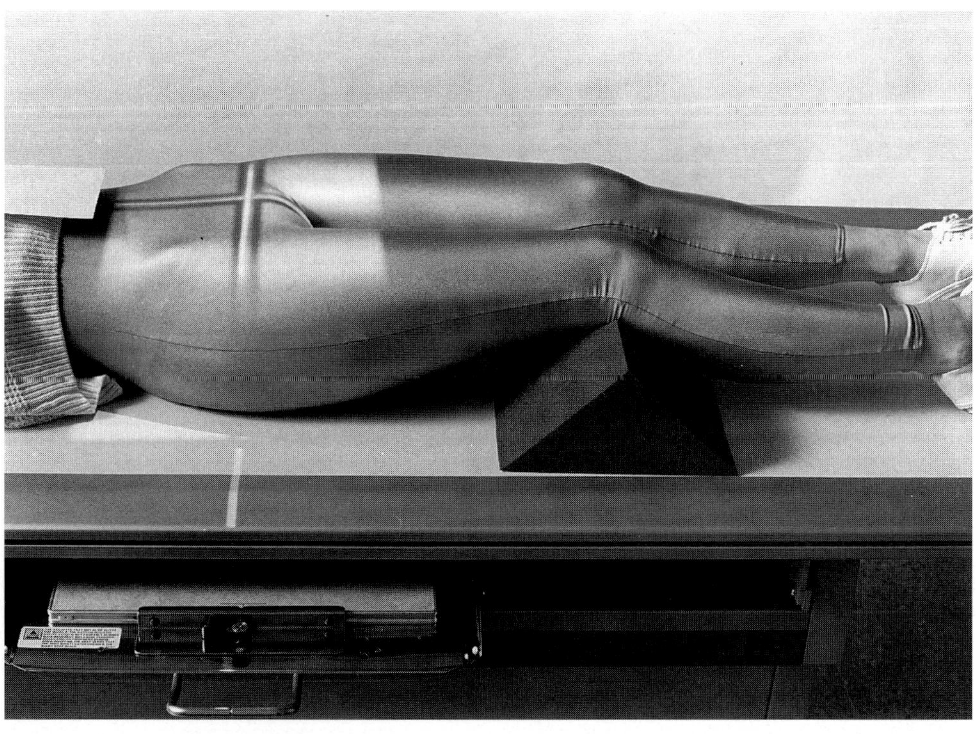

Figure 10.113. AP pelvis.

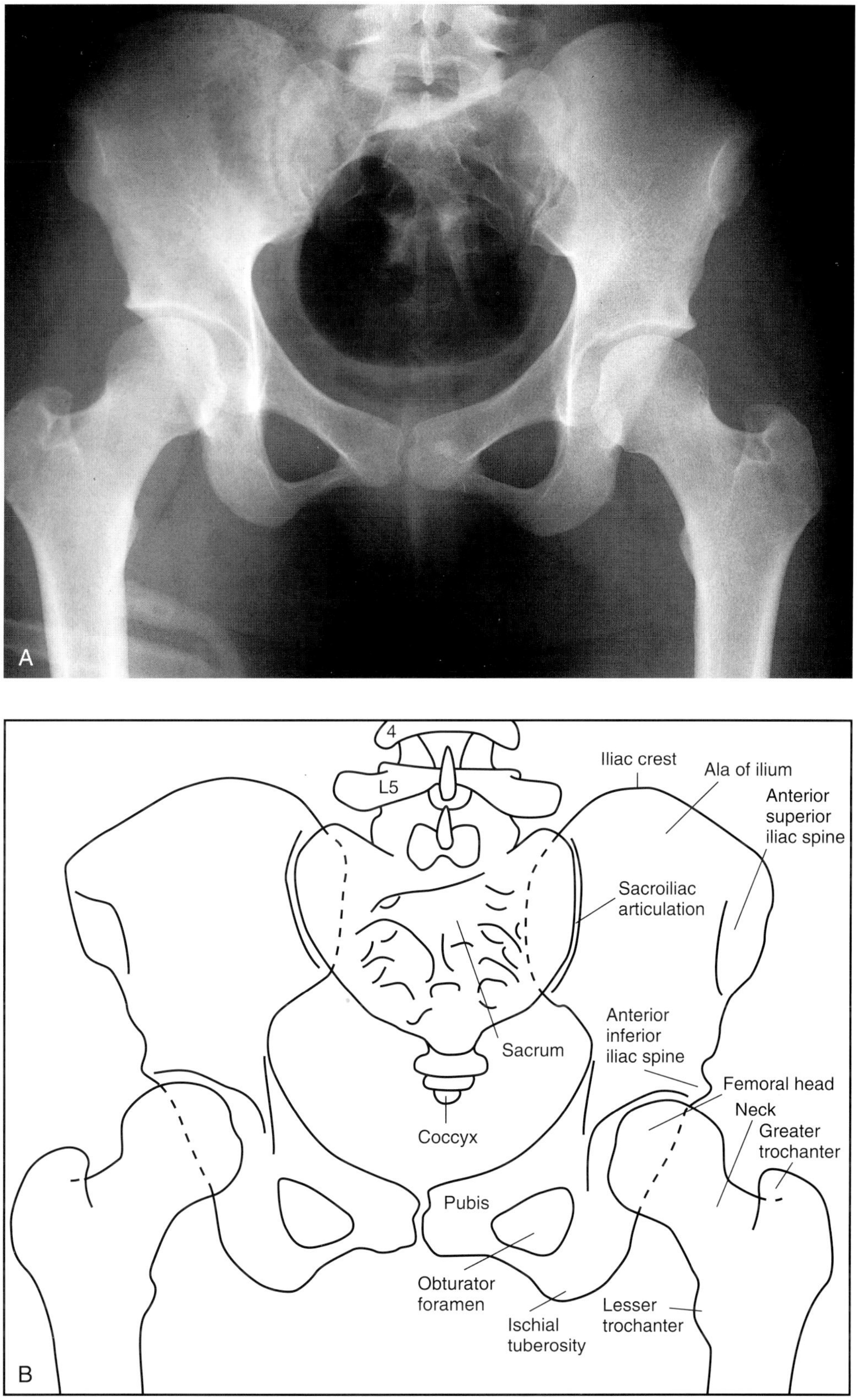

Figure 10.114. A and B, AP pelvis.

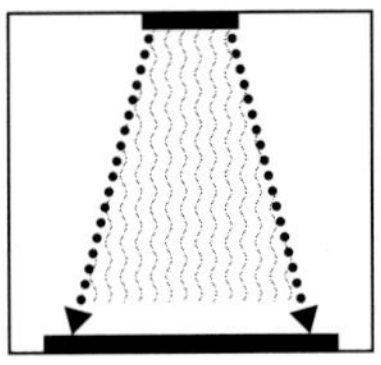

Pelvis and Upper Femora

Position/Projection

Lateral projection

Film Size:
14 × 17 inches (35 × 43 cm) lengthwise Bucky

Patient Position

Recumbent with legs extended or erect with weight equally distributed on feet (Fig. 10.115).

Part Position

Recumbent

Place patient in lateral position with legs extended. Center midaxillary plane of body to midline of the table. Be sure pelvis is in true lateral position and not rotated (ASISs should be in same vertical plane).

Erect

Place patient in lateral position with weight equally distributed on feet. Center midaxillary plane of table to midline of vertical grid.

Central Ray

Perpendicular to level of soft depression just above greater trochanter. Center midpoint of cassette to central ray.

Breathing Instructions

Respiration is suspended after full exhalation.

Structures Demonstrated

Lateral projection of upper femora, superimposed hipbones, lumbosacral junction, and sacrum and coccyx (Fig. 10.116).

Evaluation Criteria

1. Femurs should be superimposed.
2. Acetabular shadows should be superimposed.
3. Posterior margins of ischium and ilium should be superimposed.
4. Femurs should not obscure pubic arch.
5. Entire pelvis and proximal femurs should be seen.

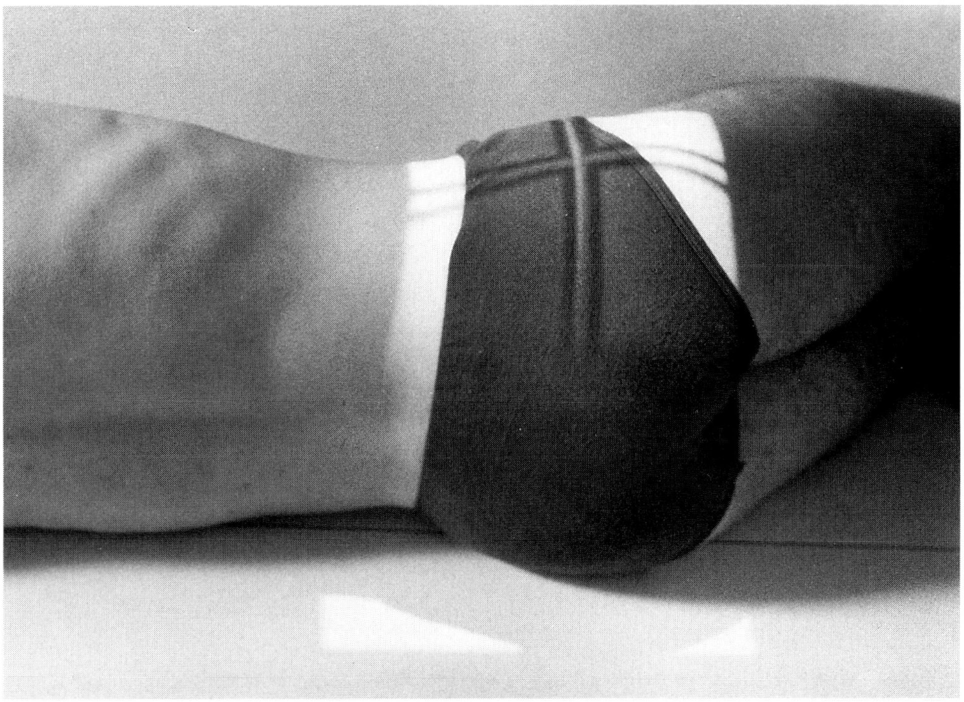

Figure 10.115. Lateral pelvis.

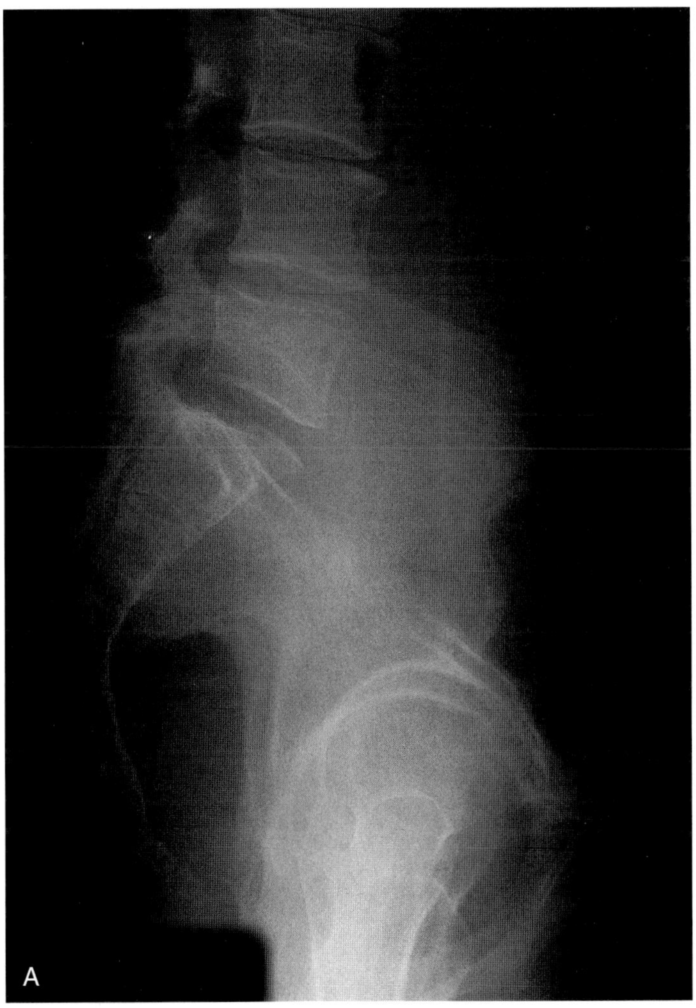

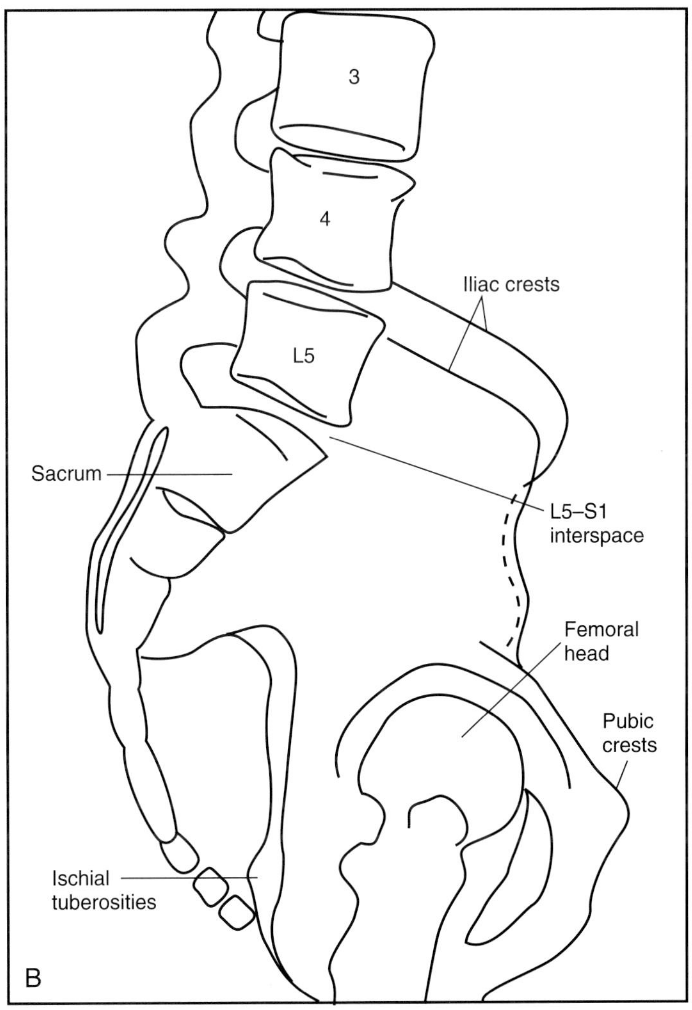

Figure 10.116. A and B, Lateral pelvis.

Pelvis and Hip Joints

Position/Projection

Axial projection—Chassard-Lapiné method

Film Size:
14 × 17 inches (35 × 43 cm) crosswise Bucky

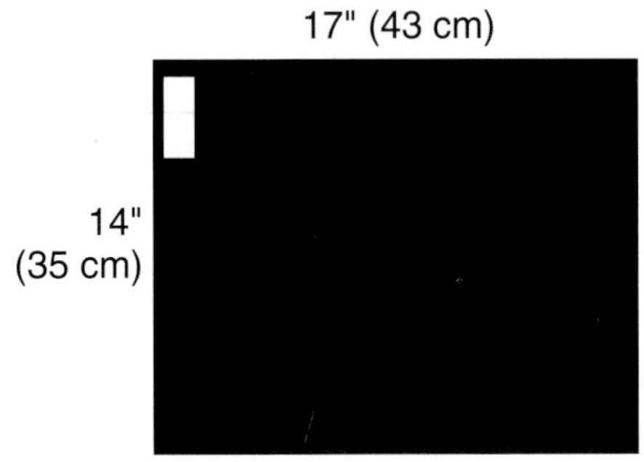

Patient Position

Sitting on side or end of table with posterior surface of knees touching edge of table (Fig. 10.117).

Part Position

Align midsagittal plane of body to midline of table if patient is sitting at end of table. Align longitudinal axis of film to midsagittal plane of body if patient is sitting on side of table. Have patient lean forward to place symphysis pubis in close contact with table (have patient grasp ankles—pelvis will be tilted forward 45°).

Central Ray

Perpendicular through lumbar region to level of greater trochanters. Center midpoint of cassette to central ray.

Breathing Instructions

Respiration is suspended after full exhalation.

Structures Demonstrated

Axial projection of pelvis. Ischial tuberosity, greater trochanter, femoral head, acetabulum, ala of ilium, and femoral shaft should be seen (Fig. 10.118).

Evaluation Criteria

1. Pelvis should not be rotated.
2. Demonstration of entire pelvis including proximal femurs.
3. Greater trochanters should be same distance from sacrum.

NOTE: The exposure technique for this projection is generally the same as for a lateral pelvis.

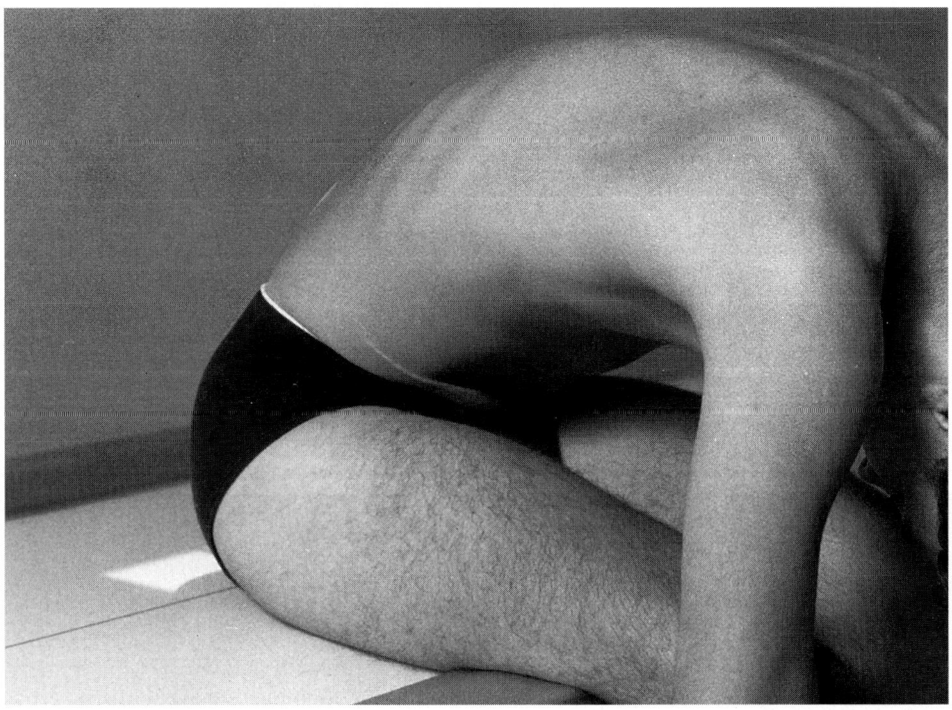

Figure 10.117. Axial pelvis (Chassard-Lapiné method).

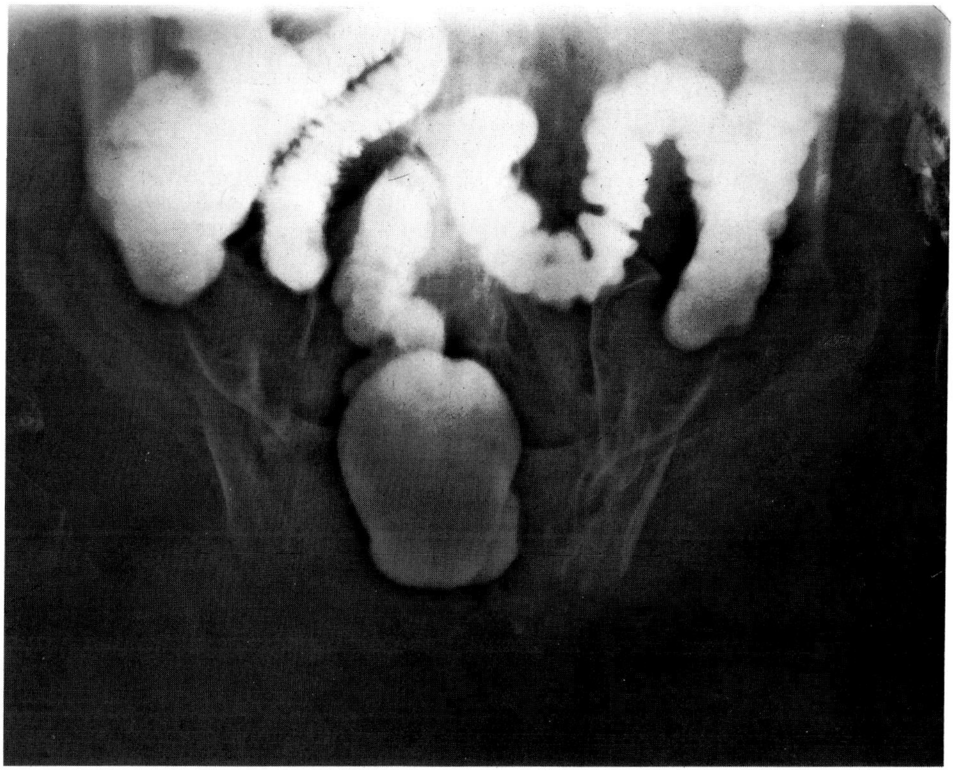

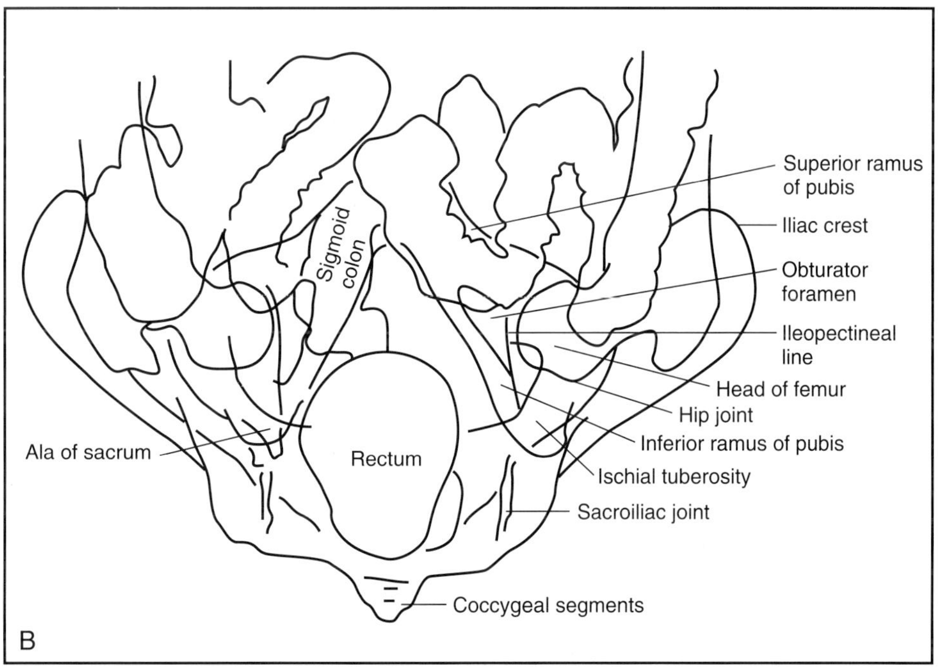

Figure 10.118. Chassard-Lapiné method. (A and B [redrawn], From Meschan I: Radiographic Positioning and Related Anatomy. 2nd ed. Philadelphia: WB Saunders, 1978, p 488.)

Pelvis and Hip Joints

Position/Projection

Lateral projection—Lauenstein's and Hickey's methods

Film Size:
10 × 12 inches (24 × 30 cm) crosswise Bucky

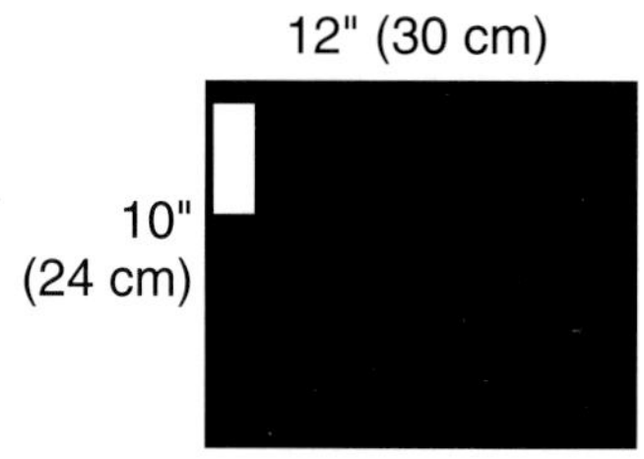

Patient Position

Supine, turn patient toward affected hip (laterally) approximately 45°. Align sagittal plane of affected hip to midline of table. Support elevated side (Fig. 10.119).

Part Position

Flex dependent knee to nearly right-angle position. Abduct affected thigh to place in contact with table.

Central Ray

Perpendicular to enter femoral neck. Hickey's method—20° to 25° cephalic angle to enter femoral neck. Center midpoint of cassette to central ray.

NOTE: To locate the femoral neck, bisect an imaginary line drawn between the ASIS and the symphysis pubis, then move down 2½ inches (6 cm).

Breathing Instructions

Respiration is suspended at end of exhalation.

Structures Demonstrated

Lateral projection of hip joint including proximal femur (Fig. 10.120).

Evaluation Criteria

1. Hip joint should be in center of radiograph with greater trochanter slightly superimposed by neck of femur.
2. Hip joint and proximal femur should be seen.

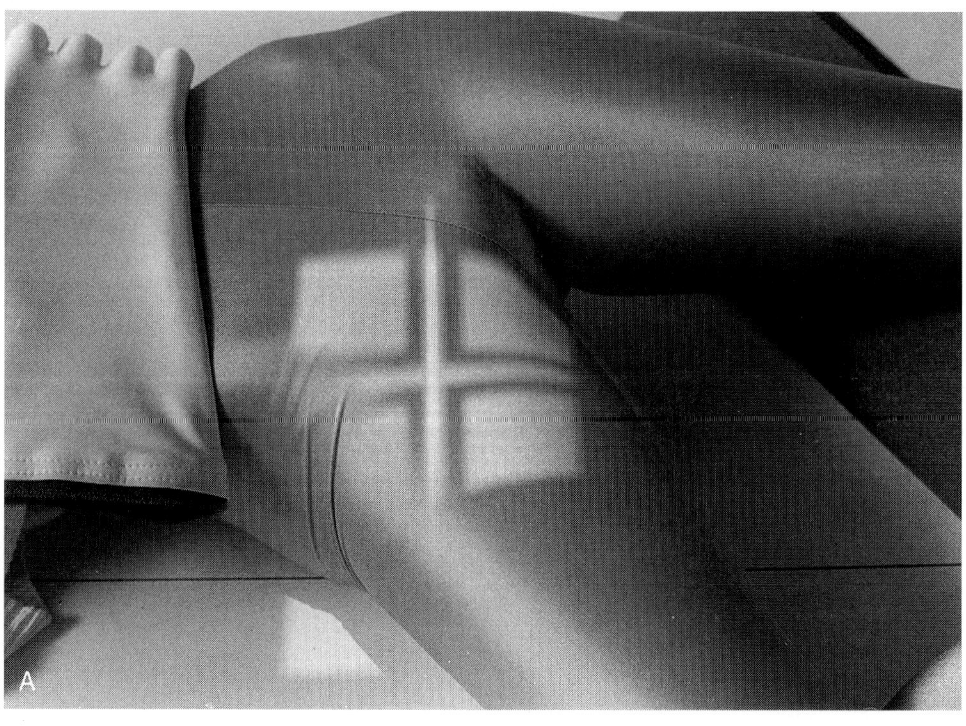

Figure 10.119. A, Lateral hip, Lauenstein's method.

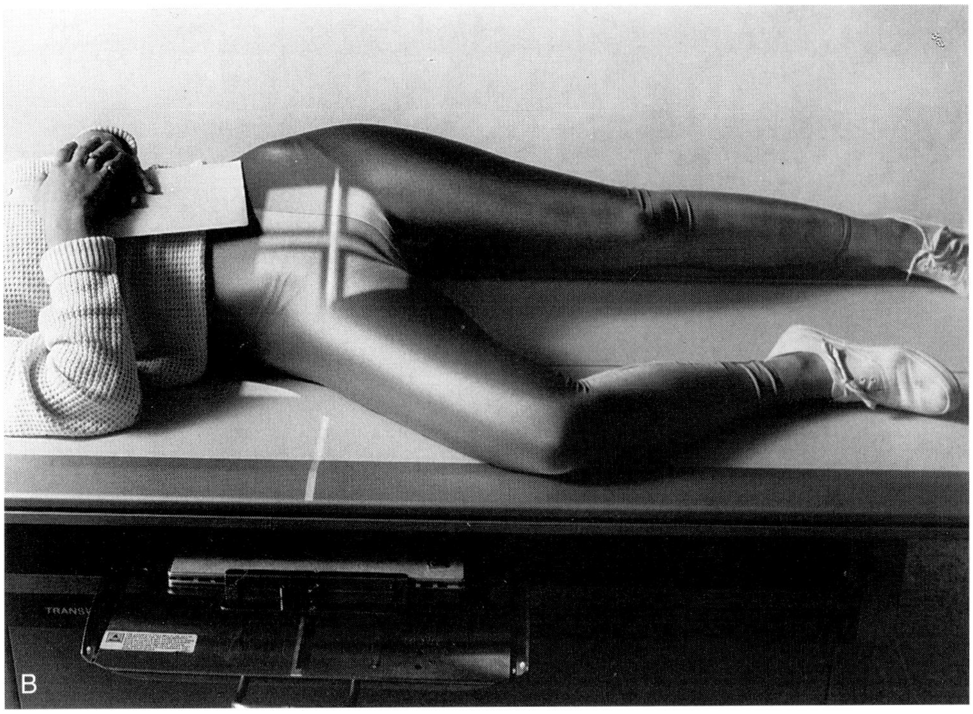

Figure 10.119 *(Continued)* B, Hickey's method.

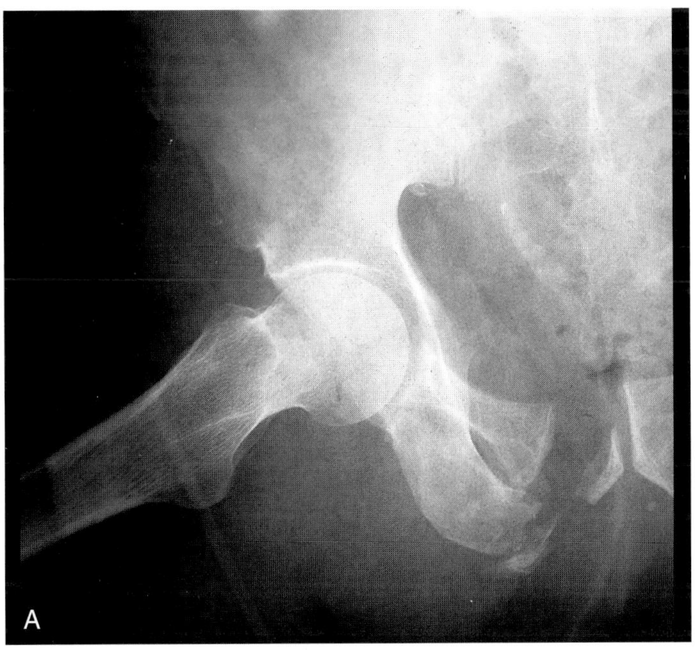

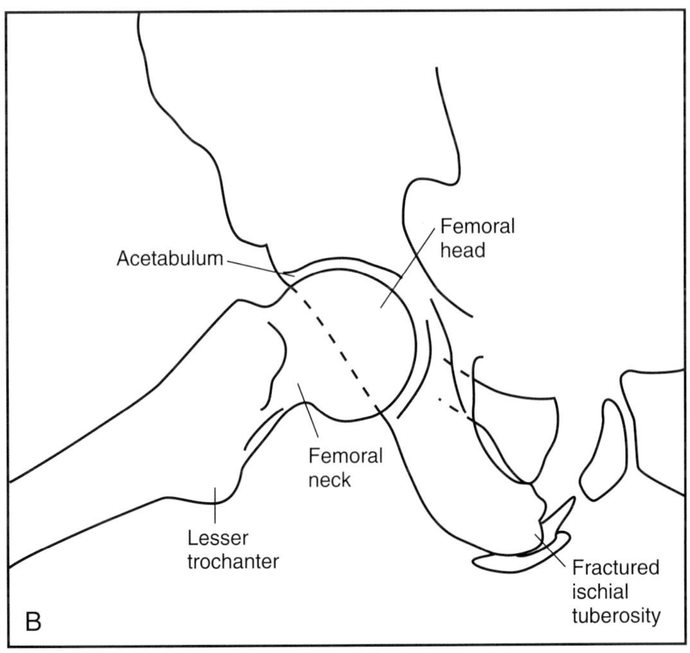

Figure 10.120. A and B, Lauenstein's method.

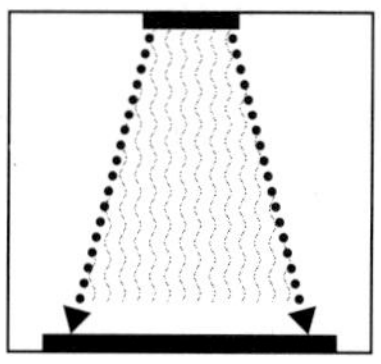

Hip

Position/Projection

AP projection

Film Size:
10 × 12 inches (24 × 30 cm) lengthwise Bucky

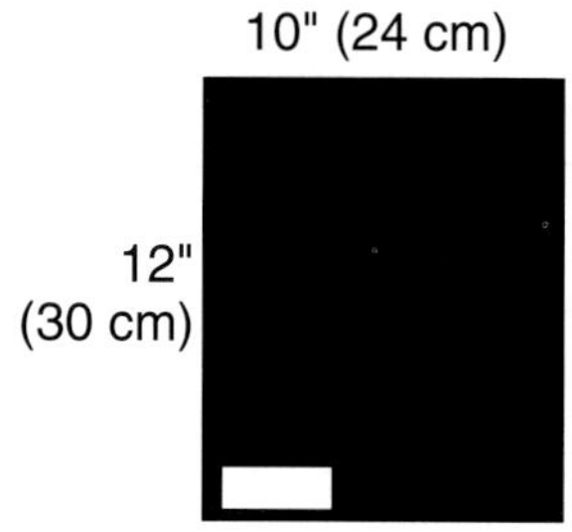

Patient Position

Recumbent (supine), with midsagittal plane parallel to midline of table. Place patient in true AP position, making sure both ASISs are equidistant from table (Fig. 10.121).

Part Position

Center sagittal plane passing 2 inches (5 cm) medial to ASIS of affected side to midline of table. Center cassette at level of soft depression just above greater trochanter. Top of cassette should be 1½ inches (4 cm) above level of iliac crest. Invert foot of affected hip 15° to overcome anteversion of affected femoral neck.

Central Ray

Perpendicular to midpoint of cassette.

Structures Demonstrated

AP projection of hip, acetabulum, and proximal femur (Fig. 10. 122).

Evaluation Criteria

1. Entire hip joint including adjacent pubic bones, ischium, and ilium.
2. No foreshortening of femoral neck.
3. Lesser trochanter should not be seen.

NOTE: If more than the tip of the lesser trochanter is seen, the leg of the affected side has not been rotated internally enough. If the radiograph is being done for hip fixation or for a prosthesis, be sure to include the complete fixation or prosthesis on the radiograph.

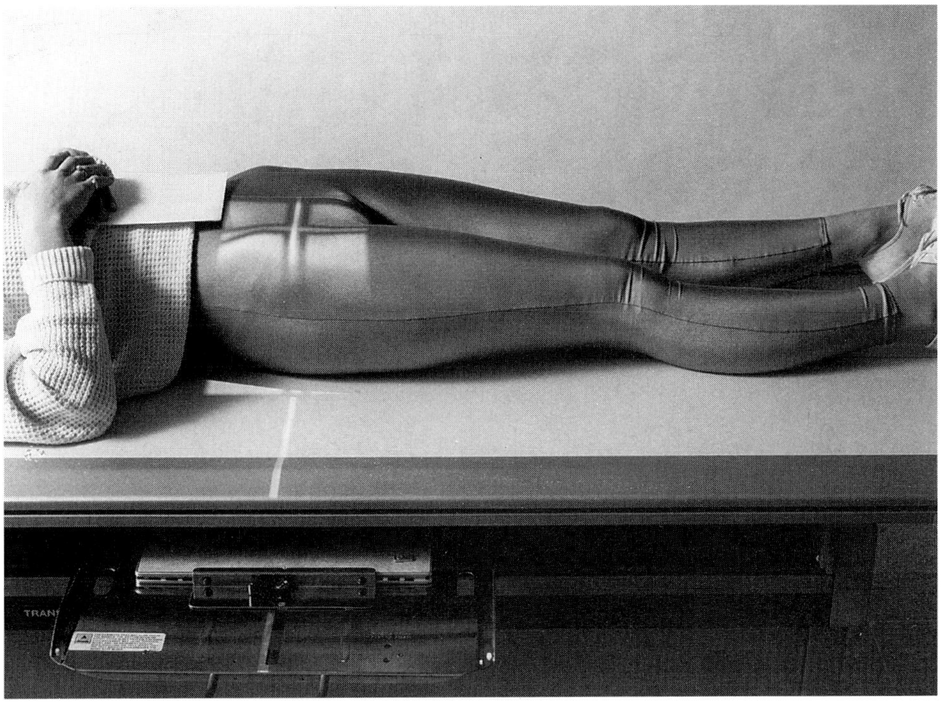

Figure 10.121. AP unilateral hip.

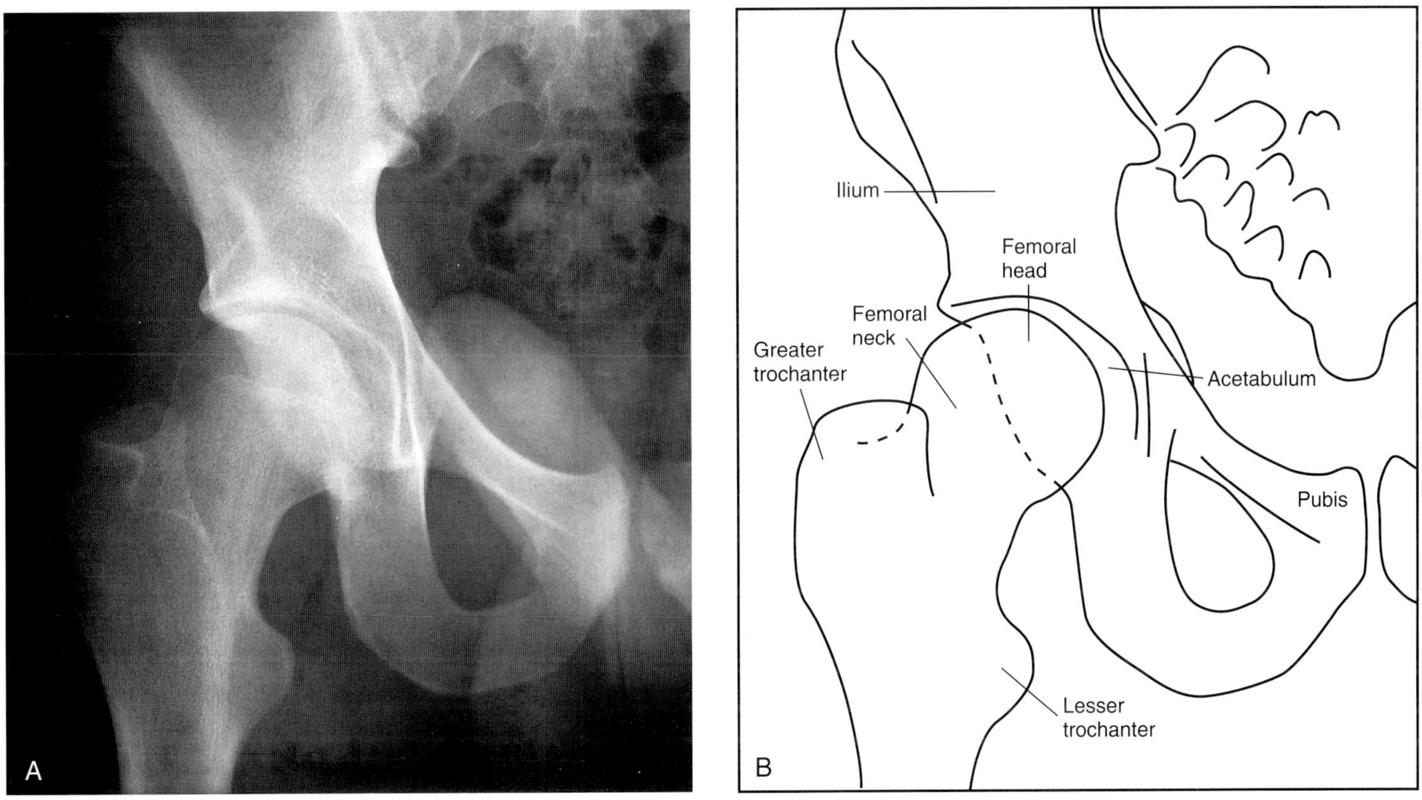

Figure 10.122. A and B, AP hip.

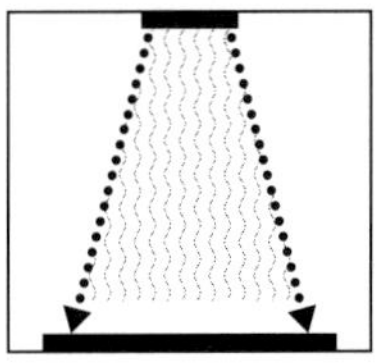

Bilateral Hips

Position/Projection

AP projection

Film Size:
14 × 17 inches (35 × 43 cm) crosswise Bucky

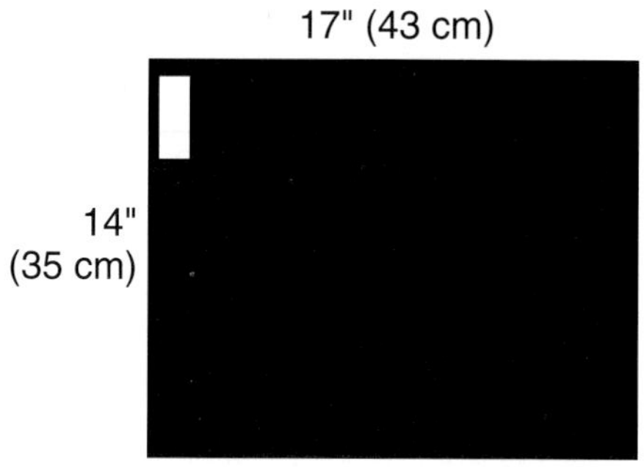

Patient Position

Supine with legs extended. Align midsagittal plane parallel to midline of table. Place patient in true AP position, making sure both anterior superior iliac spines (ASISs) are equidistant from table (Fig. 10.123).

Part Position

Invert toes of both extremities medially 15° to overcome anteversion of femoral neck.

Central Ray

Perpendicular to enter 1 inch (2.5 cm) above symphysis pubis.

NOTE: To locate the femoral neck, bisect an imaginary line drawn between the ASIS and the symphysis pubis, then come down 2½ inches (6 cm). To locate femoral head, bisect an imaginary line drawn between the ASIS and the symphysis pubis, then come down 1½ inches (4 cm).

Breathing Instructions

Respiration is suspended at end of exhalation.

Structures Demonstrated

AP projection of hip joints, acetebulum, and femoral heads, necks, greater trochanters, both hip bones, sacrum, and coccyx (Fig. 10.124).

Evaluation Criteria

1. Hip joints, adjacent ilium, pubic bone, ischium, and proximal third of femurs should be seen.
2. There should be no foreshortening of femoral necks.
3. Lesser trochanters should not be demonstrated—only tip should be free of superimposition (if more than tip is visualized, legs need to be rotated more).

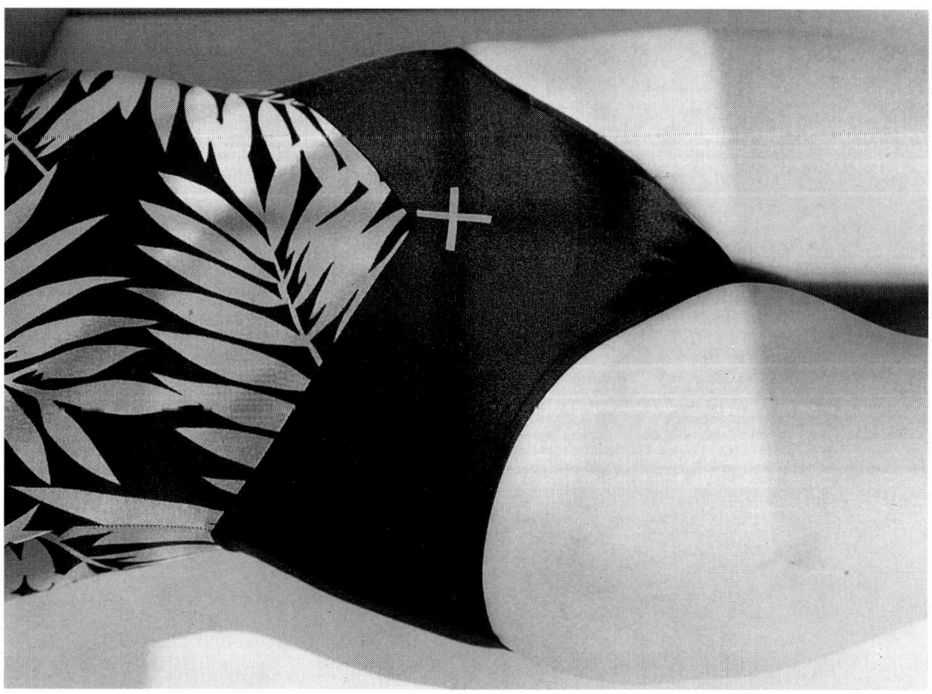

Figure 10.123. AP bilateral hip.

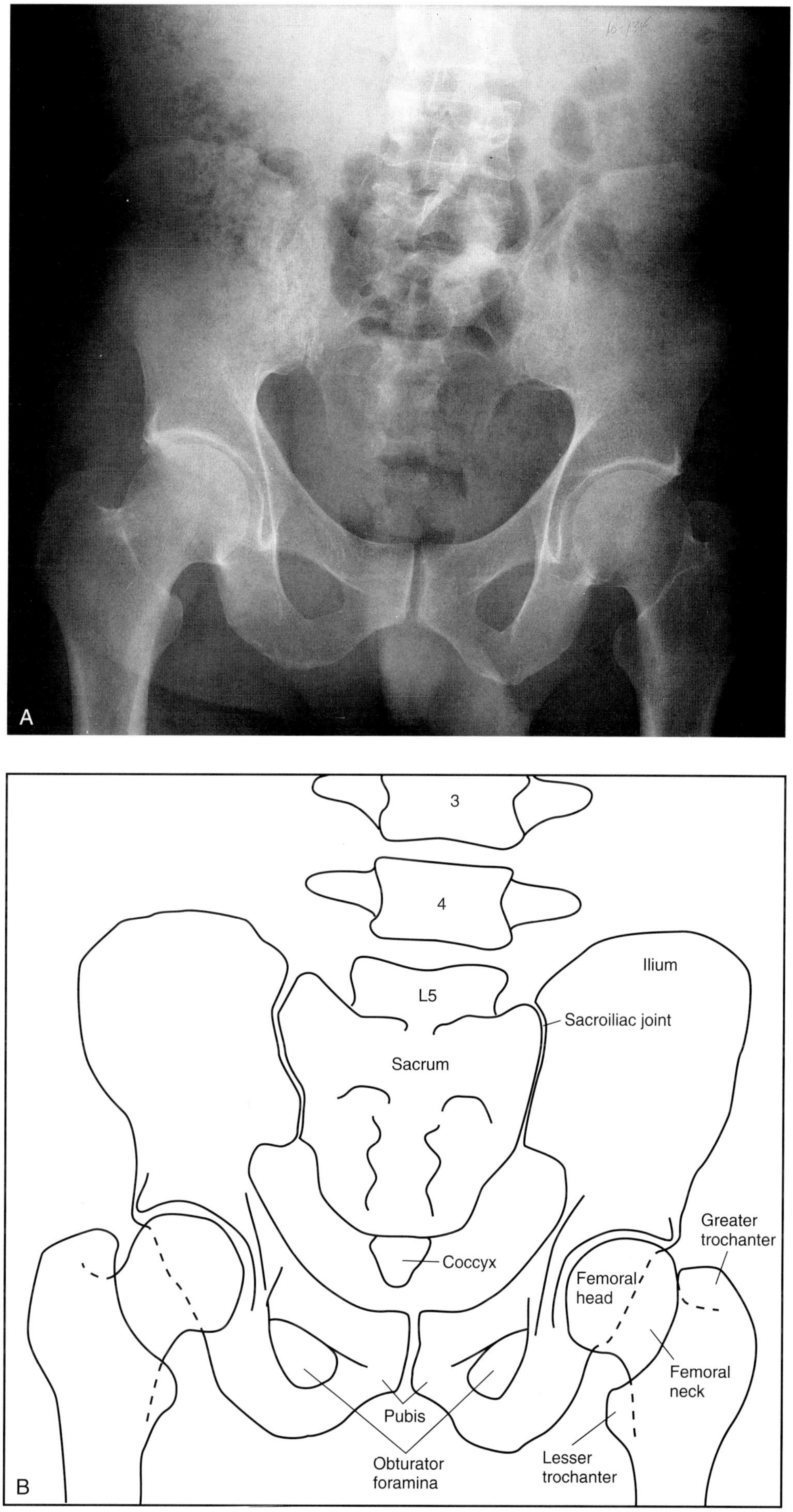

Figure 10.124. A and B, AP bilateral hip.

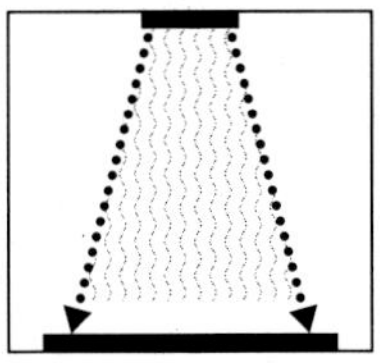

Bilateral Hips

Position/Projection

Bilateral frog-leg position—Cleaves' nontrauma position

Film Size:
14 × 17 inches (35 × 43 cm) crosswise Bucky

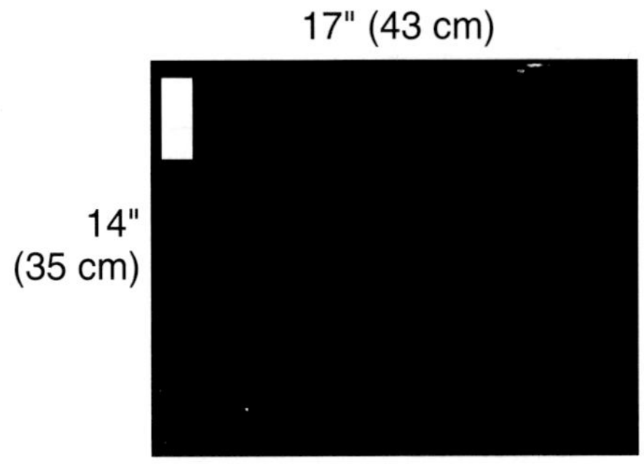

Patient Position

Supine, align MSP (midsagittal plane) to midline of table (Fig. 10.125).

Part Position

Place pelvis in true AP position with hip in same plane. Bend knees as much as possible. Abduct thighs about 40° from vertical, place femoral necks parallel with cassette, place plantar surfaces of feet together.

Central Ray

Perpendicular through symphysis pubis. Center midpoint of cassette to central ray.

Breathing Instructions

Respiration is suspended at end of exhalation.

Structures Demonstrated

Axiolateral projection of femoral necks, heads, and trochanteric areas (Fig. 10.126).

Evalution Criteria

1. No rotation of pelvis.
2. Hip joints should be seen.
3. Femoral heads and necks should be seen.
4. Should project lesser trochanters on medial surfaces of femurs.

NOTE: This projection should not be used on a patient with a recent, new, or suspected hip fracture or dislocation. This projection is done frequently on nontrauma pediatric patients to rule out possible congenital hip deformities.

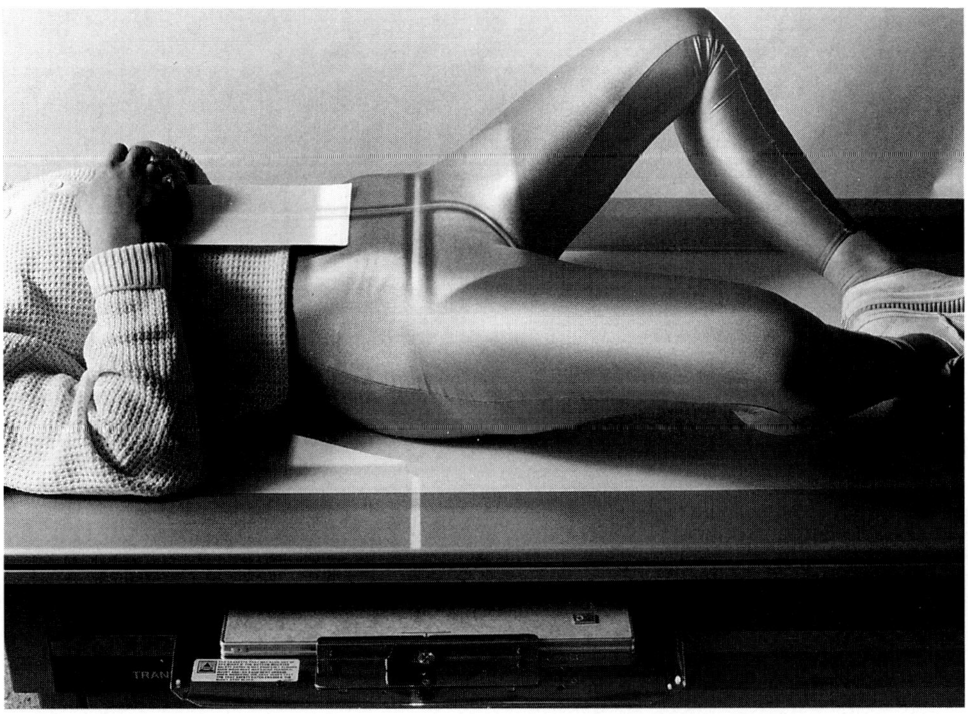

Figure 10.125. Bilateral frog-leg.

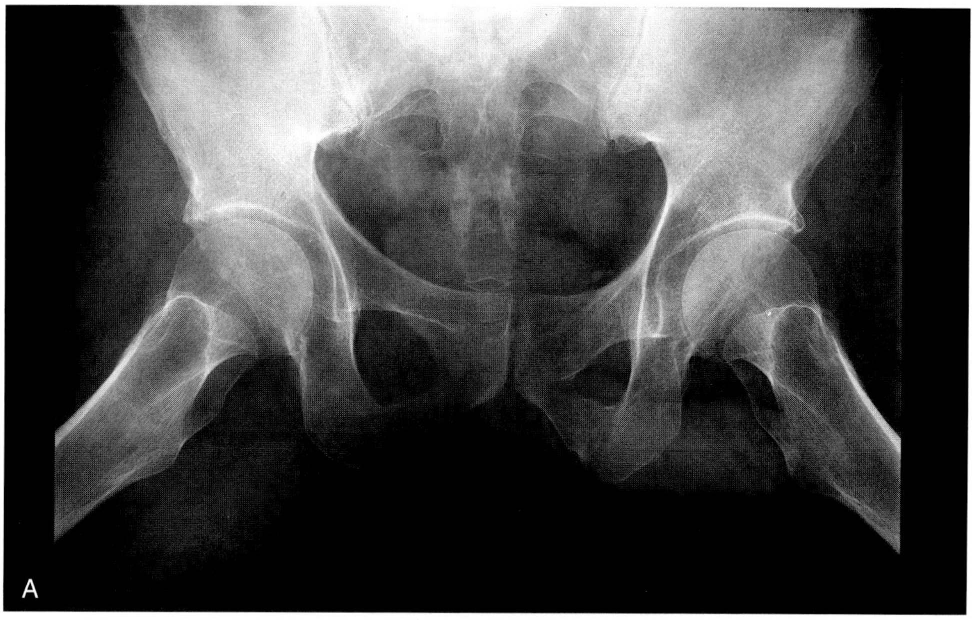

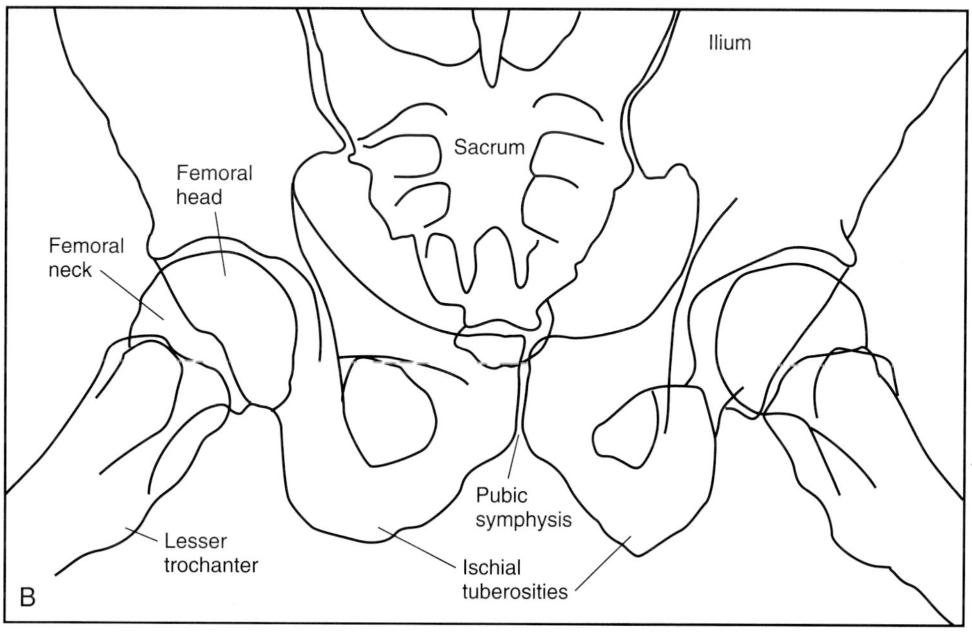

Figure 10.126. A and B, Bilateral frog-leg.

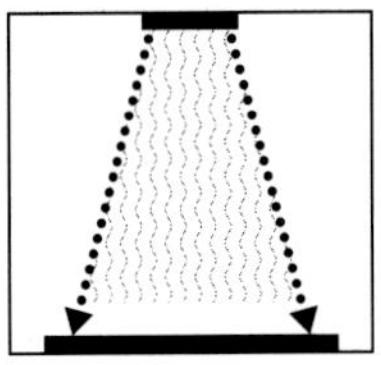

Unilateral Hip

Position/Projection

Frog-leg projection (nontrauma routine)

Film Size:
10 × 12 inches (24 × 30 cm) lengthwise Bucky

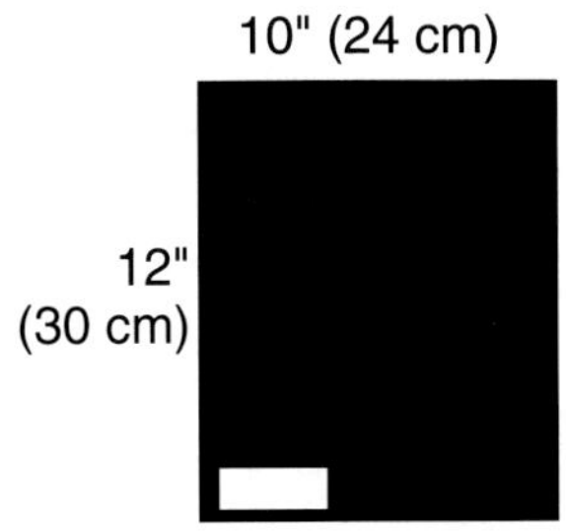

Patient Position

Supine, rolled 45° toward affected hip. Align sagittal plane of affected hip to midline of table (Fig 10.127).

Part Position

Bend affected knee as much as possible, place plantar surface of foot on table. Abduct affected thigh about 40° from vertical to place femoral neck parallel with cassette. Plantar surface touching medial lower leg of unaffected hip.

Central Ray

Perpendicular to femoral neck. Center midpoint of cassette to central ray.

NOTE: To locate the femoral neck, bisect an imaginary line drawn between the ASIS and the symphysis pubis, then move down 2½ inches (6 cm).

Breathing Instructions

Respiration is suspended at end of exhalation.

Structures Demonstrated

Lateral projection of hip joint including proximal femur (Fig. 10.128).

Evaluation Criteria

1. Hip joint, including the proximal femur, should be demonstrated.
2. Greater trochanter should be slightly superimposed by neck of femur.

NOTE: This projection should not be used on a patient with a recent, new, or suspected hip fracture or dislocation.

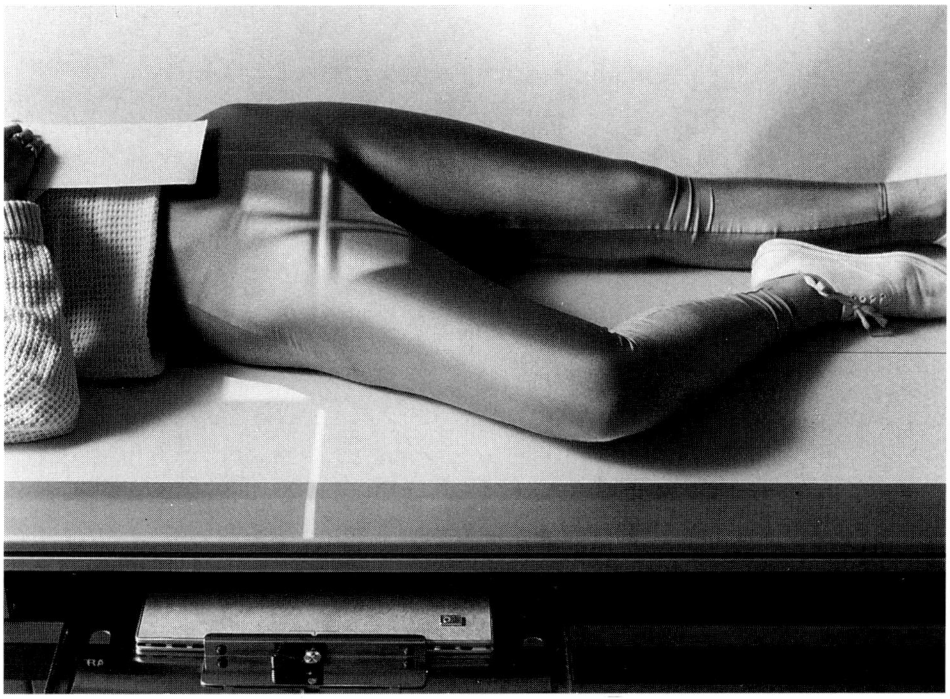

Figure 10.127. Unilateral frog-leg.

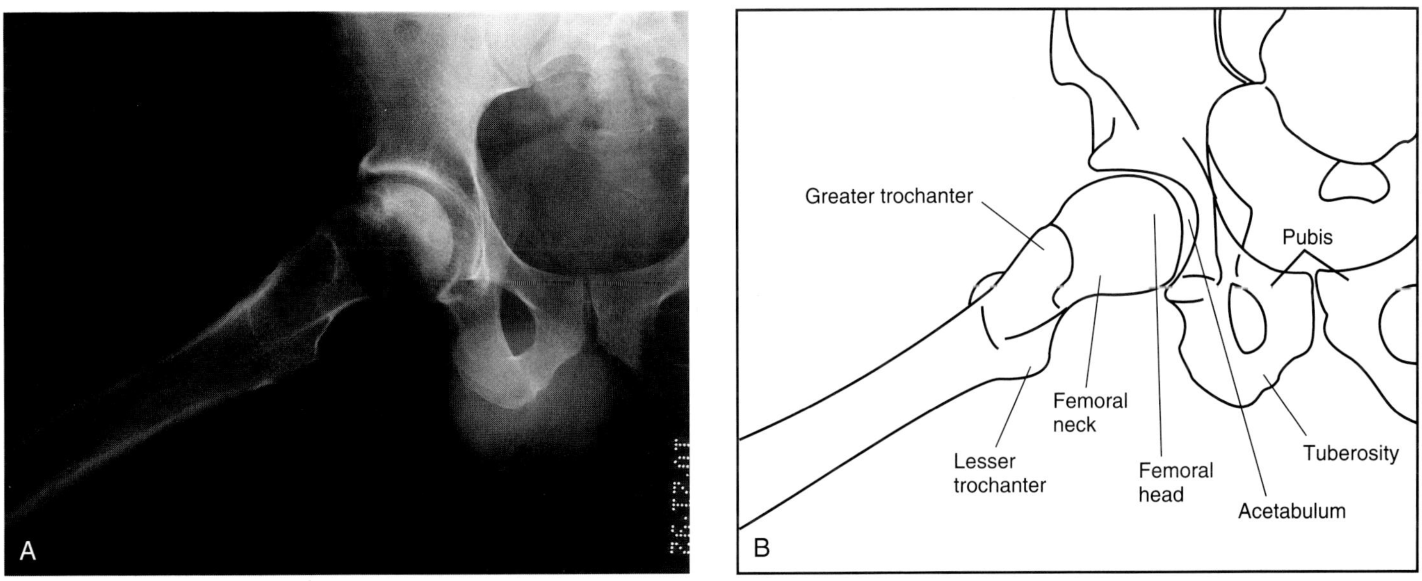

Figure 10.128. A and B, Unilateral frog-leg.

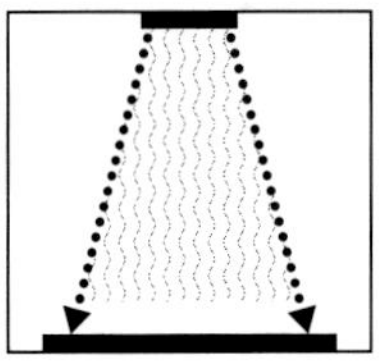

Unilateral Hip

Position/Projection

Danielus-Miller modification of Lorenz' method

Film Size:
10 × 12 inches (24 × 30 cm) lengthwise (grid or grid holder)

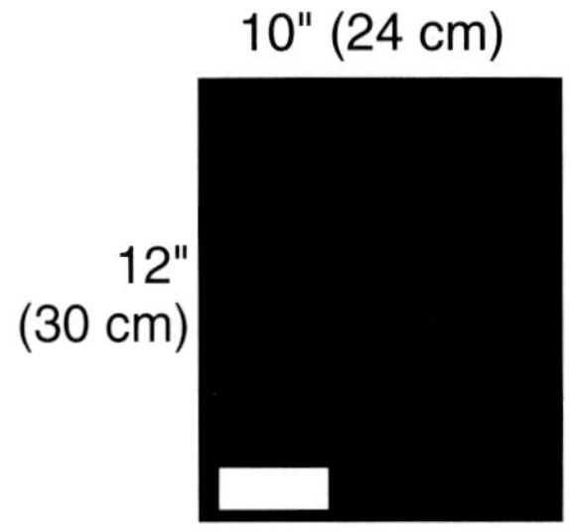

Patient Position

Supine, on table or stretcher (Fig. 10.129).

Film Position

Place upper cassette border just above level of crest of ilium of affected hip. Nameplate blocker of cassette should be placed distally. Angle lower border of cassette away from affected hip to place cassette parallel with long axis of femoral neck.

Part Position

Flex knee of unaffected hip. Raise and rest unaffected leg on suitable support so that leg will not interfere with central ray projection. Evaluation of pelvis by gluteal region and pelvic and lumbar curves is usually sufficient to allow femoral necks to be centered to midpoint of cassette. To localize long axis of femoral neck, bisect imaginary line between ASIS on affected side and upper border of symphysis pubis. Neck will be parallel to a line connecting this point to palpated lateral margin of greater trochanter of affected femur.

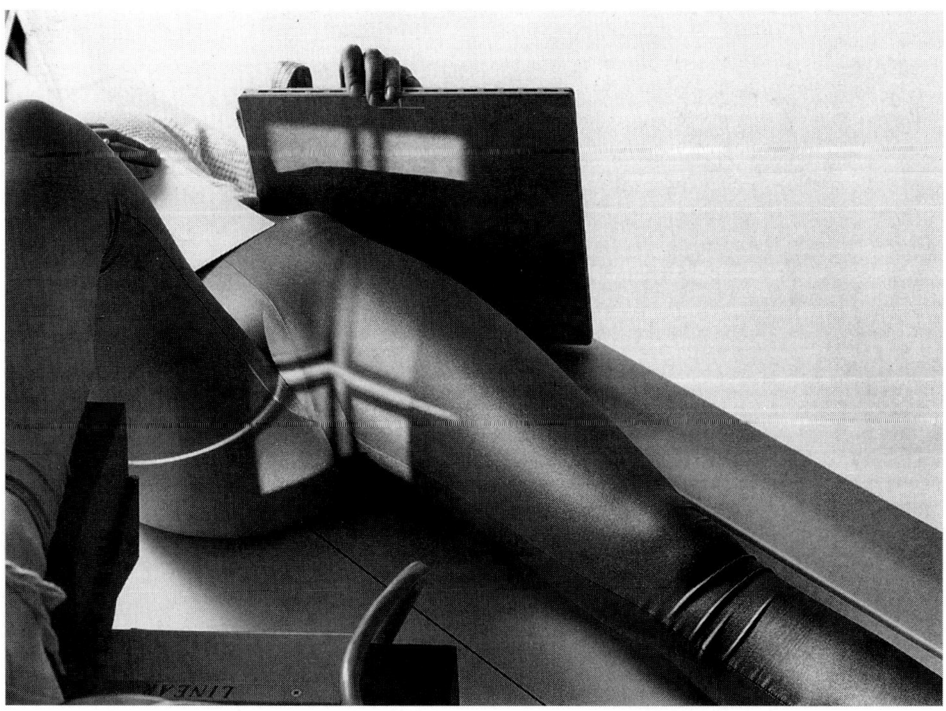

Figure 10.129. Danielus-Miller method.

Central Ray

Horizontal at right angle to long axis of femoral neck.

Breathing Instructions

Respiration is suspended at end of exhalation.

Structures Demonstrated

Axiolateral projection of head, neck, and trochanter of femur (Fig. 10.130).

Evaluation Criteria

Hip joint should be in center of radiograph with greater trochanter slightly superimposed by neck of femur.

NOTE: The affected leg should be rotated internally 15° to 20° if patient's condition permits.

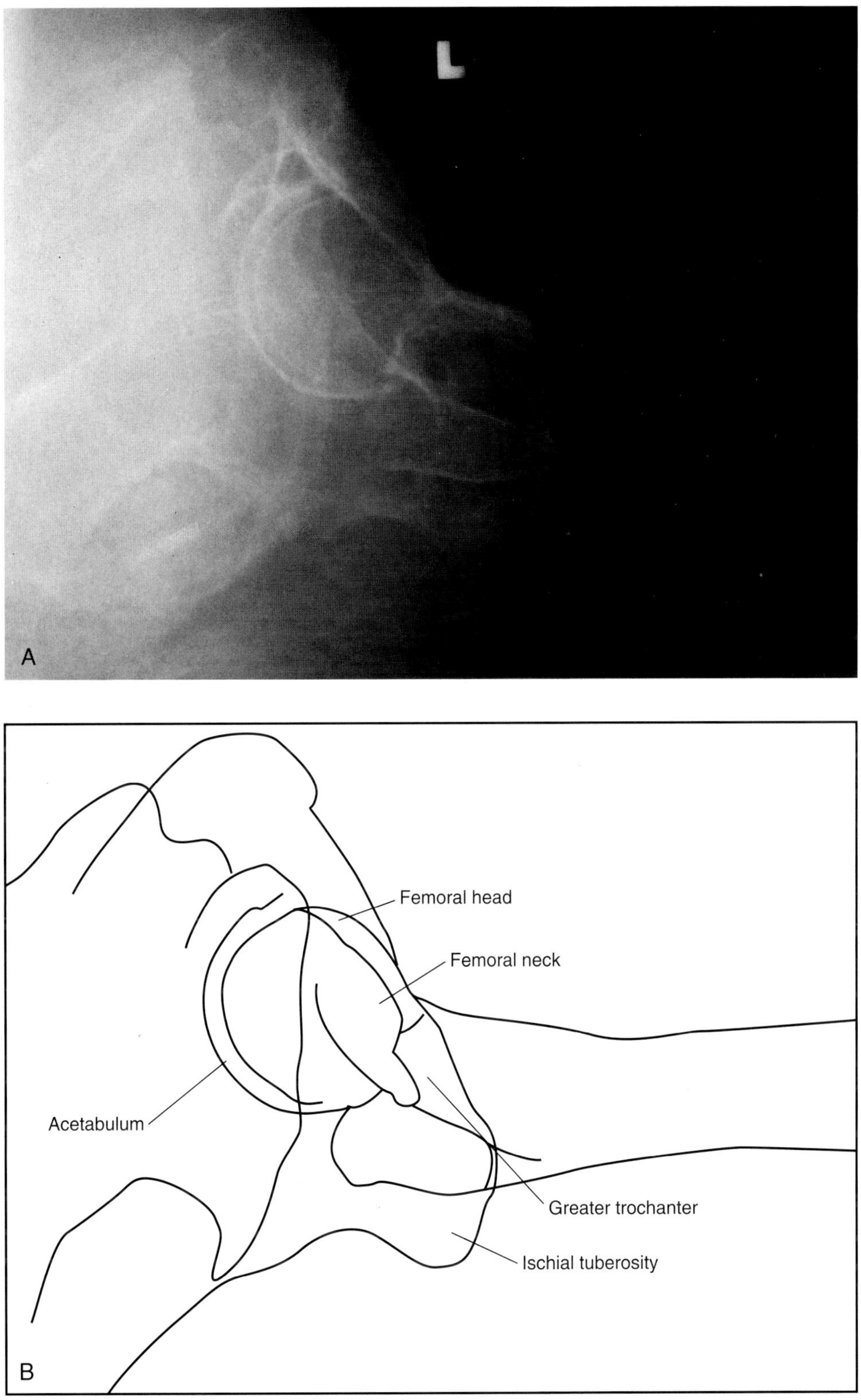

Figure 10.130. A and B, Axiolateral hip.

Acetabulum

Position/Projection

PA oblique projection—Teufel's method

Film Size:
8 × 10 inches (20 × 24 cm)
lengthwise Bucky

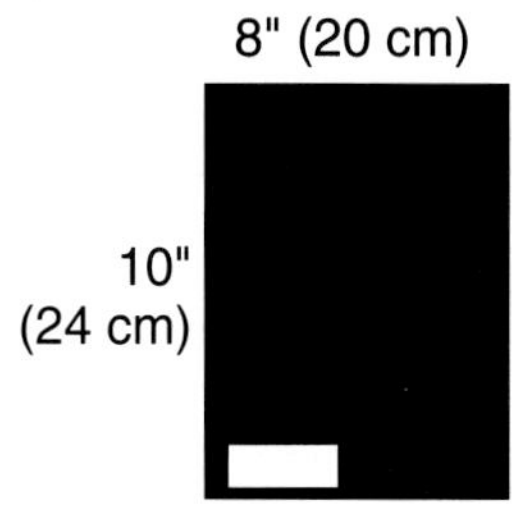

Patient Position

Prone (Fig. 10.131).

Part Position

Place affected acetabulum in midline of table (acetabulum is 2 inches [5 cm] lateral from midsagittal plane, toward affected side, at level of greater trochanter). Evaluate unaffected side 38°.

Central Ray

12° cephalic angle to exit at level of affected acetabulum. Center midpoint of cassette to central ray.

Breathing Instructions

Respiration suspended after full exhalation.

Structures Demonstrated

Acetabulum (Fig. 10.132).

Evaluation Criteria

1. Acetabulum should be in center of film.
2. Head and neck of femur should be seen.

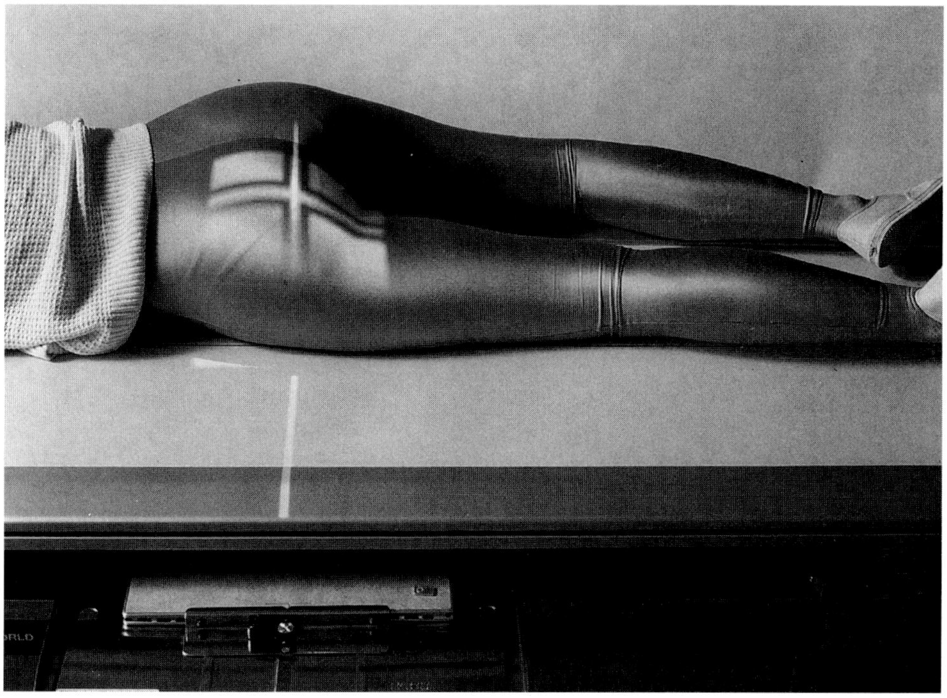

Figure 10.131. PA oblique acetabulum.

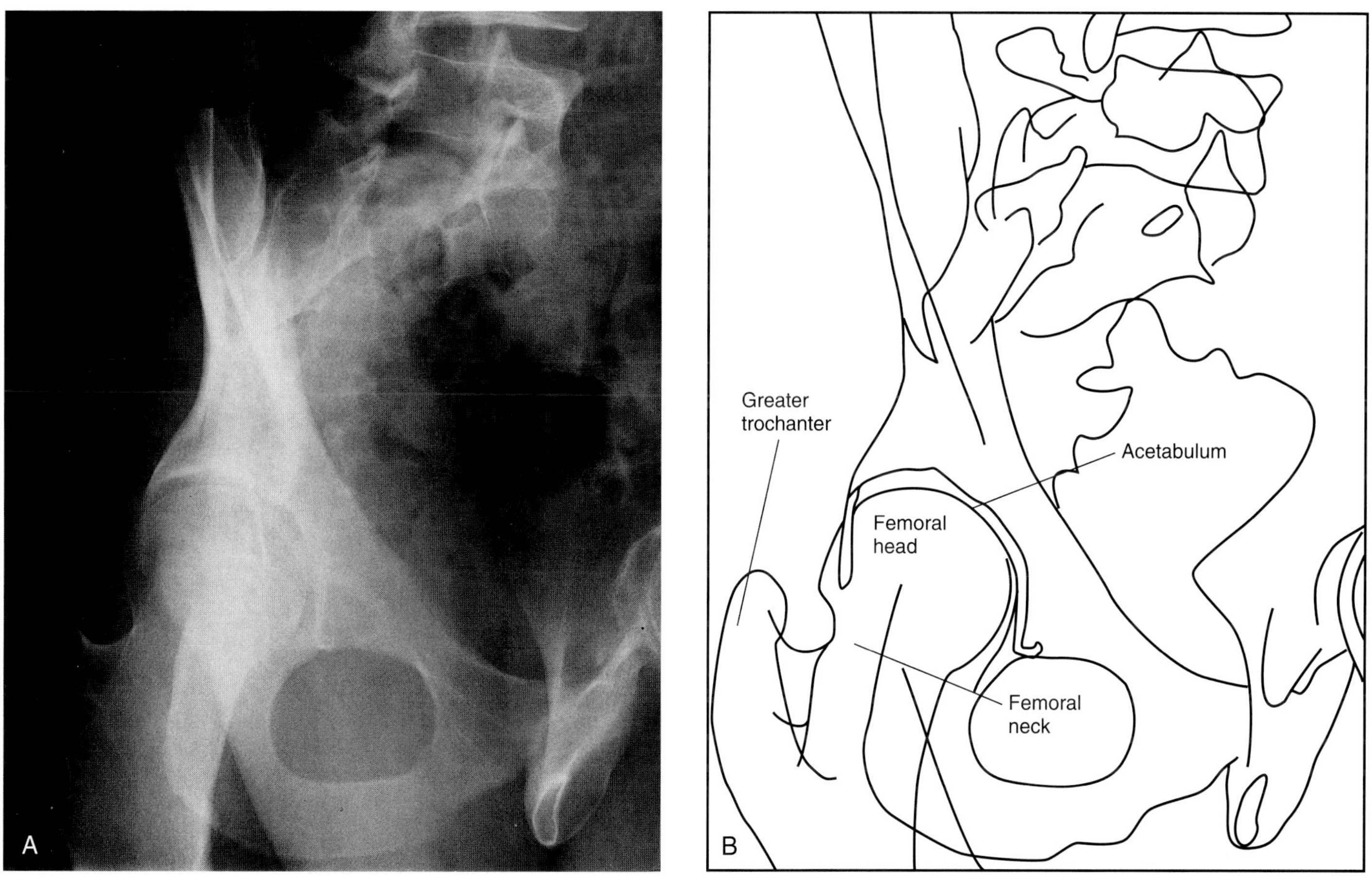

Figure 10.132. A and B, PA oblique.

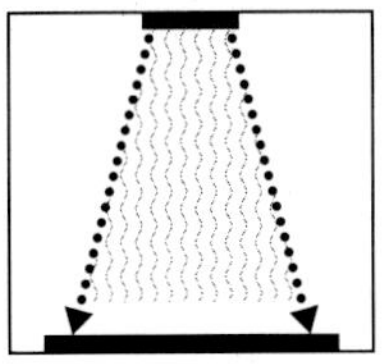

Anterior Pelvic Bones

Position/Projection

PA projection

Film Size:
8 × 10 inches (20 × 24 cm)
crosswise

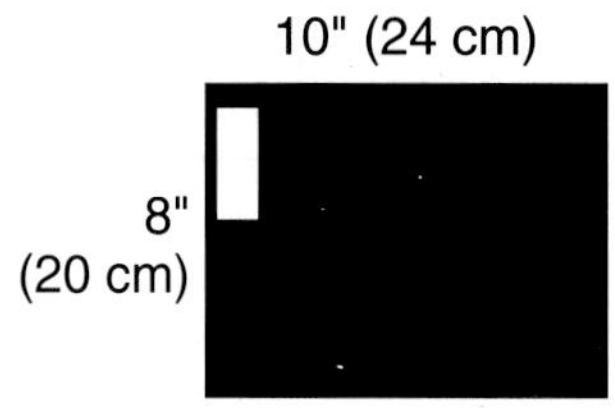

Patient Position

Prone with legs extended (Fig. 10.133).

Part Position

Align midsagittal plane of body to midline of table. Be sure pelvis is not rotated.

Central Ray

Perpendicular to level of greater trochanters (same level as symphysis pubis). Center midpoint of cassette to central ray.

Breathing Instructions

Suspend respiration after full exhalation.

Structures Demonstrated

Symphysis pubis, obturator foramina, ischial and pubic rami (Fig. 10.134).

Evaluation Criteria

1. No rotation of pelvis should be seen.
2. Symphysis pubis should be open.
3. Obturator foramina should appear oval or egg-shaped and be equal in size and shape.
4. Ischial and pubic rami should be in center of film.

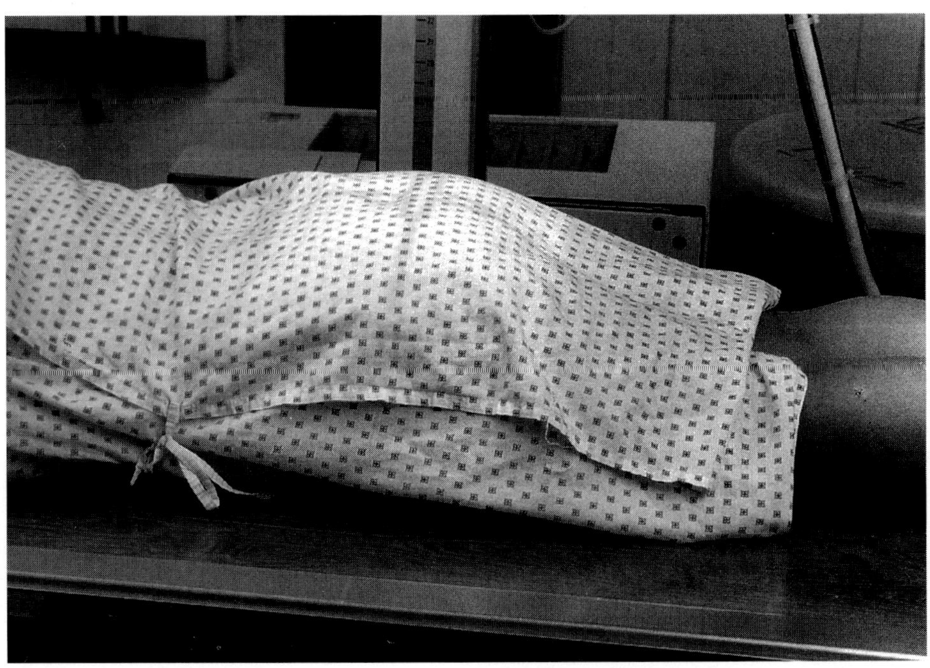

Figure 10.133. PA anterior pelvic bones.

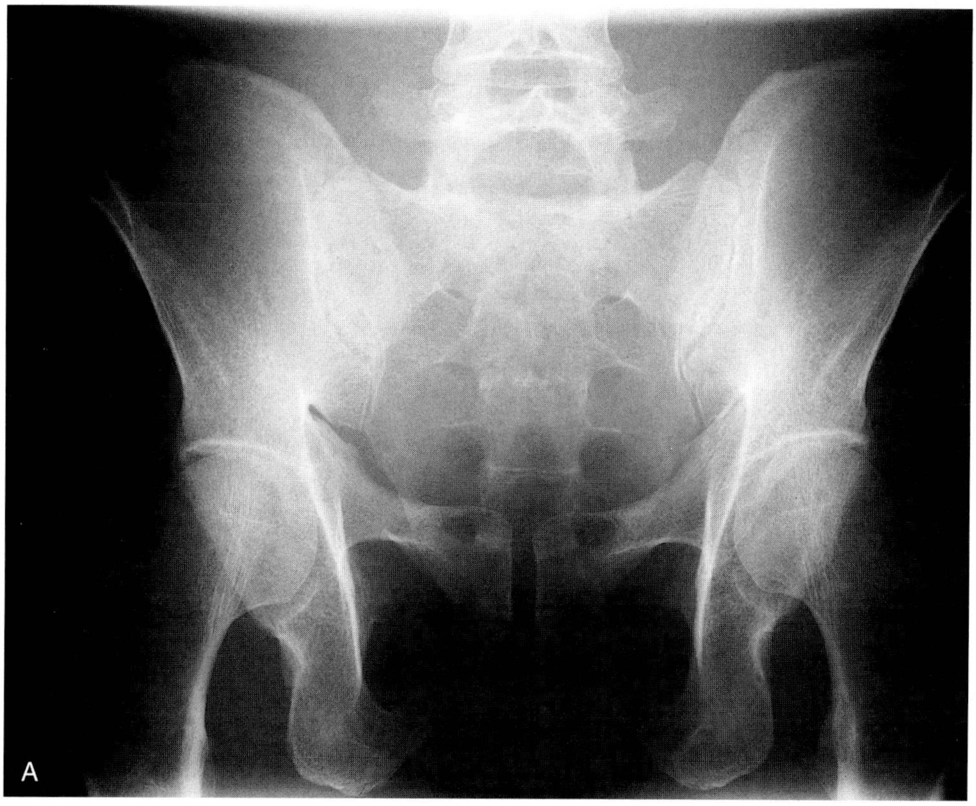

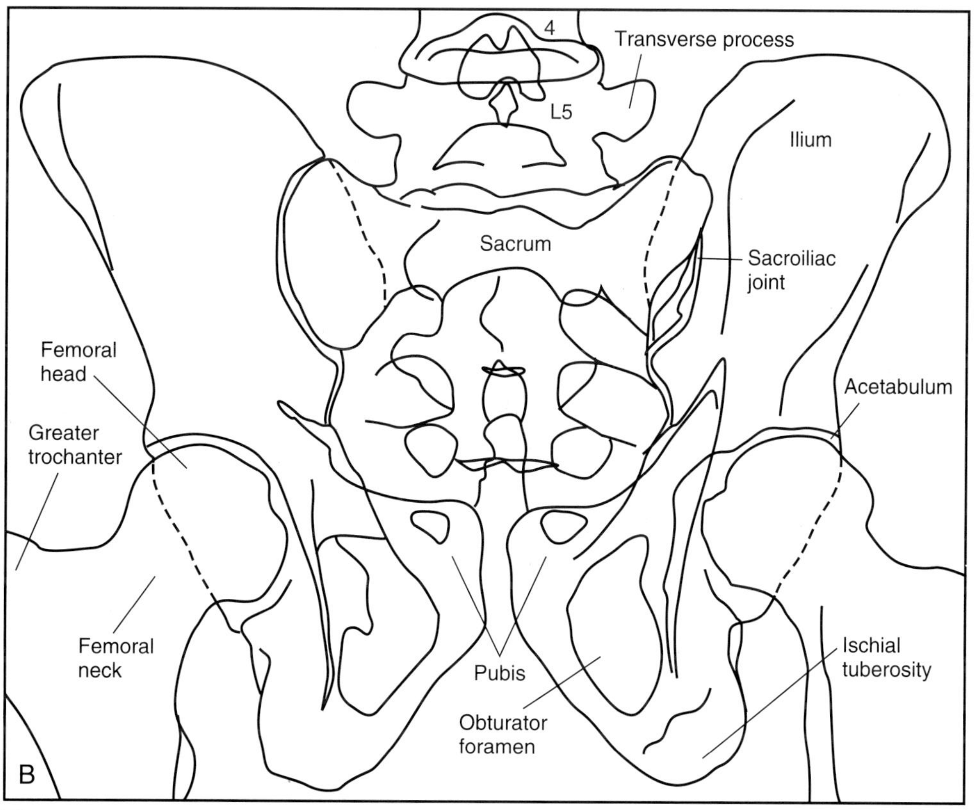

Figure 10.134. A and B, PA pelvic bones.

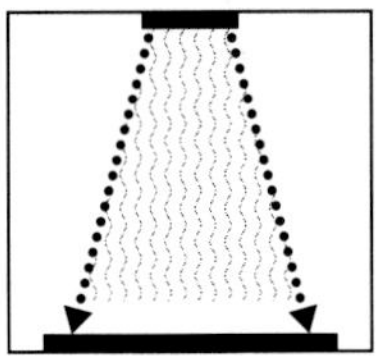

Anterior Pelvic Bones

Position/Projection

AP axial projection—Taylor's method

Film Size:
10 × 12 inches (24 × 30 cm) crosswise Bucky

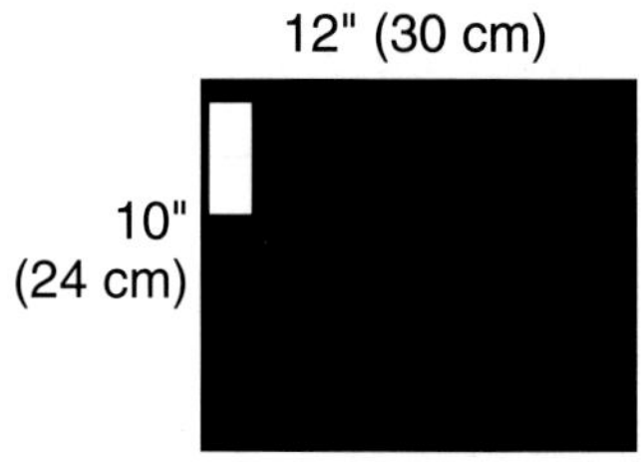

Patient Position

Supine with legs extended (Fig. 10.135).

Part Position

Align midsagittal plane of body to midline of table. Be sure pelvis is not rotated.

Central Ray

Center midpoint of cassette to central ray.

Female Pelvis
40° cephalic angle to enter 2 inches (5 cm) inferior to symphysis pubis.

Male Pelvis
25° cephalic angle to enter 2 inches (5 cm) inferior to symphysis pubis.

Breathing Instructions

Suspend respiration at end of full exhalation.

Structures Demonstrated

Ischial and pubic rami (Fig. 10.136).

Evaluation Criteria

1. No rotation of pelvis should be seen.
2. Ischial and pubic rami should be in center of film.
3. Obturator foramina should appear equally distorted.
4. Sacrum will be superimposed by part of pubic rami.

NOTE: The female pelvis is broader and shallower than the male pelvis, so more angulation is needed.

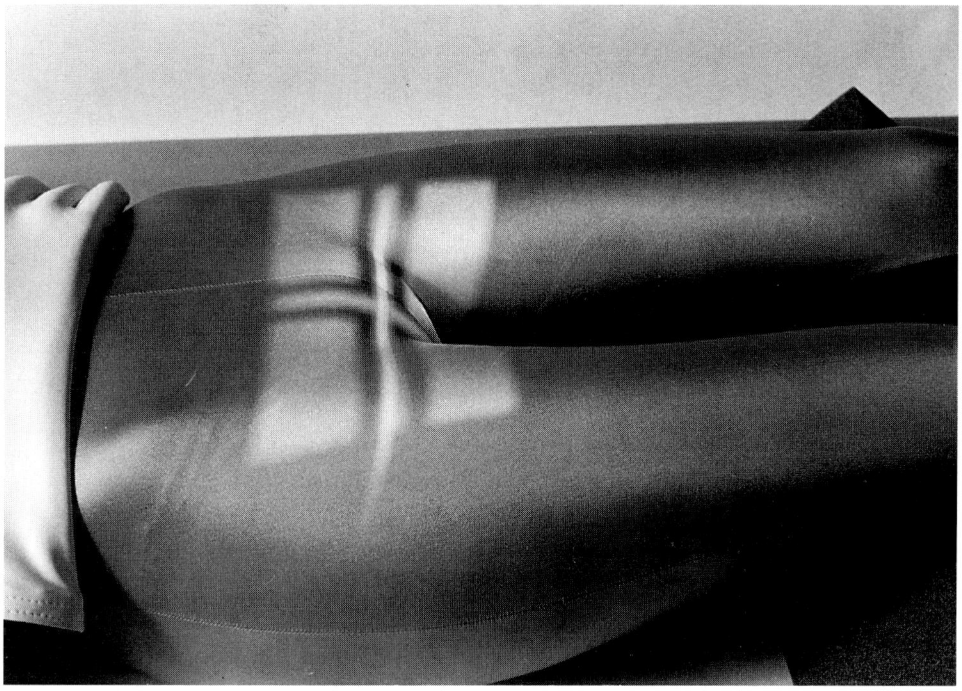

Figure 10.135. AP axial pelvic bones (Taylor's method).

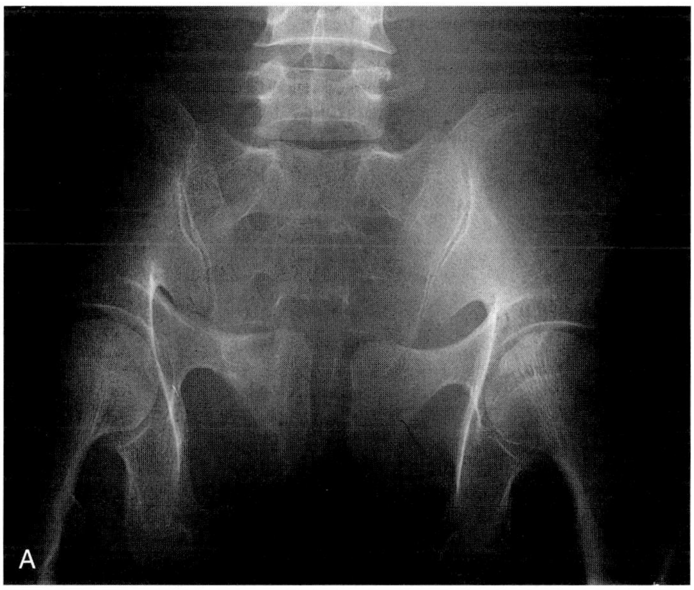

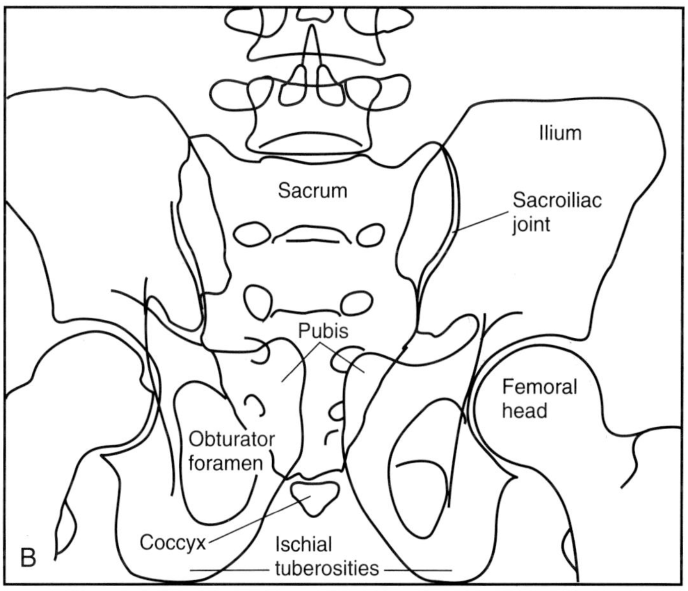

Figure 10.136. A and B, AP axial pelvic bones.

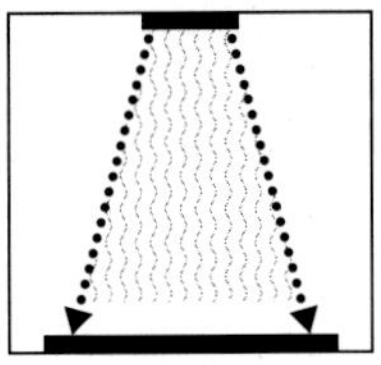

Ilium

Position/Projection

AP oblique projection

Film Size:
10 × 12 inches (24 × 30 cm) lengthwise Bucky

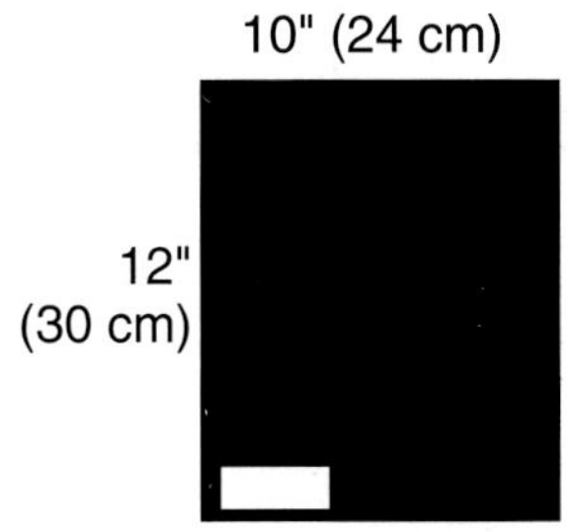

Patient Position
Supine with legs extended (Fig. 10.137).

Part Position
Elevate unaffected side 40°. Place affected ilium in midline of table (2 inches) [5 cm] medial to ASIS).

Central Ray
Perpendicular to midportion of affected ilium (level of ASIS, 2 inches [5 cm] medial to ASIS). Center midpoint of cassette to central ray.

Breathing Instructions
Respiration is suspended after full exhalation.

Structures Demonstrated
Iliac wing (Fig. 10.138).

Evaluation Criteria
Entire ilium and hip joint should be seen.

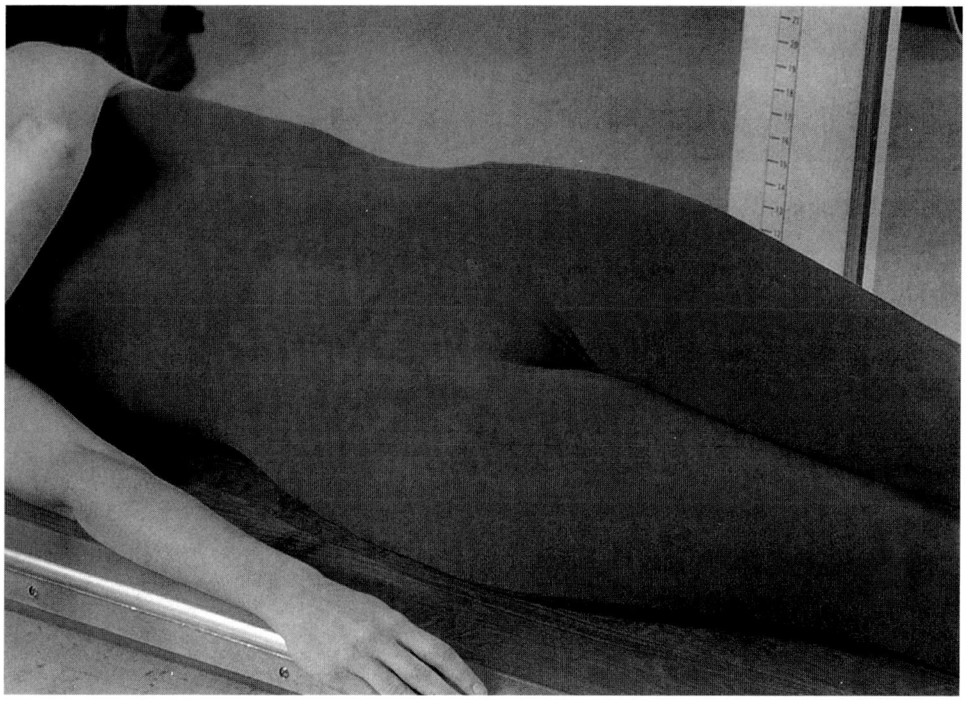

Figure 10.137. AP oblique ilium.

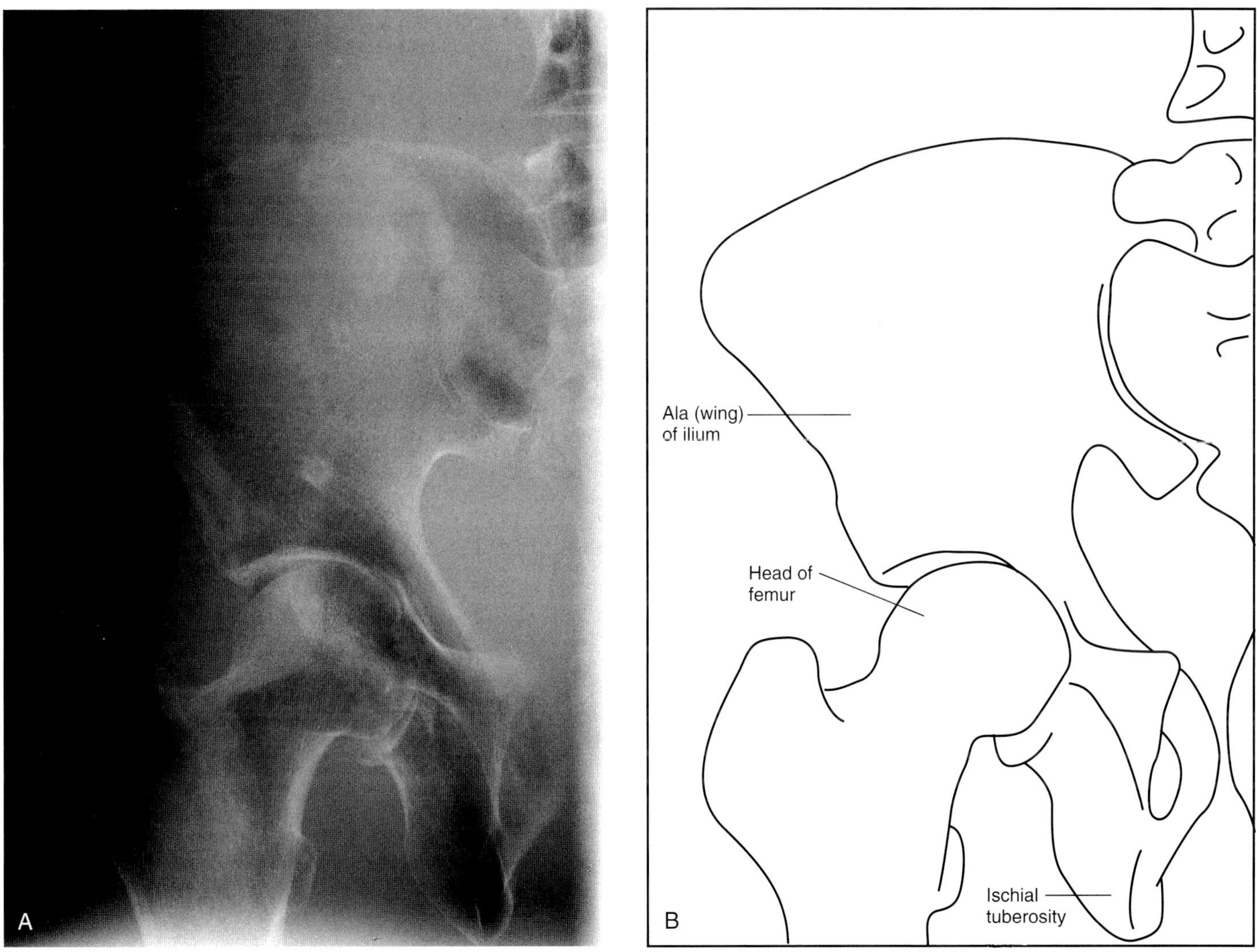

Figure 10.138. A and B, AP oblique ilium.

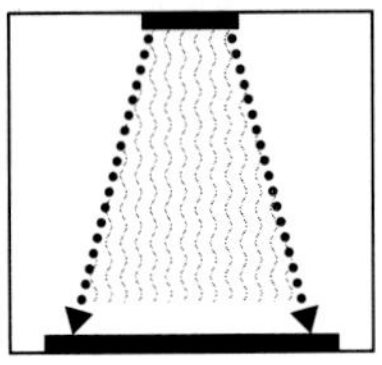

Ilium

Position/Projection

PA oblique projection

Film Size:
10 × 12 inches
(24 × 30 cm) lengthwise
Bucky

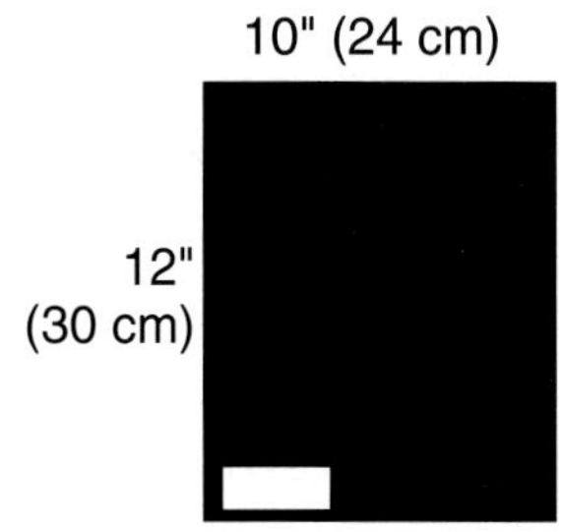

Patient Position

Prone with leg extended (Fig. 10.139).

Part Position

Elevate unaffected side 40°. Place affected ilium in midline of table (2 inches [5 cm] medial to ASIS).

Central Ray

Perpendicular to midportion of affected ilium (level of ASIS, 2 inches [5 cm] medial to ASIS). Center midpoint of cassette to central ray.

Breathing Instructions

Respiration is suspended after full exhalation.

Structures Demonstrated

Iliac wing (Fig. 10.140).

Evaluation Criteria

1. Ilium in profile should be seen.
2. Hip joint should be seen.

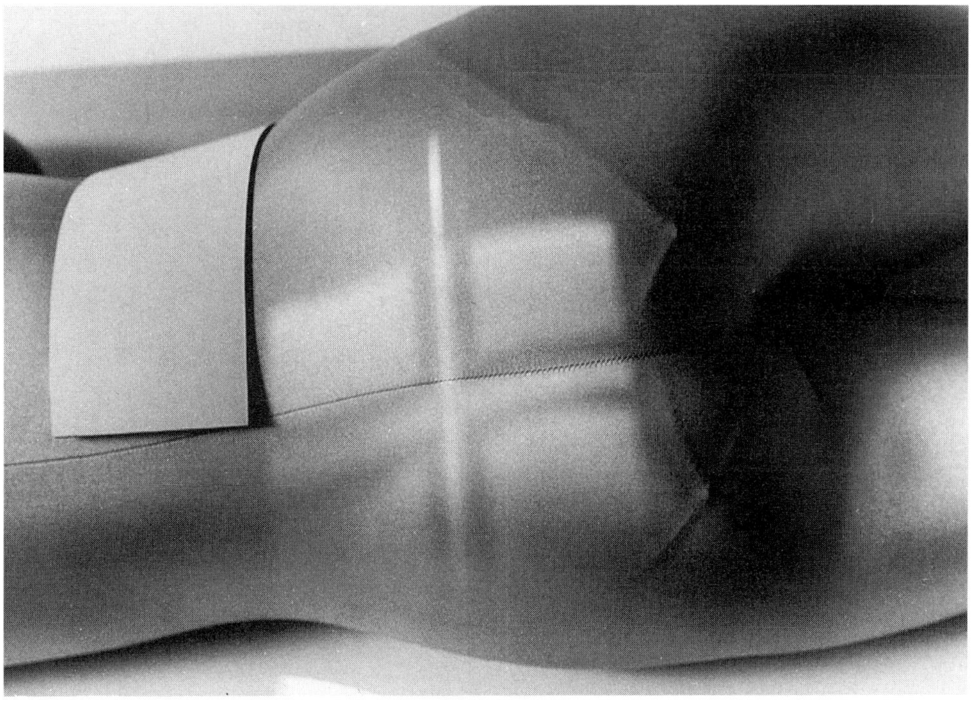

Figure 10.139. PA oblique ilium.

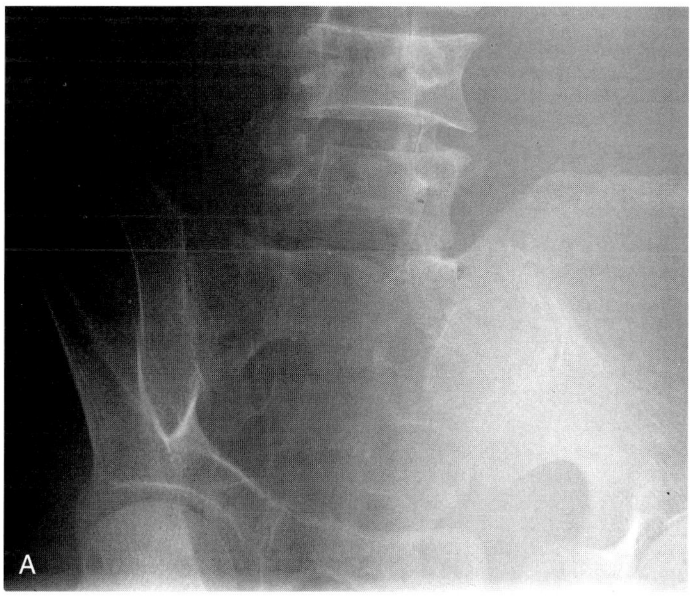

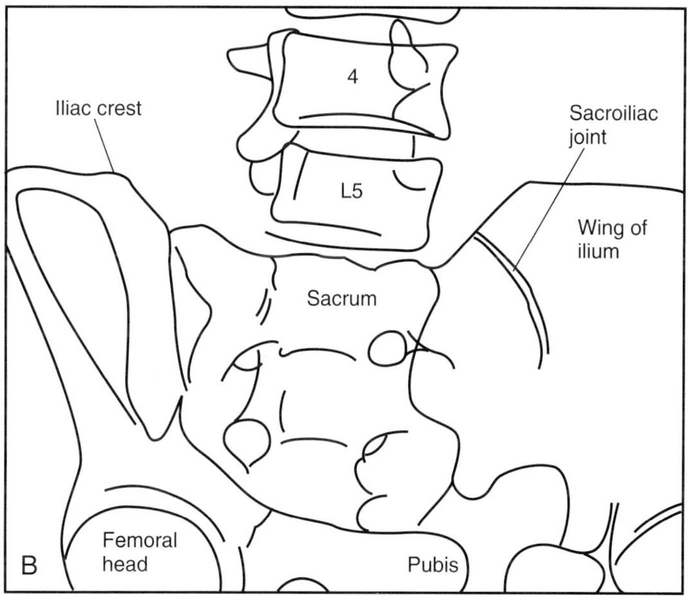

Figure 10.140. A and B, PA oblique ilium.

Bibliography

Ballinger PW: Radiographic Positions and Radiologic Procedures. 7th ed. St. Louis: Mosby–Year Book, 1991.

Bontrager KL: Radiographic Positioning and Related Anatomy. 3rd ed. St. Louis: Mosby–Year Book, 1993.

Eisenberg RL, Dennis CA, May CR: Radiographic Positioning. Boston: Little, Brown, 1989.

Fodor J, Malott JC: Magnification radiography. Radiol Technol 1987; 58:313.

Meschan I, Farrer-Meschan RM: Normal Radiographic Anatomy. 2nd ed. Philadelphia: WB Saunders, 1965.

Tortora GJ, Anagnostakos NP: Principles of Anatomy and Physiology. 4th ed. New York: Harper & Row, 1984.

Watkins GL, Moore TF: Atypical Orthopedic Radiographic Procedures. St. Louis: Mosby–Year Book, 1993.

CHAPTER 11

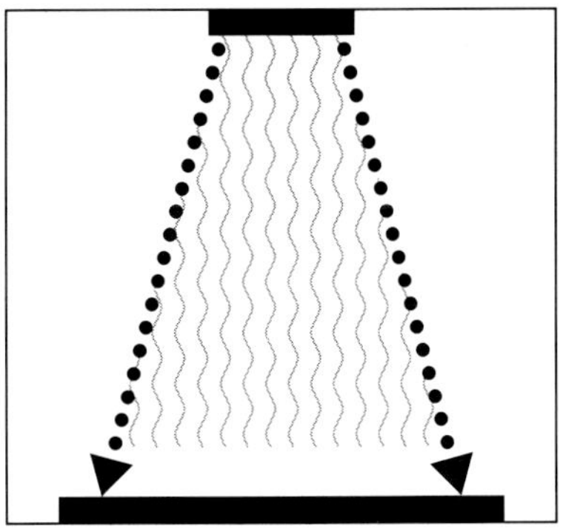

Chest and Bony Thorax

Steven B. Dowd, Ed.D., R.T.(R.)

This chapter discusses the anatomy, positioning, and radiographic film evaluation of the chest and bony thorax. The first part reviews basic anatomy of the sternum, ribs and costal joints, and thoracic viscera and lungs. The second part describes the positioning and film evaluation of positions of the chest and bony thorax. The primary underlying assumption of this entire text is that the radiographer is a professional with total control over positioning. Thus, this chapter teaches the radiographer about common procedures of the thoracic cage. It is the responsibility of the radiographer to learn the means by which these common procedures can be adapted to difficult patients.

Another underlying assumption of this text is that positioning is one means to an end; that is, it is one part of an imaging process that holistically includes positioning, patient care, technique selection, radiation protection, and initial assessment of the film by the radiographer culminating in a diagnostic film. As Cooper and Sargent note regarding the chest radiograph:

> Because a radiograph is a two-dimensional representation of a three-dimensional object, an incorrectly positioned patient creates a confusing array of overlapping structures on the resultant radiograph that often precludes accurate diagnosis.

Thus, this chapter emphasizes the role of radiographer as both film producer and *initial evaluator* of the film. The radiographer must be able to ascertain when an "abnormal" film is abnormal owing to pathology or to image production factors, for example, regardless of the fact that the radiographer is not the individual providing a specific diagnosis—the domain of the radiologist. In recent years, the nursing profession has sought to determine its role in providing nursing assessment and how this both relates to and differs from medical diagnosis, including, for example, nursing assessment from radiographs. The similarity between the production of radiographic film and the evaluation of films performed by radiologists lies in the fact that the radiographer must understand the needs of the radiologist in terms of a diagnostic film.

ANATOMY

General Anatomy

The chest consists of the respiratory system and the heart and major vessels. The four major sections of respiratory system relevant to chest radiography are (1) the larynx or voice box; (2) the trachea; (3) the right and left bronchi; and (4) the lungs (Fig. 11.1).

The heart and major vessels are contained in a section of the thoracic cavity between the lungs known as the mediastinum. The trachea, the thymus, and the esophagus are also part of the mediastinum (Fig. 11.2).

The bony thorax provides the framework and protection for the thoracic cavity (Fig. 11.3). The sternum is the anterior portion of the thorax. Twelve pairs of ribs circle the bony thorax forming a cagelike structure.

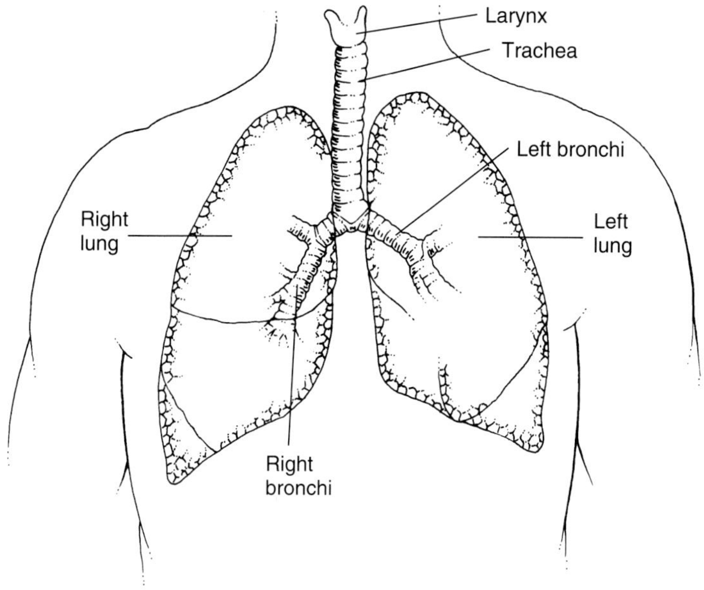

Figure 11.1. Larynx, trachea, bronchi, and lungs.

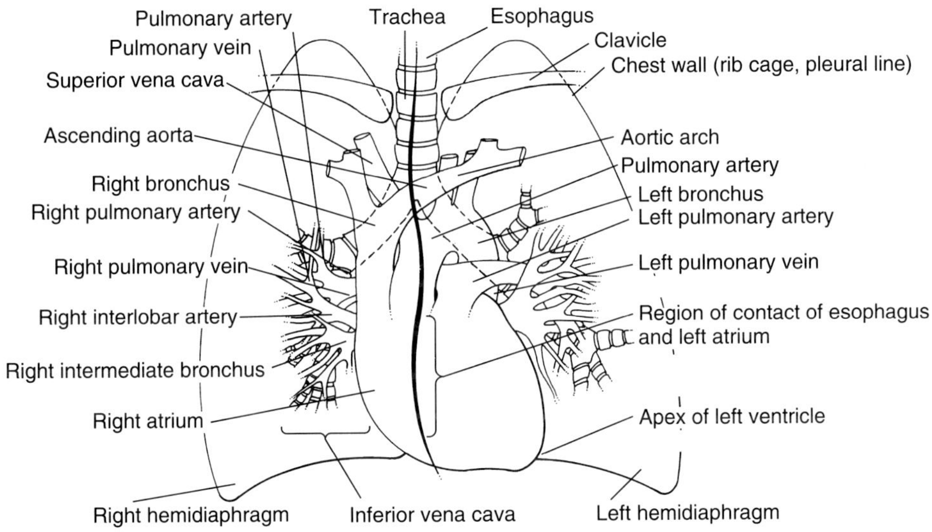

Figure 11.2. Mediastinum.

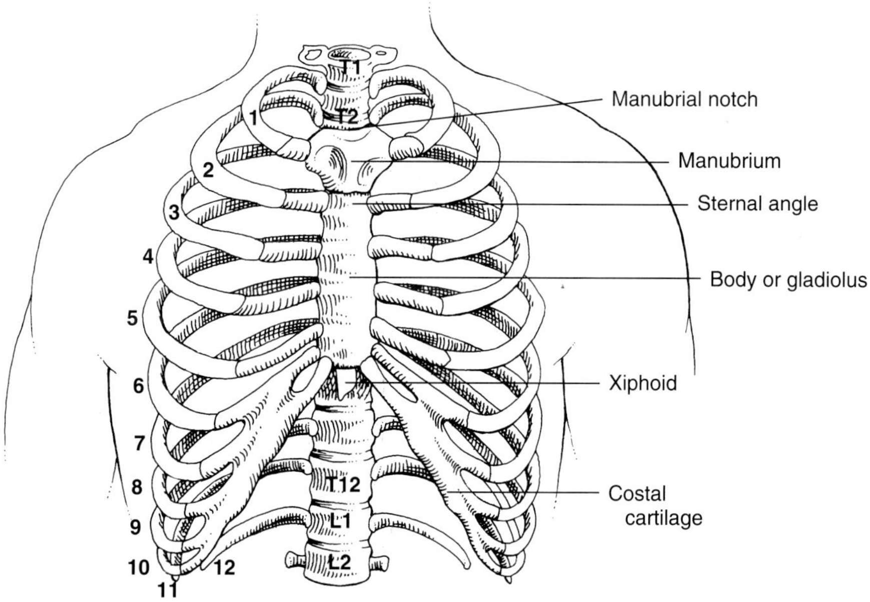

Figure 11.3. Thoracic cavity.

Sternum

The sternum (Fig. 11.4), also known as the breast bone, is a thin, narrow, flat bone divided into three sections. The upper portion is the manubrium, about 2 inches (5 cm) in length. The uppermost border of the manubrium, the suprasternal notch, is easily palpable. It is also called the manubrial notch or jugular notch. This notch is at the same level as the disk space between T2 and T3.

The joint formed by the articulation of the clavicles and the manubrium is known as the sternoclavicular joint, which forms the only bony connection between the upper extremities and the bony thorax. At the lower end of the manubrium, another palpable point, the sternal angle, is found. This angle is at the level of the disk space between T4 and T5, and forms the articulation of the manubrium with the body, or corpus. The body is the longest part of the sternum, about 4 inches (10 cm) in length. Some older texts refer to the corpus or body as the gladiolus.

The most distal and smallest portion of the sternum is the xiphoid or ensiform process. It varies in shape and partially ossifies in later life. It normally lies over the level of T10.

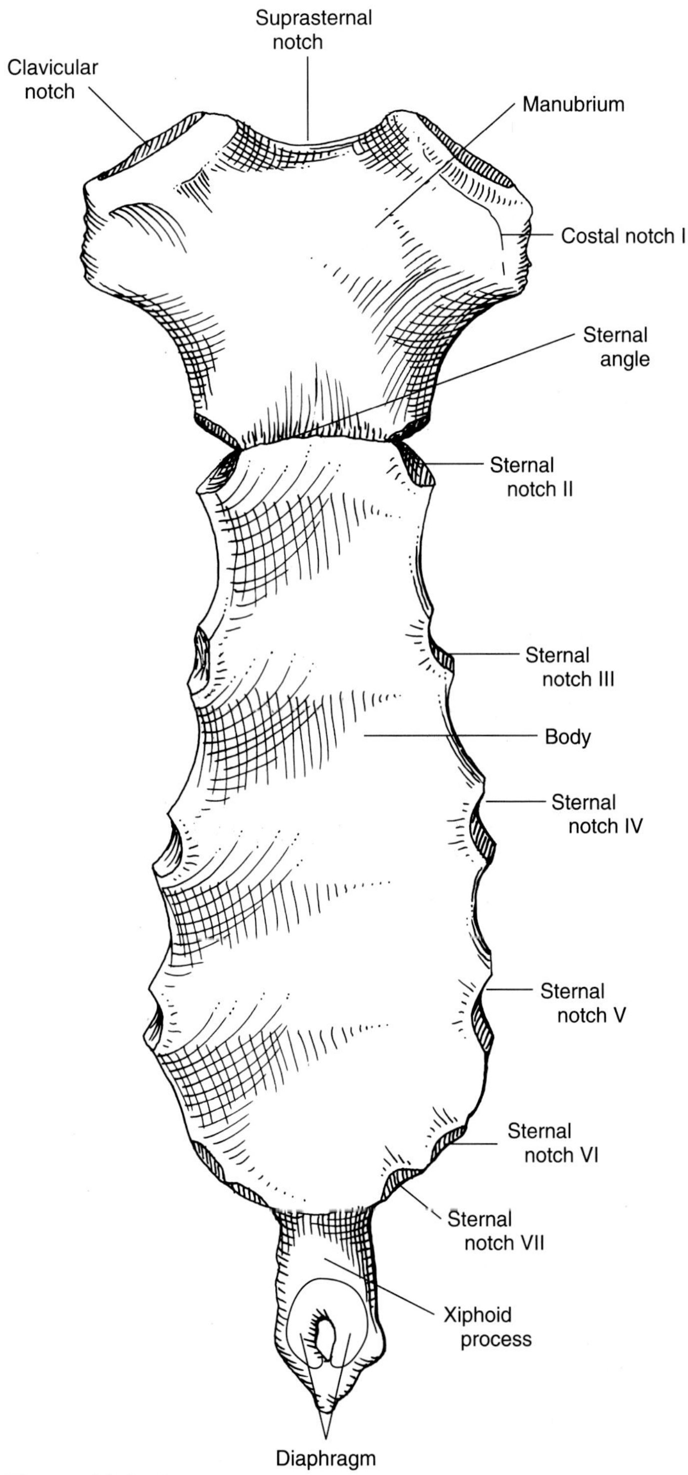

Figure 11.4. Sternum.

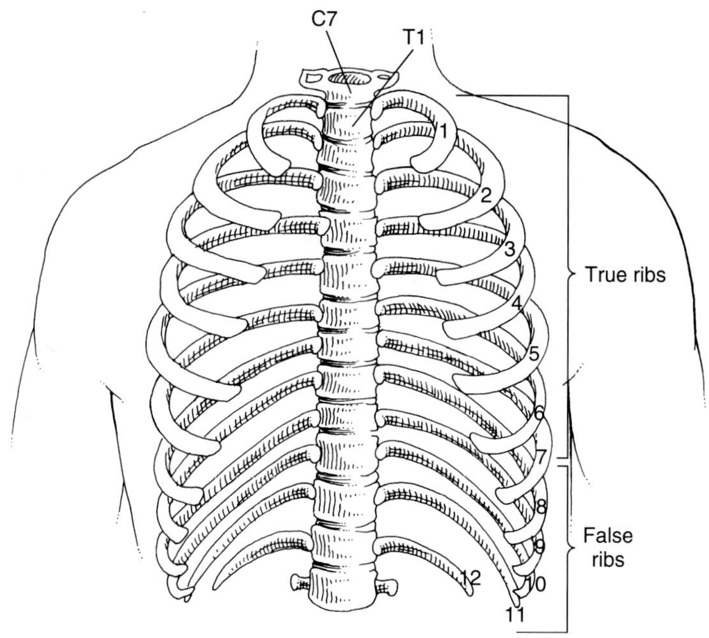

Figure 11.5. Ribs, including floating ribs.

Ribs and Costal Joints

Ribs are numbered from the top down correlating with the thoracic vertebra with which each rib attaches. The first 7 pairs of ribs are called true ribs, as they attach directly to the sternum by their own costocartilage. The first ribs are short and broad as well as the most vertical. Ribs lengthen until the 7th rib. From this point on, they shorten. The widest point of the bony thorax is at the lateral margin of the 8th or 9th rib.

The last five pairs of ribs (8 to 12) are called false ribs. Ribs 8, 9, and 10 have costocartilage, but connect to the costocartilage of the 7th rib. The last two ribs (11, 12) are called floating ribs, as they do not have costocartilage (Fig. 11.5).

Figure 11.6 shows a central rib as an example. Ribs have two ends: an anterior or sternal end and a posterior or vertebral end, consisting of a head and neck. Laterally from the neck is a tubercula that is slightly elevated, articulates with the transverse process of the vertebra, and allows for ligamentous attachment. The shaft, or body, of the ribs sits between the two ends. The angle of the ribs is its area of forward angulation. Figure 11.7 shows a posterior view of the same rib, demonstrating the costal groove, a passageway for arteries, veins, and nerves.

Thoracic Viscera

The thoracic viscera include the lungs and associated mediastinal structures: heart, thoracic aorta, pulmonary artery and veins, vena cava, thymus gland, lymph nodes, trachea, bronchi, esophagus, and thoracic duct (Fig. 11.8).

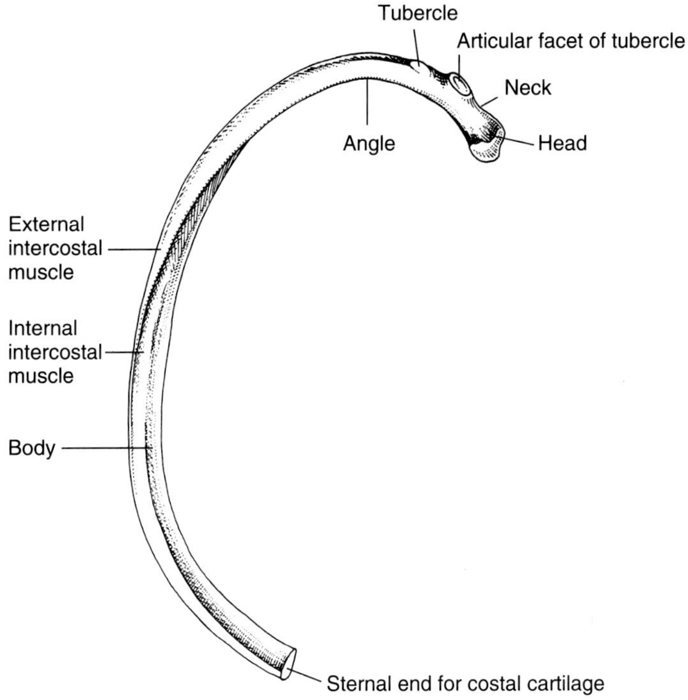

Figure 11.6. Central rib.

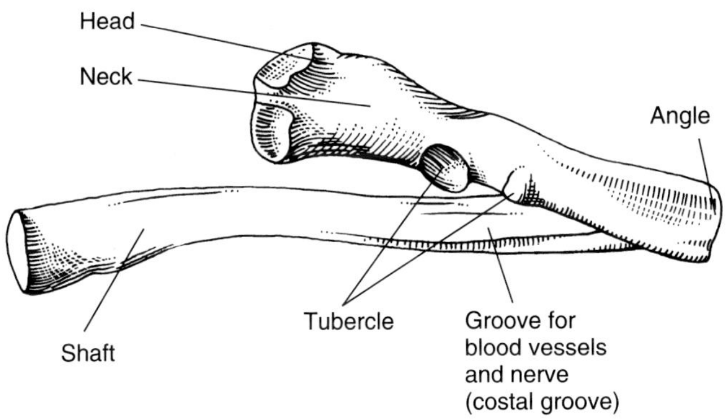

Figure 11.7. Posterior view of rib, demonstrating the costal groove.

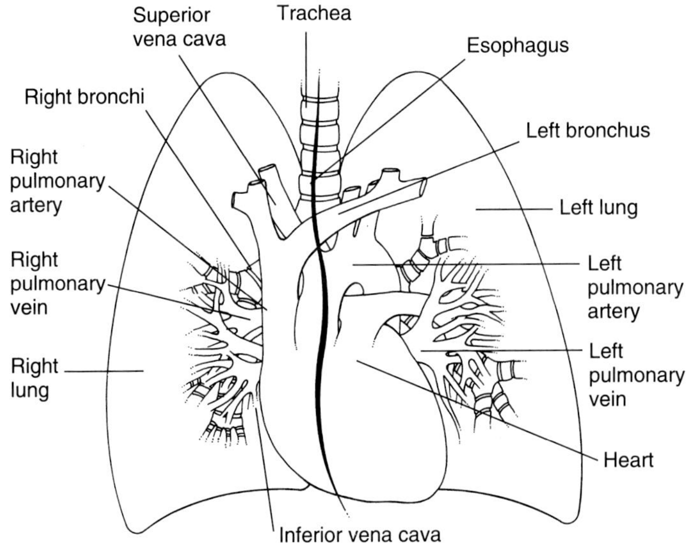

Figure 11.8. Thoracic viscera.

POSITIONING AND FILM EVALUATION

Chest

Often thought of as a "simple" examination, in actuality the chest radiograph is quite intricate and challenging to evaluate. Meschan and Ott describe the routine used by radiologists to evaluate the chest radiograph (Fig. 11.9):

1. Costophrenic sinuses.
2. Diaphragm level to include gas bubble.
3. Chest wall—axillae, pectoralis muscle, breast.
4. Neck and trachea.
5. Mediastinum, heart, major vessels, and azygos vein.
6. The three zones of the lung.

Based on Squire and Novelline's (1988) methods of teaching medical students to evaluate chest radiographs, Sanchez has developed an approach to chest film assessment for critical care nurses:

1. Compare the degrees of density.
2. Study the form of the density to compare with known anatomic structures.
3. Compare side-to-side to determine pathology. It is rare to have bilateral pathology.
4. Think three-dimensionally; look past structures such as the ribs to view the heart and lungs.
5. Always look for the abnormal last.

Cullinan has developed a similar approach for radiographers based on their role as film producer and evaluator:

1. The densities of both lung fields should be equal. If not, the cause must be ascertained—for example, pathology, unilateral grid cutoff, or artifact.
2. The scapulae must be clear of the lung fields.
3. The clavicles must be horizontal. The medial ends of the clavicles should be symmetric.
4. There should be a symmetric relationship between the sternoclavicular joints and the thoracic spine.
5. The exposure should show full inspiration.
6. Check for evidence of motion.
7. Beam collimation must be evident.
8. The radiograph must be properly identified (items 6, 7, and 8 are essential for *all* radiographs).
9. The apices and costophrenic angles are shown.
10. Is there tracheal displacement?

A chest radiograph uses technical factors (e.g., high kVp of 120 or more with a grid) that best visualize the lungs and other soft tissues. The extra penetration is useful for cases of dense opacification (breast shadows or pathology) that would obscure underlying anatomy. Automatic exposure control devices are preferred, when available, to ensure constant density, except in the case of expiration chest films, in which small pneumothoraces may be obscured.

Other technical factors in chest radiography include the use of faster-speed screens and short exposure times. This limits both voluntary and involuntary motion. The air-gap technique, described in Chapter 6, has the patient stand about 10 inches (25 cm) from the film and uses a source-to-image receptor distance (SID) of 10 feet (0.3 m) or greater to reduce the increased geometric unsharpness of the greater object-to-film distance (OFD).

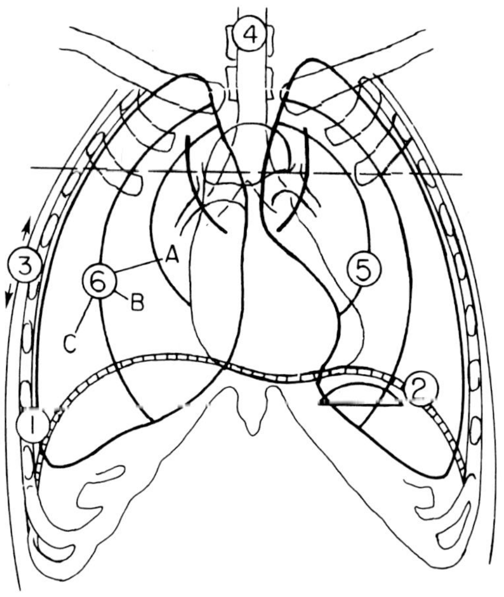

1. Costophrenic Sinuses
2. Diaphragm level (and gas bubble)
3. Chest wall (axillas, pect. mm. breast)
4. Neck and trachea
5. Mediastinum and heart and major vessels and azygos
6. 3 zones of lung

Figure 11.9. Routine for study of PA film of the chest. (From Meschan I, Ott DJ: Introduction to Diagnostic Imaging. Philadelphia: WB Saunders, 1984, p 15.)

The clavicles, scapulae, and ribs are usually well visualized; two other thoracic structures, the sternum and the thoracic vertebrae, are not. Also well visualized are the trachea and the heart, the large blood vessels, and the diaphragm. The bronchi are not usually well visualized. Table 11.1 summarizes pathological conditions in which technique must be increased (additive pathology) or decreased (destructive pathology).

Owing to variances in body habitus, three types of chest vary from the norm. Type 1 can be identified as a thick chest. This individual has a large frame (usually muscular) and is thick in build (hypersthenic; perhaps endomorphic or mesomorphic). In women, individuals of this type have a large frame and large breasts. If an automatic exposure control is not used, technical factors must be increased.

Type 2 has a thin chest. This individual has visible ribs due to a lack of surrounding tissue. When positioning the patient, the radiographer may notice that the scapulae protrude. Type 3 has a very thin chest. This individual can be identified as having a barrel-type chest. Radiography of both of these types requires a decrease in technical factors if an automatic exposure control is not used.

It is important to be able to both identify and count all 12 pairs of ribs on a PA chest radiograph. The diaphragm, on a well-aerated patient, should extend to the 10th rib, if possible. Achieving full inspiration by having the patient take in a deep breath, exhale, and then take in another deep breath minimizes the Valsalva effect, which increases intrapulmonary pressure and decreases the apparent size of the heart and proximal vessels.

Chest radiographs are taken erect at an SID of at least 72 inches (183 cm) if possible. An erect position allows the diaphragm to move further down and better shows possible air-fluid levels in the chest. The longer distance minimizes enlargement and distortion of the heart and large vessels. Compensatory filters are often used to overcome variations in tissue density.

One reason why PA projections are preferred is to limit radiation exposure to the sternum and, for female patients, the mammary glands. Another means of radiation protection is the use of mobile lead shields or waist lead rubber aprons to shield the trunk below the diaphragm.

Ribs

No single position can obtain a complete view of the ribs. Thus, oblique projections are often taken to image the axillary portion of the ribs; the AP or PA shows the shafts and sternal costal articulations. Kattan lists optimum views for the study of ribs as:

1. PA chest view.
2. Well-penetrated AP view of lower ribs.
3. Oblique views.
4. A "coned-down" view of the affected area.

A film taken on expiration is also often helpful for suspected pneumothorax.

Good (short-scale) contrast is imperative, and can be attained using a relatively low (80) kVp and *not* using the automatic exposure device (this is a preference of the author that may not correlate with recommendations of other authors*). The ribs should be seen clearly through the lungs or abdomen and have good sharpness of edges. Penetration is a key concern, as overpenetration will tend to obscure pneumothorax, yet underpenetration will result in a lack of information in the mediastinum.

Table 11.1 Chest Pathologies in which Technical Factors Must Be Increased (Additive) or Decreased (Destructive)

Additive	Destructive
Actinomycosis	Early lung abscess
Atelectasis	Emphysema
Bronchiectasis	Pneumothorax
Cardiomegaly	
Congestive heart failure	
Edema	
Empyema	
Encapsulated abscess	
Hydropneumothorax	
Malignancies	
Pleural effusion	
Pneumoconioses	
Pneumonia	
Syphilis	
Thoracoplasty	
Tuberculosis (miliary and advanced)	

The ribs are radiographed quite differently than the same anatomic area of the lungs. Since bone rather than soft tissue is of primary interest, long-scale contrast, such as is seen on a chest radiograph, is not of value. Also, the automatic exposure device is not used as these tend to even out and give grayer densities than manual timing with low kVp (author preference—see earlier). In many cases, the film-screen system used is slower for ribs than for chest, which translates into a higher exposure, shorter scale of contrast, less margin for exposure error, and better detail.

Sternum

In addition to being difficult to radiograph, the parts of the sternum are difficult to visualize on a radiograph. The RAO position provides an oblique view of the sternum that uses the heart shadow to obtain better density. The degree of angulation depends on the depth (width) of the chest. A deep chest, as is seen typically on an hypersthenic patient, requires less angulation than a shallow chest, as is seen typically on an asthenic patient.

The notches of the lateral borders of the body of the sternum must be visualized, and the entire sternum from the manubrium to the tip of the xiphoid must be included. A breathing technique is used with a low kVp and a long exposure time to blur out lung markings.

*Malott and Fodor (1993) attribute the lack of an automatic exposure control to provide adequate density on rib x-rays to the fact that the air-filled lungs will allow radiation to pass through easily, prematurely terminating the exposure. They recommend using a +1 setting for ribs.

Sternum

Position/Projection

Right PA oblique projection

Film Size:
10 × 12 inches (24 × 30 cm) lengthwise; top of film placed about 2 inches (5 cm) above level of sternoclavicular notch

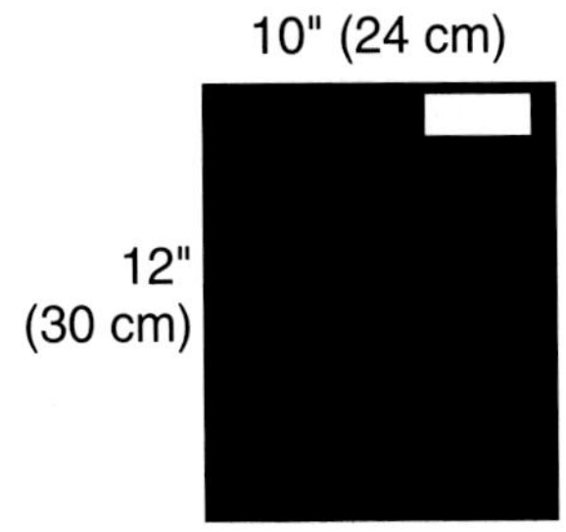

Patient Position

Semiprone in an RAO position. Obliquity is about 15–30°, depending on anterior to posterior measurement of thorax. Asthenic patient with shallow thorax will require greater obliquity than hypersthenic patient with deep thorax. Patient may use arm and knee for support (Fig. 11.10).

Part Position

Long axis of sternum is centered to film. Sternum should superimpose heart shadow. Obliquity shifts vertebral column to right of sternum.

Central Ray

Directed perpendicular to midsternum. FFD: 40 inches (102 cm).

Breathing Instructions

Breathing technique (shallow)—works best with older patients and heavy smokers to obliterate pulmonary markings.

If nonbreathing technique is used, breath is held at end of expiration.

Structures Demonstrated

PA sternum with slight obliquity (Fig. 11.11).

Evaluation Criteria

1. Entire manubrium and xiphoid tip should be visible.
2. Sternum should be free from vertebral column, in heart shadow.
3. Obliquity should be sufficient to avoid superimposition of thoracic spine and sternum, but not too much, otherwise sternum will move out of heart shadow.
4. There should be no rotation of sternum.

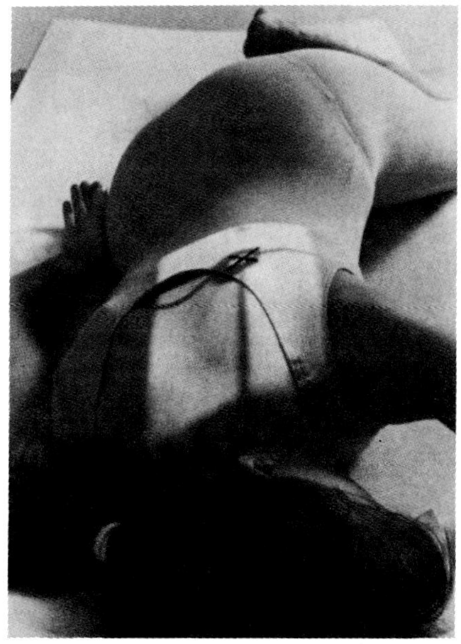

Figure 11.10. Right PA oblique (RAO) sternum. (From Hagler MJ: The Pocket Rad Tech. Philadelphia: WB Saunders, 1993, p 35.)

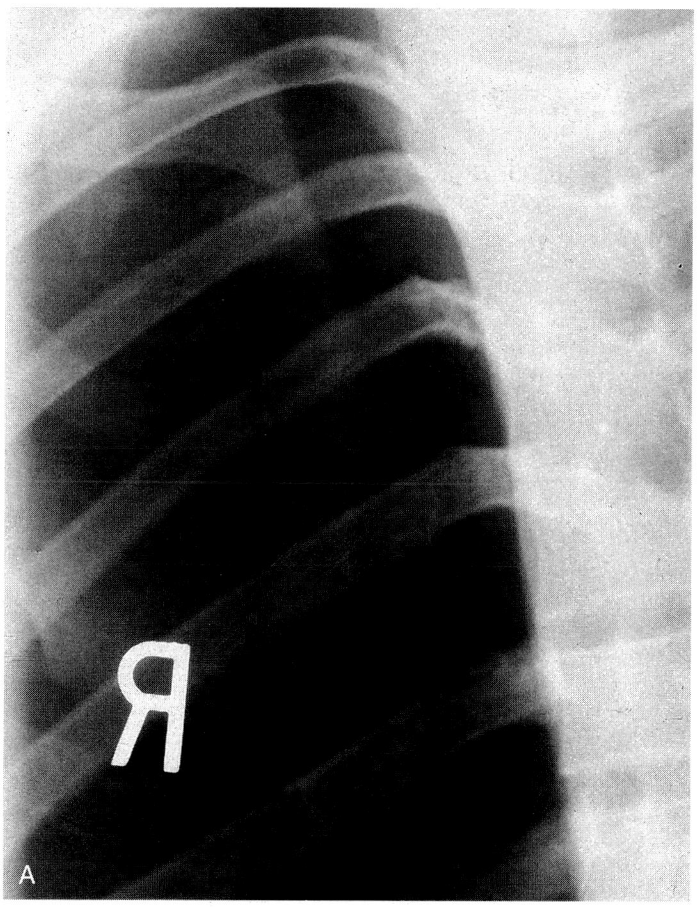

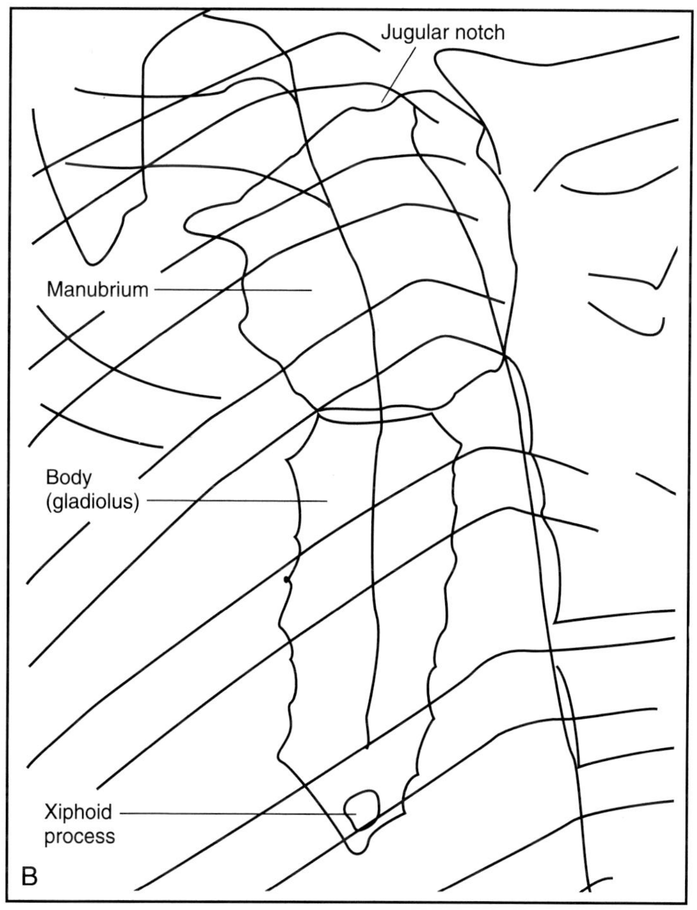

Figure 11.11. A and B, Right PA oblique sternum.

Sternum

Position/Projection

Lateral projection

Film Size:
10 × 12 inches (24 × 30 cm) lengthwise (8 × 10 inches [20 × 24 cm] for lateral sternoclavicular region)

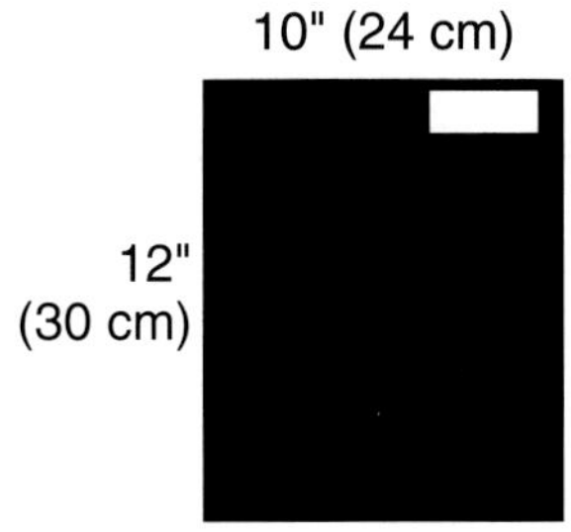

Patient Position

Lateral, upright or recumbent. Midsagittal plane vertical (Fig. 11.12).

Part Position

Upright standing or sitting. Shoulders and arms pulled back; if recumbent, ensure arms are out of way. Body and sternum should be true lateral.

Central Ray

Perpendicular to midsternum. FFD, 40 inches (102 cm). 72 inches (183 cm) may be used to reduce magnification.

Breathing Instructions

Suspend respiration at deep inhalation. This gives sharper contrast.

Structures Demonstrated

Lateral projection of sternum, sternoclavicular joints superimposed (Fig. 11.13).

Evaluation Criteria

1. Entire lateral sternum shown in uniform density.
2. Ensure that shoulder soft tissue shadows do not obscure manubrium.
3. Breast shadows may obscure lower portion of sternum. Compensating filter or second radiograph may be necessary.

NOTE: A modification of this position is the dorsal decubitus position, usually used with a multiple trauma patient.

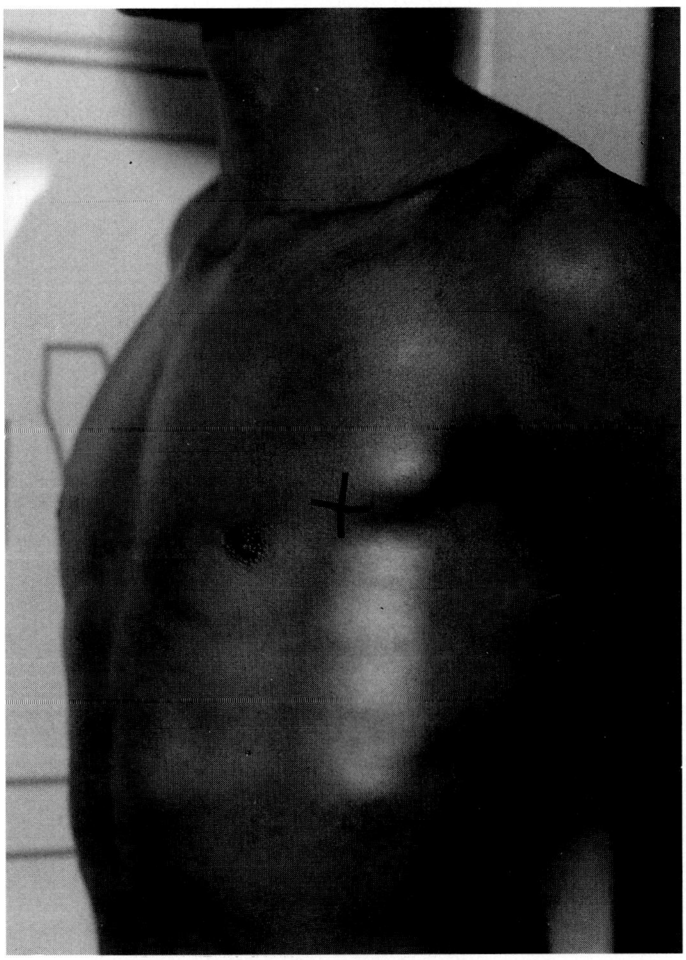

Figure 11.12. Lateral sternum.

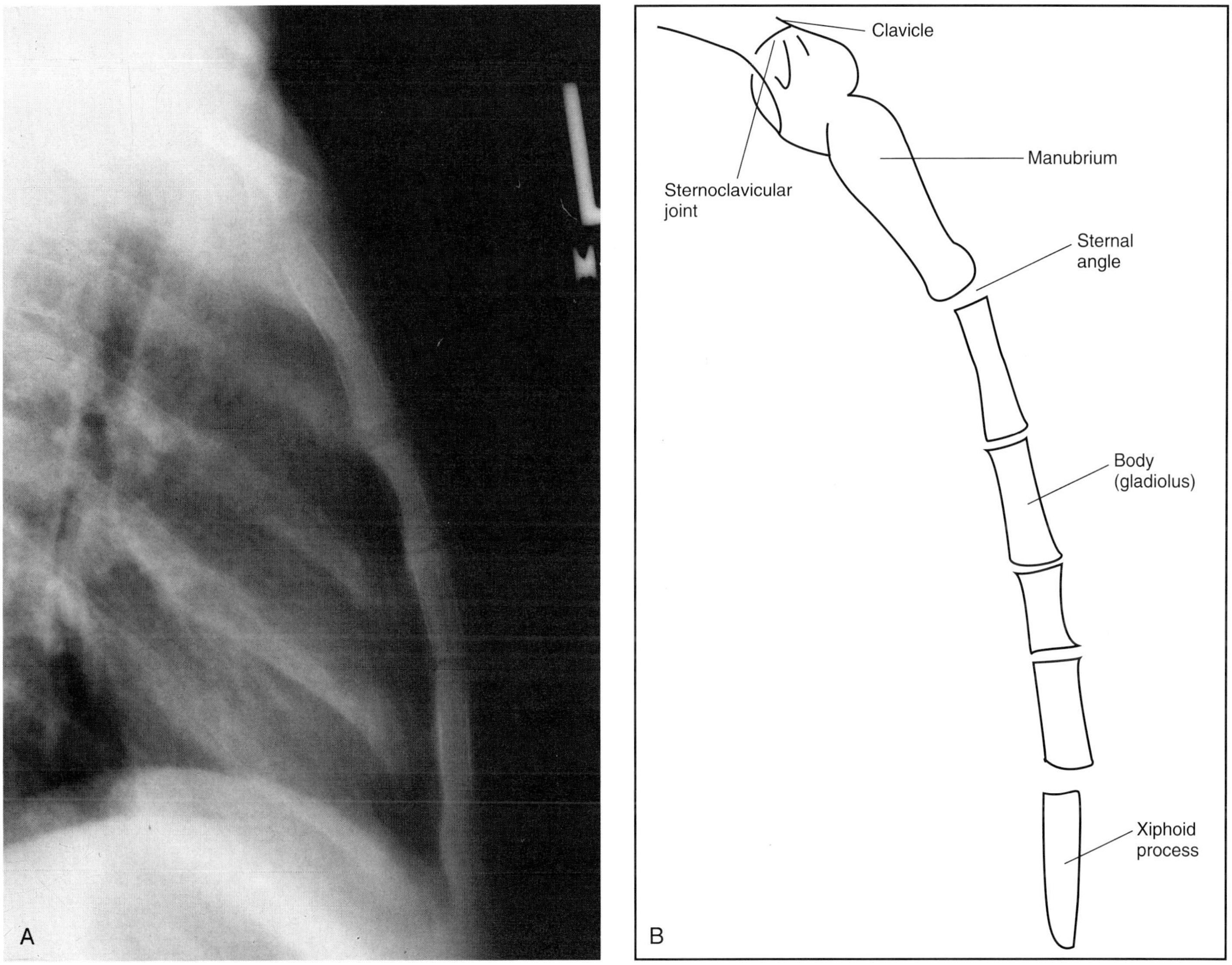

Figure 11.13. A and B, Lateral sternum.

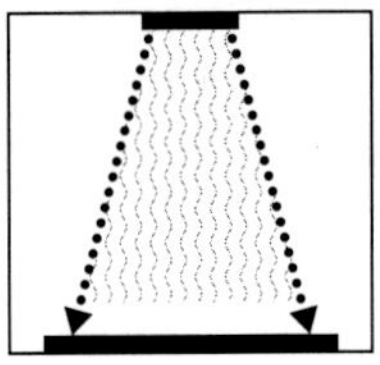

Sternoclavicular Articulations

Position/Projection

PA projection

Film Size:
8 × 10 inches (20 × 24 cm)
crosswise

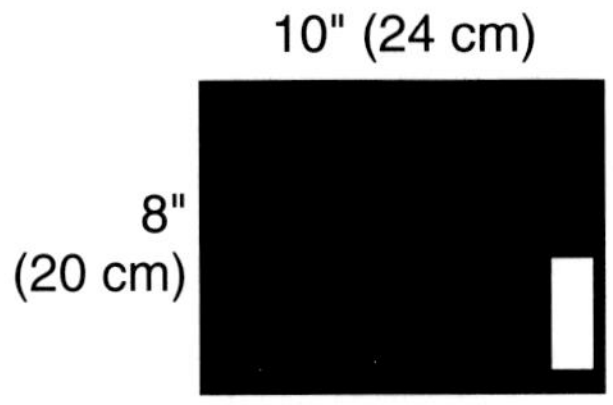

Patient Position

Prone, arms along sides of body with palms facing film.

Bilateral

Rest patient's head on chin and place midsagittal plane vertical (Fig. 11.14*A*).

Unilateral

Turn patient's head toward affected side, letting head rest on cheek. This movement moves spine away from side bing examined, giving a better picture of lateral portion of manubrium (Fig. 11.14*B*).

Central Ray

Perpendicular to T3 spinous process or to manubrial notch.

Breathing Instructions

Respiration is suspended at end of exhalation to obtain more uniform density.

Structures Demonstrated

Presents PA projection of sternoclavicular joints and medial portions of clavicles. Demonstrates both sternoclavicular joints and medial ends of clavicles. Joints are seen through superimposing vertebral and rib shadows (Fig. 11.15).

Evaluation Criteria

1. No rotation present on bilateral, slight rotation present on unilateral.
2. Ensure that medial ends of clavicles are demonstrated.

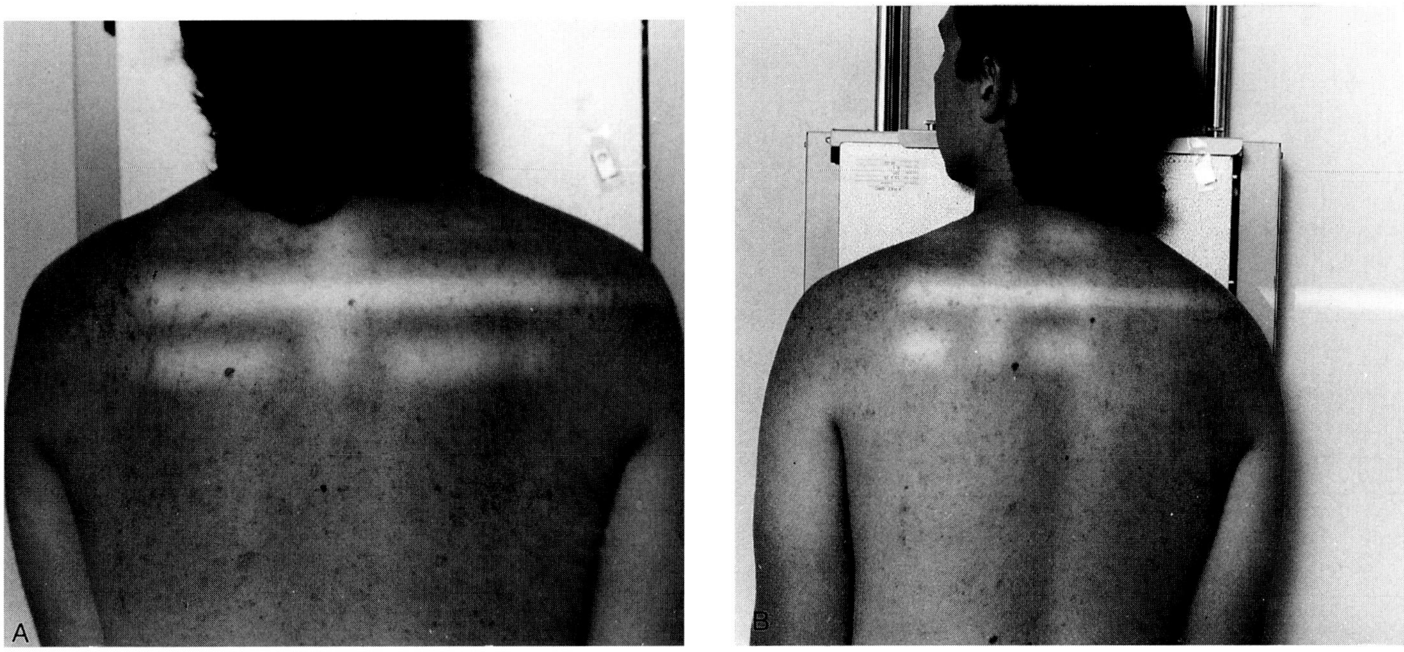

Figure 11.14. Sternoclavicular articulations, PA projection. A, Bilateral. B, Unilateral.

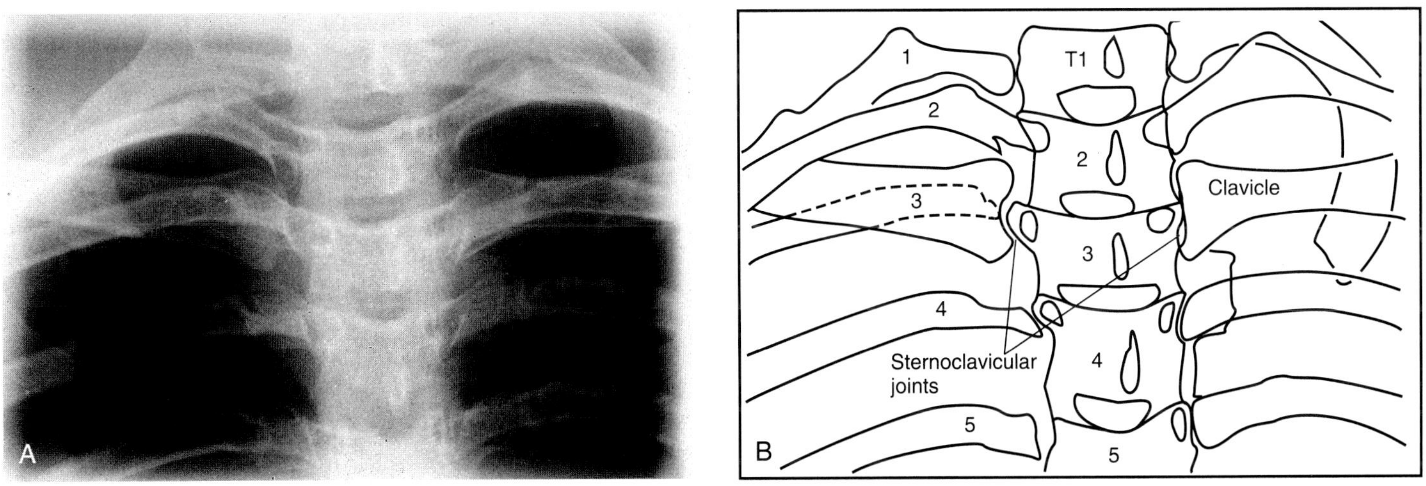

Figure 11.15. A and B, PA projection, sternoclavicular articulations.

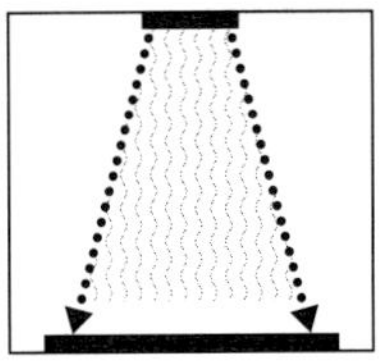

Sternoclavicular Articulations

Position/Projection

PA oblique projections (LAO and RAO)

Film Size:
8 × 10 inches (20 × 24 cm)
crosswise

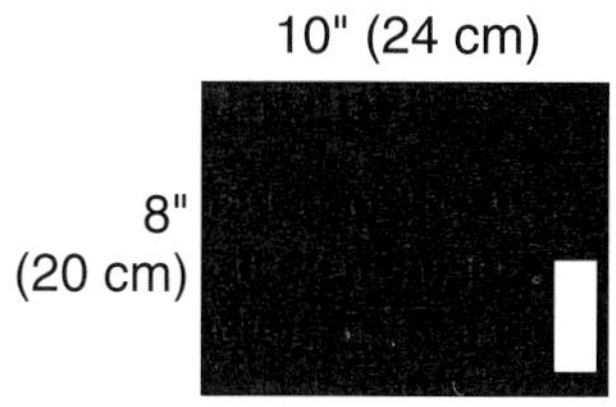

Patient Position

Prone or seated upright (Fig. 11.16)

Part Position

Patient obliqued enough to throw vertebral shadow behind sternoclavicular joint. Side being demonstrated is up.

Central Ray

Perpendicular to T3 spinous process or manubrial notch.

Breathing Instructions

Suspend breathing.

Structures Demonstrated

Shows slightly oblique projection of sternoclavicular joint. Demonstrates sternoclavicular joint of interest, manubrium, and medial end of clavicle (Fig. 11.17).

Evaluation Criteria

1. Sternoclavicular joints should be directly in front of vertebral column and should be visible through superimposing rib and lung fields.
2. Sternoclavicular joint space should be open.

NOTE: An alteration of this method involves a prone patient, using a nongrid or portable grid technique (Fig. 11.18). The cassette is centered to the affected sternoclavicular joint. Arms are down at sides and palms are up. A 15° angle of the central ray from the side being examined toward the midsagittal plane of the body is used.

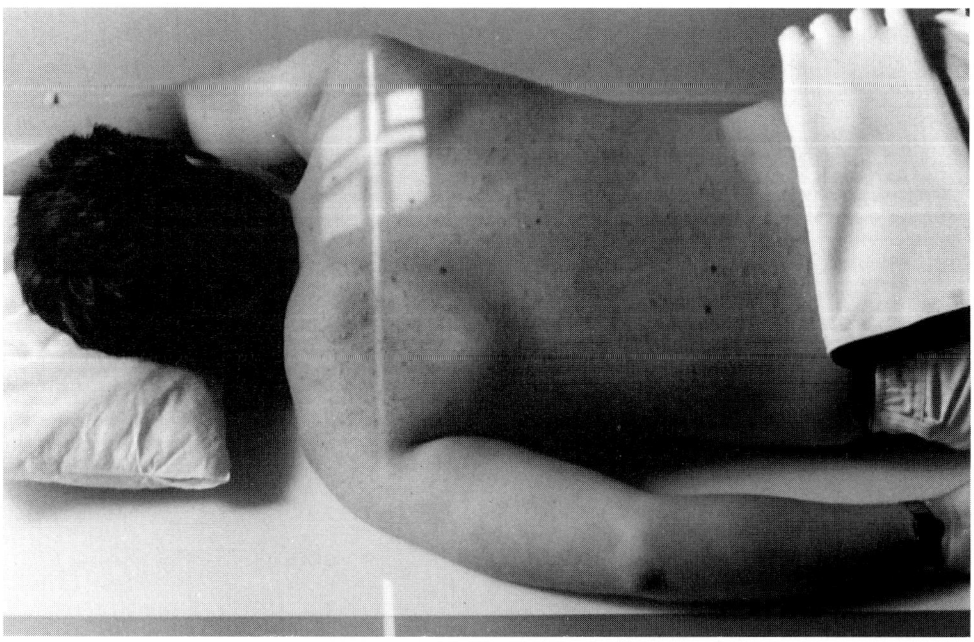

Figure 11.16. PA oblique projection (RAO), sternoclavicular articulations.

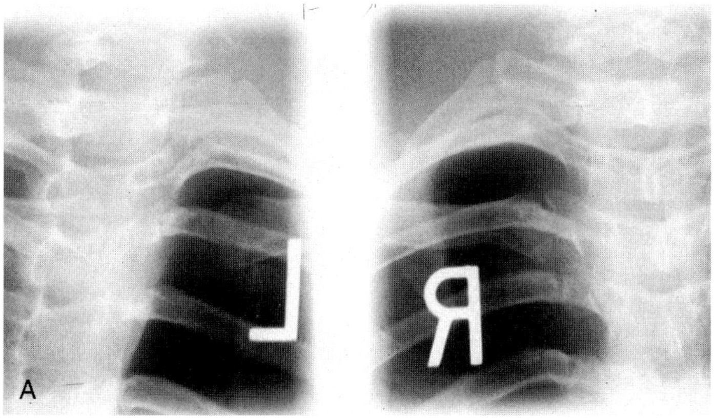

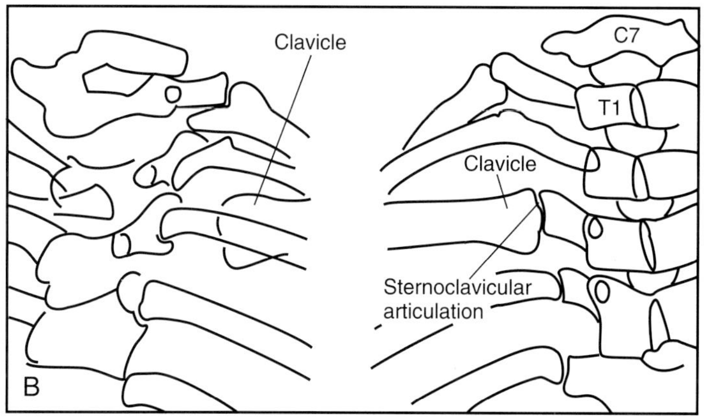

Figure 11.17. A and B, PA oblique, sternoclavicular articulation.

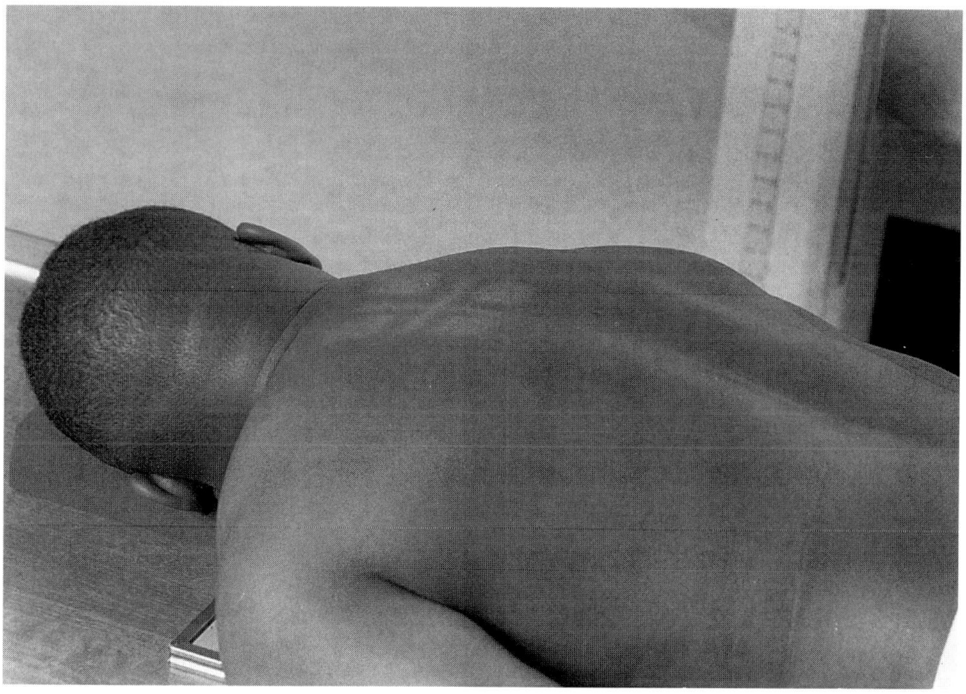

Figure 11.18. Alternate to Figure 11.16.

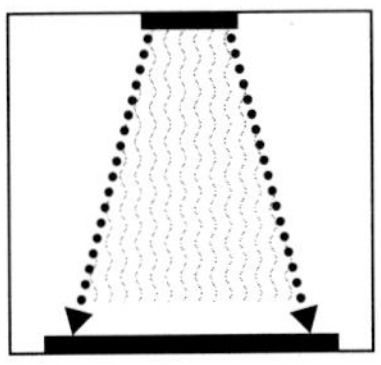

Sternoclavicular Articulations

Position/Projection

Lateral projection—Kurzbauer's method

Film Size:
8 × 10 inches (20 × 24 cm)
lengthwise

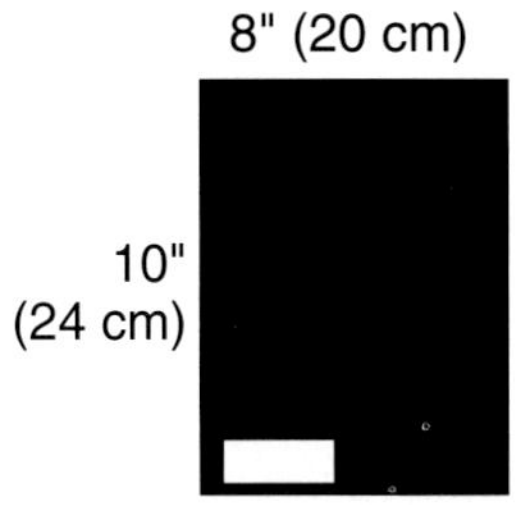

Patient Position

Lateral recumbent position with side being examined down. Flex knees and hips to comfortable position. Extend dependent arm above head and then place uppermost arm along side of body, grasping hip and depressing shoulder (Fig. 11.19).

Central Ray

15° caudad through lowermost sternoclavicular joints.

Breathing Instructions

Suspend breathing at end of full inhalation.

Structures Demonstrated

Shows unobstructed lateral projection of sternoclavicular articulation. Demonstrates sternoclavicular joint of interest (Fig. 11.20).

Evaluation Criteria

Shoulders should not superimpose sternoclavicular joint.

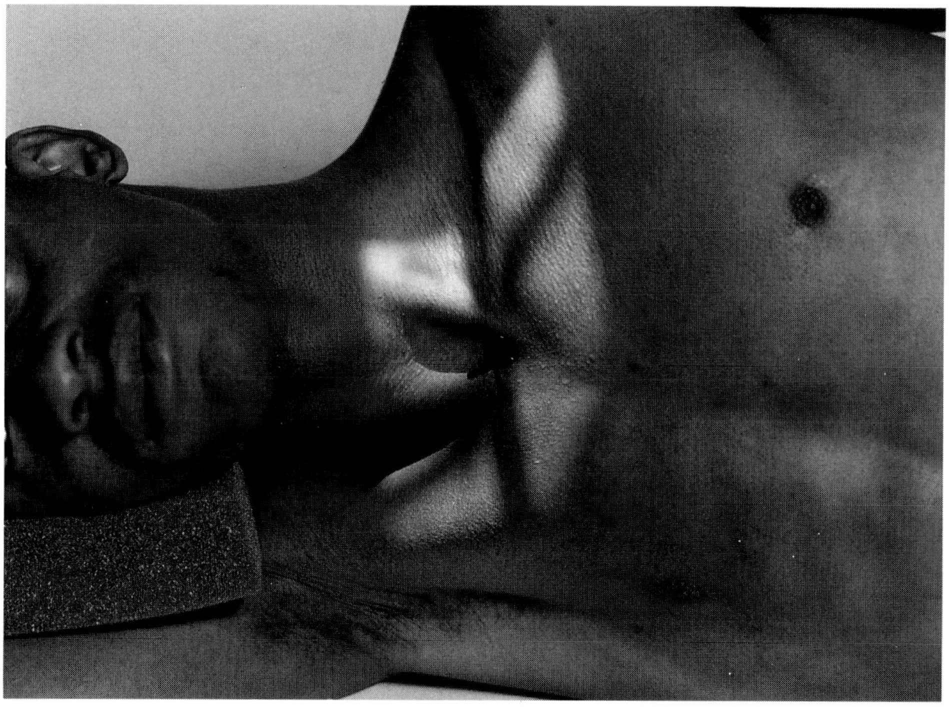

Figure 11.19. Kurzbauer's method—lateral projection.

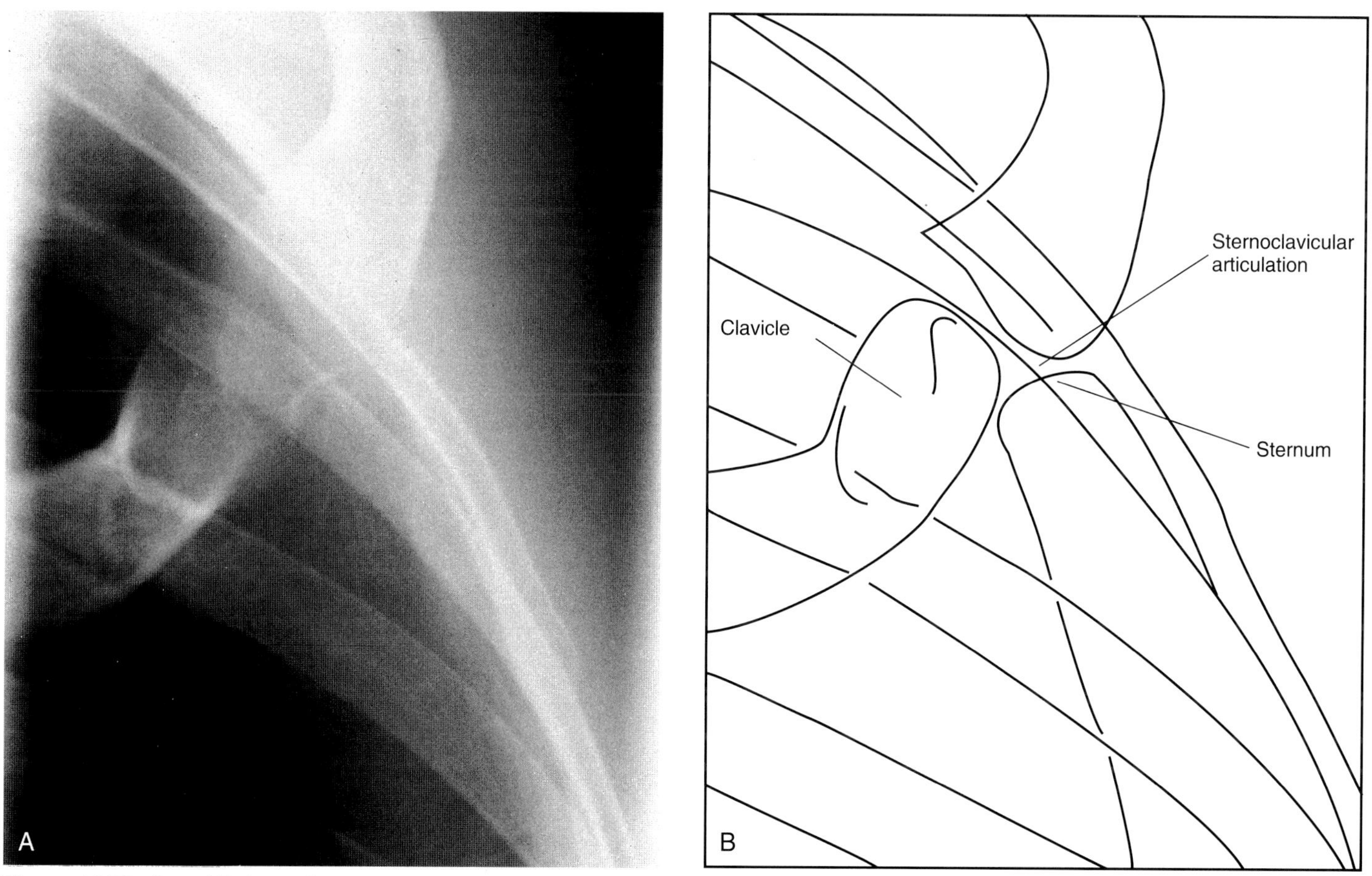

Figure 11.20. A and B, Lateral projection, sternoclavicular articulations—Kurzbauer's method.

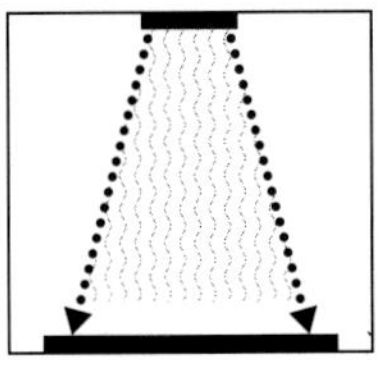

Ribs

Position/Projection

Ribs bilateral PA

Film Size:
14 × 17 inches (35 × 43 cm) lengthwise or crosswise in Bucky

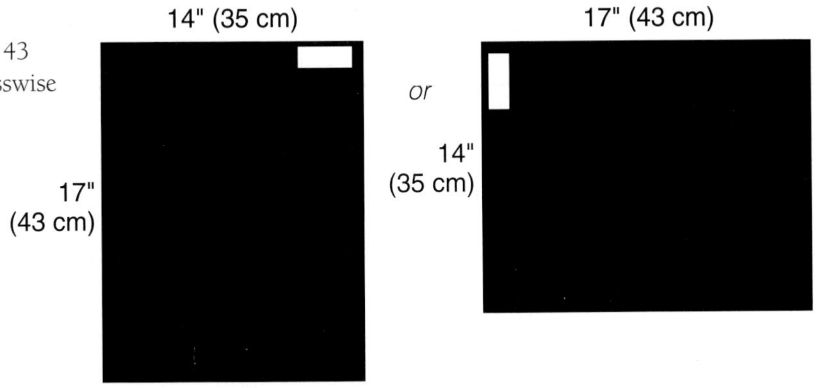

Patient Position

PA, preferably erect. Patient should face cassette with arms abducted and flexed elbows encircling film cassette *or* when erect hands should be against hips with palms turned outward to rotate scapulae away from rib cage. If patient is prone, rest head on chin and adjust midsagittal plane vertical with arms at sides (Fig. 11.21).

Part Position

Midsagittal plane of body should be centered to grid. Cassette should be placed 1.5 to 2 inches (4 to 5 cm) above upper border of shoulder.

Central Ray

Perpendicular to film and centered to midpoint of film to T6 or T4.

Breathing Instructions

For posterior ribs, when no movement during quiet respiration, long exposure time with low MA may be used to diffuse lung shadows and show posterior ribs in greater detail. Exposure should otherwise be taken on full inspiration to depress diaphragm as much as possible. Expiration is used to demonstrate small pneumothoraces.

Structures Demonstrated

PA projection demonstrates ribs above diaphragm. Upright projection demonstrates pneumothorax or hemothorax (Fig. 11.22).

Evaluation Criteria

Ideally 1st through 10th; minimally 1st through 9th anterior ribs should be demonstrated.

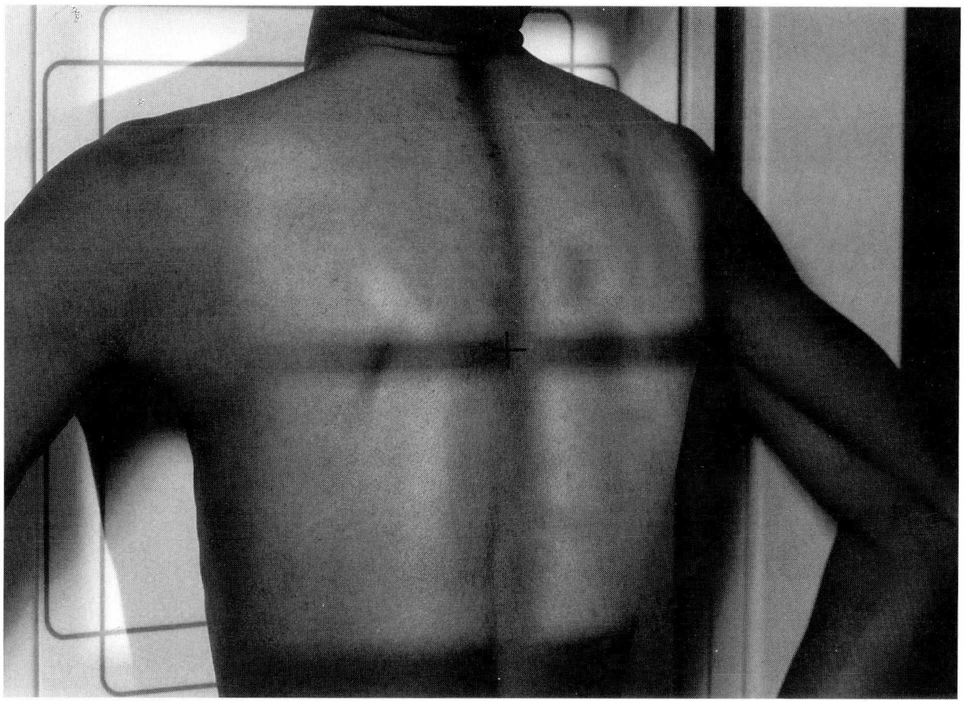

Figure 11.21. Bilateral PA ribs.

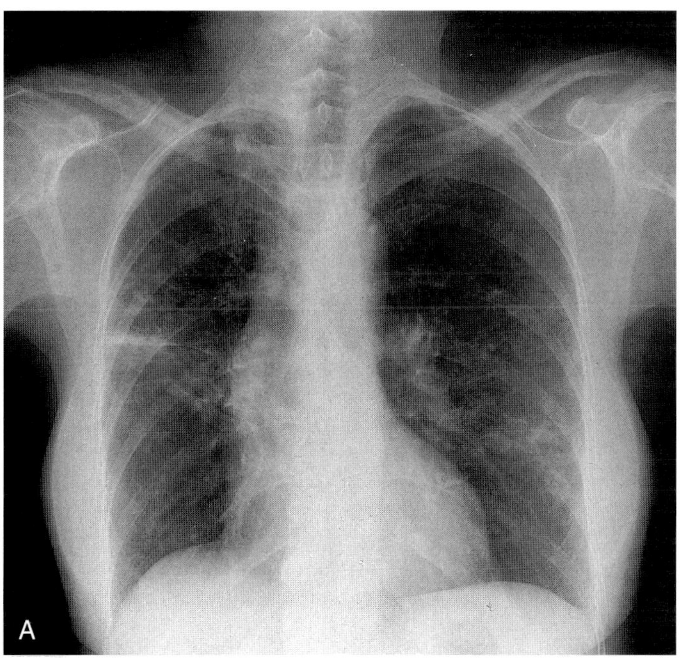

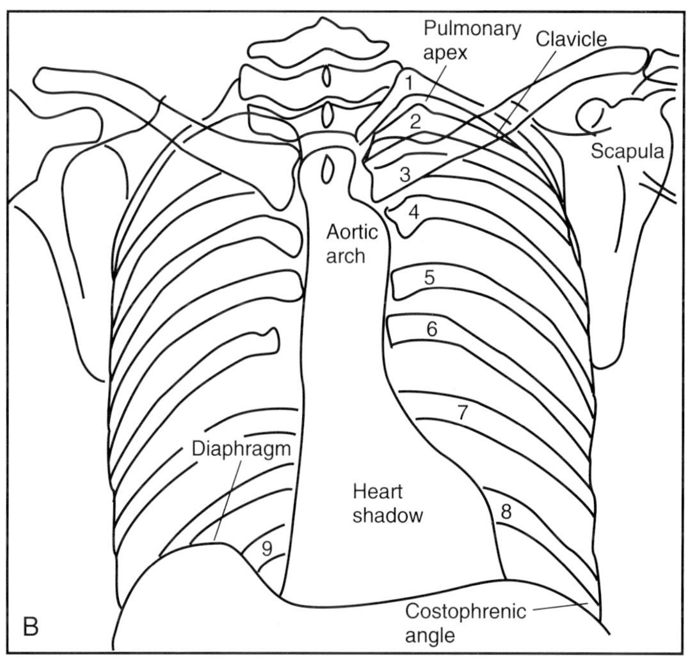

Figure 11.22. A and B, Bilateral PA, posterior ribs.

Ribs

Position/Projection

Posterior ribs (above diaphragm) AP Position

Film Size:
14 × 17 inches (35 × 43 cm) crosswise or lengthwise

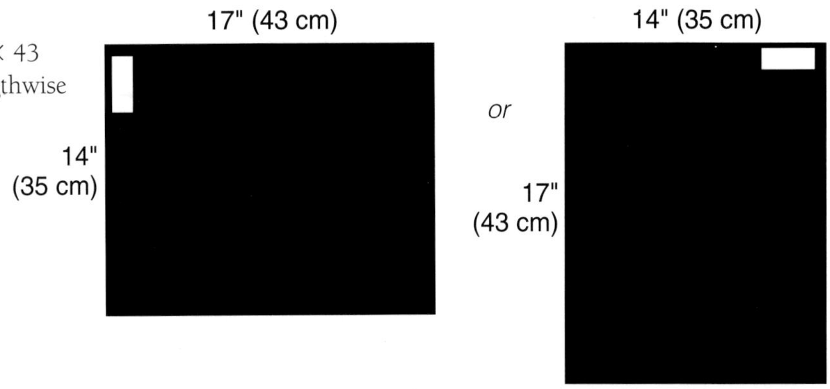

Patient Position

AP position, erect if possible (Fig. 11.23).

Part Position

Place patient in contact with Bucky so that midsagittal plane is perpendicular to film with flash just above right shoulder. Arms are extended, and shoulders are rotated forward.

Central Ray

Perpendicular and centered to film to level of T7.

Breathing Instructions

To better lower diaphragm, exposure should be taken on second full inspiration.

Structures Demonstrated

Posterior ribs above diaphragm (Fig. 11.24).

Evaluation Criteria

First 10 posterior bilateral ribs should be well demonstrated above diaphragm.

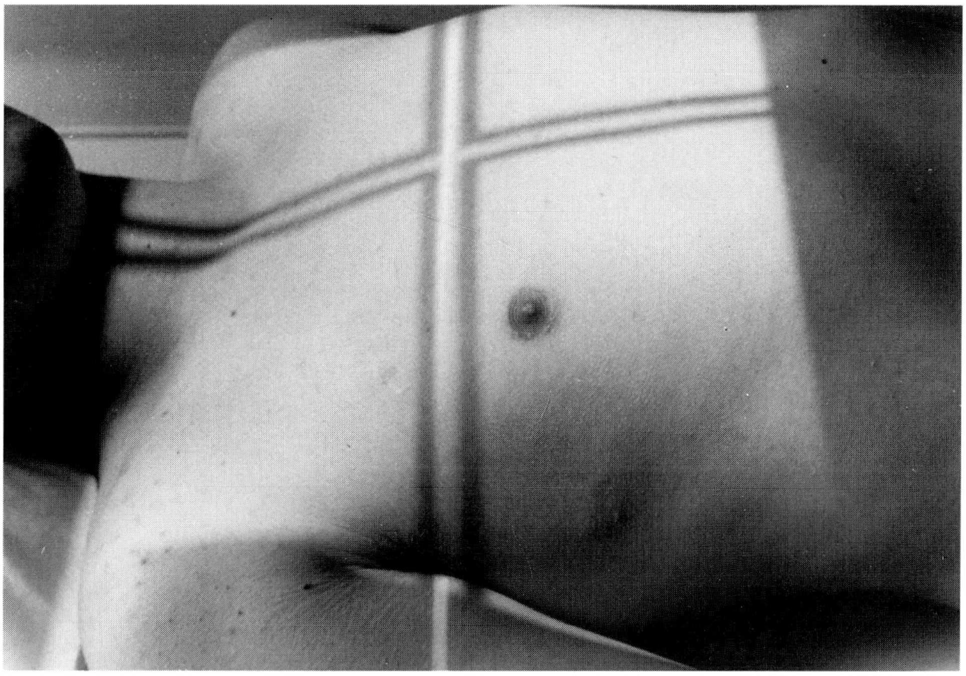

Figure 11.23. AP position, posterior ribs, above diaphragm.

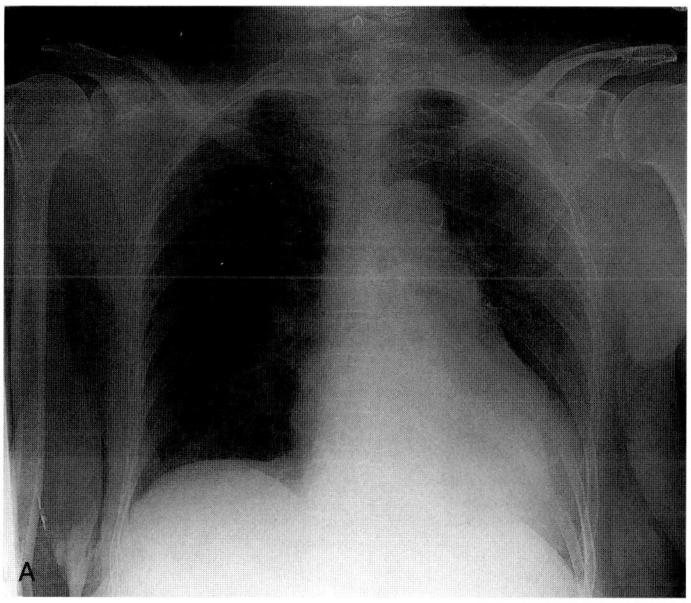

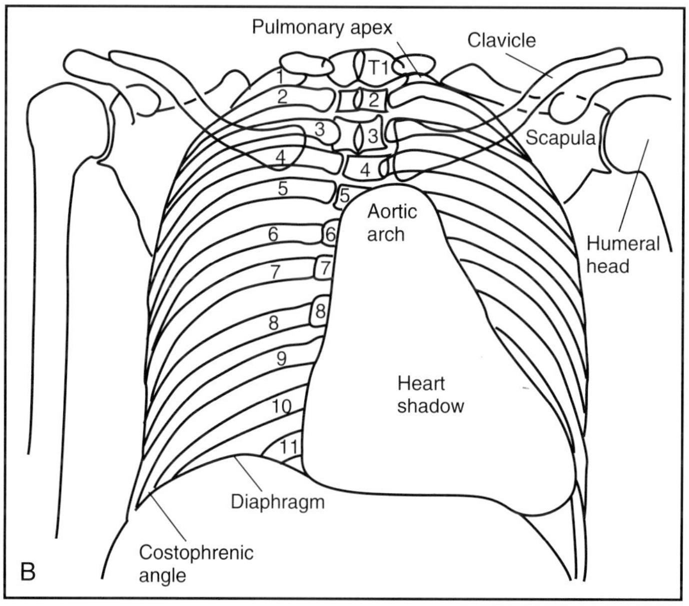

Figure 11.24. AP position, A and B, posterior ribs, above diaphragm.

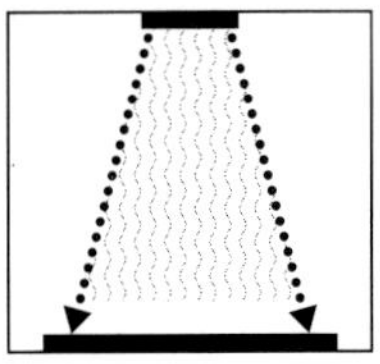

Ribs

Position/Projection

Posterior ribs (below diaphragm) AP position

Film Size:
14 × 17 inches (35 × 43 cm) crosswise or lengthwise

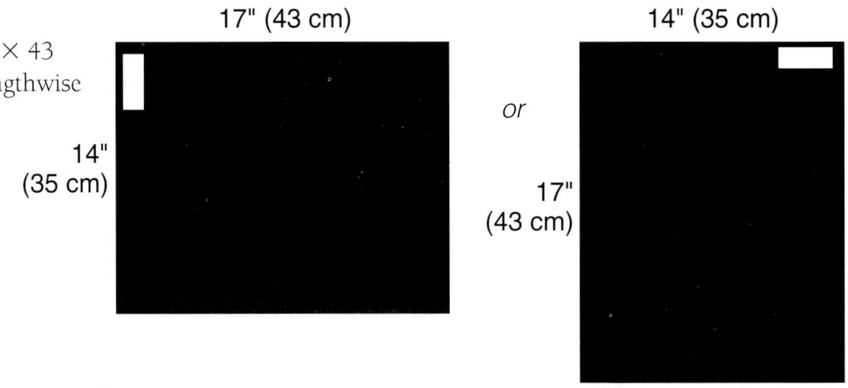

Patient Position

AP position, erect if possible (Fig. 11.25).

Part Position

Place patient's back against Bucky so that midsagittal plane is perpendicular to film. Caudal edge of cassette is placed at level of crest of ilium.

Central Ray

Perpendicular and centered to film. Direct central ray to T12 for crosswise cassette; T10 for lengthwise.

Breathing Instructions

To better lower diaphragm, exposure should be taken on second full inspiration.

Structures Demonstrated

Posterior ribs below diaphragm (Fig. 11.26).

Evaluation Criteria

8th through 12th posterior ribs on both sides seen below diaphragm bilaterally.

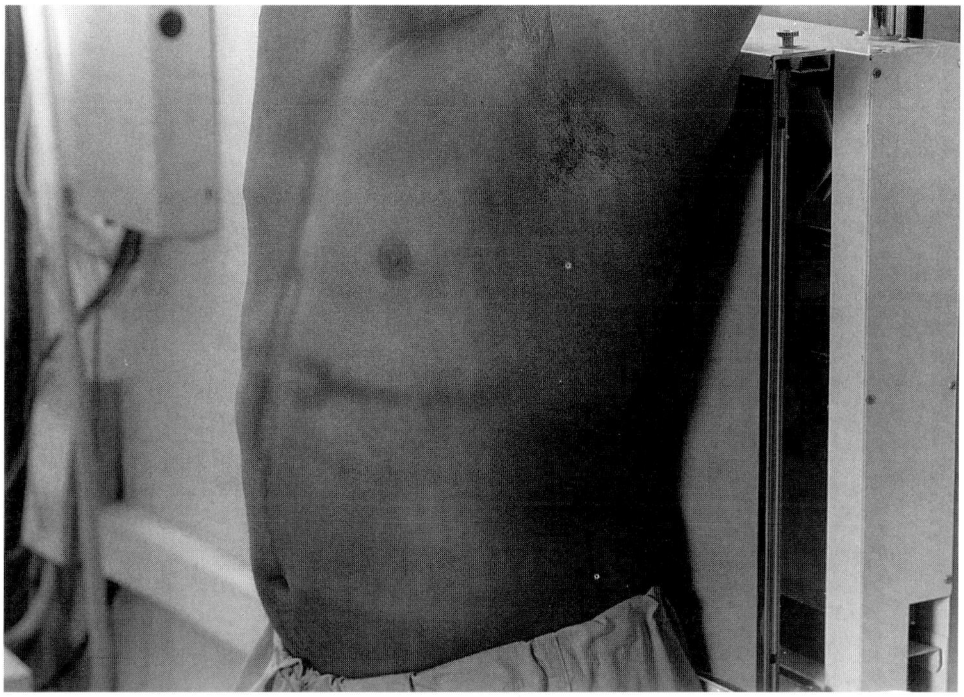

Figure 11.25. AP position, posterior ribs, below diaphragm.

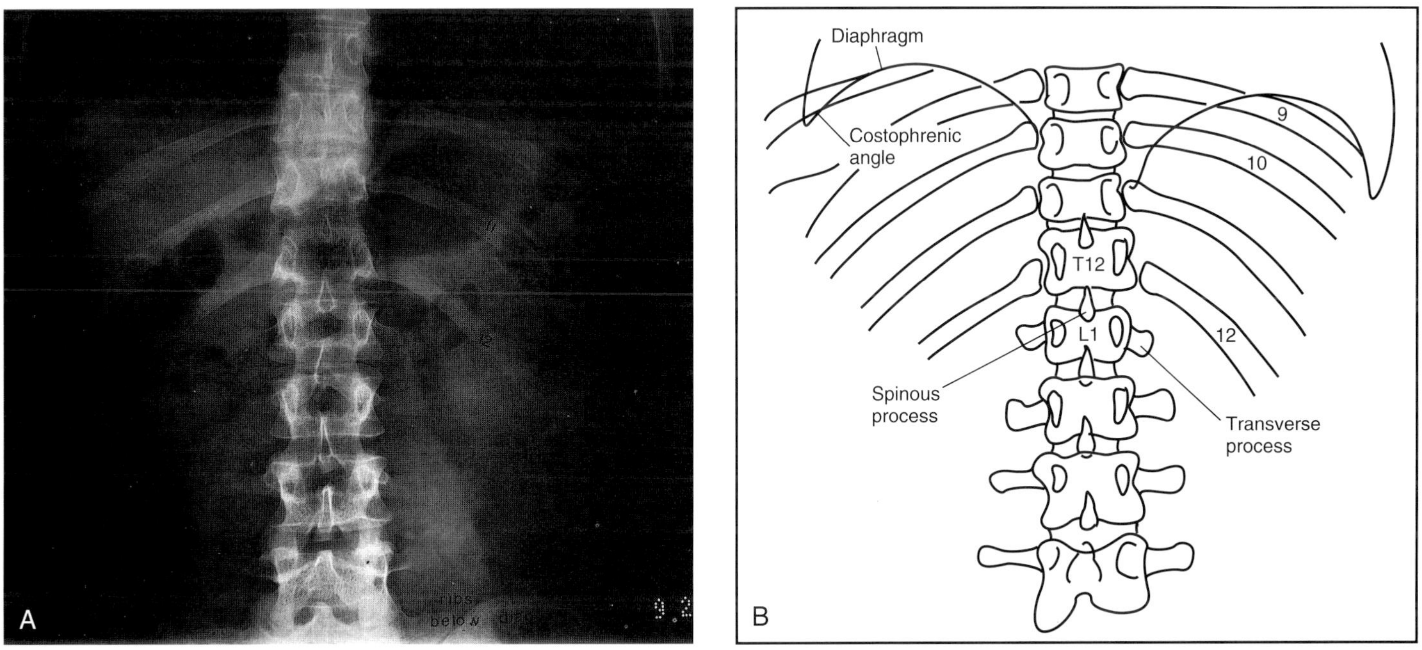

Figure 11.26. A and B, AP position, posterior ribs, below diaphragm.

Ribs

Position/Projection

Oblique position/projection

Film Size:
14 × 17 inches lengthwise
(35 × 43 cm)

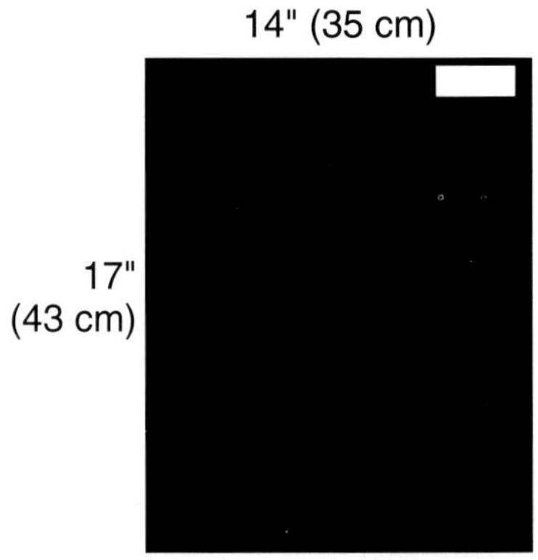

Patient Position

Semisupine, semiprone, or upright. Body rotated 45° (Figs. 11.27 to 11.30).

Part Position

Spine rotated away from ribs of interest. For right ribs, perform RPO/LAO. For left ribs, LPO/RAO. For bilateral study, perform both obliques (RPO and LPO *or* RAO and LAO). Posterior obliques have affected side closest to film, anterior obliques have affected side away from film.

Central Ray

Perpendicular to level of T7 for ribs above diaphragm; T12 for ribs below diaphragm.

Breathing Instructions

Suspend respiration at end of deep exhalation for ribs below diaphragm. Respiration is suspended at end of full inhalation for ribs above diaphragm.

Structures Demonstrated

Ribs, especially axillary portions, free of bony superimposition (Figs. 11.31 and 11.32).

Evaluation Criteria

1. Above diaphragm (upper ribs) 1st through 10th ribs are shown.
2. For below diaphragm (lower) ribs, 8th through 12th ribs are shown.
3. Ribs should be seen clearly through lungs or abdomen.
4. Twice distance between vertebral column and outer border of the ribs should be seen on affected side as opposed to unaffected side.

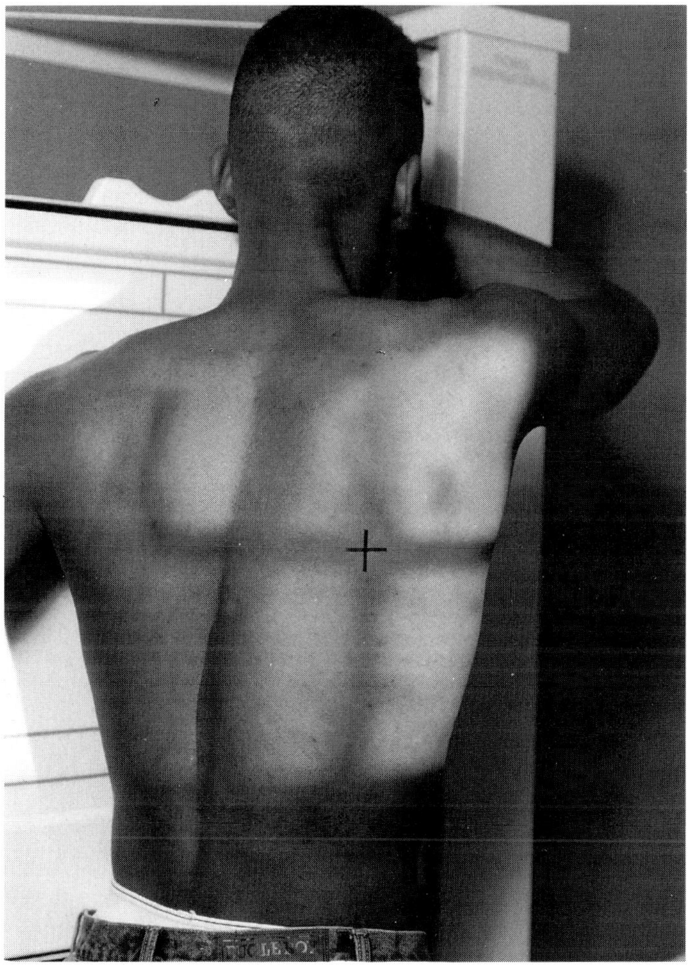

Figure 11.27. LAO ribs.

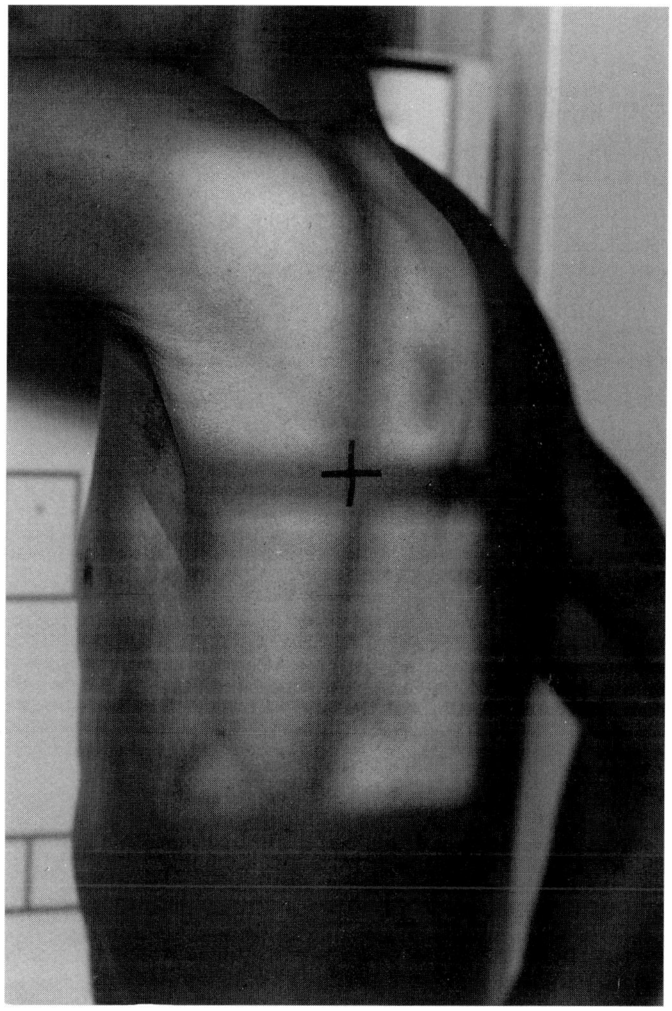

Figure 11.28. RAO ribs (unilateral for left side).

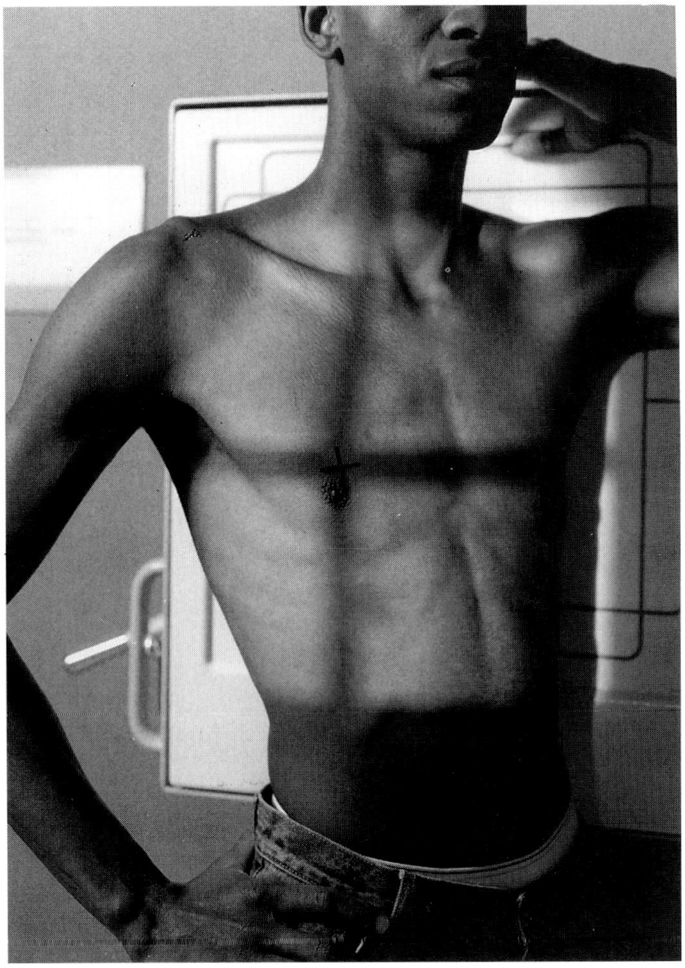

Figure 11.29. LPO ribs.

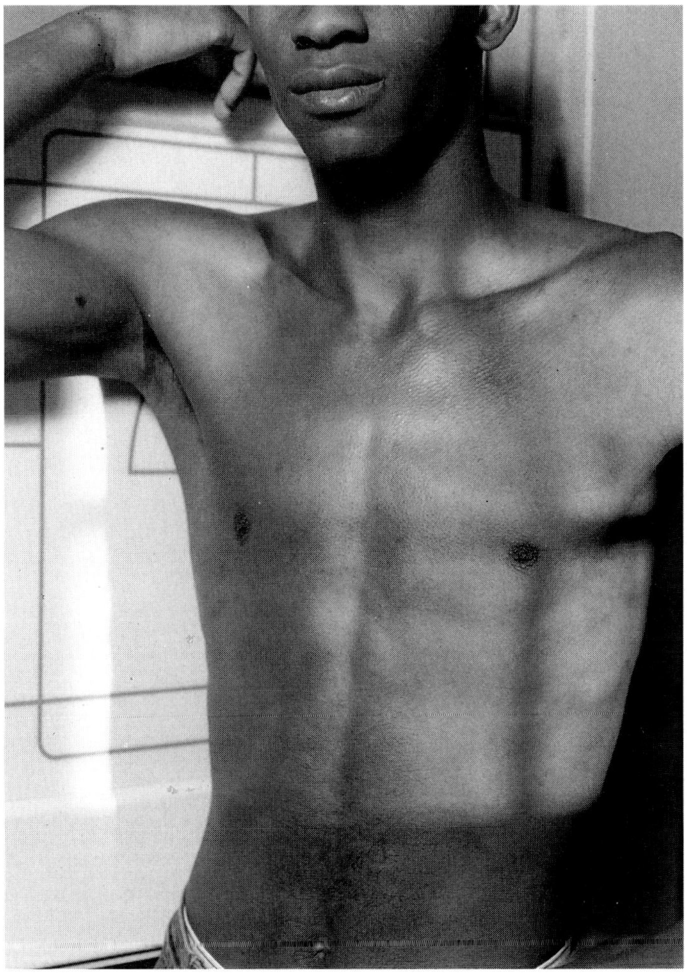

Figure 11.30. RPO ribs.

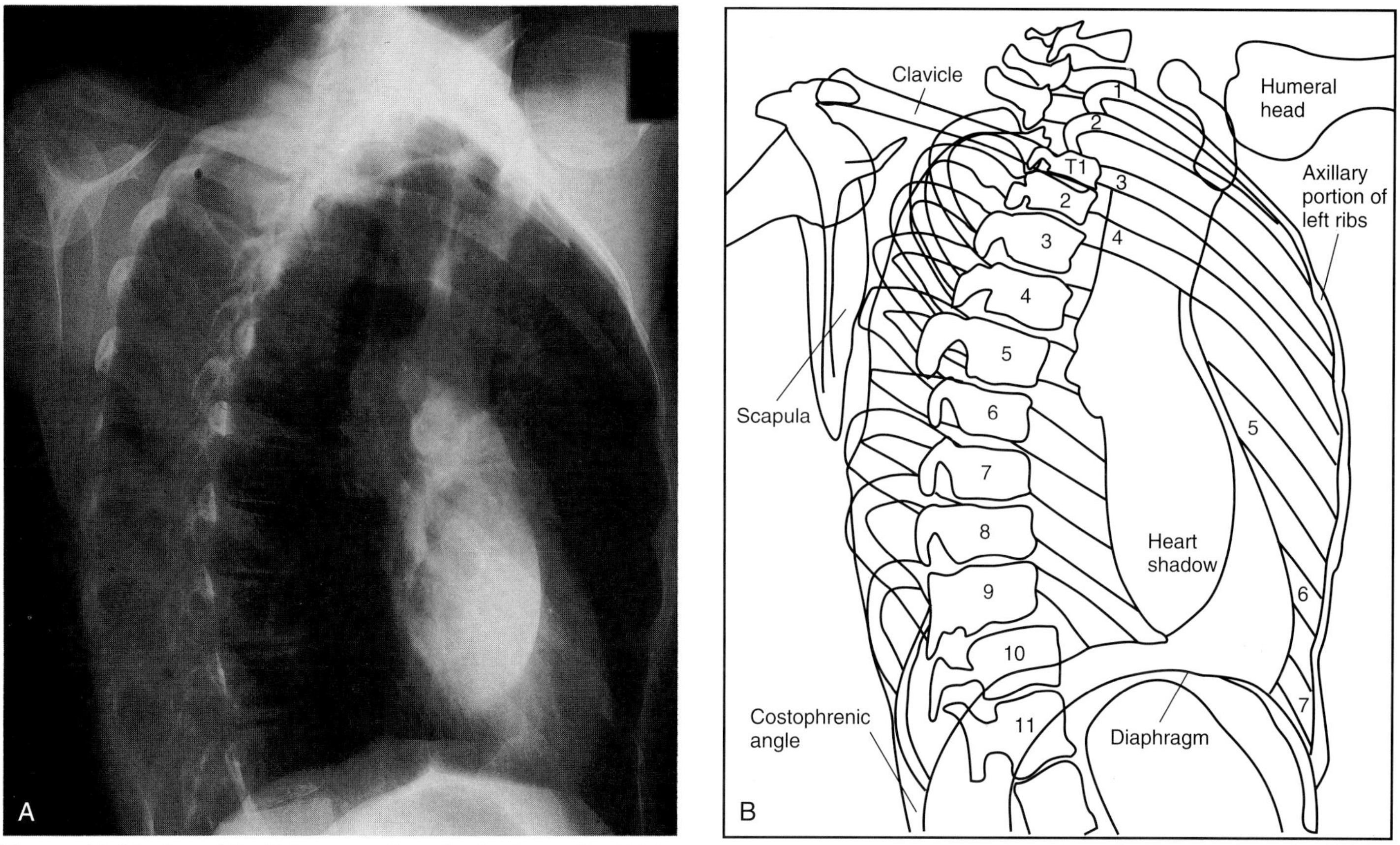

Figure 11.31. A and B, Oblique positions/projections, ribs RAO.

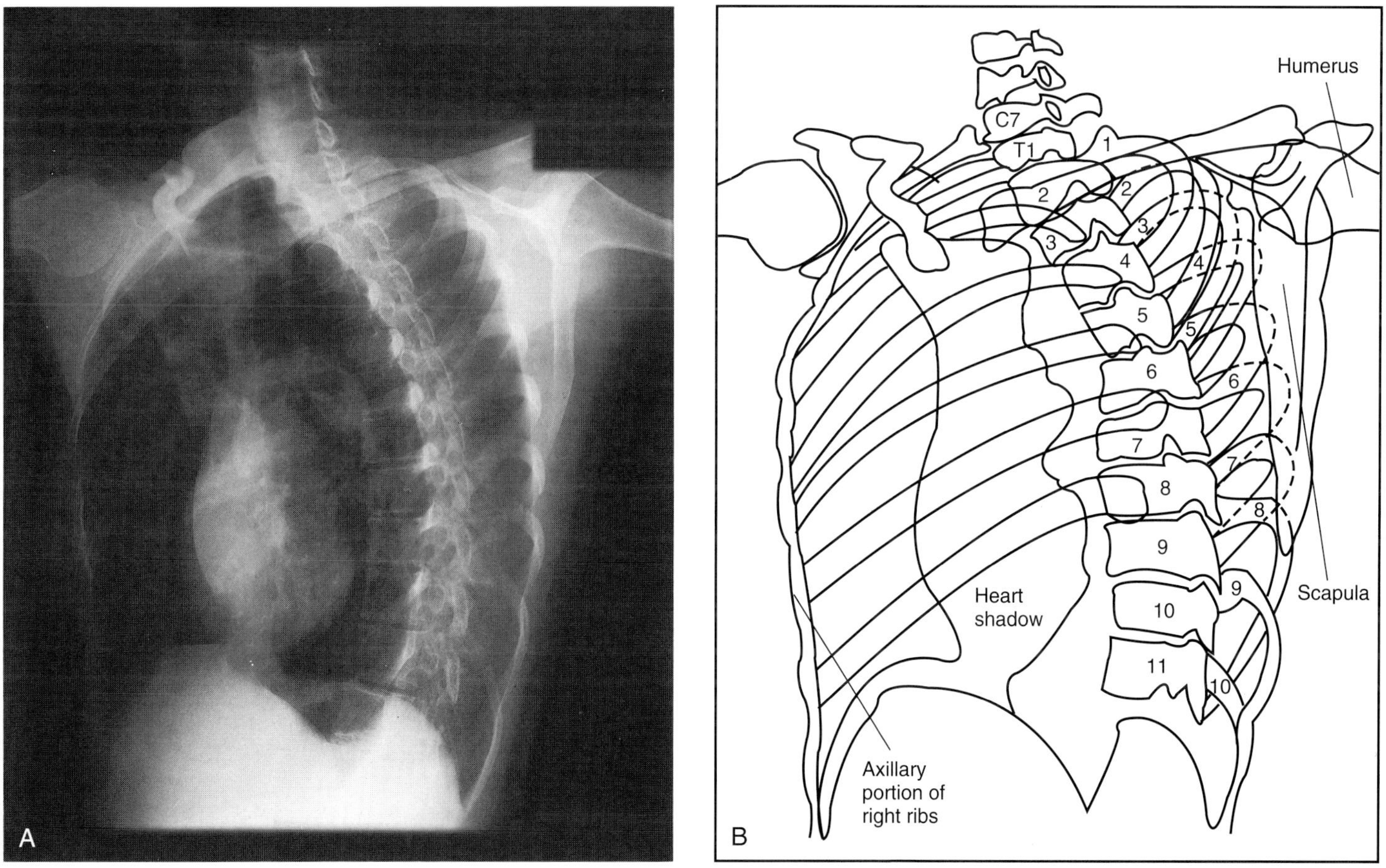

Figure 11.32. A and B, Oblique positions/projections, ribs LPO.

Costal Joints

Position/Projection

AP axial projection

Film Size:
11 × 14 inches (28 × 35 cm) lengthwise

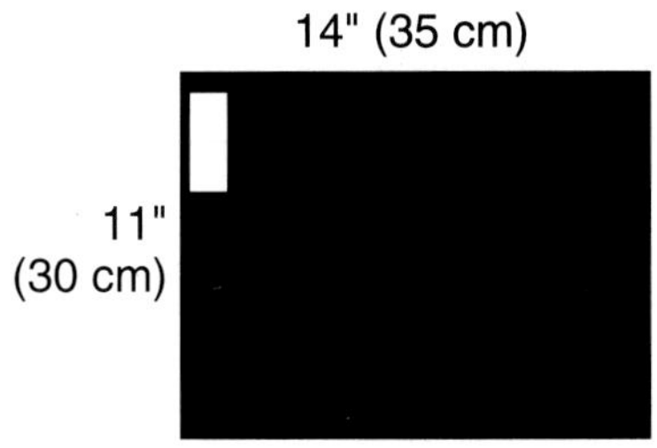

Patient Position

Supine with head resting on table (Fig. 11.33).

Part Position

True AP with midsagittal plane centered to midline of table. Larger patients may require two views to demonstrate costovertebral joints. 10° medial angle of body will best demonstrate elevated side. Arms are placed alongside body unless patient has large amount of kyphosis. Then, arms are extended over head.

Central Ray

Directed through T6 at 20° cephalad angle. Some authors recommend 30–40° angle. Angulation is increased when patient has large dorsal kyphosis.

Breathing Instructions

Respiration is suspended at end of full inspiration.

Structures Demonstrated

Costovertebral and costotransverse joints (Fig. 11.34).

Evaluation Criteria

1. Primary use is demonstration of costal joints for patients with rheumatoid spondylitis.
2. Open costovertebral and costotransverse joints.

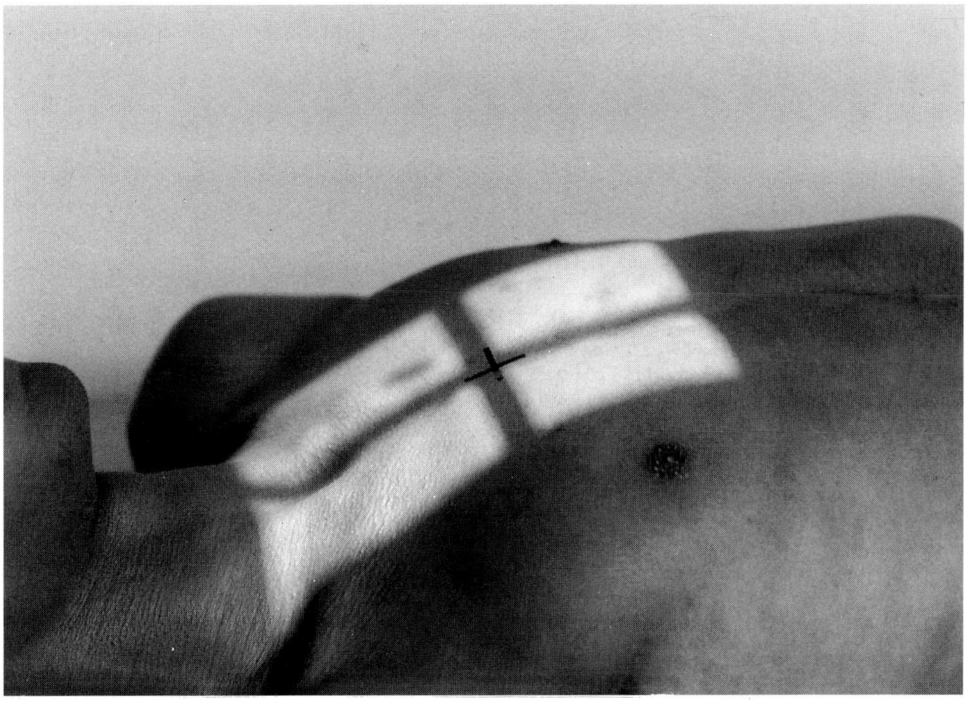

Figure 11.33. AP axial, costal joints.

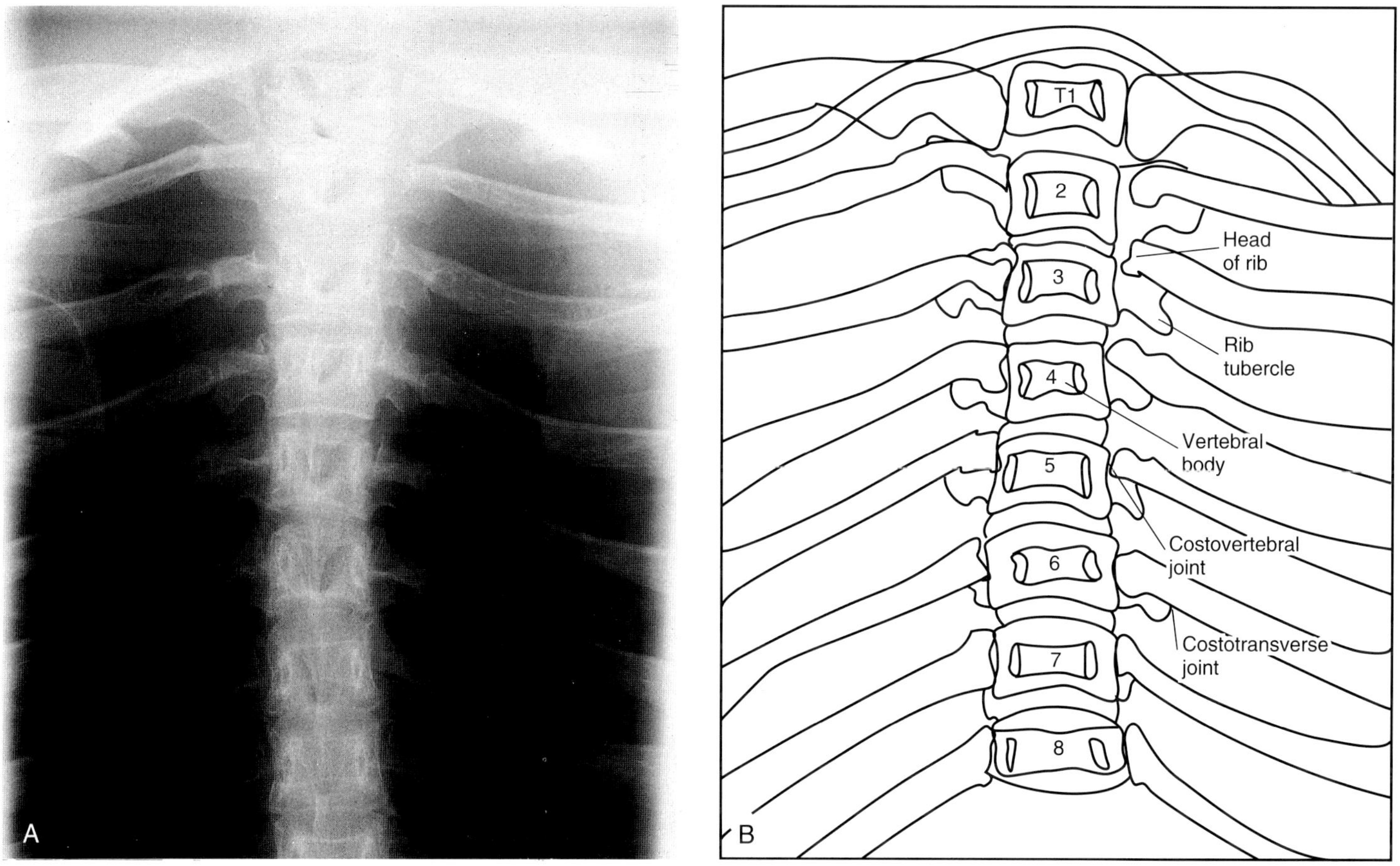

Figure 11.34. A and B, AP axial projection, costal joints.

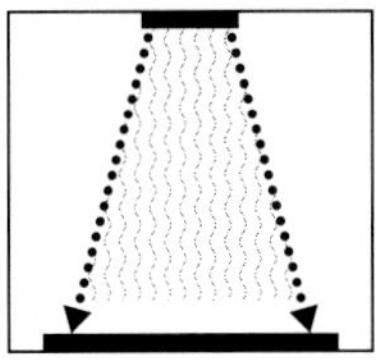

Thoracic Viscera

Position/Projection

AP projection of trachea

Film Size:
10 × 12 inches (24 × 30 cm) lengthwise

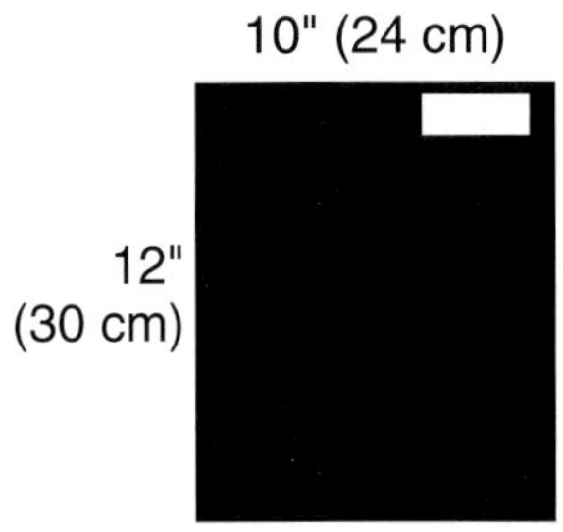

Patient Position
Supine or erect (Fig. 11.35).

Part Position
Midsagittal plane is perpendicular to plane of film.

Central Ray
Perpendicular through manubrium.

Breathing Instructions
Patient inhales slowly during exposure. In some cases, exposure is made on forced expiration.

Structures Demonstrated
Shows AP projection of air-filled trachea (Fig. 11.36).

Evaluation Criteria
1. Include from midcervical to midthoracic region.
2. Should not be rotated.
3. Air-filled trachea should be demonstrated.

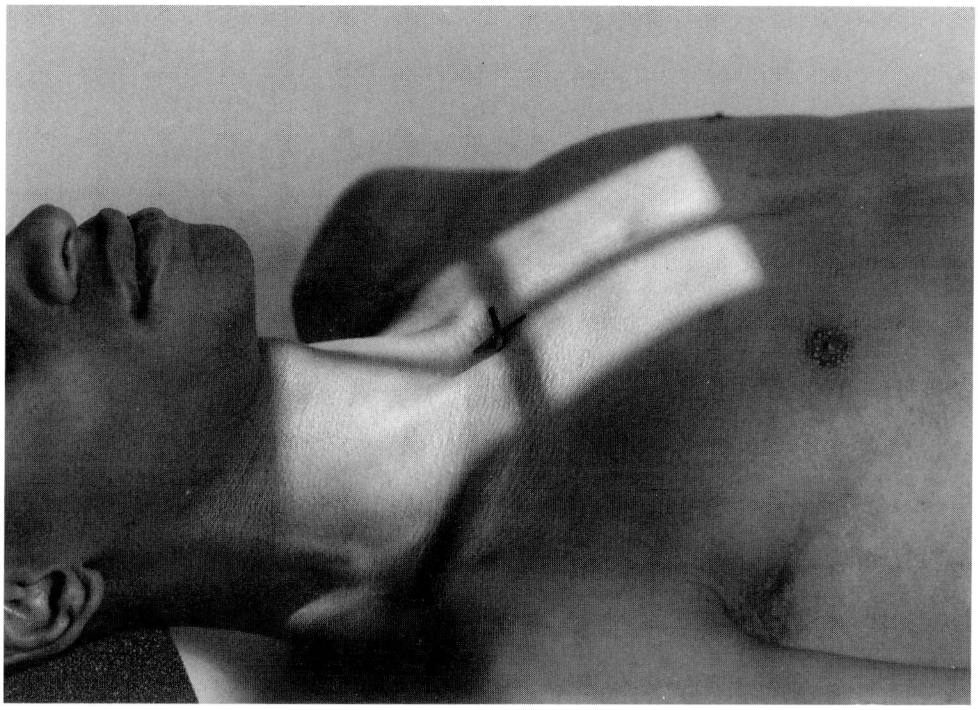

Figure 11.35. AP, trachea.

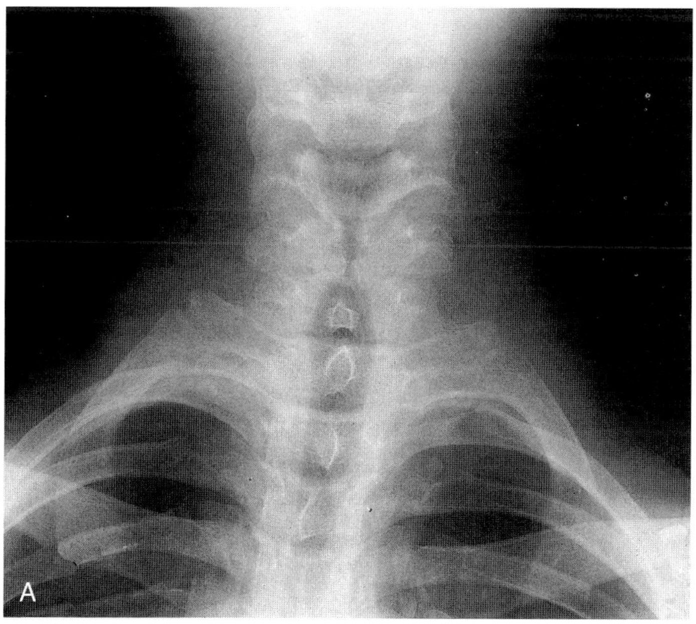

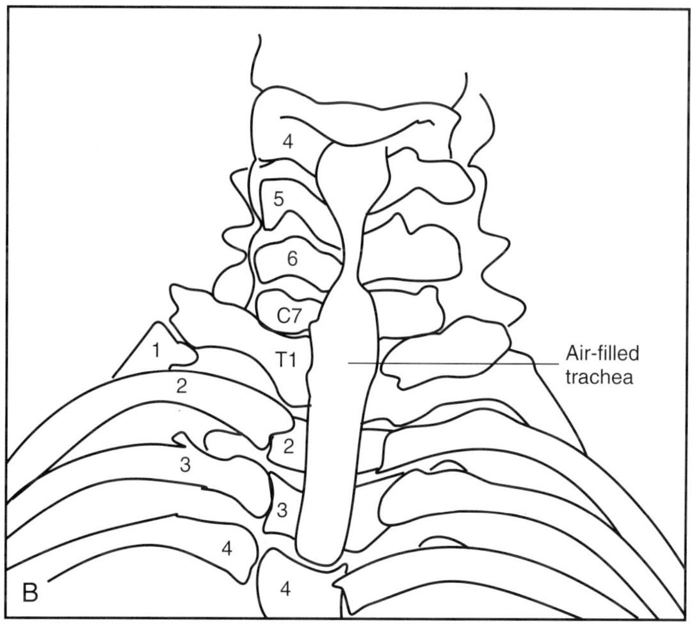

Figure 11.36. A and B, AP projection, trachea.

Thoracic Viscera

Position/Projection

Lateral projection of trachea and superior mediastinum

Film Size:
10 × 12 inches (24 × 30 cm) or larger lengthwise to include from lower pharynx to lower end of trachea at level of sternal angle

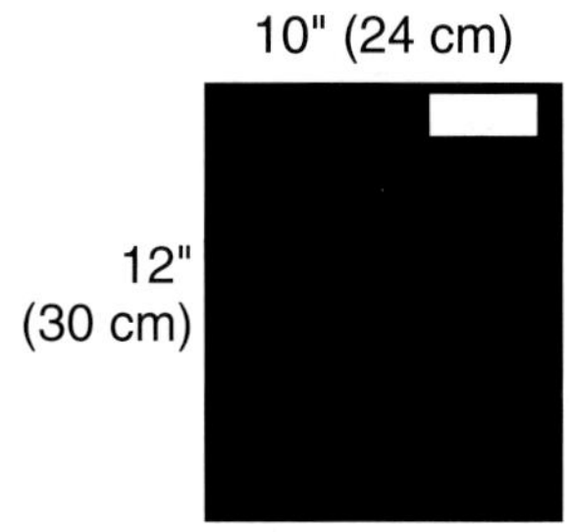

Patient Position

Lateral, sitting or erect (Fig. 11.37).

Part Position

Rotate shoulders posteriorly; extend head slightly. Midsagittal plane is parallel to plane of film. This position can be aided by having patient clasp hands behind back and pulling arms backward.

Central Ray

Through point midway between manubrial notch and anterior border of humeral head for superior mediastinal structures and 4 to 5 inches (10 to 13 cm) lower for the entire chest.

Breathing Instructions

Make exposure during deep inhalation to fill trachea with air.

Structures Demonstrated

Shows lateral projection of air-filled trachea (Fig. 11.38).

Evaluation Criteria

1. Include from midcervical to midthoracic region.
2. Make sure trachea is filled with air and well demonstrated.

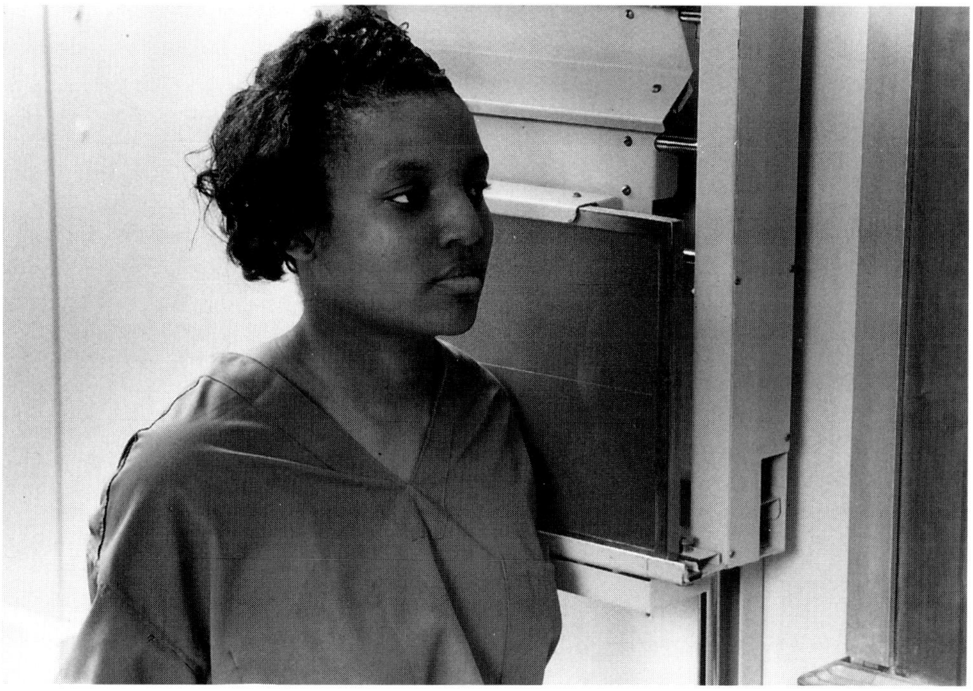

Figure 11.37. Lateral trachea.

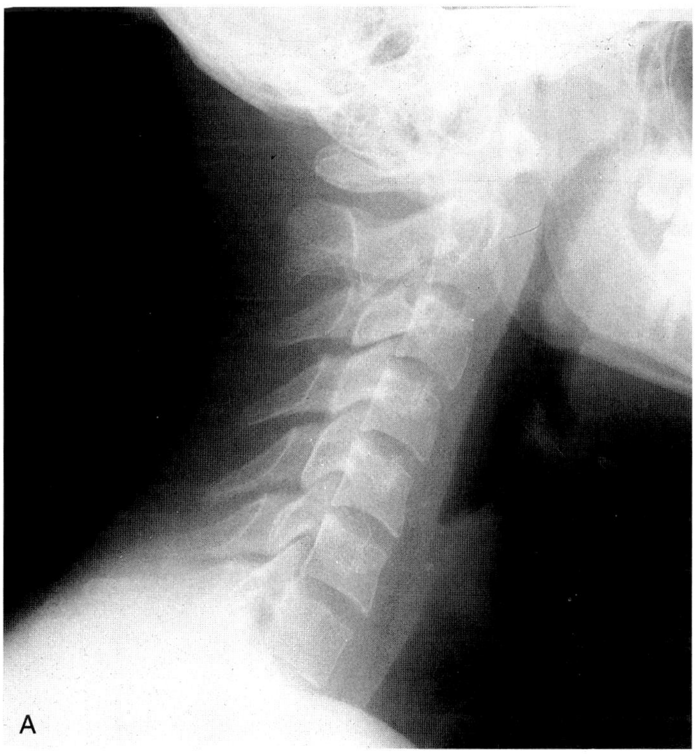

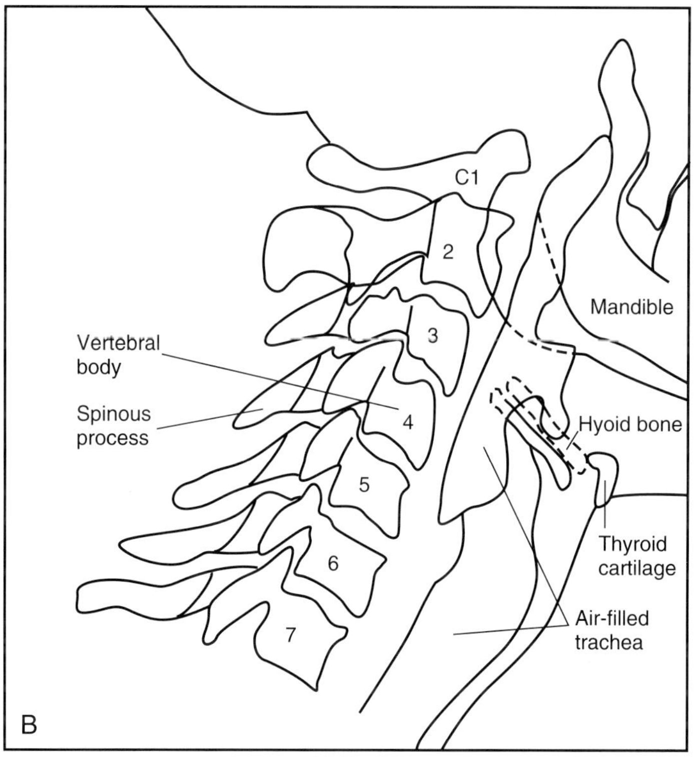

Figure 11.38. A and B, Lateral projection, trachea.

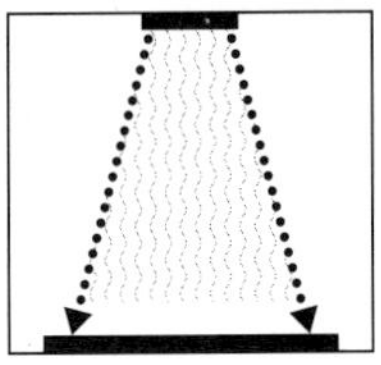

Thoracic Viscera

Position/Projection

Transshoulder lateral projection of trachea and pulmonary apex—Twining's method

Film Size:
10 × 12 inches (24 × 30 cm) lengthwise

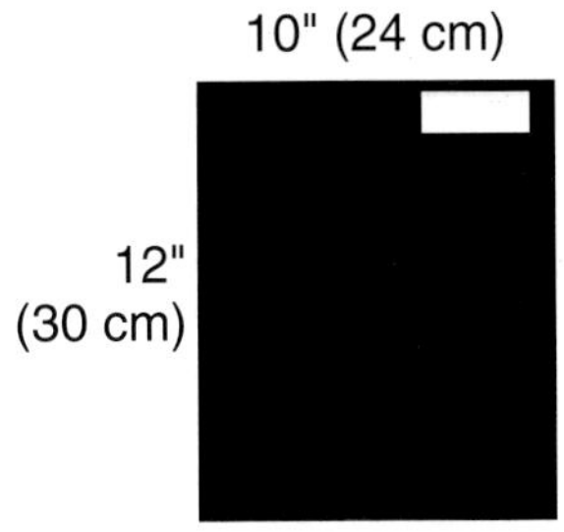

Patient Position

Standing or seated, with affected side to cassette. With body in true lateral position, flex elbow to place forearm behind head (Fig. 11.39).

Central Ray

Directed 15° caudally through supraclavicular fossa to exit axilla.

Breathing Instructions

Inhale slowly during exposure. For apex of lung, make exposure at full inhalation.

Structures Demonstrated

Shows lateral projection of air-filled trachea and apex of lung closest to film (Fig. 11.40).

Evaluation Criteria

1. Trachea full of air.
2. No rotation, shoulders well separated.
3. Include from midcervical to midthoracic region.

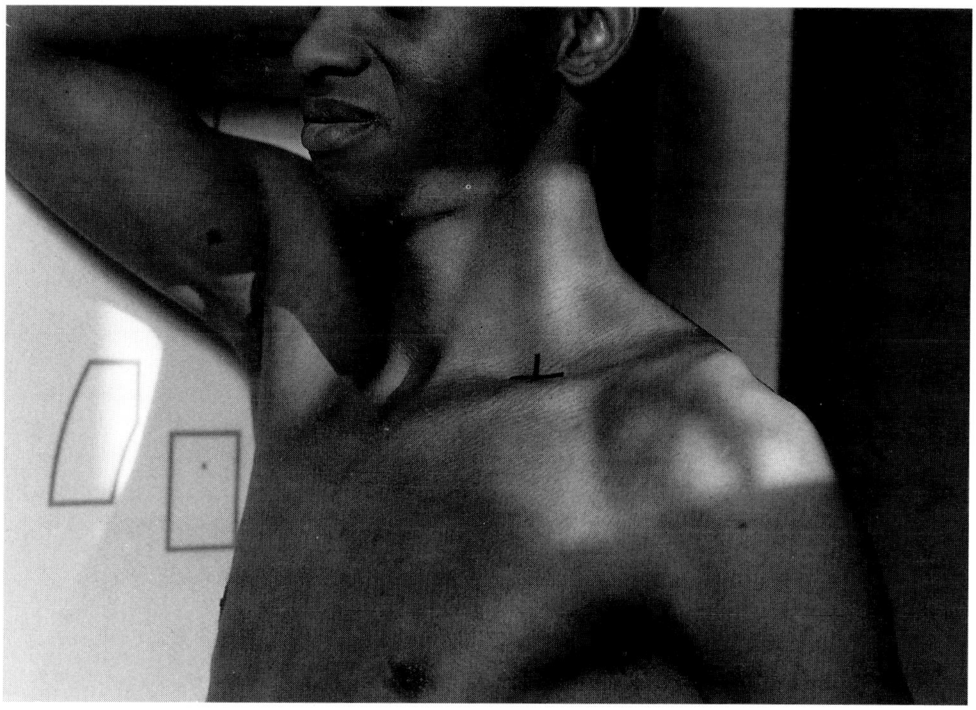

Figure 11.39. Twining's method.

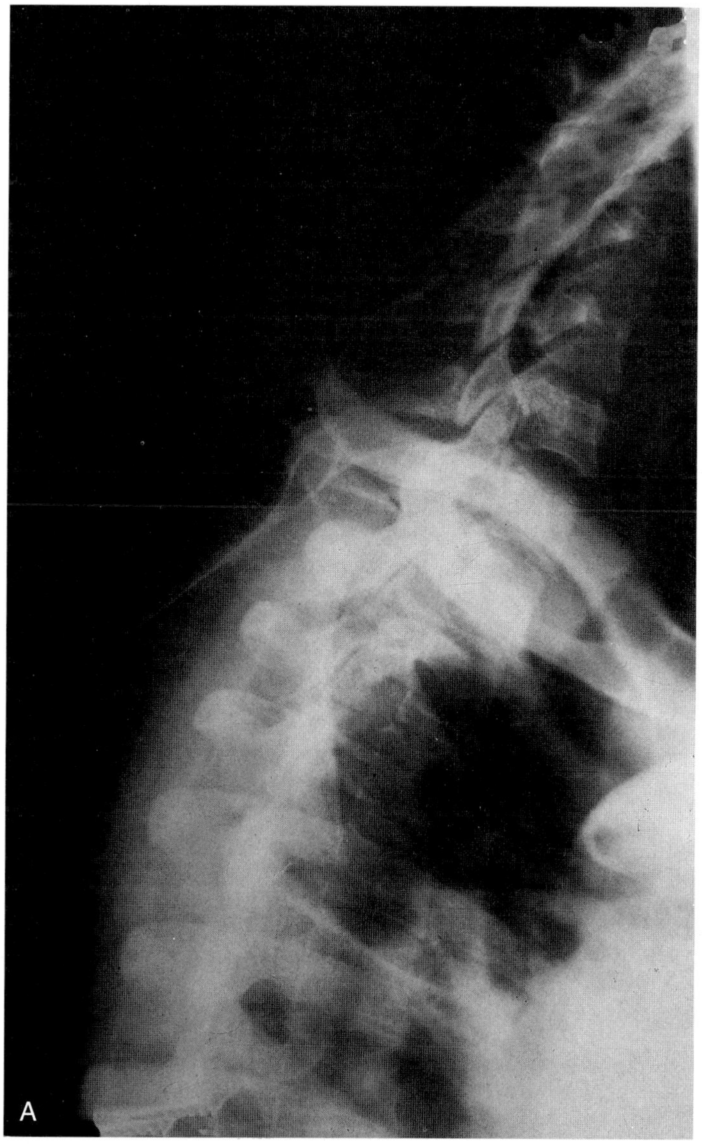

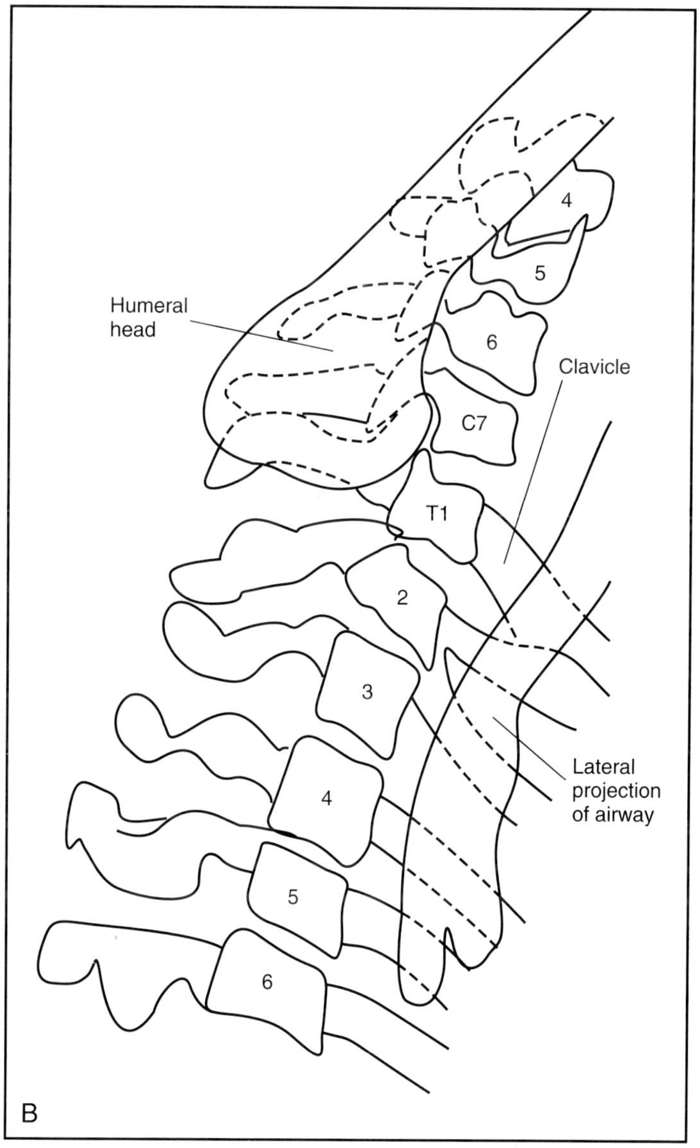

Figure 11.40. A and B, Twining's method.

Chest

Position/Projection

PA projection—erect

Film Size:
14 × 17 inches (35 × 43 cm) lengthwise, Bucky preferred; place top of film 2 inches (5 cm) higher than shoulders. *Exception*: For hypersthenic patients, place film crosswise at level of shoulders

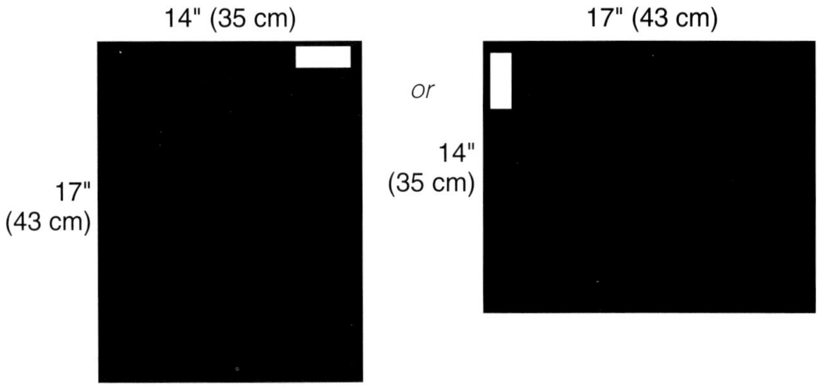

Patient Position

Erect, facing Bucky (Fig. 11.41).

Part Position

Roll shoulders forward, putting hands on hips, palms up, to move scapulae from lung field.

Central Ray

Perpendicular to film at level of T6 for emphasis of heart (midway down length of sternum or 1 inch [2.5 cm] above tip of scapula); FFD: 72 inches (183 cm).

Breathing Instructions

Patient to hold breath on the *second* inhalation. Full expiration is sometimes used (Valsalva's maneuver) to increase size of small pneumothorax, to demonstrate effects of foreign body obstructing air passage to segment of lung, and to show movement of diaphragm. Here, kVp is increased by 5.

Structures Demonstrated

Entire chest cavity with lung field and mediastinal area clearly demonstrated (Fig. 11.42).

Evaluation Criteria

1. Exposure should clearly penetrate and show lung field. 10 posterior ribs should be seen above diaphragm.
2. 1 to 2 inches (2.5 to 5 cm) of lung apex should be seen above clavicles. Heart and diaphragm should show sharp outlines.
3. Costophrenic angles must be included.

NOTE: The PA projection can also be achieved with the patient sitting on a cart (stretcher) (Fig. 11.43). Ideally, a chest unit is used for patient support and the arms are extended around the unit; a cassette held by the patient and elevated with padding on the legs can also be used.

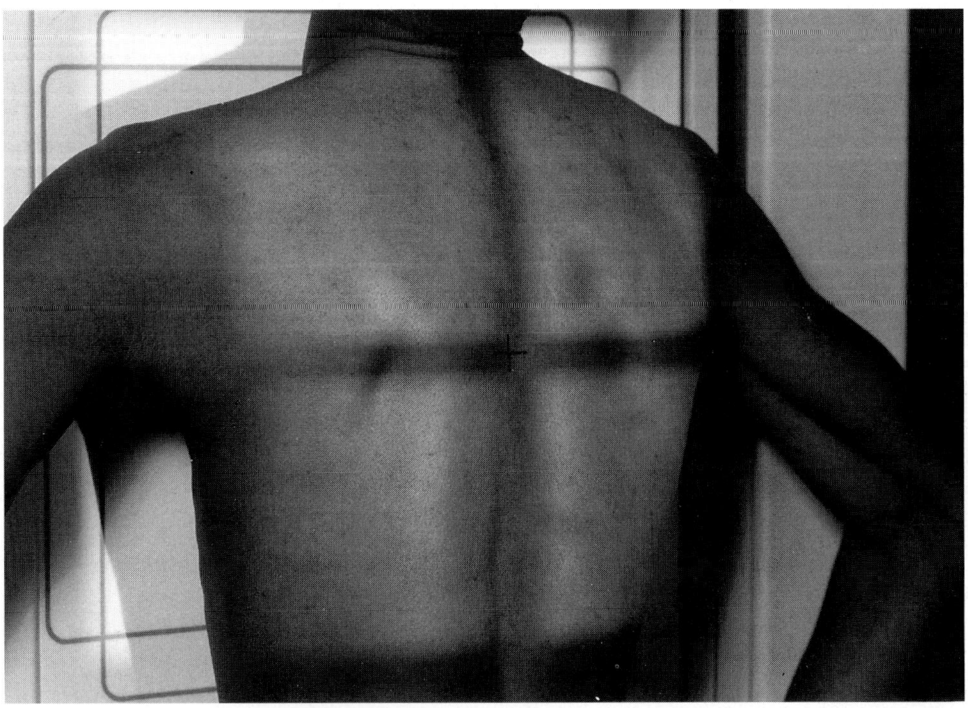

Figure 11.41. PA chest.

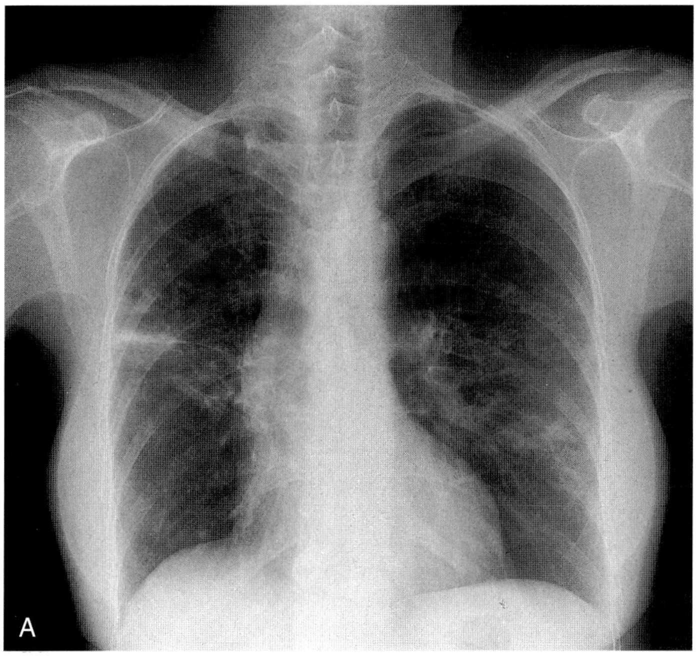

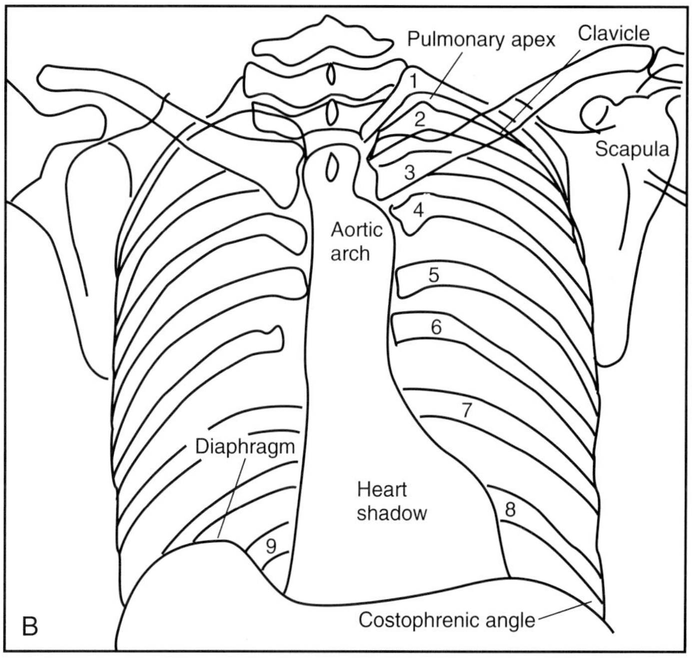

Figure 11.42. A and B, PA chest.

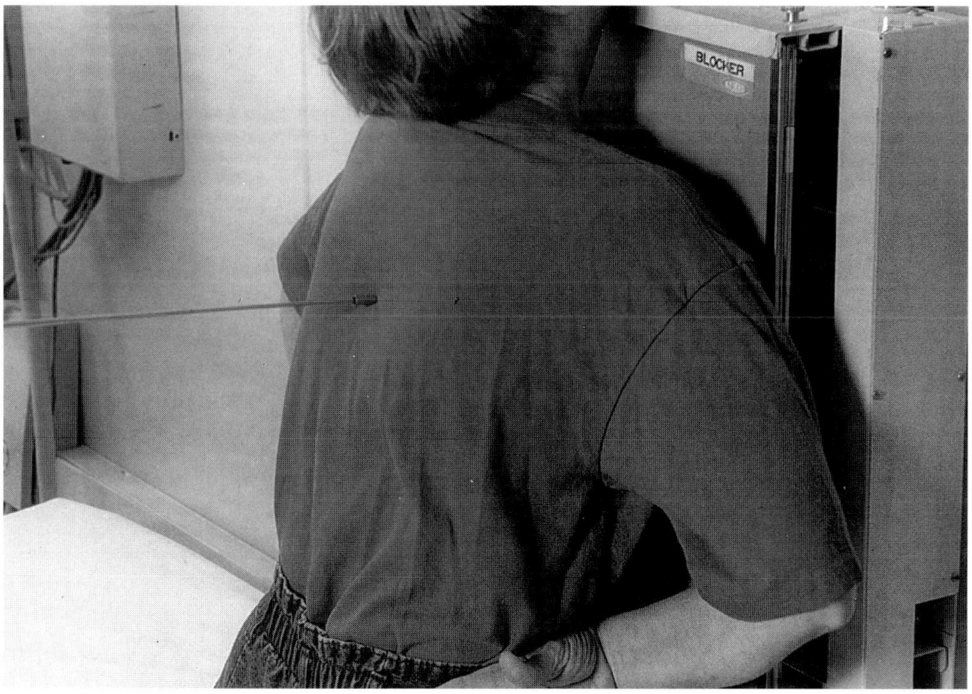

Figure 11.43. PA chest on cart.

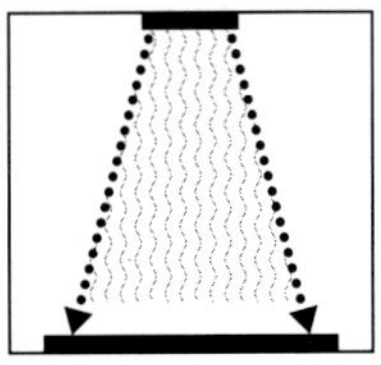

Chest

Position/Projection

AP projection—nonambulatory
Either portable or manual technique with no Bucky

Film Size:
14 × 17 inches (35 × 43 cm) lengthwise

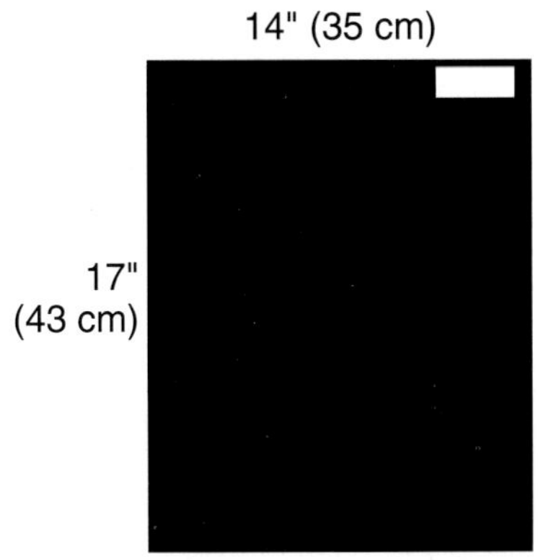

Patient Position

Usually supine (Fig. 11.44).

Part Position

Bring patient as close to erect as condition of patient allows to help demonstrate any pleural effusion. Try to bring shoulders downward and forward with backs of hands below hips, and elbows well forward, if possible. If not, scapulae become superimposed on lateral chest margins increasing radiation absorption.

Central Ray

Perpendicular to film at level of T4 (sternal angle) or T6 (midway length of sternum).

Breathing Instructions

Exposure made on second inhalation. If patient is unresponsive or on respirator, make exposure at fullest stage of inspiration using shortest possible exposure time.

Structures Demonstrated

Similar to PA Chest (Fig. 11.45).

Evaluation Criteria

1. Same criteria as for PA Chest.
2. One additional criterion usually necessary is evaluation to ensure that central ray is perpendicular to film.

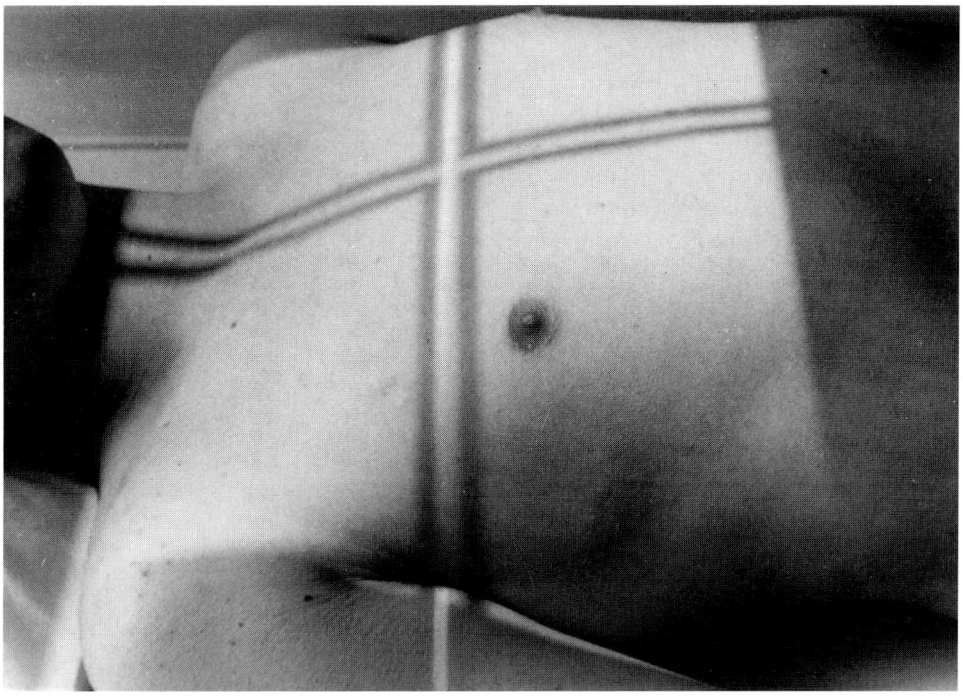

Figure 11.44. AP chest supine.

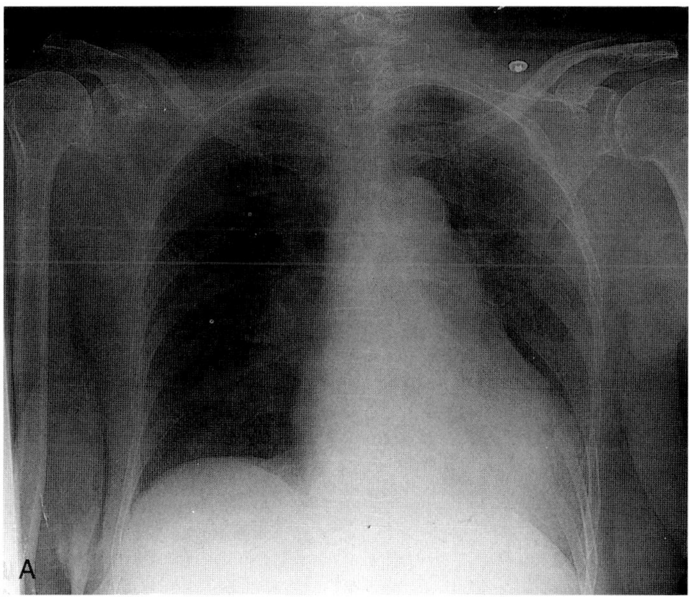

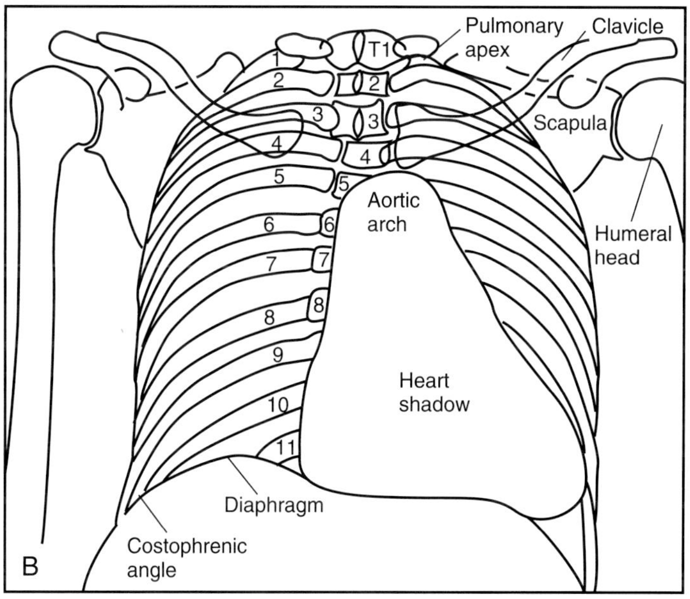

Figure 11.45. A and B, AP chest.

Chest

Position/Projection

Lateral projection—erect

Film Size:
14 × 17 inches (35 × 43 cm) lengthwise

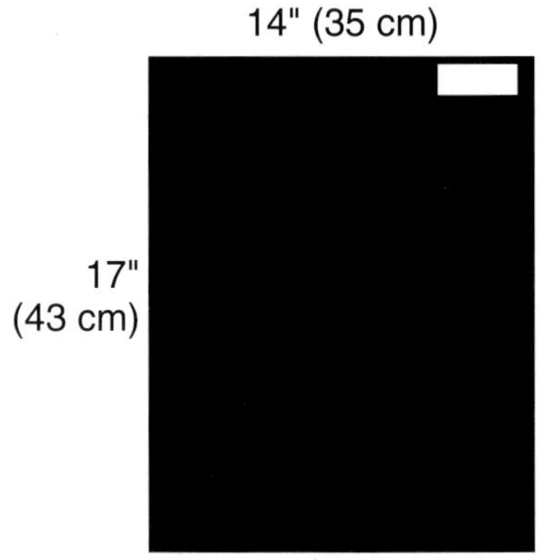

Patient Position

Lateral erect, with left side against vertical grid. Use right side only when demonstrating right lung or if physically impossible to use left side. Place upper border of cassette 1½ inches (4 cm) above shoulders (Fig. 11.46).

Part Position

Have the patient stand squarely with pelvis straight and adjacent shoulder resting against grid. Have patient extend arms up over head and out of thoracic region. Patient may hold on to railing, rest arms on or alongside head, or (less preferred) have arms held up by individual to increase steadiness. Thorax should be centered to midline of grid. Check that all portions of chest will be on film.

Central Ray

Horizontal and perpendicular centered to film at level of T6.

Breathing Instructions

Exposure is made at end of second full inspiration.

Structures Demonstrated

Routinely used to demonstrate heart and aorta and left lung field. Use right lateral to demonstrate right lung field. Demonstrates various lobes and interlobar fissures (Fig. 11.47).

Evaluation Criteria

1. Arm and its soft tissue should be out of upper lung field.
2. Ribs posterior of the vertebral column should be superimposed.
3. Sternum should be truly lateral.
4. Apices and costophrenic angles must be included.
5. Technique should be sufficient to correctly penetrate heart and lung fields.

NOTE: This position can also be performed erect or semierect with the patient sitting on a cart. This position is more easily achieved if the patient can hang her or his legs over the edge of the cart; patient safety must be secured if the procedure is performed in this manner.

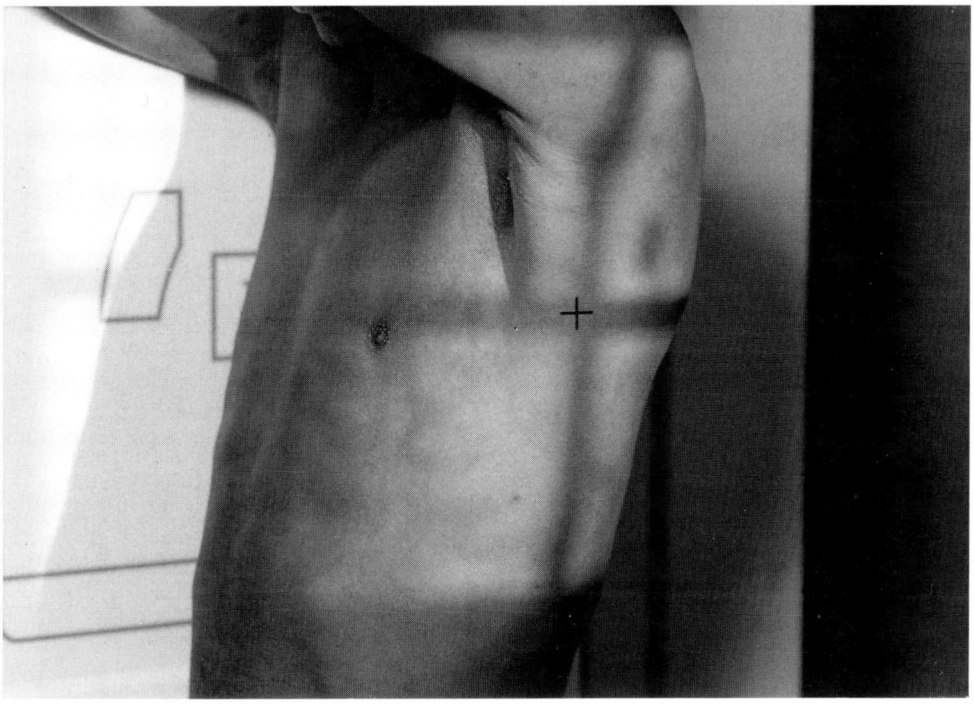

Figure 11.46. Lateral chest.

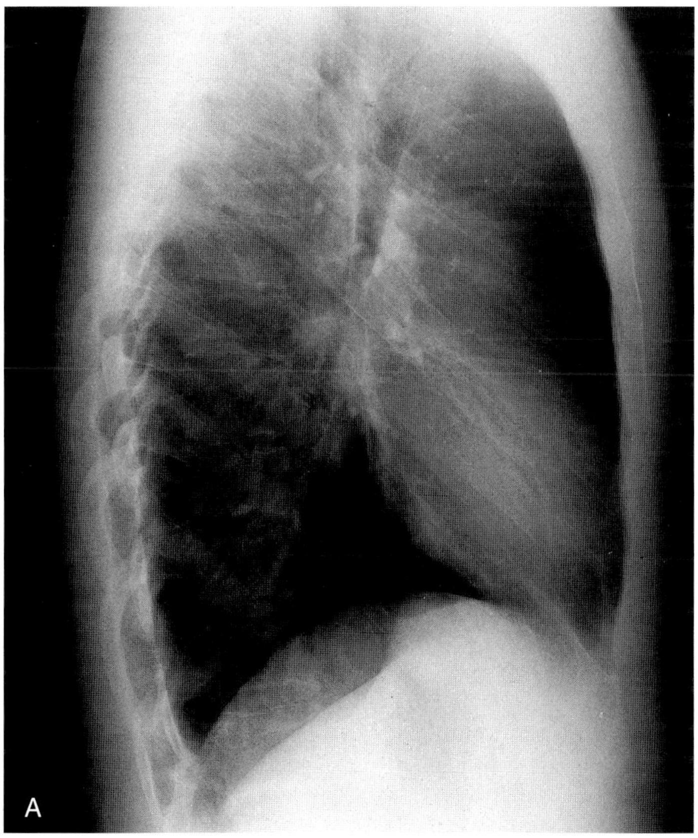

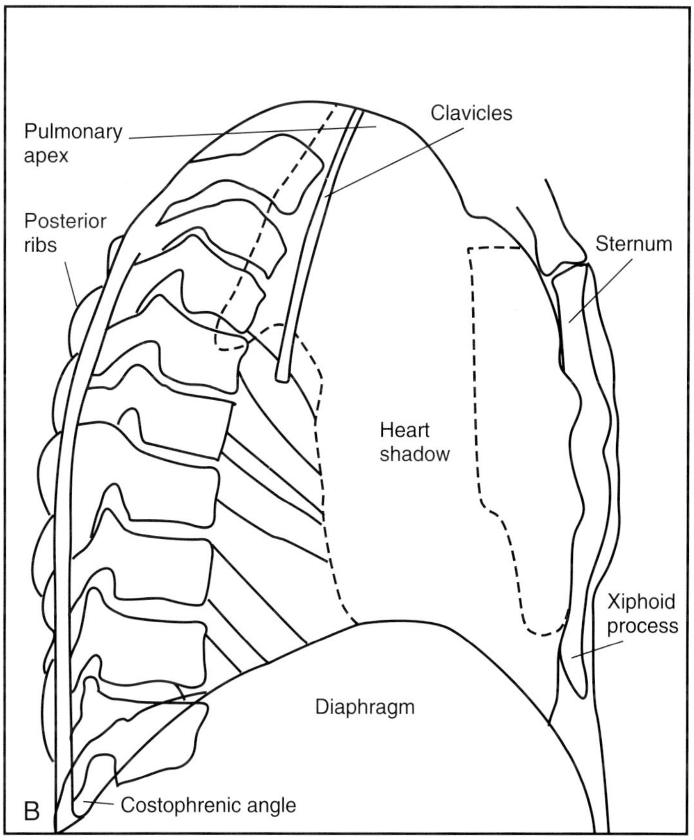

Figure 11.47. A and B, Lateral chest.

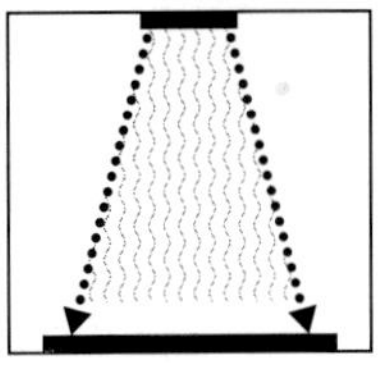

Chest

Position/Projection

Lateral projection—nonambulatory

Film Size:
14 × 17 inches (35 × 43 cm) crosswise

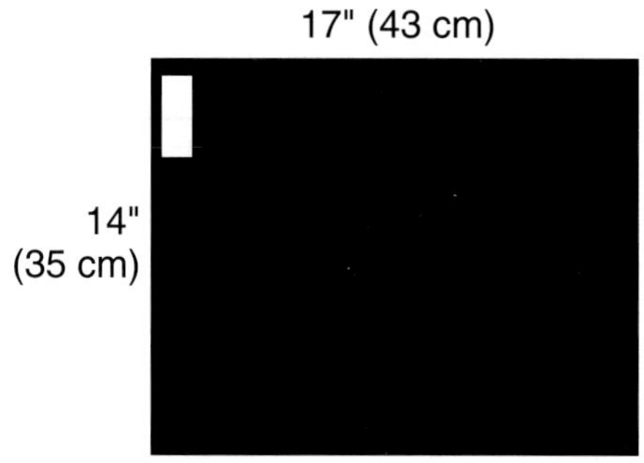

Patient Position

Supine or prone, on film pad or sheets to elevate thorax (Fig. 11.48).

Part Position

Thorax is centered to grid with affected side against grid. Extend arms over patient's head and out of lung fields. Place affected side of thorax as close to grid as possible. Cassette is centered to midaxillary line.

Central Ray

Horizontal and perpendicular to T6.

Breathing Instructions

Same as for Regular Lateral.

Structures Demonstrated

Same as for Regular Lateral and to demonstrate air/fluid levels. If automatic exposure device is used, be sure to center chest to automatic exposure control (Fig. 11.49).

Evaluation Criteria

1. Entire lung fields should be included.
2. Technique should be sufficient to correctly penetrate heart.
3. Evaluation criteria similar to Regular Lateral is used.

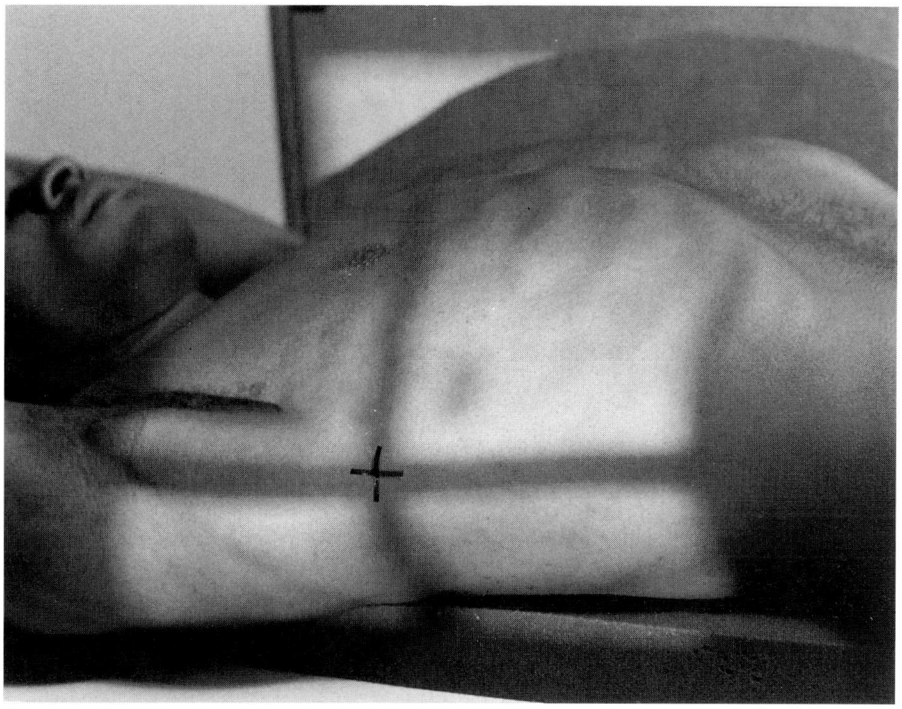

Figure 11.48. Nonambulatory lateral chest.

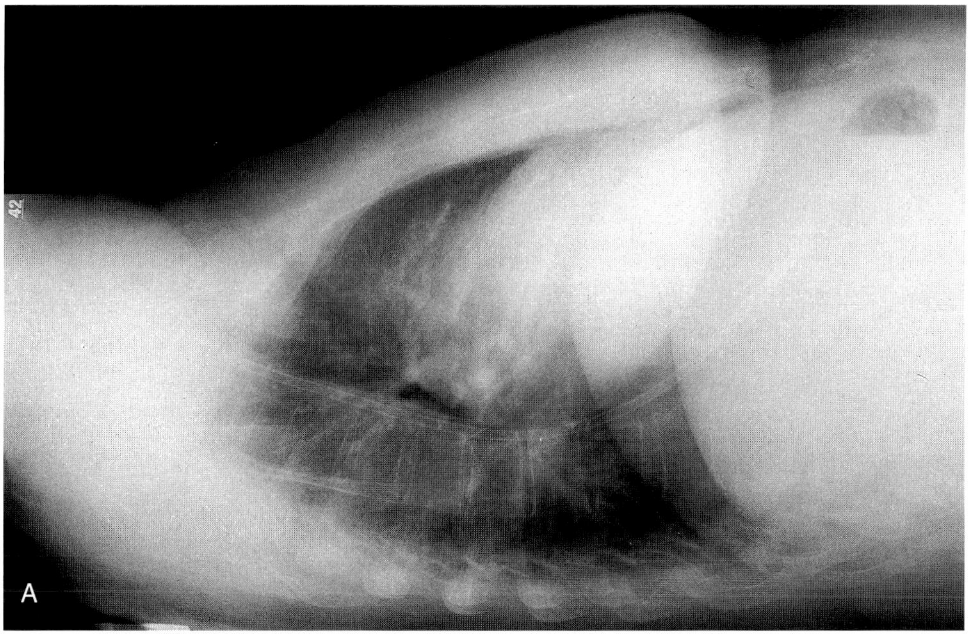

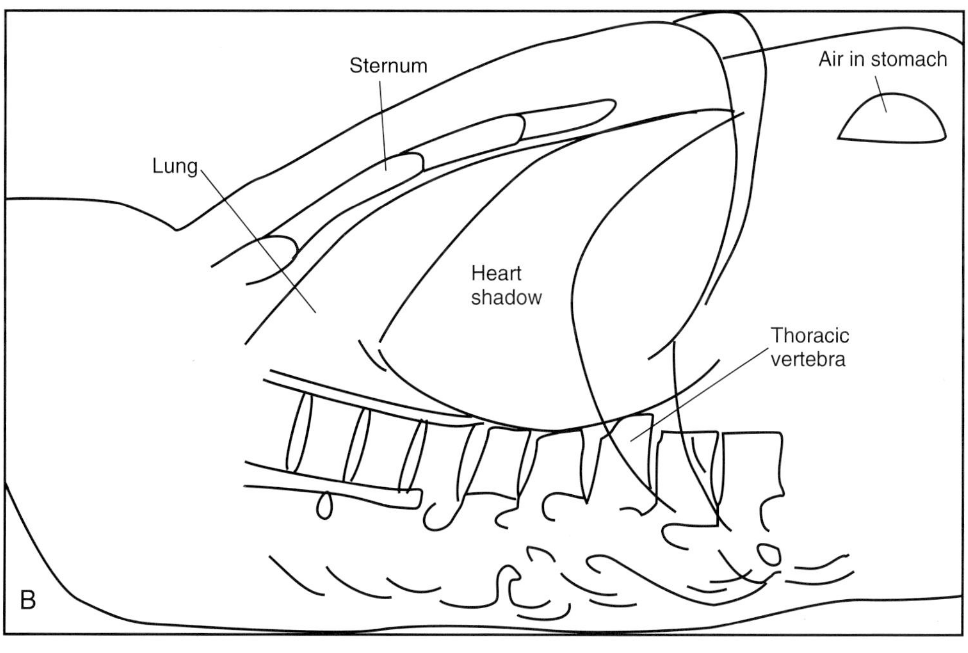

Figure 11.49. A and B, Nonambulatory lateral chest.

Chest

Position/Projection

LAO and RAO PA oblique projections

Film Size:
14 × 17 inches (35 × 43 cm) lengthwise in Bucky

Patient Position

LAO
Start with patient in PA upright position against Bucky. Oblique patient 45° with left anterior side of chest closest to film (Fig. 11.50).

RAO
Start with patient in PA upright position against Bucky. Oblique patient 45° with right anterior side of chest closest to film (Fig. 11.51).

For Both Radiographs
Flex arm closest to film with hand on hip and palm forward. Raise opposite arm and place on patient's head. For obese patients, raise both arms over head to prevent superimposition of soft tissue of arms over costopleural margins.

Part Position

For both projections, position film so its top is 2 to 3 inches (5 to 7.6 cm) above patient's shoulders.

Central Ray

Perpendicular to T6; FFD: 72 inches (183 cm)

Breathing Instructions

Exposure is on full inspiration.

Structures Demonstrated

LAO
Left lung, trachea, bony thorax with heart and aorta in front of vertebral column (Fig. 11.52).

RAO
Right lung, trachea, bony thorax with heart and aorta in front of vertebral column (Fig. 11.53).

Evaluation Criteria

1. On both projections, distance between vertebral column and outer portion of ribs, of dependent side, should be doubled.
2. Both lungs should be demonstrated on each radiograph.

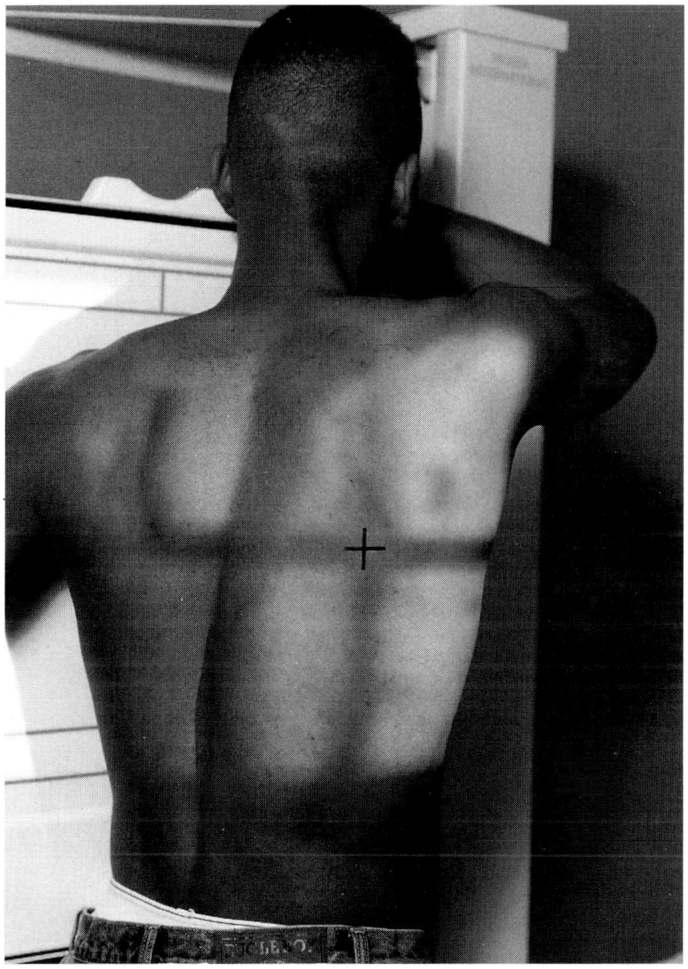

Figure 11.50. PA oblique chest LAO.

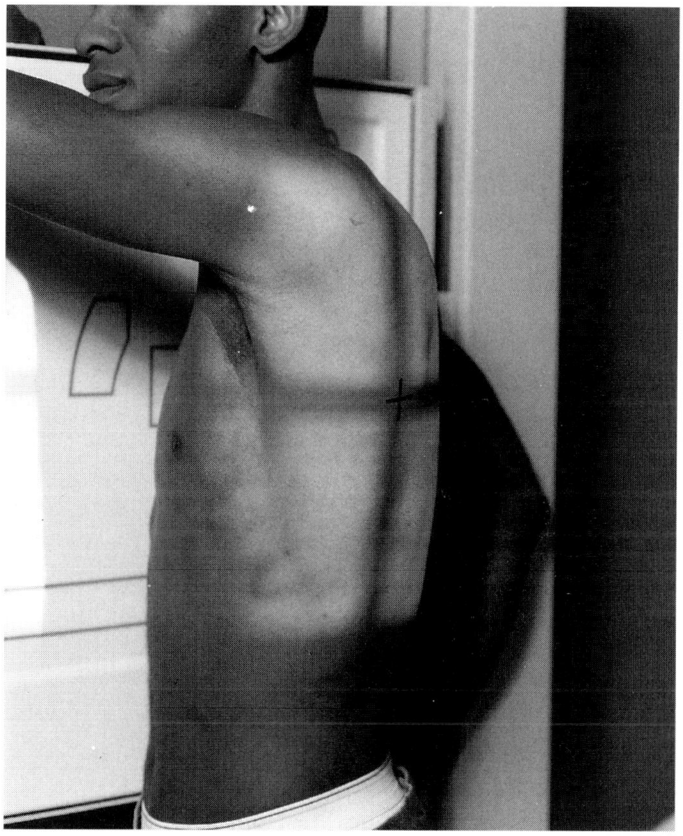

Figure 11.51. PA oblique chest RAO.

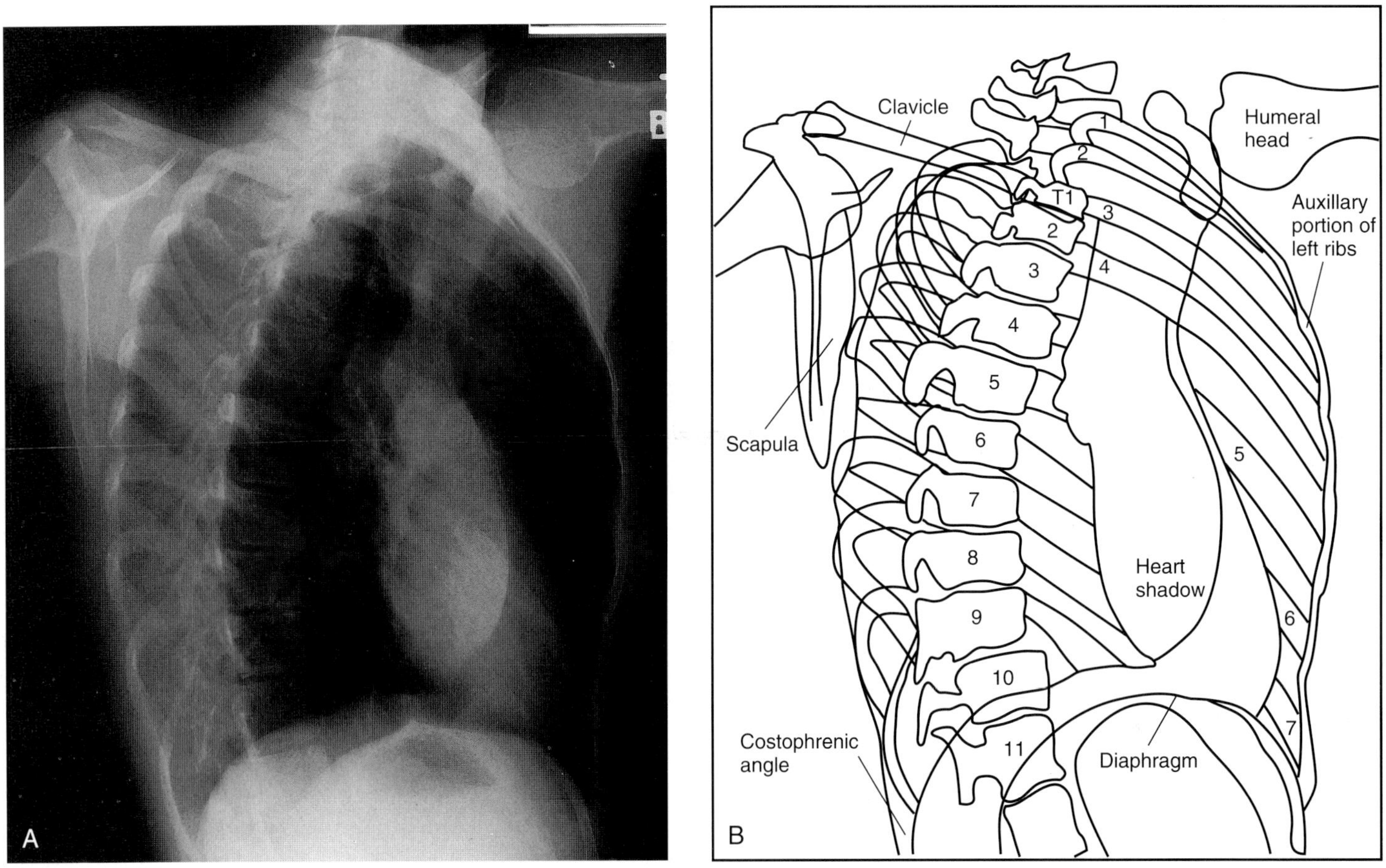

Figure 11.52. A and B, RAO chest.

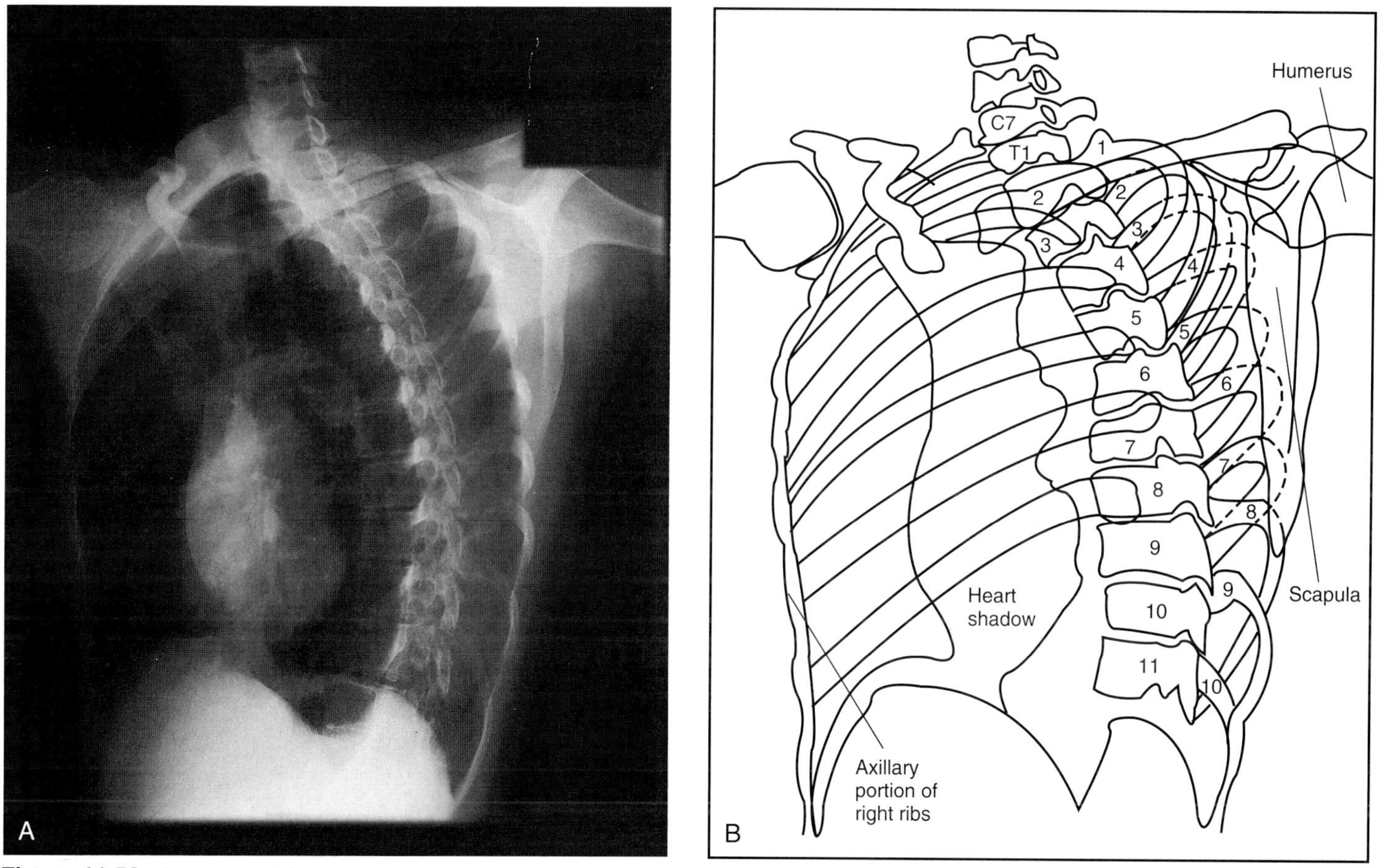

Figure 11.53. A and B, LAO chest.

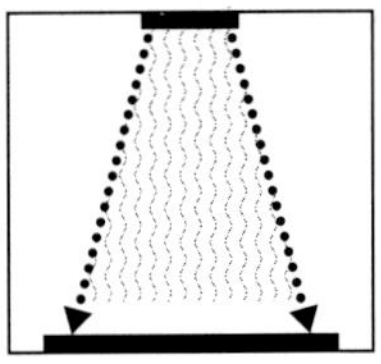

Chest

Position/Projection

LPO and RPO AP oblique projections

Film Size:
14 × 17 inches (35 × 43 cm) lengthwise in Bucky

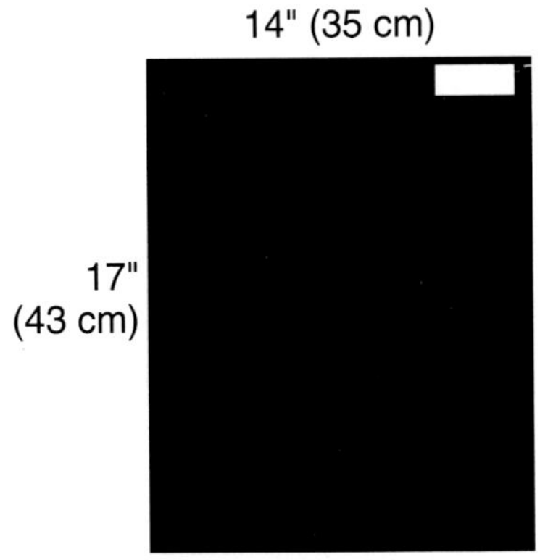

Patient Position

LPO
Start with patient in AP upright position against Bucky. Oblique patient 45° with left posterior shoulder closest to film (Fig. 11.54).

RPO
Start with patient in AP upright position against Bucky. Oblique patient 45° with right posterior shoulder closest to film (Fig. 11.55).

For Both Radiographs
Have patient raise arm adjacent to film device, flex elbow, and rest hand on device.

Part Position

For both projections, position film so its top is 2 to 3 inches (5 to 7.6 cm) above patient's shoulders.

Central Ray

Perpendicular to T6; FFD: 72 inches (183 cm).

Breathing Instructions

Exposure is on full inspiration.

Structures Demonstrated

LPO
Left lung, trachea, bony thorax with heart and aorta in front of vertebral column (Fig. 11.56).

RPO
Right lung, trachea, bony thorax with heart and aorta in front of vertebral column (Fig. 11.57).

Evaluation Criteria

1. On both projections, distance between vertebral column and outer portion of ribs, or dependent side, should be doubled.
2. Both lungs should be demonstrated on each radiograph.

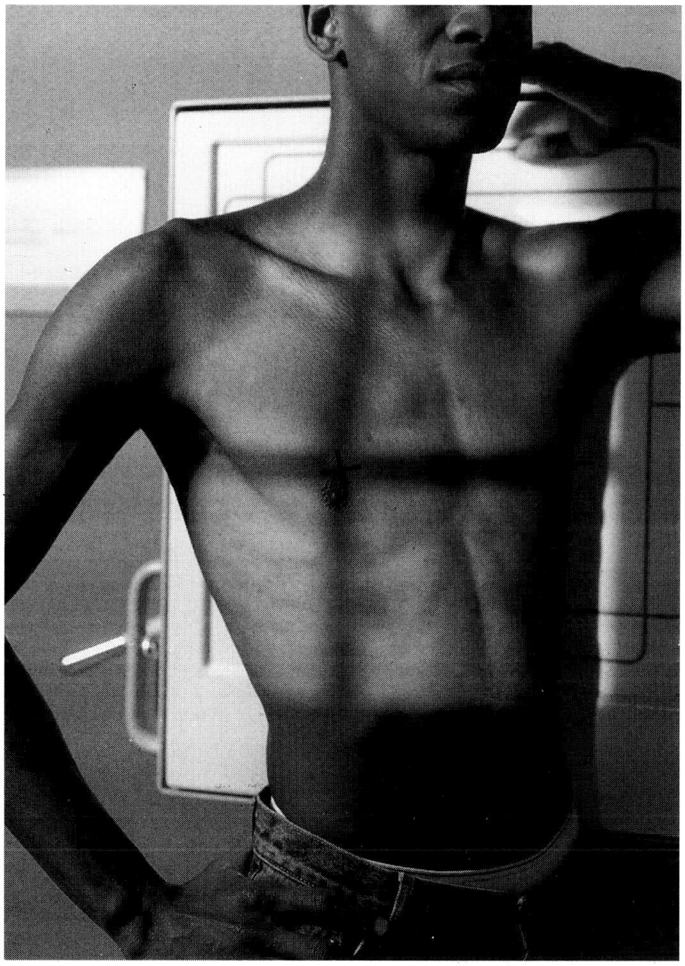

Figure 11.54. AP oblique chest LPO.

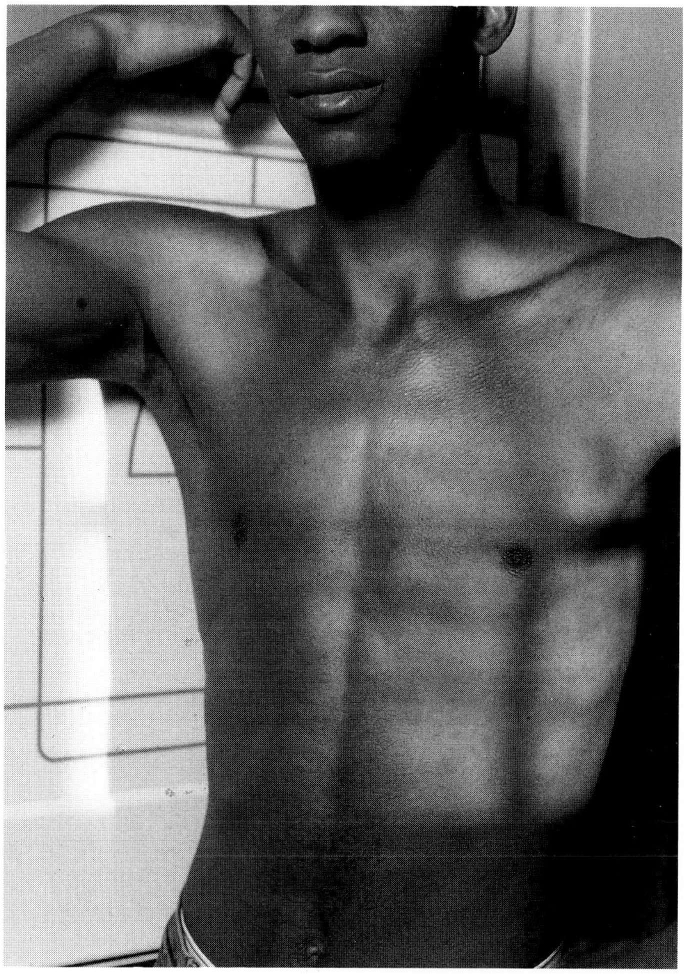

Figure 11.55. AP oblique chest RPO.

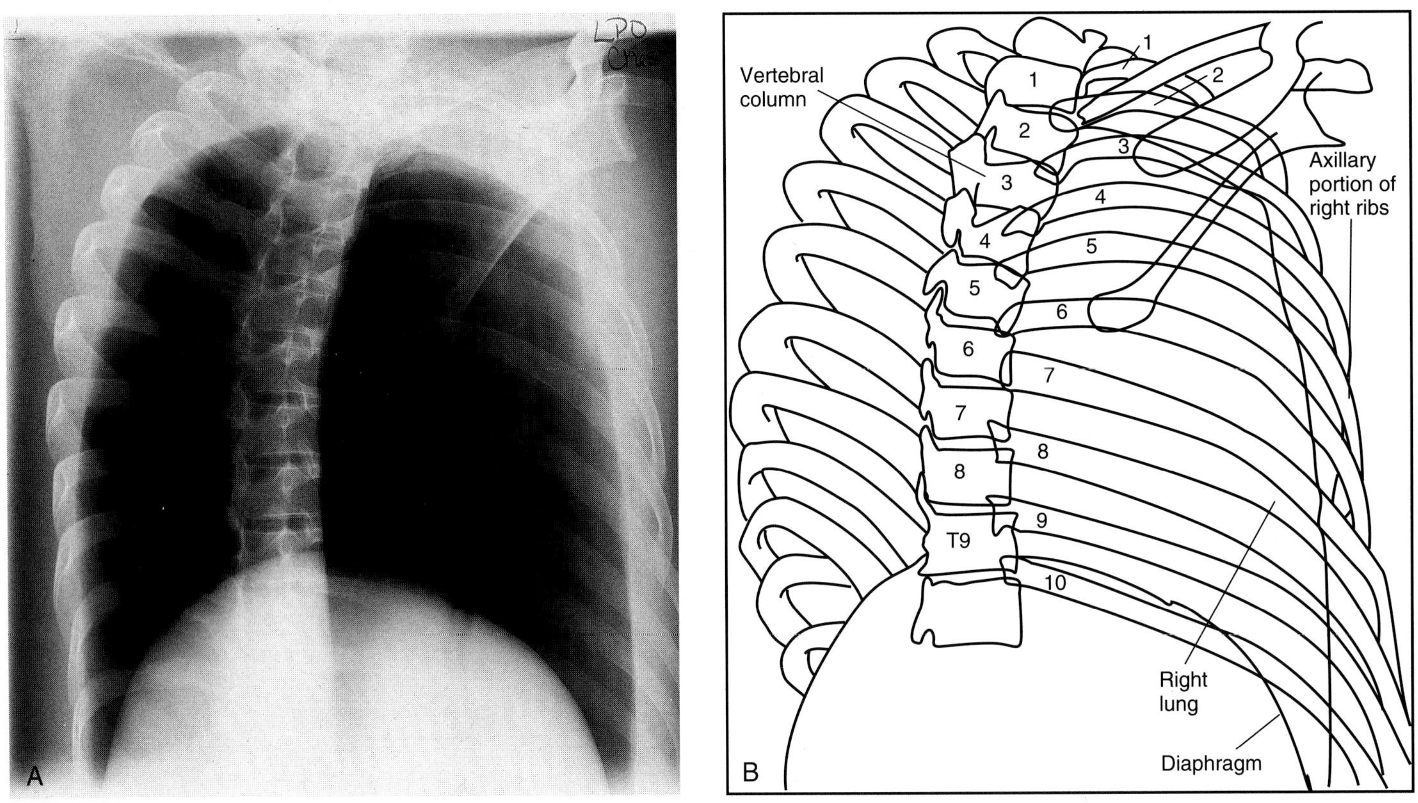

Figure 11.56. A and B, LPO chest.

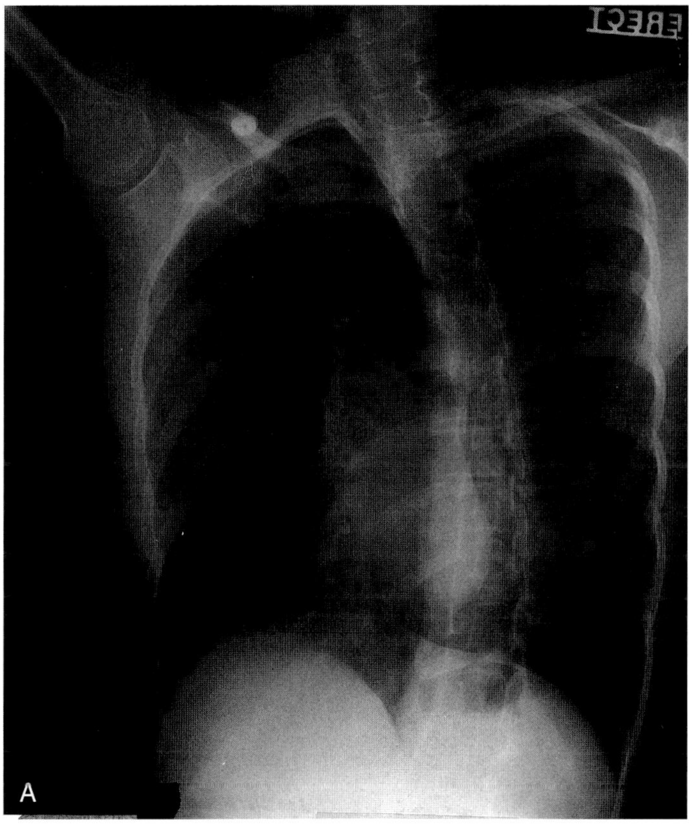

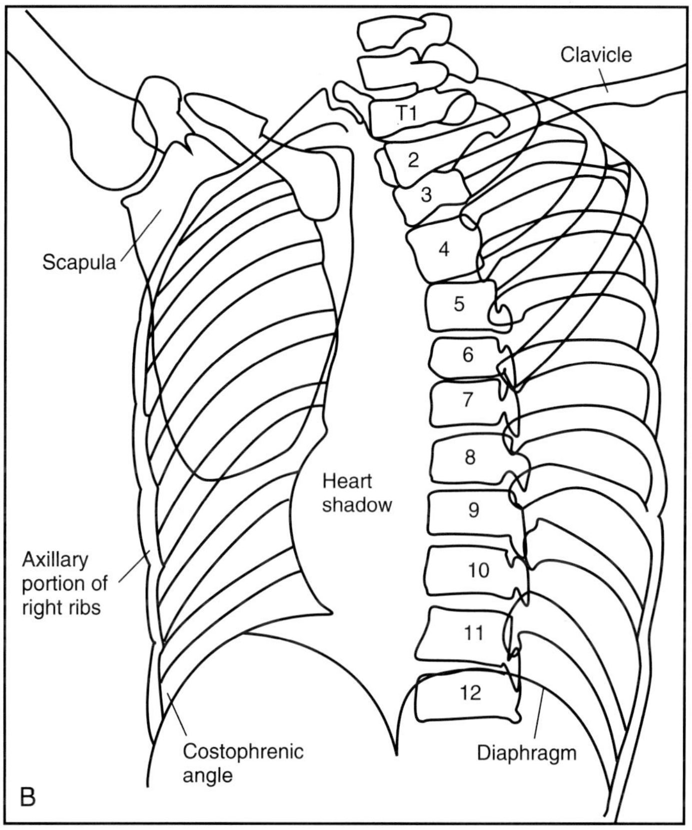

Figure 11.57. A and B, RPO chest.

Cardiac Barium Studies

Position/Projection

PA projection; left lateral projection; RAO projection; LAO projection

Film Size:
14 × 17 inches (35 × 43 cm) lengthwise

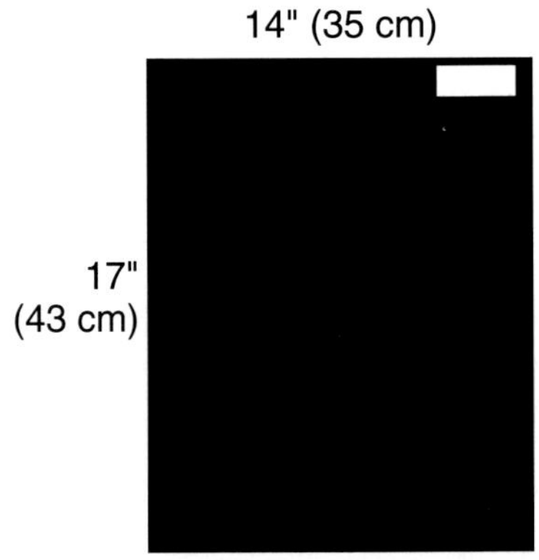

NOTE: Barium swallows are performed using a thickened mixture of barium sulfate. The thick consistency is used so that the mixture will adhere to the walls of the esophagus, permitting it to descend slowly. Any pathological disease that results in the enlargement of the heart or aorta will produce abnormal impressions on the esophagus (shown as a thinning or flattened area on a barium-filled esophagus). Also, the enhanced esophagus better demonstrates heart borders. Therefore, different borders of the heart can be seen depending on the position used. PA oblique positions demonstrate the side farthest from the film. The PA and left lateral positions are performed as described for regular chest radiography.

Patient Position

Upright, seated or standing. If routine chest or separation of aorta and spine are desired, place patient in PA position and have him or her rotate body so that thorax is 45° from plane of film with desired side away from film. However, if heart and great vessel are of interest, adjust rotation of patient to 55 or 60° (Figs. 11.58 and 11.59).

Part Position

Have patient relax and drop arm closest to film while elevating other arm (on side of interest). Be sure to have patient sit or stand as straight as possible, distributing his or her weight evenly. To ensure proper centering, adjust the film cassette so that it projects about 2 inches (5 cm) above upper margin of shoulders.

Central Ray

Directed midway between spine and outside of body (side farthest from film) at level of T6 (heart).

Breathing Instructions

In advance, instruct patient to take several rapid swallows of barium mixture, holding third mouthful in mouth without swallowing. Instruct patient to take one deep breath, hold it on full inspiration, and then swallow. Exposure is made as patient swallows (Fig. 11.60).

Structures Demonstrated

RAO

RAO demonstrates esophagus' anterior border, aortic arch, pulmonary artery, left main bronchus, left atrium, trachea, entire left branch of bronchial tree and anterior portion of apex of left verticle (Fig. 11.61).

LAO

LAO demonstrates trachea and its bifurcation, right branch of bronchial tree, descending aorta, aortic arch, pulmonary artery, and foreshortened right lung.

Evaluation Criteria

1. Lungs should be fully expanded and included in their entirety.
2. Lung markings should be clearly demonstrated.
3. Lung closest to film should be foreshortened.
4. Side farthest from film should have twice the distance from its outer border to spine as is seen on side closest.

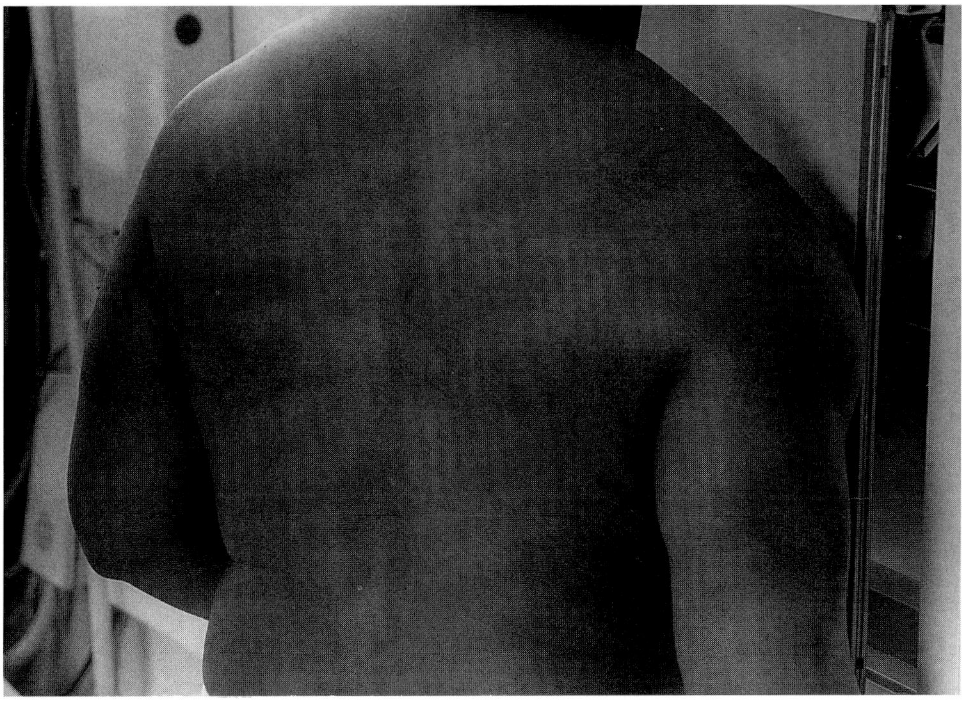

Figure 11.58. RAO cardiac study.

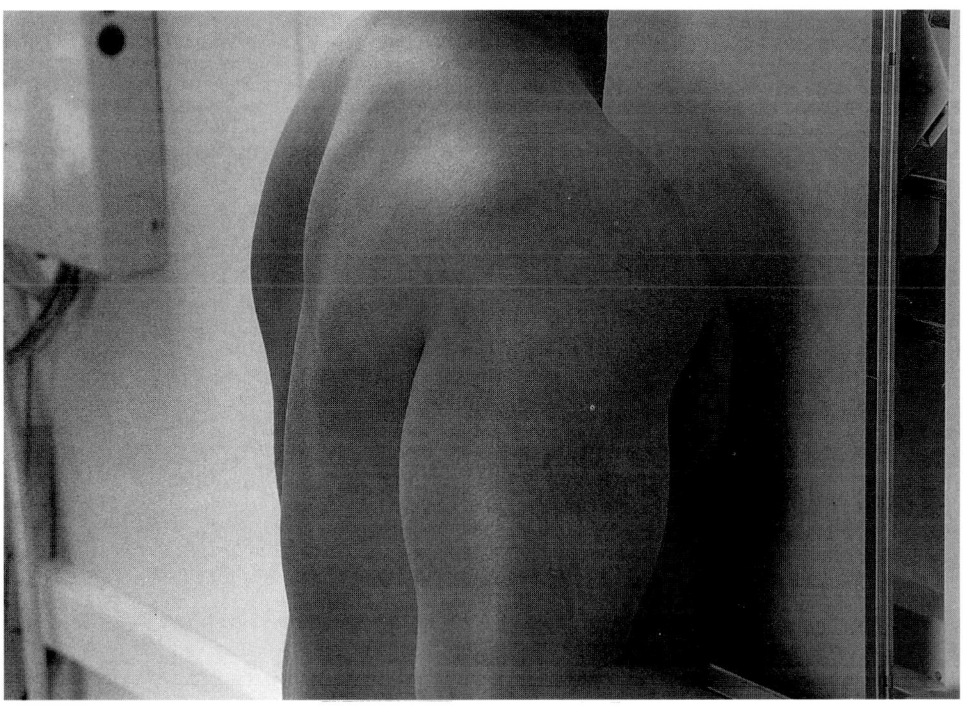

Figure 11.59. LAO cardiac study.

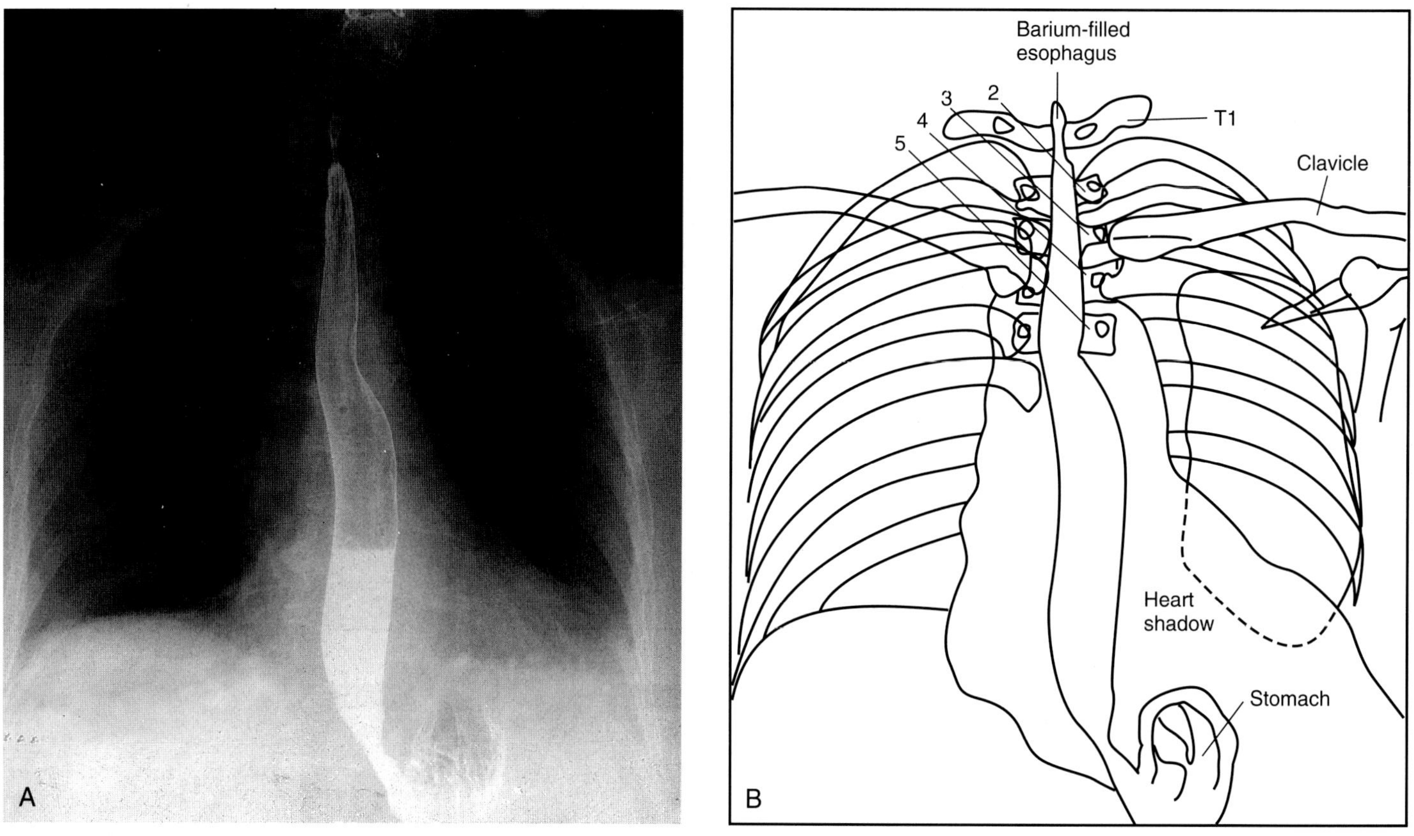

Figure 11.60. A and B, PA chest with barium.

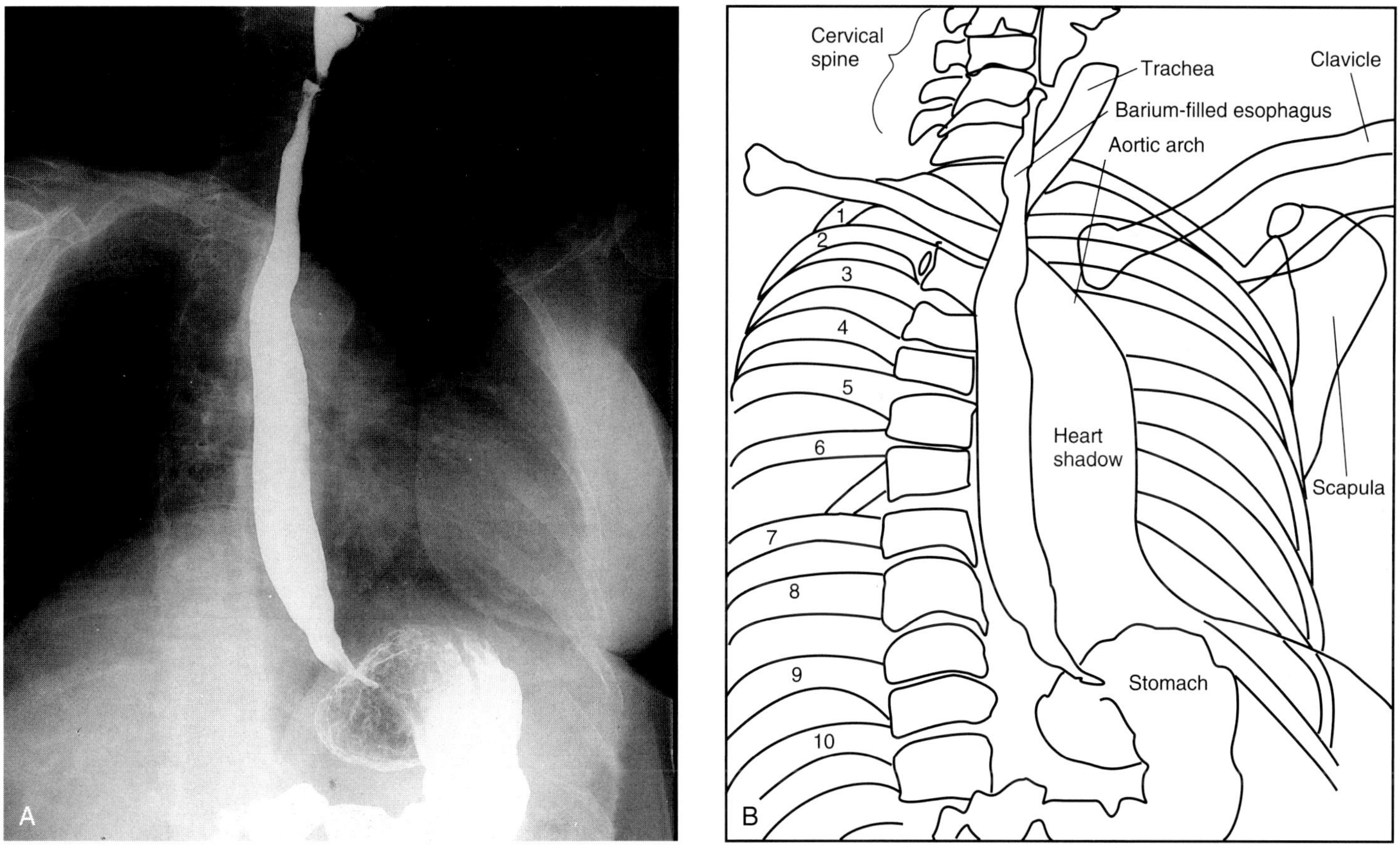

Figure 11.61. A and B, RAO chest with barium.

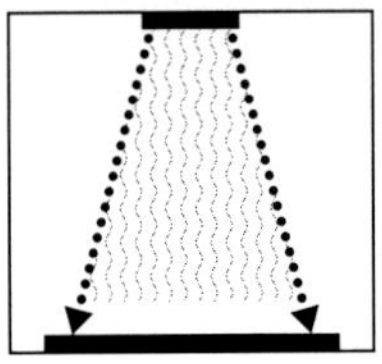

Pulmonary Apices

Position/Projection

PA axial projection

Film Size:
10 × 12 inches (24 × 30 cm) crosswise in Bucky

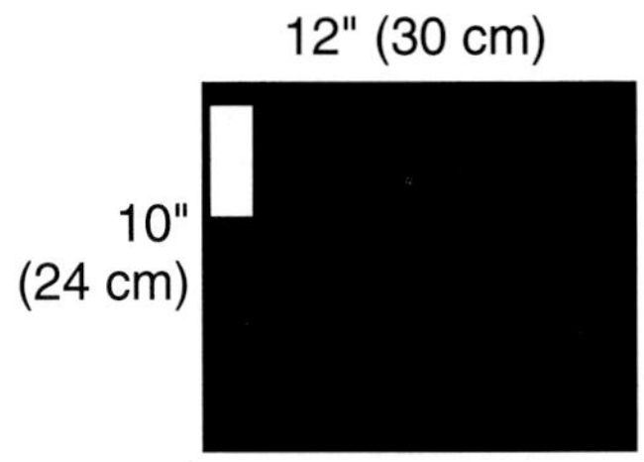

Patient Position

Erect and prone against upright Bucky (Fig. 11.62).

Central Ray

Directed at 15° cephalad angle to T3. FFD: 72 inches (183 cm).

Breathing Instructions

Expose on full inhalation.

Structures Demonstrated

On PA projection, demonstrates apices above clavicles. Good projection to detect tumors or masses in upper chest region (Fig. 11.63).

Evaluation Criteria

1. Apices should be well visualized (penetrated). Manual technique preferred.
2. Clavicles should lie below apices.
3. Only upper lung region needs to be demonstrated.
4. Be sure there is no rotation by having medial portions of clavicles equidistant from each other.

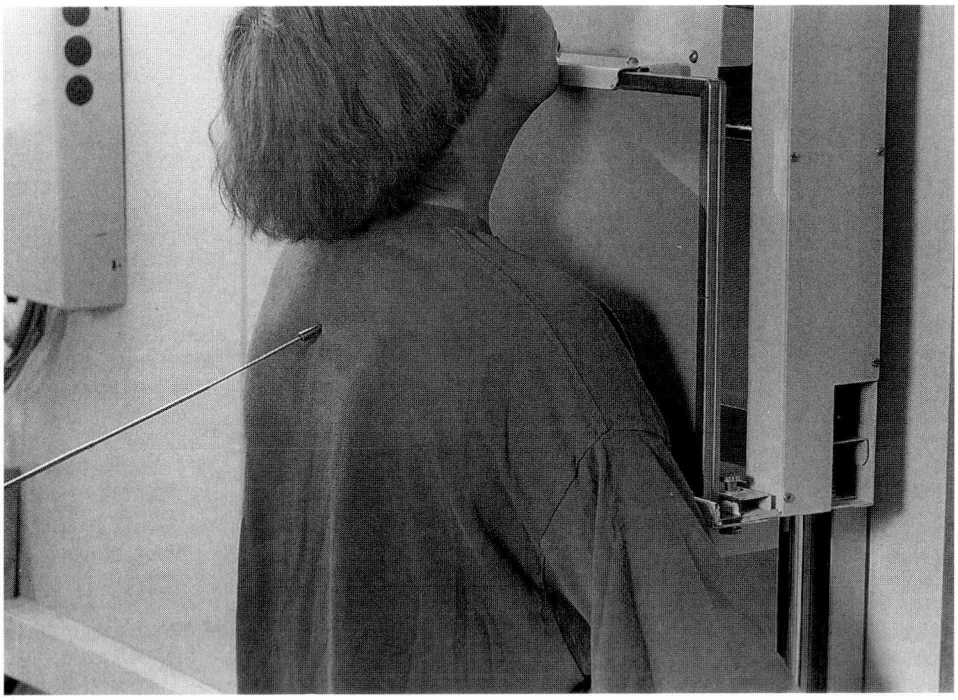

Figure 11.62. PA axial pulmonary apices.

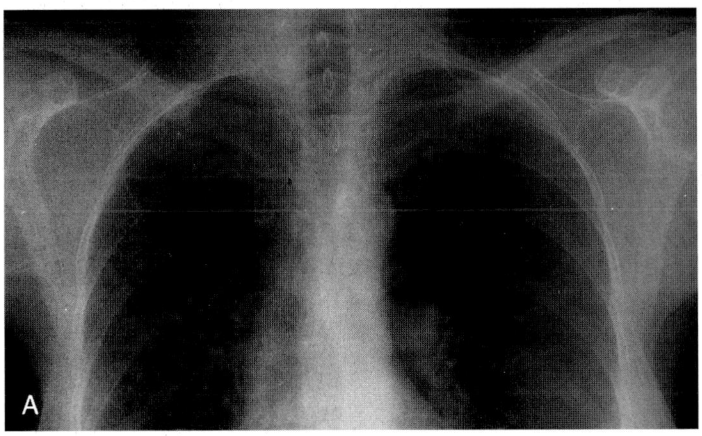

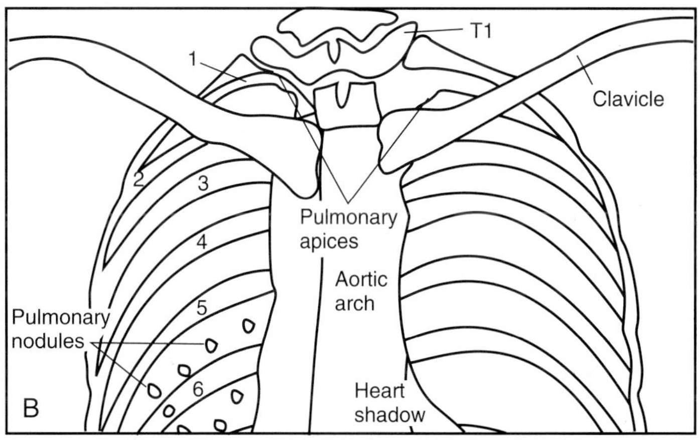

Figure 11.63. A and B, PA axial projection for pulmonary apices.

Pulmonary Apices

Position/Projection

AP axial projection

Film Size:
10 × 12 inches (24 × 30 cm) crosswise in Bucky

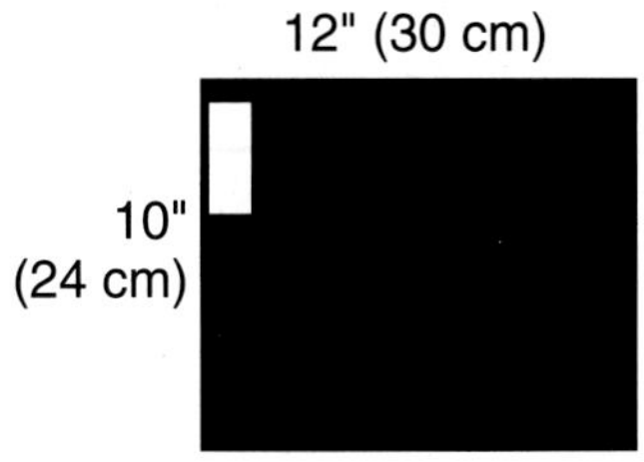

Patient Position

Erect and supine against upright Bucky (Fig. 11.64).

Central Ray

Directed 15° cephalad to T3. FFD: 72 inches (183 cm).

Breathing Instructions

Expose on full inhalation.

Structures Demonstrated

On AP projection, demonstrates apices below clavicles (Fig. 11.65).

Evaluation Criteria

1. Same as for PA projection except that clavicles are above apices, superimposing 1st and 2nd ribs.
2. Ribs should have distorted look.

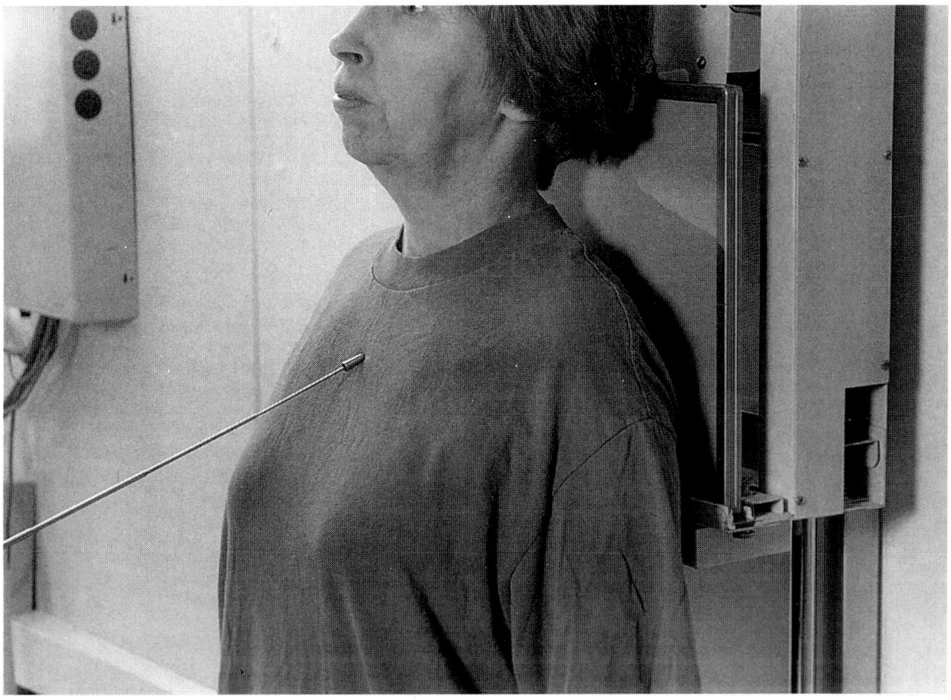

Figure 11.64. AP axial pulmonary apices.

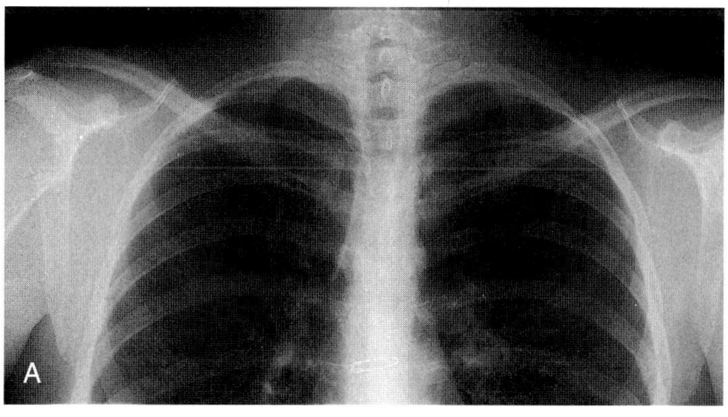

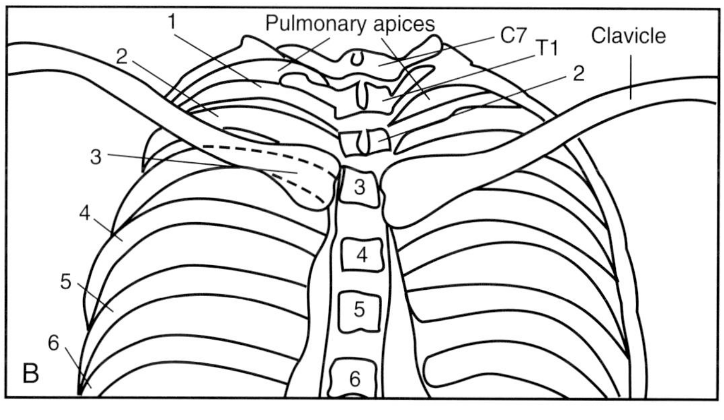

Figure 11.65. A and B, AP axial projection for pulmonary apices.

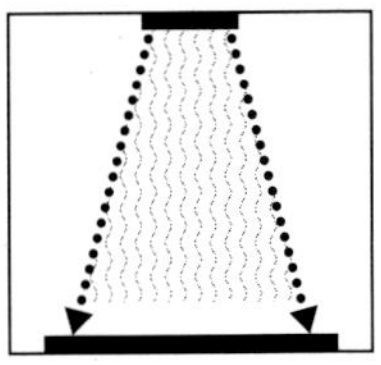

Lungs

Position/Projection

AP lordotic projections—Lindblom's method

Film Size:
14 × 17 inches (35 × 43 cm) film lengthwise

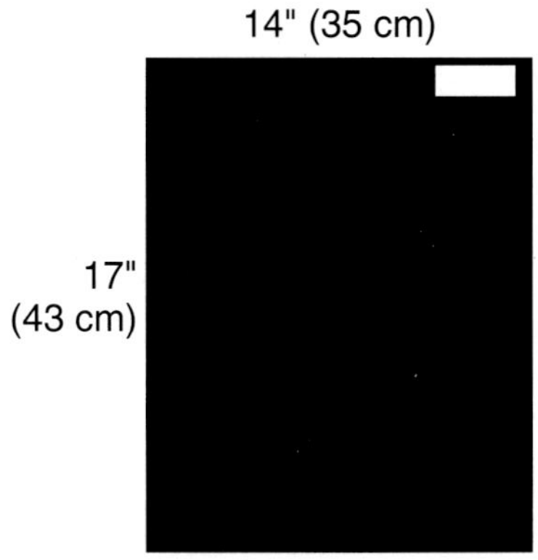

Patient Position

AP position, 1 foot (30 cm) in front of vertical grid device. Adjust height of cassette so upper margin of film is about 1½ inches (4 cm) above upper border of shoulders when patient is adjusted in lordotic position (Figs. 11.66 and 11.67).

Part Position

Adjust patient in AP position, with midsagittal plane centered to midline of grid. Have patient flex elbows and place hands, palms out, on hips. Have patient lean backward in extreme lordosis and rest shoulders against vertical grid device.

Breathing Instructions

Make exposure at end of full inhalation.

Central Ray

Directed horizontally, centered to midsternum.

Structures Demonstrated

AP axial to demonstrate apices and such conditions as interlobar effusions (Figs. 11.68 and 11.69).

Evaluation Criteria

1. Clavicles should lie superior to apices.
2. Sternal ends of clavicles should be equidistant.
3. Apices and lungs should be included in their entirety.

NOTE: Another AP lordotic method involves placing the patient flat against the grid, using a 20° cephalic angle centered midsagittally at the level of the sternoclavicular notch at T2–T3.

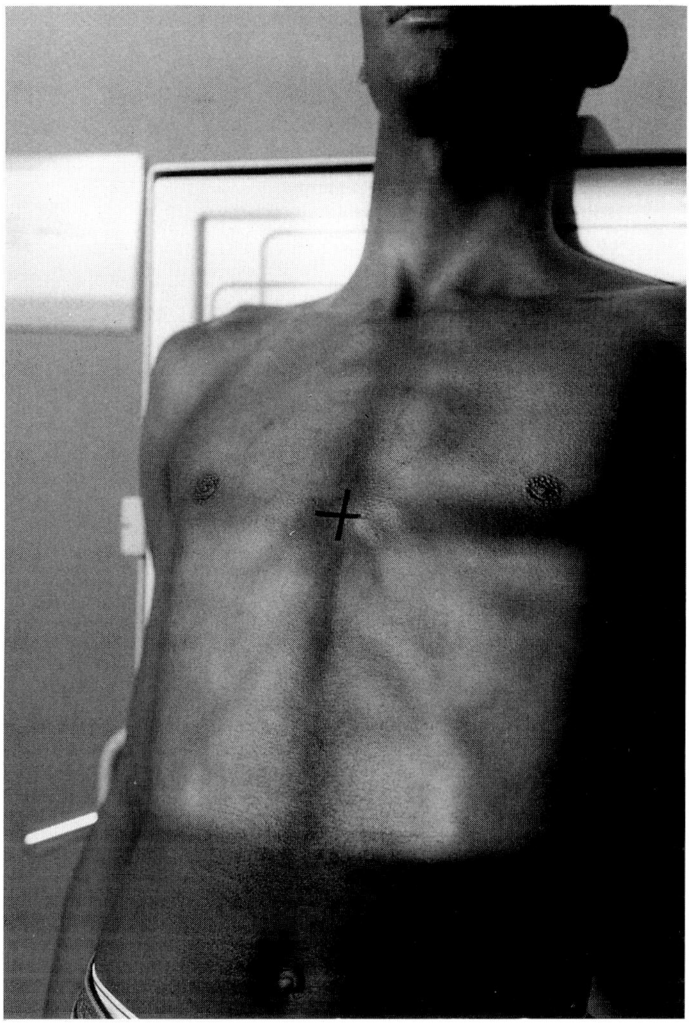

Figure 11.66. AP lordotic — Lindblom's method.

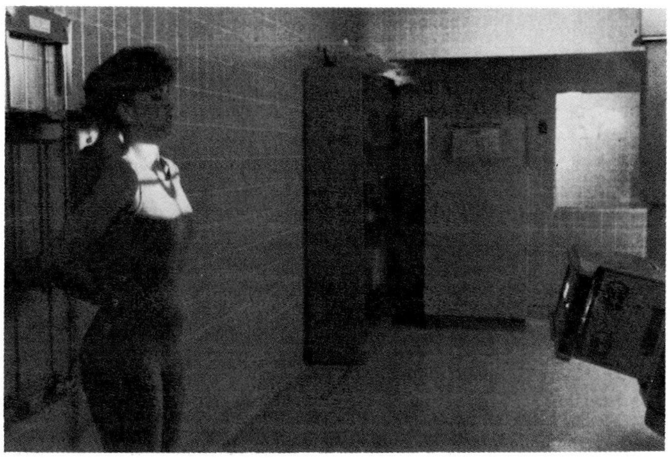

Figure 11.67. Alternate to Figure 11.66. (From Hagler MJ: The Pocket Rad Tech. Philadelphia: WB Saunders, 1993, p 29.)

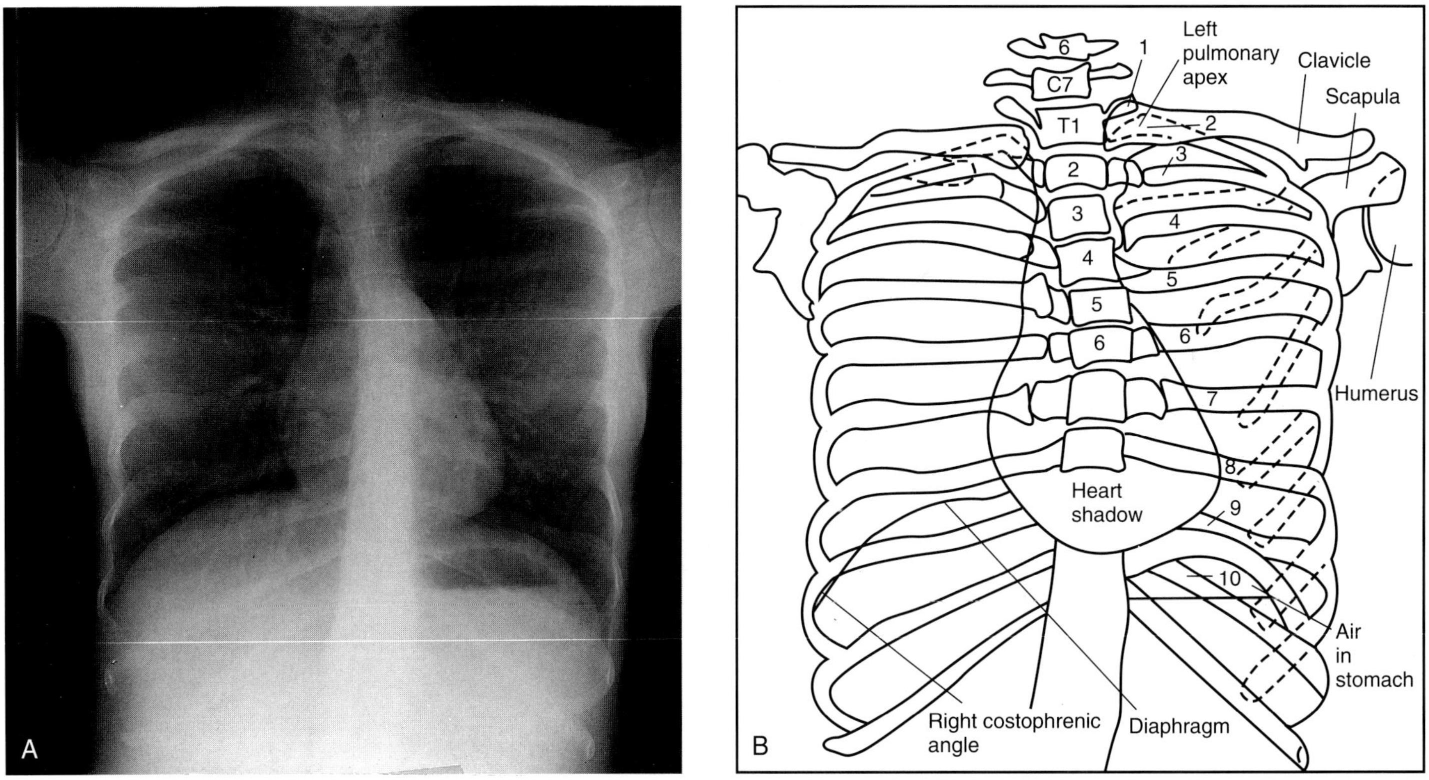

Figure 11.68. A and B, AP lordotic.

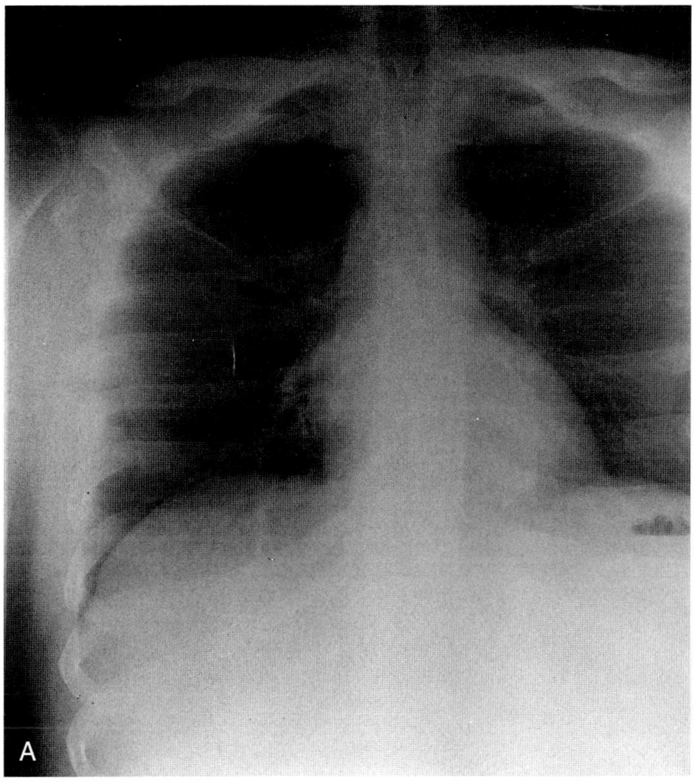

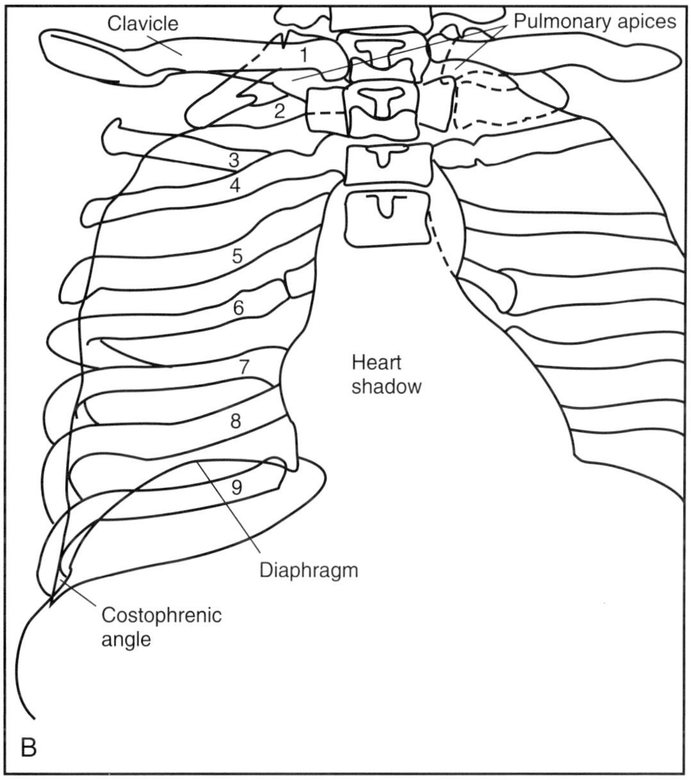

Figure 11.69. A and B, AP lordotic—modified.

Lungs

Position/Projection

PA lordotic projection—Fleischner's method

Film Size:
14 × 17 inches (35 × 43 cm) lengthwise

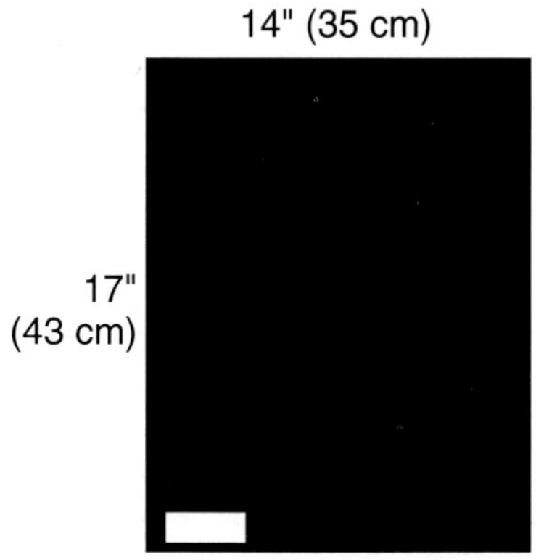

Patient Position

PA position before vertical grid device. Adjust height of cassette so upper margin of film is about 1 inch (2.5 cm) below upper borders of shoulders when patient is standing upright. With patient in lordotic position, lung should be correctly projected (Fig. 11.70).

Part Position

Center midsagittal plane of body to midline of grid. Have patient grasp grid device, brace abdomen against it and then lean backward in extreme lordosis. Thorax should be inclined posteriorly approximately 45°.

Central Ray

Directed horizontally to T4.

Breathing Instructions

Make exposure at end of full inhalation.

Structures Demonstrated

PA projection of lungs demonstrates magnified interlobar effusion (Fig. 11.71).

Evaluation Criteria

1. Clavicles should lie superior to apices.
2. Sternal ends of clavicles should be equidistant from vertebral column.
3. Apices and lungs should be included in their entirety.

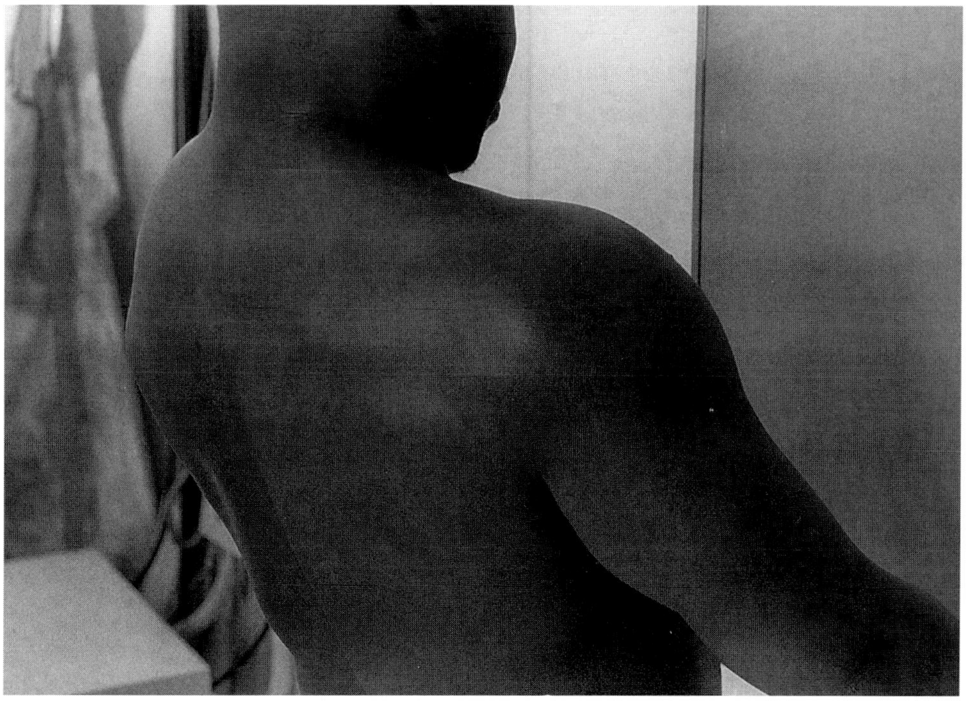

Figure 11.70. PA lordotic—Fleischner's method.

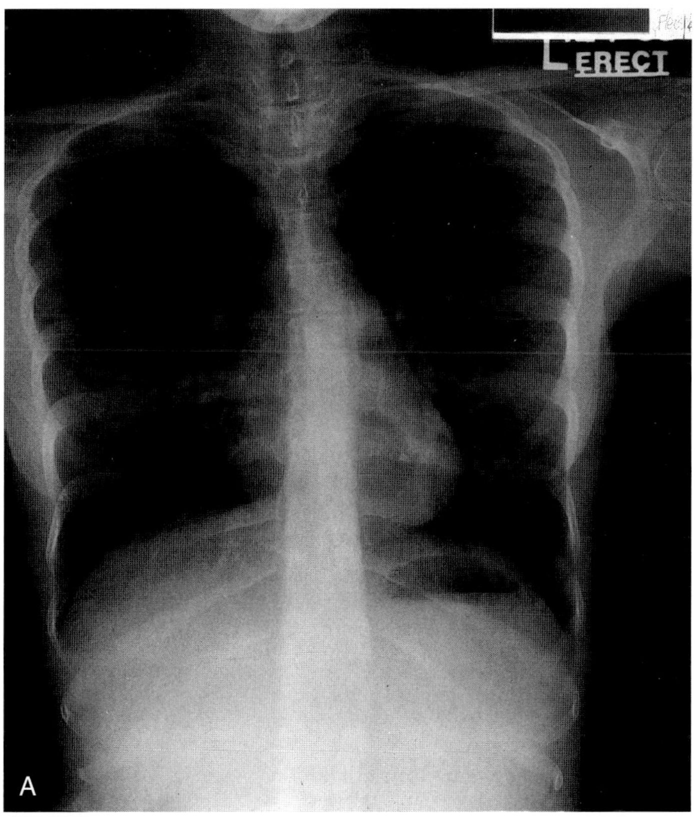

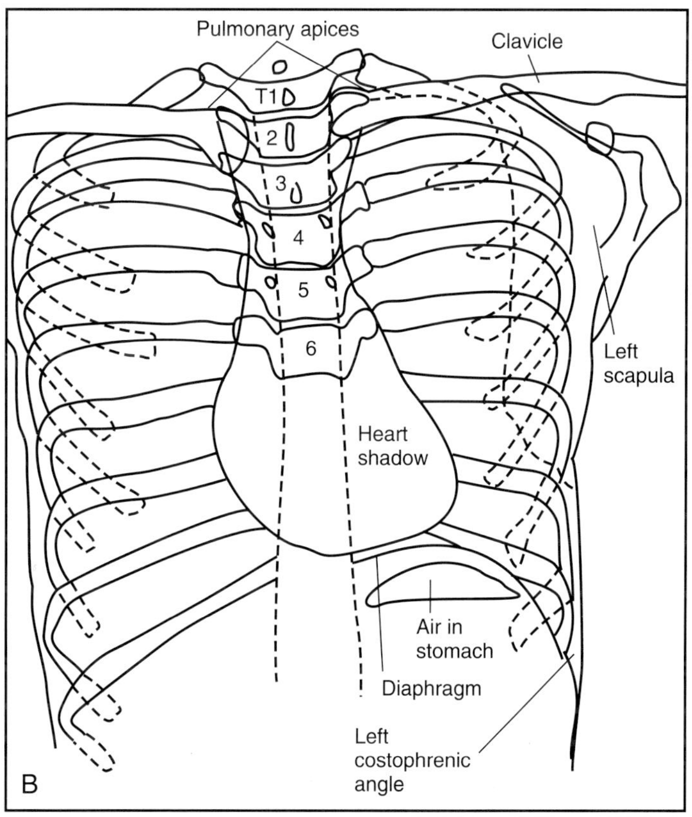

Figure 11.71. A and B, PA lordotic—Fleischner's method.

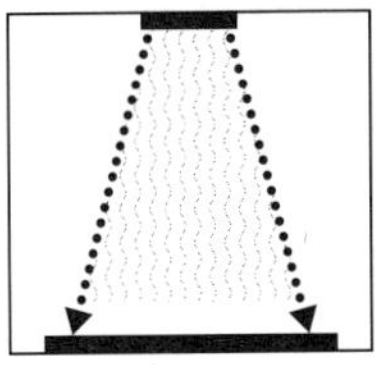

Lungs and Pleurae

Position/Projection

Frontal projections in lateral decubitus position for fluid levels and small pneumothoraces

Film Size:
14 × 17 inches (35 × 43 cm) lengthwise

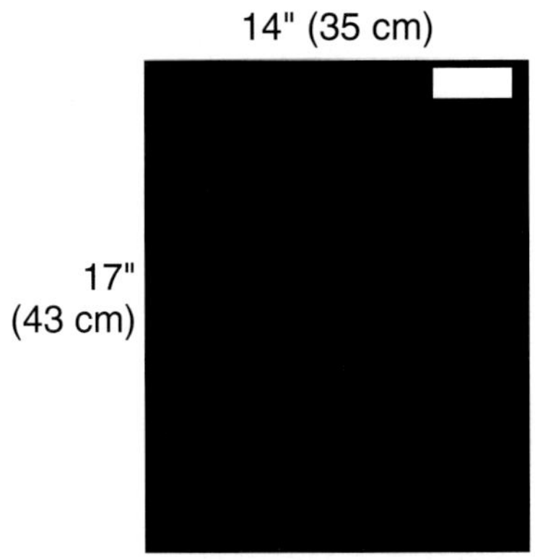

Patient Position

Lateral recumbent position on affected or unaffected side. Fluid is best shown by having patient lie on affected side. Free air is best shown by having patient lie on unaffected side (Fig. 11.72).

Part Position

Body should be elevated 4 to 5 inches (10 to 13 cm) if patient is on affected side as fluid drops, and entire bottom of thorax must be seen. Arms should be well above head and thorax in true lateral position. Chest is placed against vertical grid, with cassette 2 inches (5 cm) above shoulders.

Central Ray

Perpendicular through T4 or T7, depending on part of interest.

Breathing Instructions

Exposure is made after full inspiration.

Structures Demonstrated

Fluid levels in lungs and presence of any free air (Fig. 11.73).

Evaluation Criteria

1. Apices and affected side should be on film.
2. Radiograph should be free from any superimposition by arm.
3. Mark film to indicate as decubitus position.

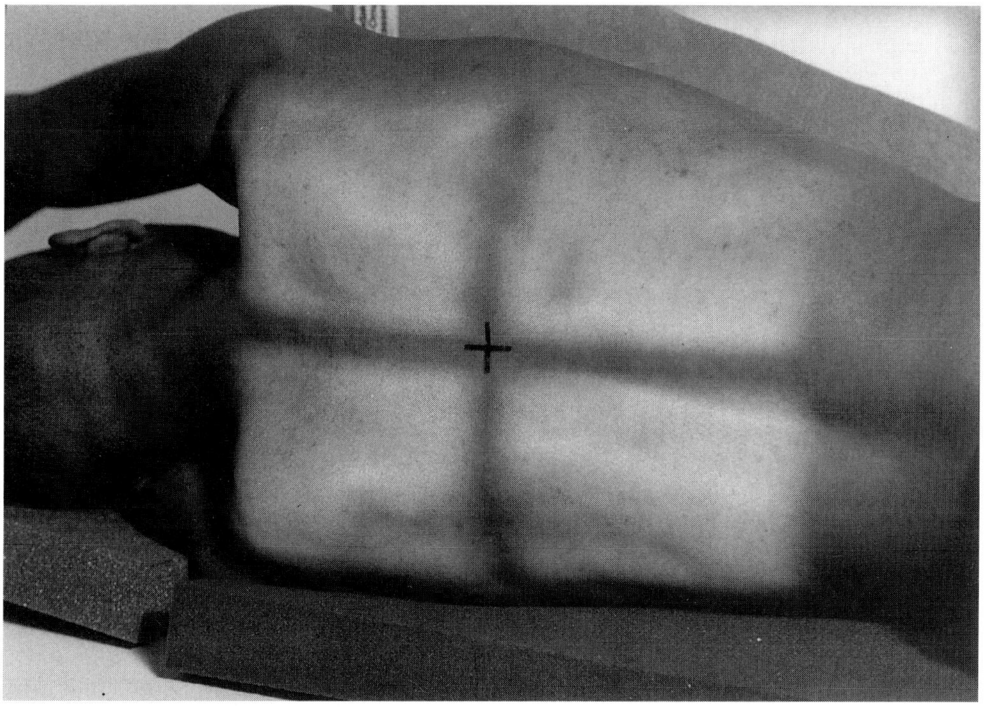

Figure 11.72. Frontal projection, lateral decubitus.

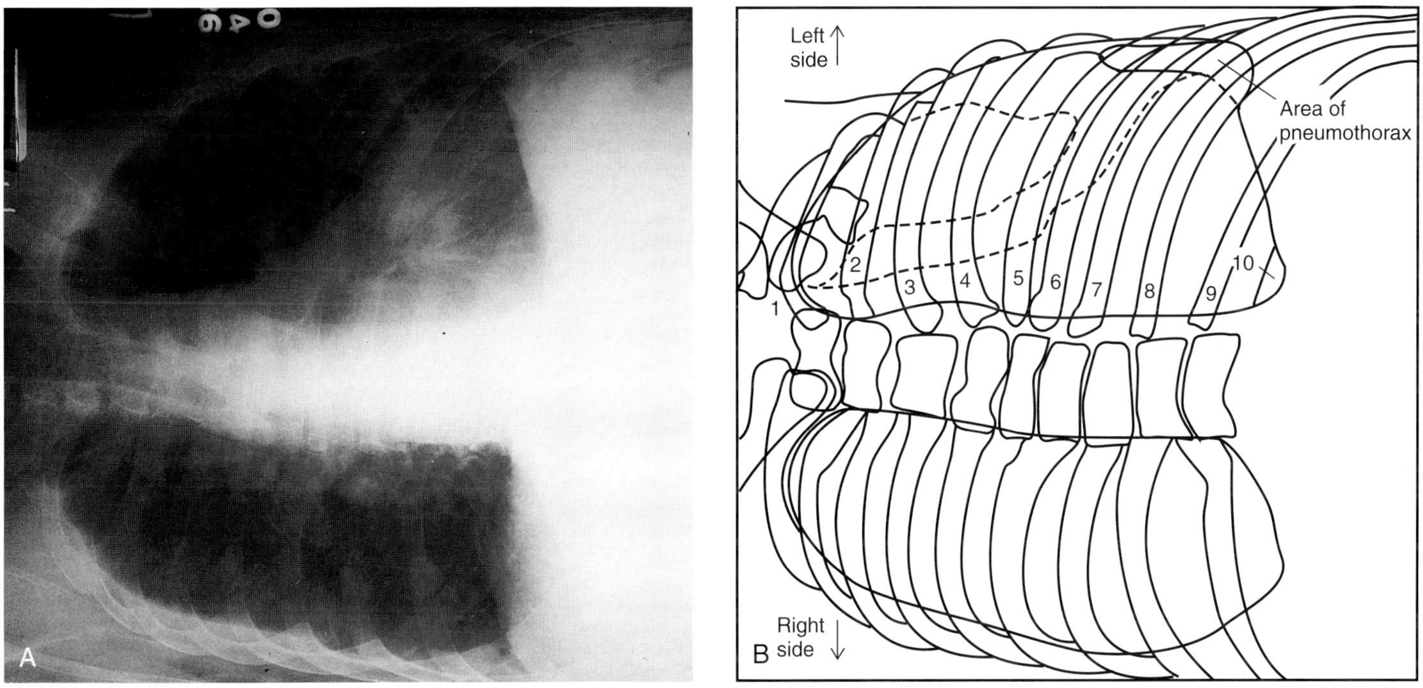

Figure 11.73. A and B, Frontal projection in lateral decubitus position.

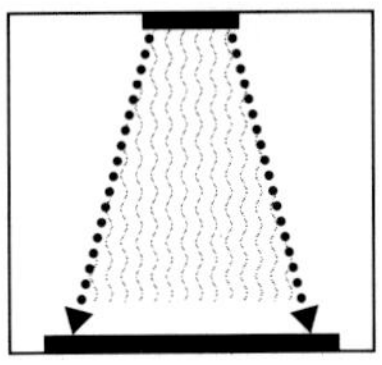

Lungs and Pleurae

Position/Projection

Ventral projections for fluid levels—ventral and dorsal decubitus positions

Film Size:
14 × 17 inches (35 × 43 cm) lengthwise

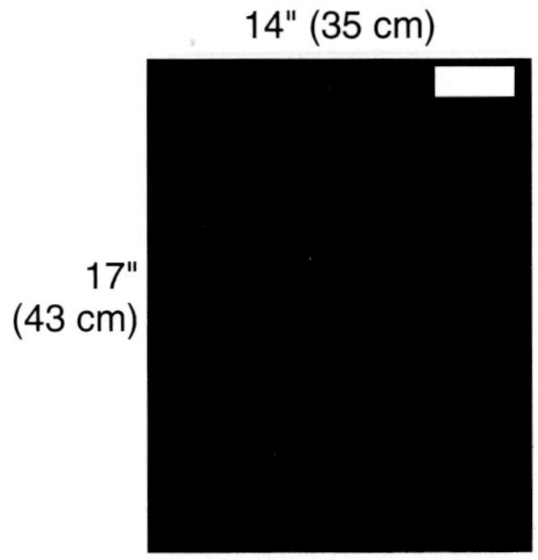

Patient Position

Prone or supine; thorax is elevated 2 to 3 inches (5 to 7.6 cm) on firm padding (Fig. 11.74).

Part Position

Arms extended well over head; place affected side against vertical grid. Adjust grid so it extends to level of laryngeal prominence.

Central Ray

Directed horizontally and perpendicularly to cassette and centered to level of T6.

Structures Demonstrated

Lateral view shows changes in fluid position and areas obscured by fluid in standard projections (Fig. 11.75).

Evaluation Criteria

1. Entire lung field should be demonstrated, including posterior and anterior surfaces.
2. Ensure that thorax is truly lateral and that arms do not obscure upper lung field.

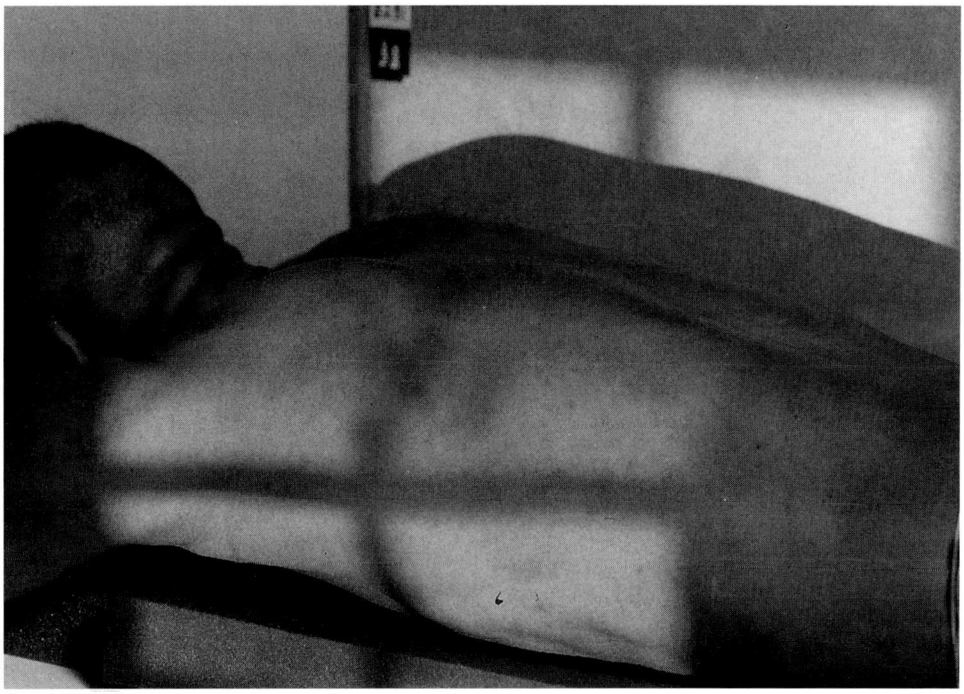

Figure 11.74. Ventral decubitus position.

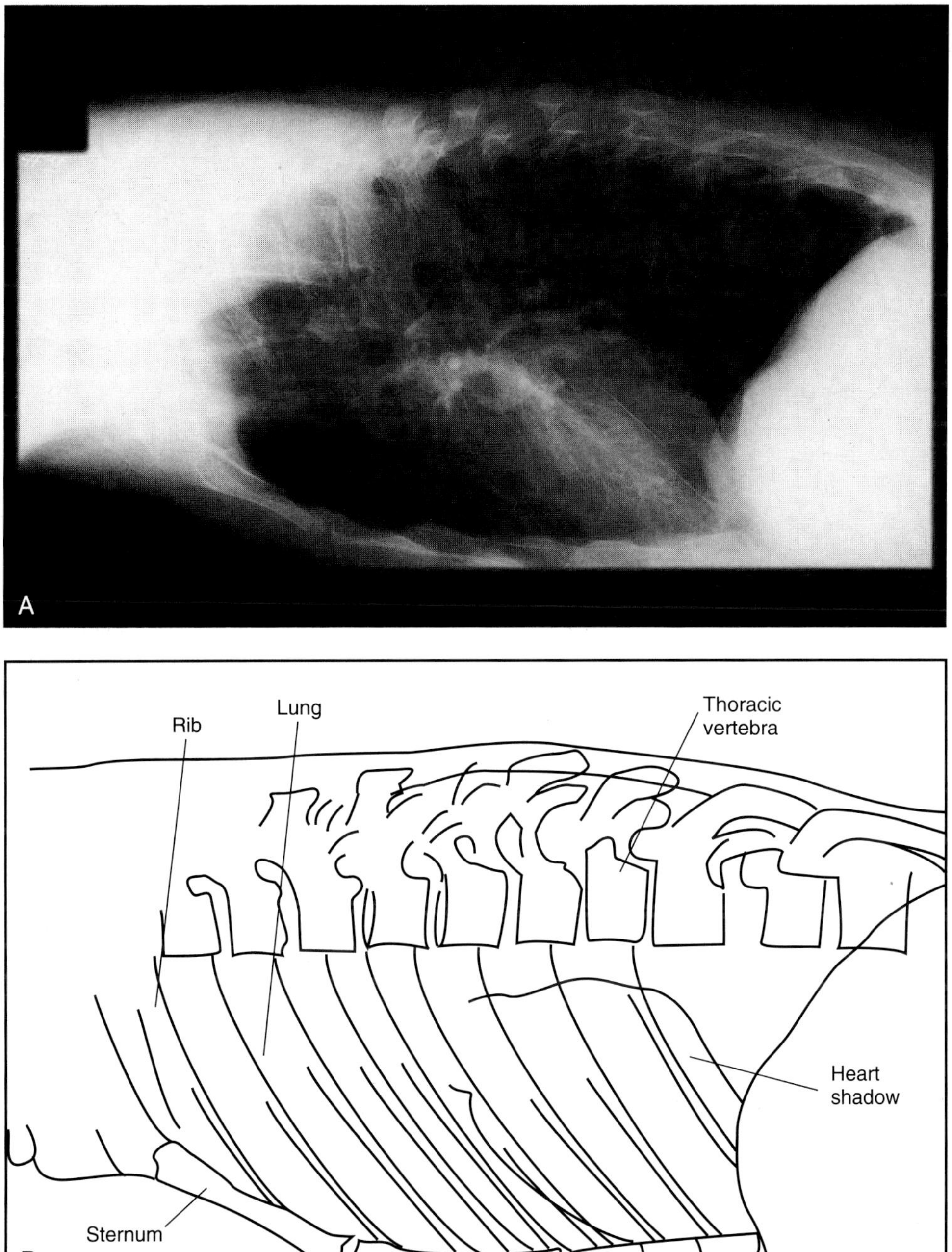

Figure 11.75. A and B, Ventral decubitus position.

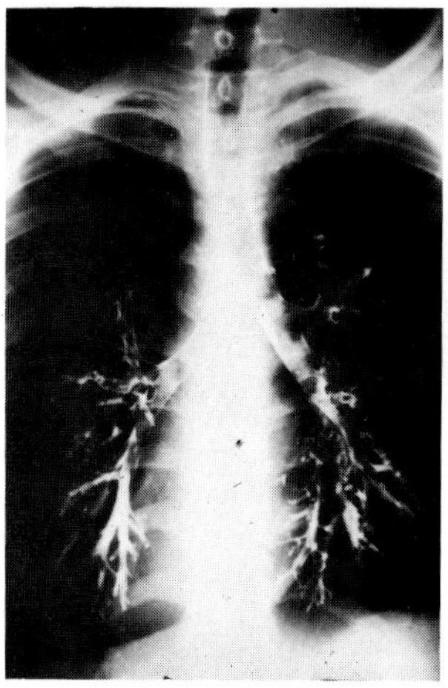

Figure 11.76. Routine bronchographic film, AP projection. (From Snopek AM: Fundamentals of Special Radiographic Procedures. 3rd ed. Philadelphia, WB Saunders, 1992, p 307.)

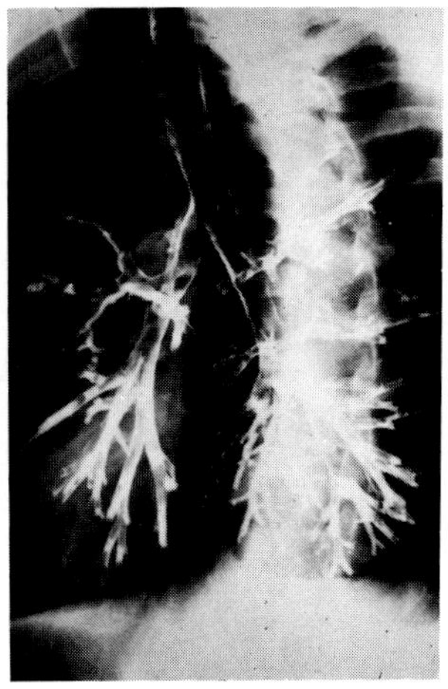

Figure 11.78. Routine bronchographic film, anterior oblique projection. (From Snopek AM: Fundamentals of Special Radiographic Procedures. 3rd ed. Philadelphia: WB Saunders, 1992, p 307.)

BRONCHOGRAPHY

Bronchography is a special technique that uses an opaque contrast medium to examine the lungs and bronchial tree (Figs. 11.76 to 11.78). It is no longer in wide use owing to computed tomography and fiberoptic bronchoscopy. However, it is still a useful procedure for bronchiectasis and in situations for which computed tomography is not useful.

The contrast medium used in bronchography can be aqueous or oily. Oily media made of iodized poppy seed oil or suspensions of propyliodone in peanut oil are the most widely used. A variety of methods exist for introducing contrast, including catheterization and aspiratino bronchography. If the media is not introduced by a catheter, gravity must be used to distribute the contrast media.

Fluoroscopy is used as a localizer to position the catheter tip and follow contrast media. Patient positions for bronchography are the same as those used for chest radiography (Table 11.2). Technical factors must be increased for postprocedural films to penetrate the contrast media.

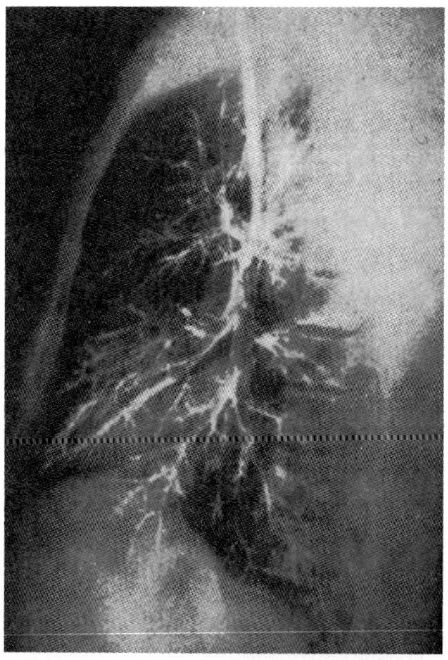

Figure 11.77. Routine bronchographic film, lateral projection. (From Lehman JS, Crellin JA: Medical Radiology and Photography. Heidelberg: Springer-Verlag, 1955, p 31.)

OTHER SPECIAL PROCEDURES

Nasopharyngography

Indications for nasopharyngography are choanal atresia, a congenital bony or membranous occlusion of one or both of the paired openings between the nasal cavity and the nasopharynx; and nasopharyngeal tumors. Dionosil Oily is the contrast medium usually used. The patient receives atropine 0.6 mg intravenously, 30 minutes prior to the procedure.

Preliminary films taken are a lateral, centered to the lower border of the zygoma, and a submentovertical projection (see Chapter 14), centered midway between the angles of the mandible.

The patient lies supine with the head on the skull unit and the neck hyperextended. With a catheter, contrast medium is instilled into each nostril. The patient is asked not to swallow and to indicate when he or she feels the need to. Films are taken at this point using the same projections as in the preliminary films. In infants with suspected choanal atresia, films are taken when contrast medium fills the nose.

Laryngography

Indications for laryngography include staging of laryngeal tumors, especially determining their inferior extension; laryngeal trauma; and laryngeal strictures. If the patient has poor respiratory reserve, the procedure is not indicated because contrast medium will enter the lungs. The contrast medium used is Dionosil Aqueous 10 to 15 ml.

The patient can take nothing by mouth for 5 hours before the procedure. Atropine 0.6 mg intravenous, 30 minutes, is administered prior to the procedure, followed by amethocaine lozenge.

Preliminary films include two lateral neck (soft tissue exposure) films, one in arrested deep inspiration and another during a Valsalva maneuver; and an AP or PA (chin raised) in deep inspiration.

During the procedure, the pharynx and larynx are further anesthetized with lidocaine (Xylocaine) spray. Contrast medium is instilled into the larynx by one of two methods: (1) With the patient sitting, using a curved laryngeal syringe. (2) With the patient erect or sitting in front of a vertical fluoroscopy unit. A polythene catheter is passed through the nose so that its tip lies above the epiglottis. Films are taken either with the patient supine, using

Table 11.2 Projections Used in Bronchography

Projection	Patient Position	Central Ray	Anatomy
PA	Patient erect, facing filmholder, median sagittal plane to center of cassette, acromion process 3 inches (7.6 cm) below top of cassette, chin resting on cassette holder, shoulders rolled forward, hands on hips; exposure on inspiration	Directed horizontally and at right angle to center of cassette; SID: 72 inches (183 cm)	Anterior view of mediastinum and its structures, contrast-filled tracheobronchial tree in anterior view
Anterior oblique (right or left)	Patient erect, facing filmholder; rotate filled side approximately 35° away from cassette, center on point midway between lateral margin of chest wall and vertebral column of side being examined; arm of filled side abducted with elbow flexed, hand resting on top of filmholder; exposure on inspiration	Directed horizontally and at right angle to center of cassette; SID: 72 inches (183 cm)	Contrast-filled right bronchial tree (LAO); contrast-filled left bronchial tree (RAO)
Lateral	Patient erect, side to be examined against filmholder, arms above head, patient centered to cassette; adjust to true lateral position	Directed horizontally and at right angle to center of film; SID: 72 inches (183 cm)	Contrast-filled bronchial tree (unilateral); lateral view of both contrast-filled lungs superimposed (bilateral)

From Snopek AM: Fundamentals of Special Radiographic Procedures. 3rd ed. Philadelphia: WB Saunders, 1992.
SID, source-to–image receptor distance.

the overhead tube, or with the patient standing in front of the fluoroscopy unit.

Films taken include AP or PA and laterals: (1) Mouth closed, nasal inspiration; (2) during a phonation "eee"; (3) during a Valsalva maneuver (forced expiration against a closed epiglottis); and (4) during a modified Valsalva maneuver (forced expiration with the mouth closed). Additional films taken include: 45° obliques—valuable for demonstrating spread of tumor across the anterior commissure; reversed phonation; and possibly AP tomography.

Percutaneous Lung Biopsy

Indications for a percutaneous lung biopsy include:

1. Investigating a pulmonary opacity when other diagnostic techniques have failed to make a diagnosis.
2. Investigating a new chest lesion in a patient with a known malignancy.
3. Obtaining material for culture when other techniques have failed to identify the causative organism in a patient with persistent consolidation.

Contraindications to the procedure include:

1. Bleeding diathesis, or concurrent administration of anticoagulants; contralateral pneumonectomy.
2. Presence of bullae.
3. Suspected hydatid disease.
4. Suspected vascular lesion.
5. Seriously impaired respiratory function such that a pneumothorax could not be tolerated.

Patient preparation usually includes premedication with diazepam. However, the patient must remain cooperative so that a consistent breathing pattern can be maintained during the procedure. The procedure may be performed on an outpatient basis, but a bed should be available in case of complications. Preliminary films taken are a PA and a lateral chest.

With posterior lesions, the patient lies prone; if the scapula is obscuring the lesion, the arm can be dangled over the side of the table to move the scapula laterally. If the lesion is anterior, the patient lies supine. Fluoroscopy is used to localize the mass. The puncture site is marked vertically above the lesion. With the plain films, the approximate distance to the lesion can be measured. With an aseptic technique, local anesthetic is infiltrated down to the pleura. The needle is inserted under screen control, with suspended respiration, using forceps (or manufacturer's holder, if provided, so that the operator's hand is not irradiated).

If a specialized core biopsy is used, then the manufacturer's instructions are followed to obtain tissue. With small-bore cell aspiration needles (e.g., 22-gauge spinal), maximum suction is applied with a 20-mg syringe while the needle is rotated and advanced through the lesion. Suction is released prior to withdrawing the needle to avoid contaminating the sample. It is extremely helpful if a pathologist can be present to check that there are sufficient cells in the aspirate for diagnostic purposes. If the lesion is necrotic, the most profitable site for biopsy is the margins of the lesion. Up to three passes may be performed to obtain tissue.

A chest x-ray in expiration is usually taken after the procedure. Fifteen to 35 percent of patients experience a subsequent pneumothorax. Other postprocedural complications include local pulmonary hemorrhage (10 percent) and hemoptysis (2 to 5 percent).

Bibliography

Allison DJ, Hemingway AP: Percutaneous needle biopsy of the lung. Br Med J 1981; 282:875–878.

Ballinger P: Merrill's Atlas of Radiographic Positions and Radiologic Procedures. 7th ed. Vols 1 and 2. St. Louis: CV Mosby, 1991.

Bontrager KL, Anthony BT: Textbook of Radiographic Anatomy and Related Anatomy. Denver: Multi-Media, 1982.

Carlton R: Quality assurance in radiology. *In* Gurley LT, Callaway W (eds): Introduction to Radiologic Technology. 2nd ed. St. Louis: CV Mosby, 1986.

Chapman S, Nakielny R: A Guide to Radiologic Procedures. 2nd ed. Philadelphia: WB Saunders, 1986.

Cooper SJ, Sargent EN: Positioning. *In* Sargent EN (ed): Technique for Chest Radiography for Pneumoconiosis. Chicago: American College of Radiology, 1982.

Cullinan AM: Producing Quality Radiographs. Philadelphia: JB Lippincott, 1987.

Jaquith S: Chest x-ray interpretation: Implications for nursing intervention. Dimens Crit Care Nurs 1986; 5(1):8–19.

Jing BS, McGraw JP: Contrast nasopharyngography in the diagnosis of tumors. Arch Otolaryngol 1965; 81:365–371.

Kattan KR: What to look for in rib fractures and how. JAMA 1980; 243(3):262–264.

Kowalcyzk N: Pathology and technical radiographic considerations of the heart and great vessels. *In* Frank ED (ed): Postgraduate Advances in Radiologic Technology. Berryville, VA: Forum Medicum, 1991.
Lauer OG, Mayes JB, Thurston RP: Evaluating Radiographic Quality: The Variables and Their Effects. Mankato, MN: Burnell, 1990.
Malott JC, Fodor J: The Art and Science of Medical Radiography. 7th ed. St. Louis: CV Mosby, 1993.
Meschan I, Ott DJ: Introduction to Diagnostic Imaging. Philadelphia: WB Saunders, 1984.
Momose KJ, Macmillan AS: Roentgenological investigations of the larynx and trachea. Radiol Clin North Am 1978; 16(2):321–341.
Sanchez F: Fundamentals of chest x-ray interpretation. Crit Care Nurse 1986; 5(3):41–62.
Snopek AM: Fundamentals of Special Radiographic Procedures. 3rd ed. Philadelphia: WB Saunders, 1992.
Squire LF, Novelline RA: Fundamentals of Radiology. Cambridge, MA: Harvard University Press, 1988.
Swallow RA, Naylor E (eds): Clark's Positioning in Radiography. 11th ed. Rockville, MD: Aspen, 1986.

CHAPTER 12

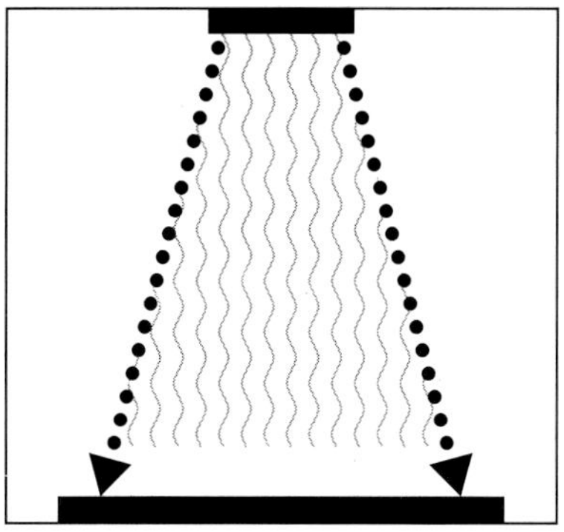

Abdomen

Patricia W. Enos, R.T.(R.)

Steven B. Dowd, Ed.D., R.T.(R.)

Radiographic examination of the abdomen is dependent on the expertise of the radiographer, specific pathological conditions affecting the patient, patient preparation, and particular anatomic considerations. All these factors affect the final product—the diagnostic radiograph. This radiograph is the product of the competent professional radiographer who must also consider the selection of optimum technical factors, patient care and communication, radiation protection, and the needs of the clinician and radiologist. This responsibility should be taken seriously and with consideration for the patient.

This chapter discusses the anatomy of the abdomen, routine positions of abdominal radiography, technical considerations, patient positioning, and factors to be considered in film evaluation.

ANATOMY

The abdominopelvic cavity (Fig. 12.1) consists of muscles, organs of the digestive system, and accessory organs of digestion. The cavity itself is lined with peritoneum. The peritoneum is divided into the parietal peritoneum, that portion adhering to the abdominopelvic cavity, and the visceral peritoneum, which surrounds the organs of the abdomen. The space formed between these two layers is called the abdominal cavity. Mesentery connects the posterior wall of the abdomen to specific abdominal organs. Retroperitoneal structures are those located behind the peritoneum. Examples of such structures are the aorta, inferior vena cava, kidneys, ureters, adrenal glands, pancreas, and duodenum. The two major muscles of the abdomen are the diaphragm and the paired psoas muscles.

The digestive system includes the mouth, pharynx and esophagus, stomach, small intestine, and large intestine or colon (Fig. 12.2). The basic functions of digestion are ingestion, absorption, and egestion. Radiographic demonstration of these functions is covered specifically in Chapter 15. The mouth serves as the entry into the gastrointestinal tract. The pharynx has a dual function—it allows air to enter the larynx and food to enter the esophagus. The tubular esophagus measures approximately 10 inches (25 cm) long. It originates posteriorly at the level of C6 and terminates at the entrance to the stomach.

The stomach (Fig. 12.3) is often described as a J-shaped organ. The radiographer must consider the patient's overall body habitus, patient position, respiratory phase, status of the stomach, and any possible pathology. The small intestine (Fig. 12.4) extends from the pylorus of the stomach to the ileocecal valve. The three divisions of the small intestine are the proximal portion, or duodenum; the jejunum; and the distal portion, the ileum. The large intestine (Fig. 12.5) is approximately 5 feet (152 cm) long and includes the cecum, colon, rectum, and anus. The colon comprises four parts: sigmoid, descending, transverse, and ascending colons. The configuration of each part of the large intestine depends on body habitus, bowel content, pathology, respiratory phase, and patient position.

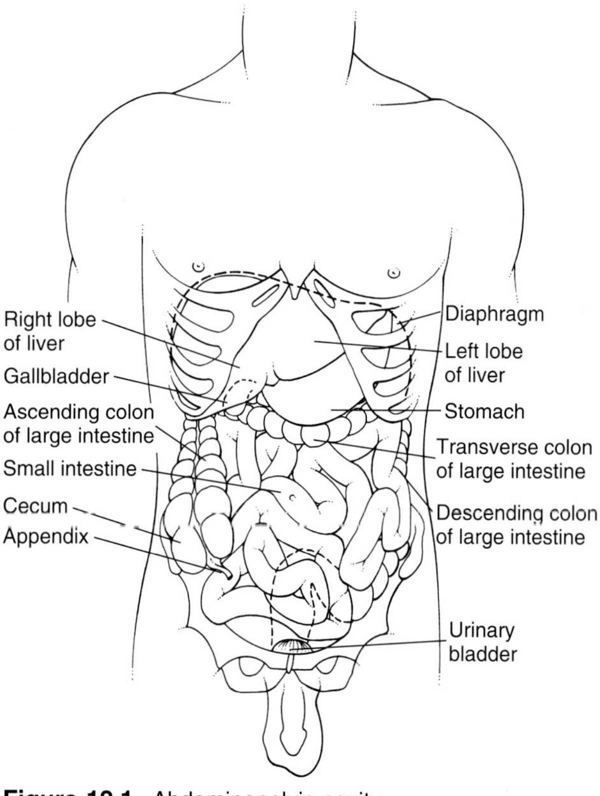

Figure 12.1. Abdominopelvic cavity.

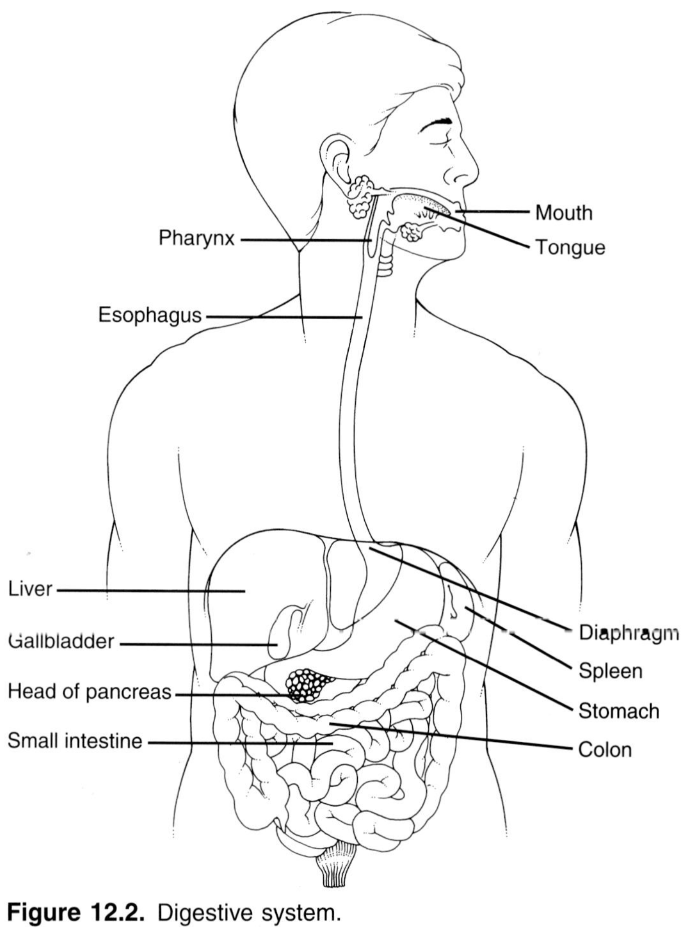

Figure 12.2. Digestive system.

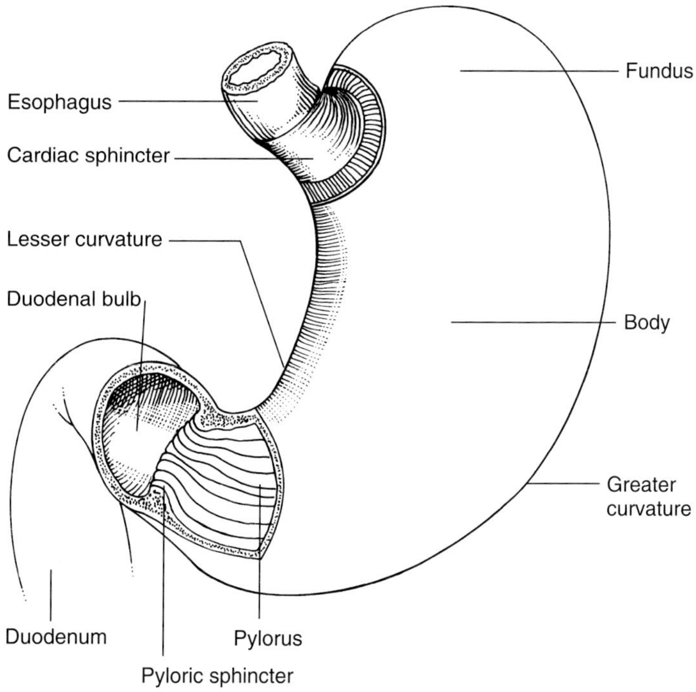

Figure 12.3. Stomach.

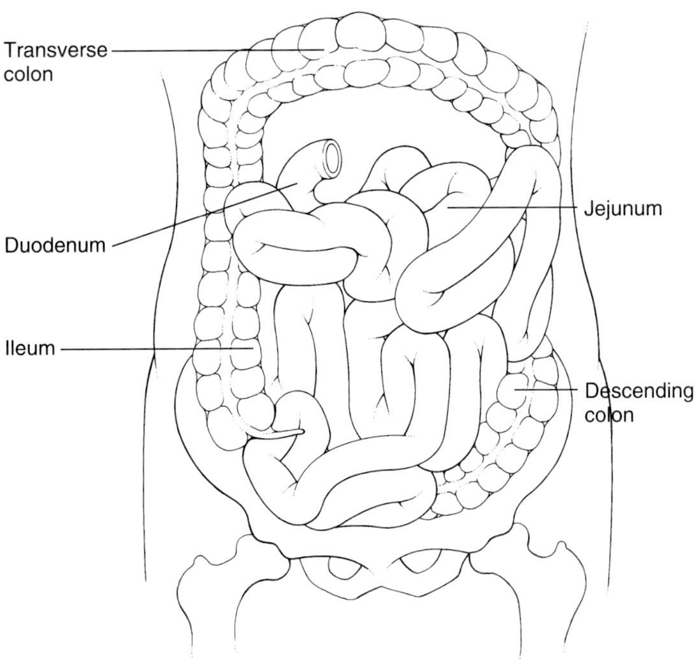

Figure 12.4. Small intestine.

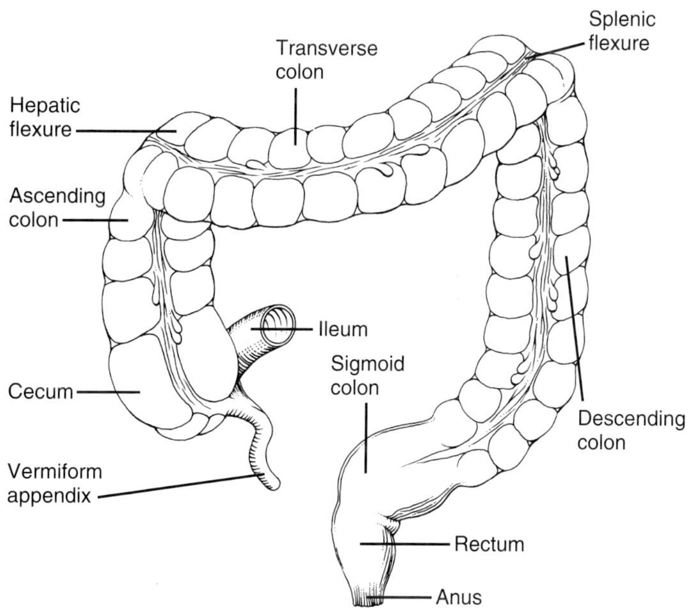

Figure 12.5. Large intestine.

The abdomen includes several accessory organs of digestion: liver, pancreas, and gallbladder. The liver (Fig. 12.6) has the distinction of being the largest gland in the human body. Its primary function is the production of bile. The bile is either transported to the gallbladder and stored until needed for digestion or conveyed into the common bile duct via the cystic duct and ultimately into the duodenum. The liver consists of two main lobes and occupies the right hypochondrium and most of the epigastrium. The liver is a homogeneous structure that plays an important role radiographically when considering the right lateral decubitus position. This is discussed subsequently in the section dealing with the positioning of the Acute Abdomen.

The pancreas is divided into lobes and is composed of cells that secrete the enzymes insulin and glucagon. The material secreted contains amylase, which aids in the digestion of fats and starches.

The gallbladder (Fig. 12.7) is located under the liver; it is pear-shaped. The gallbladder serves as a reservoir for bile secreted from the liver, contracts to stimulate the secretion of the hormone cholecystokinin, and absorbs salts and water from the concentrated bile. The gallbladder is composed of a neck, a body, and a fundus.

Detailed descriptions of abdominal anatomy and organ functions are discussed in Chapter 15.

TECHNICAL FACTORS

Abdominal radiography is performed using a grid at a moderate (70 or higher) peak kilovoltage (kVp). A common mistake made by beginning radiographers is to assume that increased abdominal girth requires increases in kVp. However, increases in abdominal measurement are usually due to increased amounts of abdominal fat; thus, increases in kVp will lengthen the contrast scale on the radiograph, which is undesirable.

One means of shortening the scale of contrast in abdominal radiography is through the use of a compression band across the patient's abdomen. Compressing the abdomen reduces the amount of scatter produced, resulting in a shorter scale of contrast.

The radiographer must be aware of the need to immobilize the diaphragm and must consider technical factors that will allow ready identification of the lateral borders of the psoas muscles on the radiograph. A short exposure time is needed to detect free air under the diaphragm by reducing the effects of diaphragmatic motion.

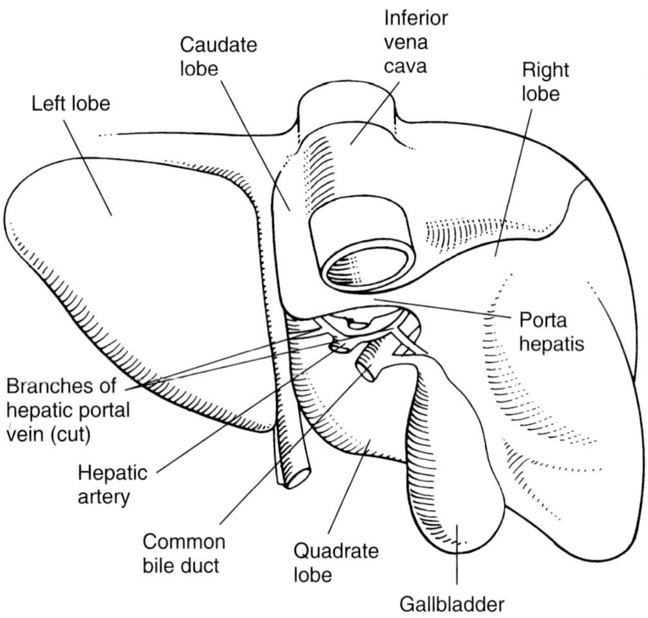

Figure 12.6. Liver.

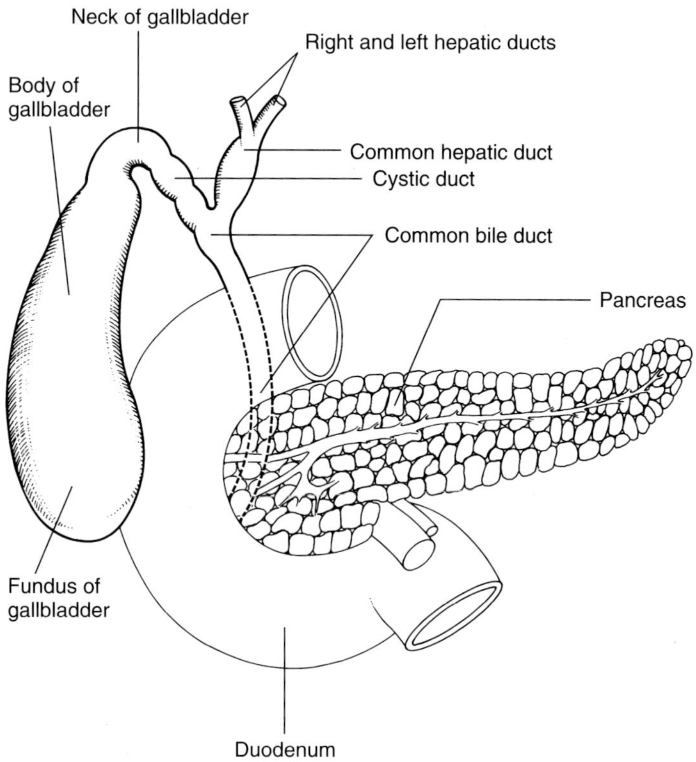

Figure 12.7. Gallbladder.

Abdomen

Projection

AP

Film Size:
14 × 17 inches (35 × 43 cm) lengthwise

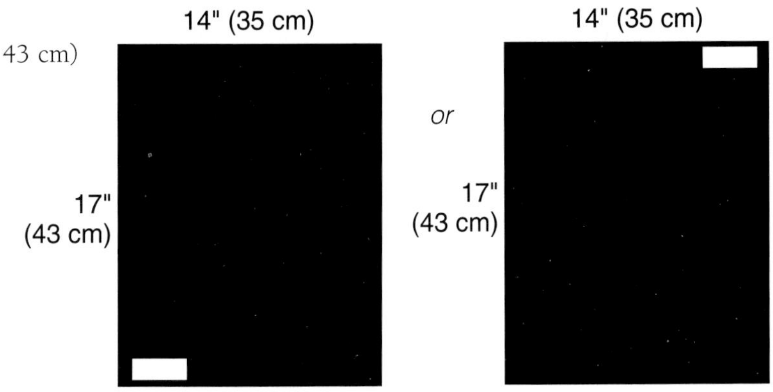

Patient Position

Supine. Midsagittal plane centered to midline of table/film. Legs fully extended. Arms at sides out of radiographic field. Shoulders level and relaxed, lying in same transverse plane (Fig. 12.8).

Part Position

No rotation of pelvis or trunk.

Central Ray

Perpendicular to midsagittal plane and centered to iliac crests or slightly above as required by procedure.

Breathing Instructions

Exhale and suspend respiration.

Structures Demonstrated

Kidneys, liver, spleen, diaphragm, outline of psoas muscles, abnormal calcifications, and tumor masses (Fig. 12.9).

Evaluation Criteria

1. Symphysis pubis included.
2. Domes of diaphragm visible.
3. Vertebral column centered.
4. No rotation of pelvis, hips, ribs, and vertebral bodies.
5. Appropriate markers visible.
6. No evidence of motion.
7. Psoas muscles visible bilaterally.
8. Lower margin of liver visible.
9. Kidney shadows visible.
10. Inferior ribs visible.

NOTE: Two crosswise films may be necessary, depending on body habitus or clinician's needs. Immobilization may be required to prevent voluntary and involuntary movement. Radiation protection may not be possible, given the required visibility of anatomy.

NOTE: This projection is still often called the KUB, which stands for *k*idneys, *u*reters, and *b*ladder, or "flat plate of the abdomen," referring to patient's position and the former use of glass plates as an imaging medium in radiology. In nonemergency situations, the patient may require bowel preparation to eliminate gas and fecal shadows that tend to obscure soft tissue detail and bony detail in the spine and pelvis.

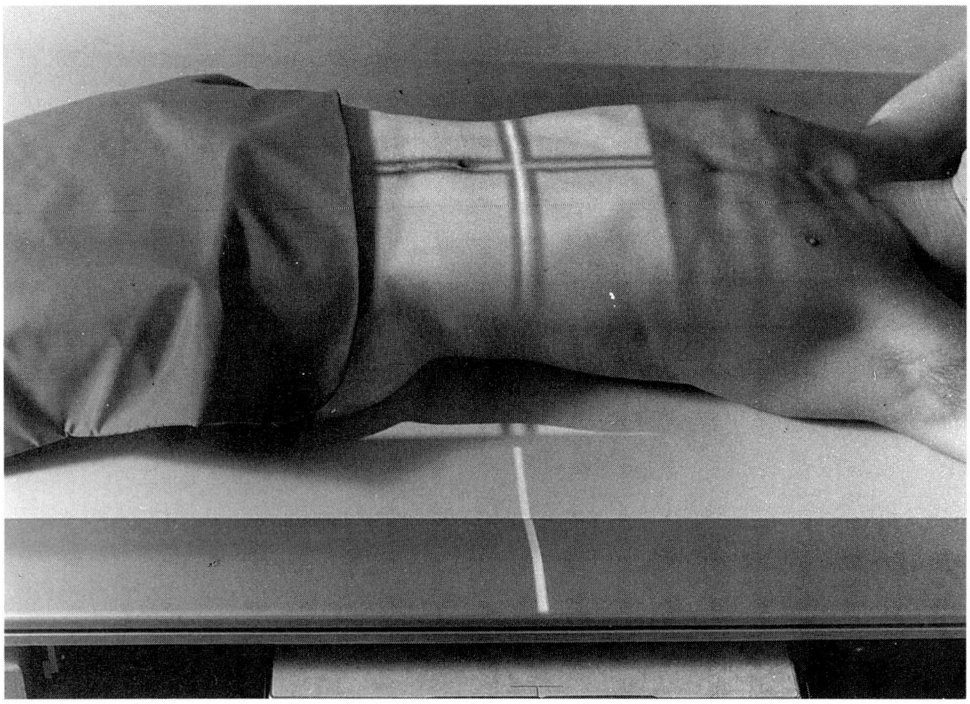

Figure 12.8. AP projection.

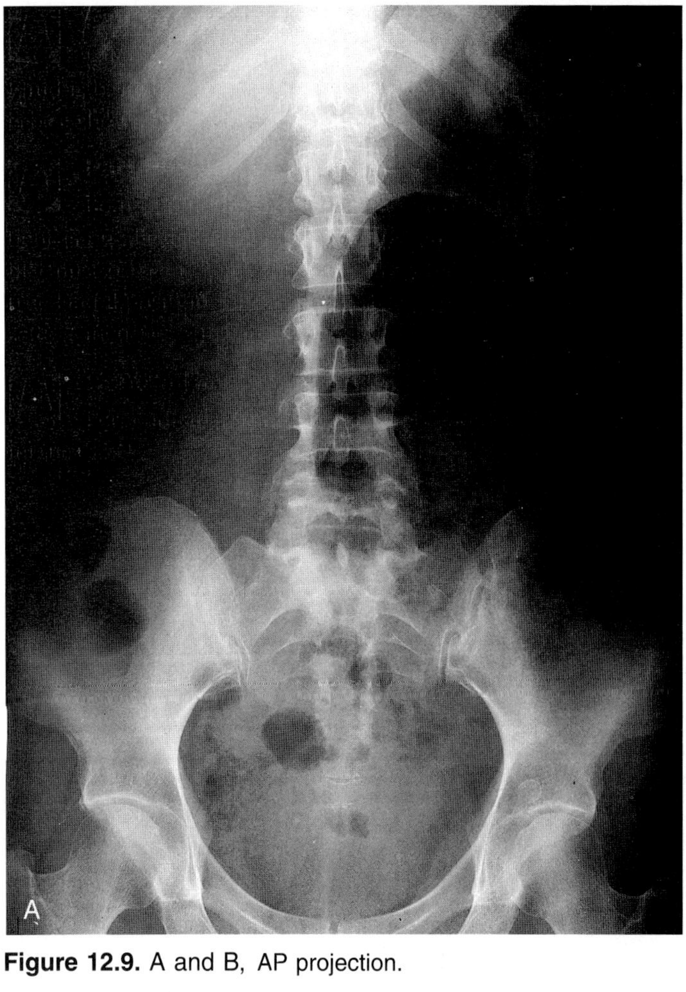

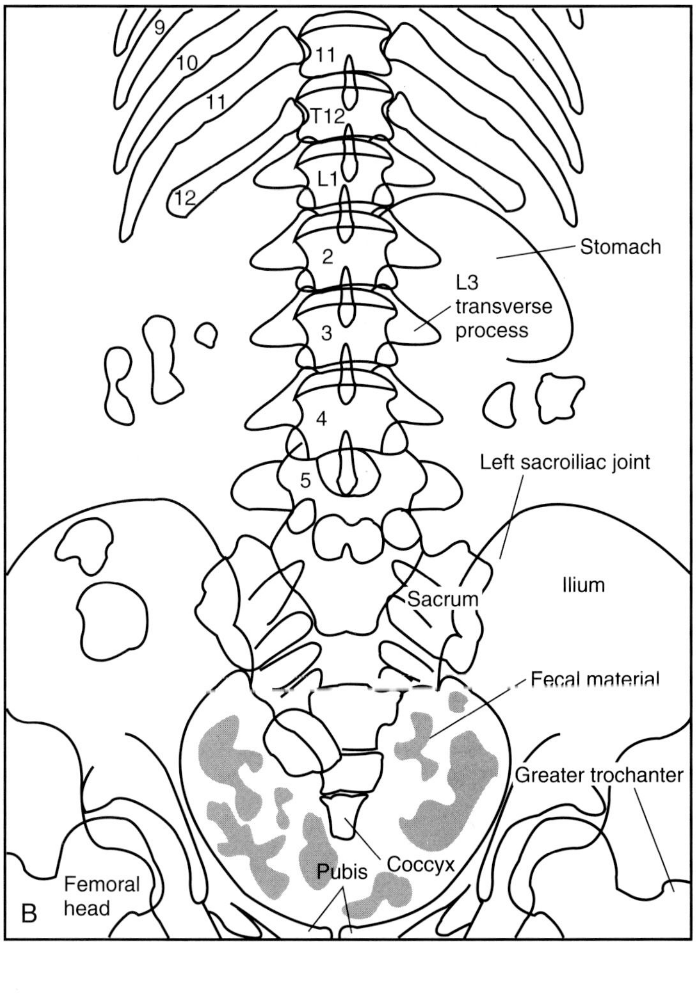

Figure 12.9. A and B, AP projection.

Abdomen

Projection

AP erect

Film Size:
14 × 17 inches (35 × 43 cm) lengthwise

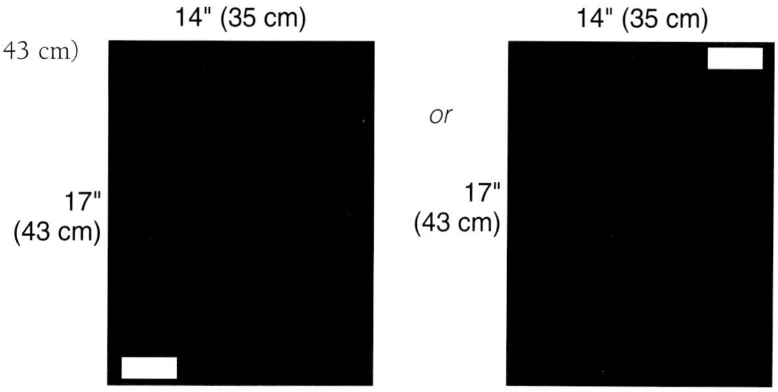

Patient Position

Erect. Midsagittal plane centered to midline of table/film/upright Bucky. Weight equally distributed on both feet. Arms at side, out of radiographic field. Shoulders level and relaxed lying in same transverse plane (Fig. 12.10).

Part Position

No rotation of pelvis or trunk.

Central Ray

Perpendicular to iliac crests if bladder must be visible. Perpendicular to level 2 to 3 inches (5 to 7.6 cm) above iliac crests if diaphragm must be visible.

Breathing Instructions

Exhale and suspend respiration.

Structures Demonstrated

Same as AP/PA recumbent (Fig. 12.11).

Evaluation Criteria

1. Domes of diaphragm visible.
2. Vertebral column centered.
3. No rotation of pelvis, hips, ribs, and vertebral bodies.
4. Appropriate markers visible.
5. No evidence of motion.
6. Psoas muscles visible bilaterally.
7. Lower margin of liver visible.
8. Kidney shadows visible.
9. Inferior ribs visible.

NOTE: Symphysis pubis may not be included if the domes of the diaphragm are a priority. Radiation protection should be evidenced if lower third of the abdomen is not required. Immobilization may be required if the patient's safety is compromised in the erect position secondary to dizziness, shortness of breath, or any other acute situation.

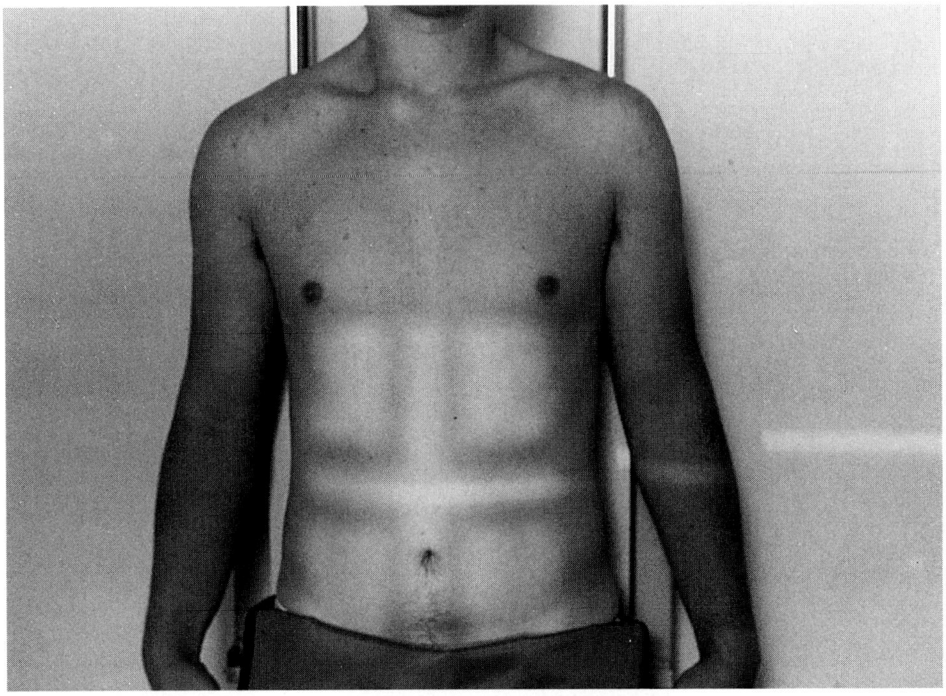

Figure 12.10. AP erect.

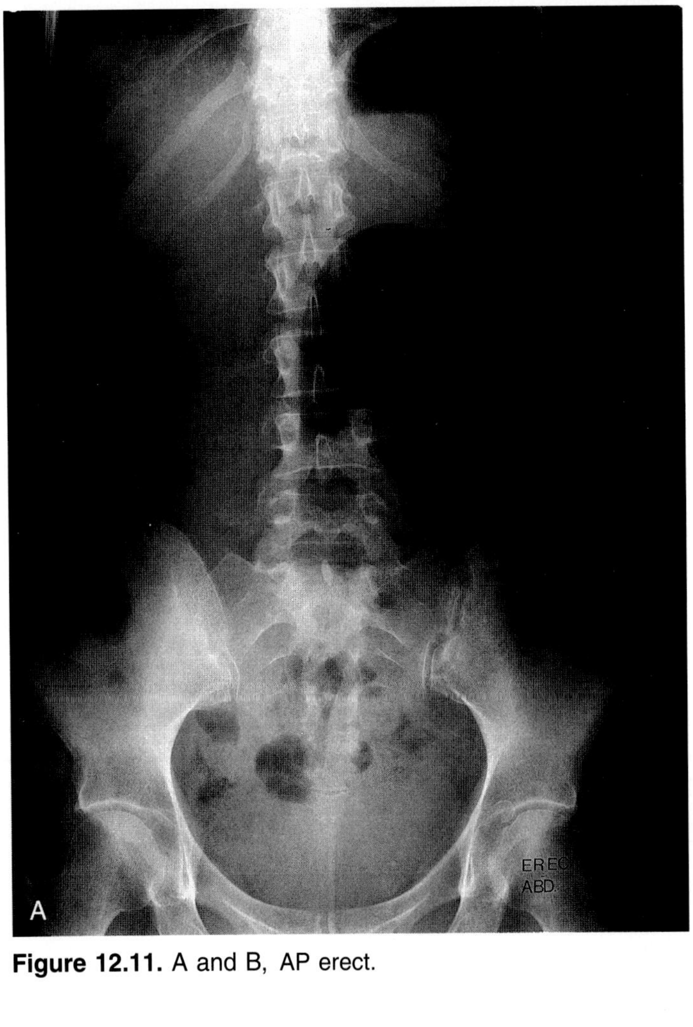

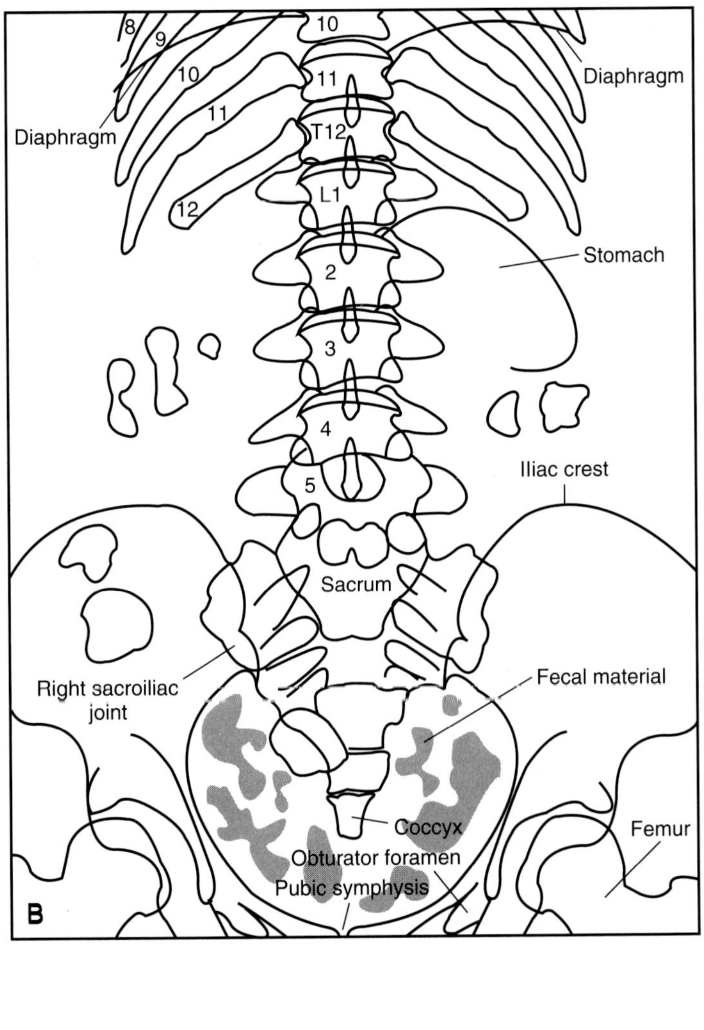

Figure 12.11. A and B, AP erect.

Abdomen

Position

Lateral

Film Size:
14 × 17 inches (35 × 43 cm)
Bucky or grid cassette, lengthwise

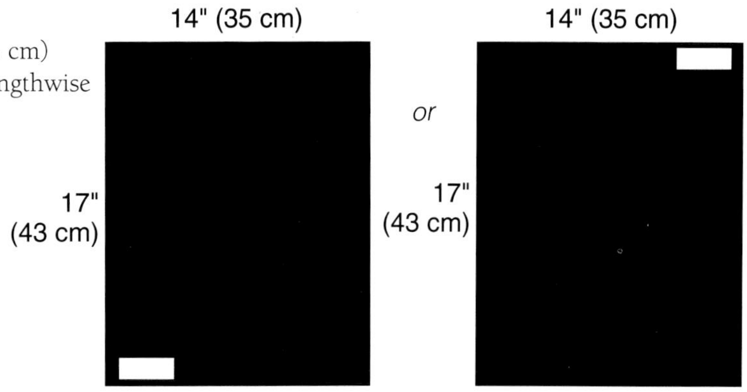

Patient Position

Recumbent/erect. Right or left side down as directed or as indicated by procedure. Arms over head with elbows flexed. Legs superimposed with knees flexed for comfort and immobilization (Fig. 12.12).

Part Position

Midaxillary plane centered to midline of table/film/upright Bucky. Adjust body so lateral position is achieved.

Central Ray

Perpendicular to level of iliac crests and approximately 2 inches (5 cm) anterior to midaxillary plane.

Breathing Instructions

Exhale and suspend respiration.

Structures Demonstrated

Lateral projection of abdominal structures. Abdominal aorta if calcified. Other abdominal structures if calcified. Tumor masses. Lateral vertebral bodies (Fig. 12.13).

Evaluation Criteria

1. Superimposition of iliac crests.
2. No rotation of abdomen and its structures.
3. Lateral aspect of vertebral bodies.

NOTE: Radiation protection as permitted by the procedure and its required visible anatomy. Immobilization techniques as necessary for patient comfort, safety, and diagnostic value of the resultant radiograph.

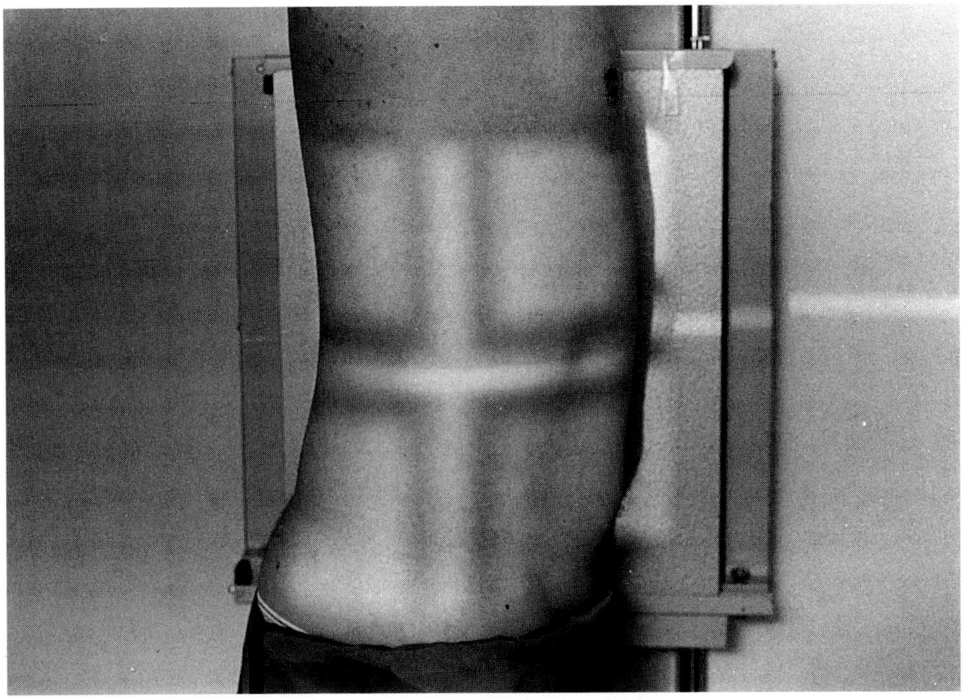

Figure 12.12. Lateral.

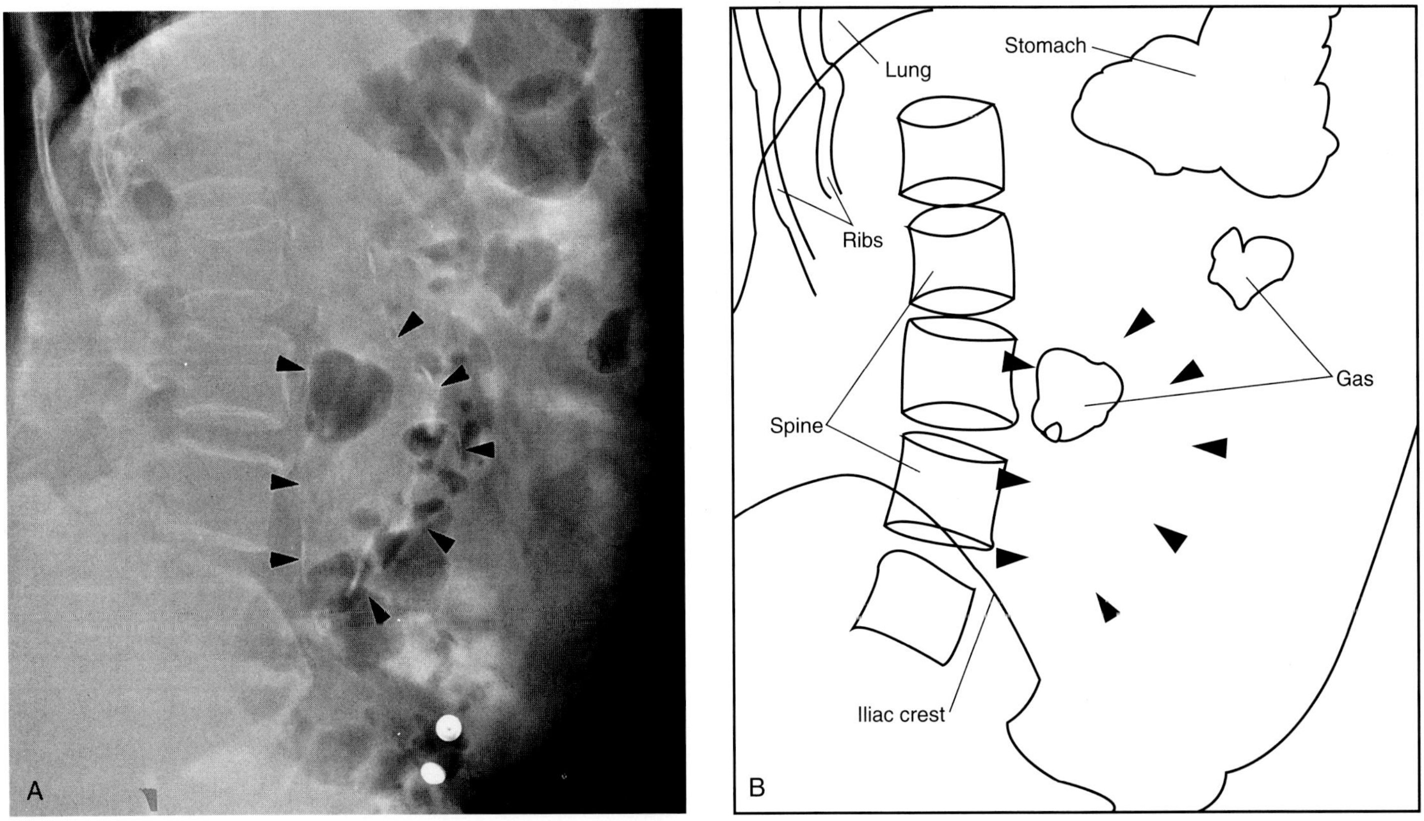

Figure 12.13. A and B, Lateral (recumbent) radiograph showing calcified wall with *arrows* indicating abdominal aortic aneurysm. (*A*, From Long BW: Radiographic Features of the Acute Abdomen, Albuquerque, NM: American Society of Radiologic Technologists, 1992.)

Abdomen

Position

Lateral decubitus

Film Size:
14 × 17 inches (35 × 43 cm)
Upright Bucky or grid cassette, lengthwise

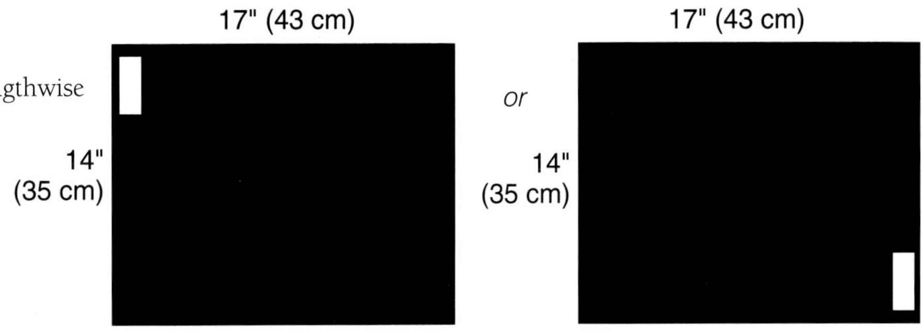

Patient Position

Lateral recumbent. Left and/or right side down. Arms over head with elbows flexed. Legs superimposed with knees flexed for comfort and immobilization (Fig. 12.14).

Part Position

Adjust body so lateral position is achieved. Midsagittal plane centered to long axis of film.

Central Ray

Horizontal to level of iliac crests and midsagittal plane. Perpendicular to film/upright Bucky.

Breathing Instructions

Exhale and suspend respiration.

Structures Demonstrated

Liver, spleen, and kidneys outlined. Air/fluid levels within abdomen. Free intra-abdominal air patterns (Fig. 12.15).

Evaluation Criteria

1. Diaphragm visible.
2. Right and left sides of abdomen visible.
3. Up side clearly demonstrated.
4. No rotation of abdomen in true AP/PA projection.
5. No rotation of alae of ilium.
6. Up side correctly marked left/right, so as not to compromise visibility of anatomy.
7. No evidence of motion.

NOTE: If manual collimation is utilized, collimate to size of film. Radiograph is correctly identified as follows: Right side up/left lateral decubitus; left side up/right lateral decubitus. Right side up decubitus will optimally demonstrate free air owing to the homogeneity of the liver.

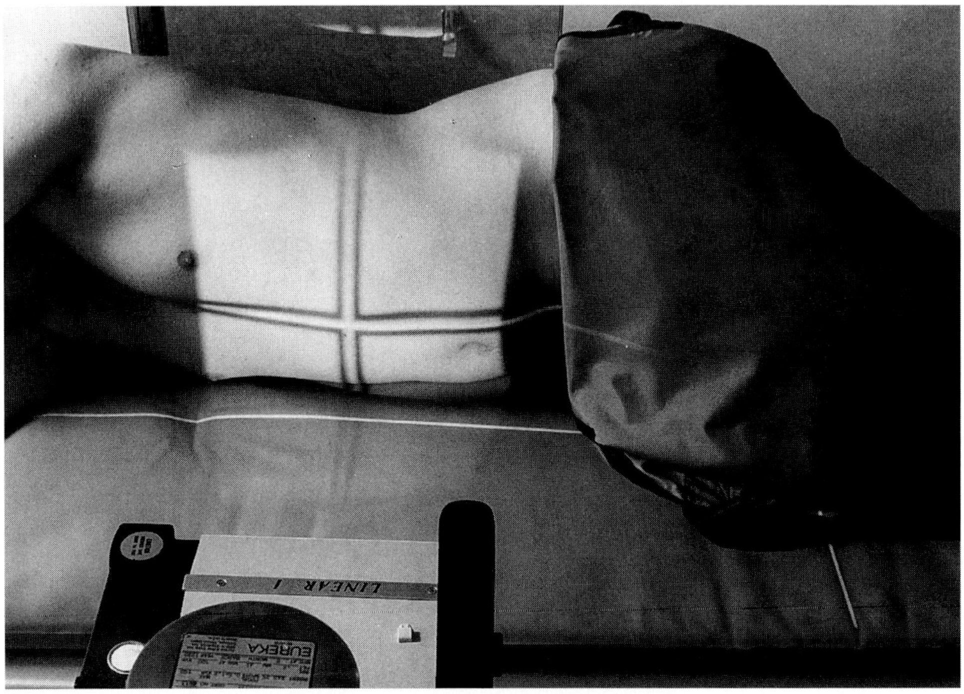

Figure 12.14. Lateral decubitus.

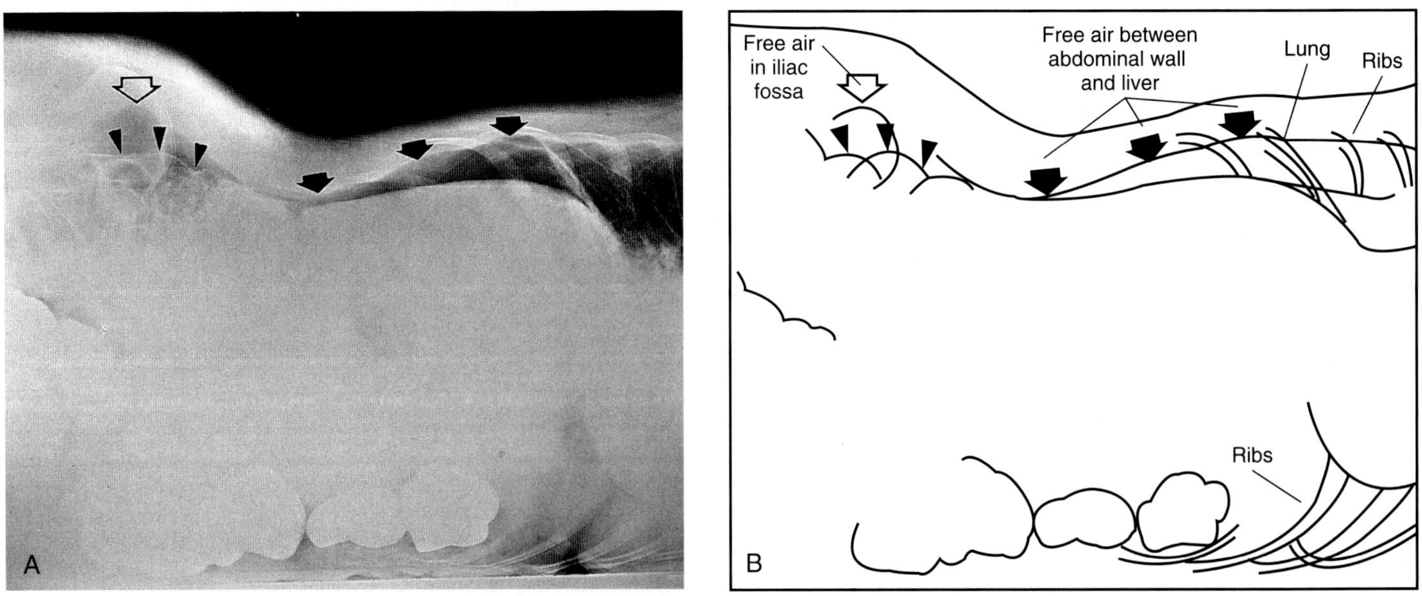

Figure 12.15. A and B, Left lateral decubitus showing free air between the abdominal wall and the liver (*closed arrows*) as well as within the iliac fossa (*arrowheads*). Note the very low radiographic density used to optimally visualize free air. (*A*, From Long BW: Radiographic Features of the Acute Abdomen, Albuquerque, NM: American Society of Radiologic Technologists, 1992.)

Abdomen

Position

Dorsal decubitus

Film Size:
14 × 17 inches (35 × 43 cm)
Upright Bucky/grid cassette, lengthwise

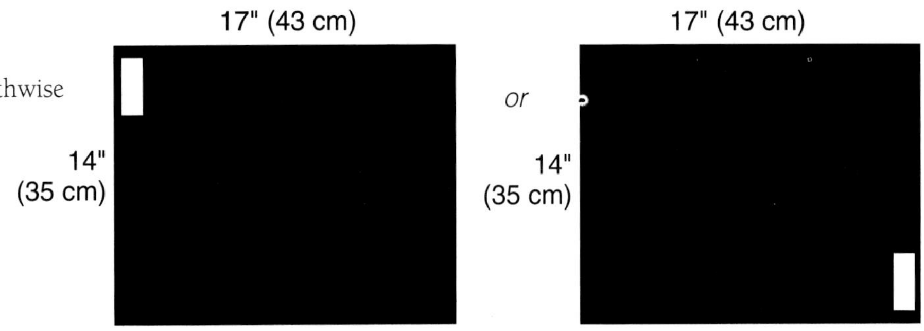

Patient Position

Supine. Arms over head or placed comfortably resting on chest and out of field. Legs fully extended (Fig. 12.16).

Part Position

Adjust trunk so as to maintain AP perspective. No rotation of hips, pelvis, or shoulders.

Central Ray

Option #1

Horizontal beam perpendicular to film. Direct to a point 2 inches (5 cm) anterior to midaxillary plane and 2 inches (5 cm) above iliac crests.

Option #2

Horizontal beam perpendicular to film. Directed to level of iliac crests and midaxillary plane.

Breathing Instructions

Exhale and suspend respiration.

Structures Demonstrated

Antevertebral accumulation of air. Intra-abdominal air/fluid levels. Umbilical hernias. Abdominal masses. Fistula/sinus tracts (Fig. 12.17).

Evaluation Criteria

1. Lateral image of abdomen.
2. Entire abdomen visible on film.
3. Diaphragm visible, especially if Option #1 utilized.
4. No evidence of motion.
5. Identifying markers correctly placed so as not to obscure anatomy or pathology.

NOTE: Collimate anterior abdomen. Selection of Option #1 or #2 is based on specific request or clinical diagnostic need(s) of patient/clinician.

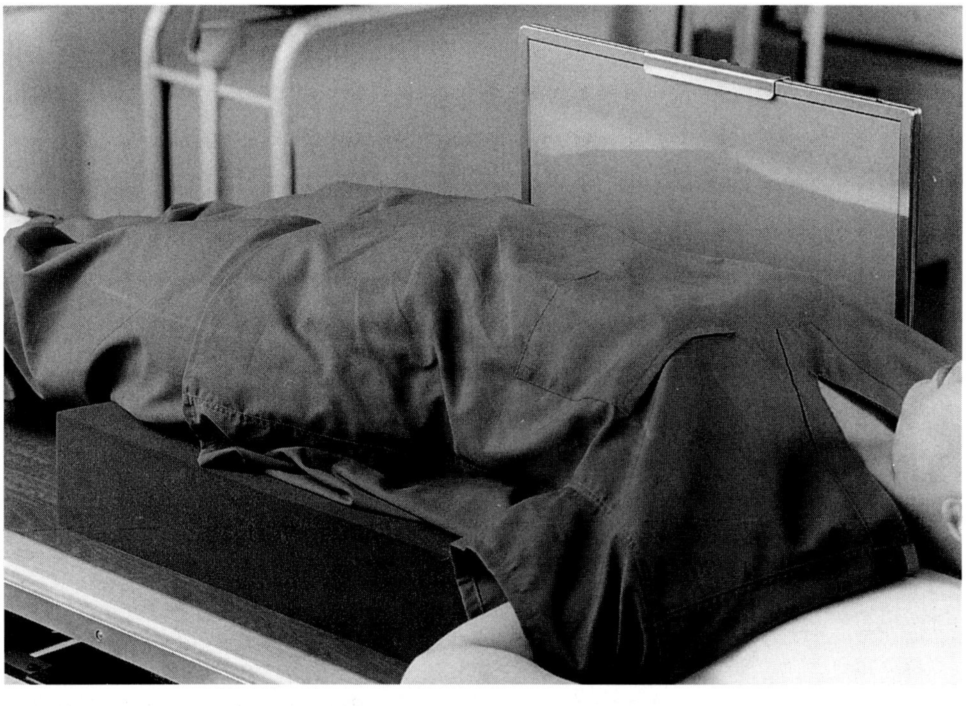

Figure 12.16. Dorsal decubitus.

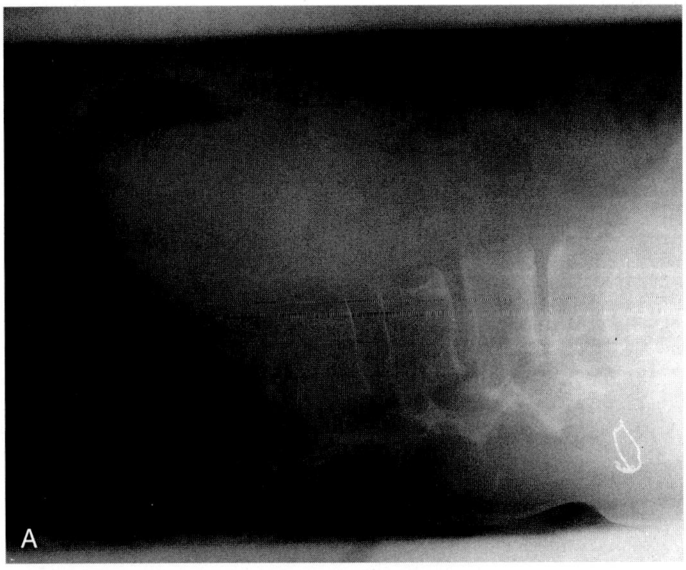

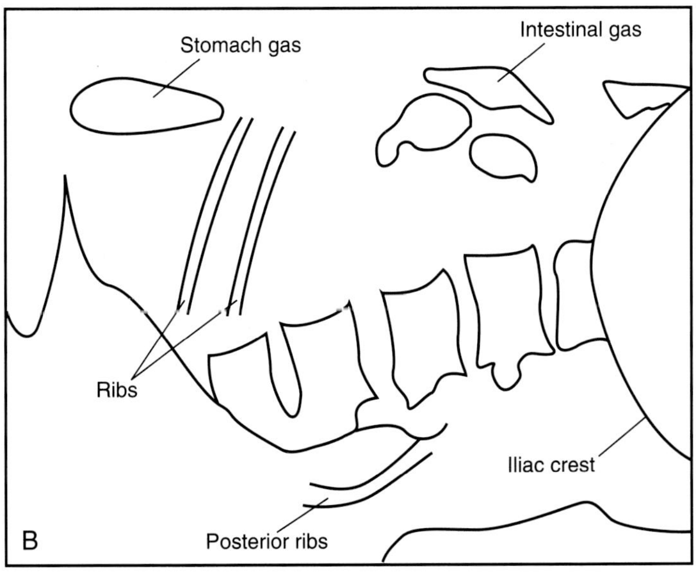

Figure 12.17. A and B, Dorsal decubitus.

Table 12.1 Findings on the Plain Radiograph in Acute Abdomen

Radiographic Appearance	Indication
RUQ calculi	Cholecystitis
RLQ fecalith RLQ segmental bowel loop	Appendicitis
Small bowel loops	Small bowel obstruction
Distended colon	Large bowel obstruction Toxic megacolon Pseudo-obstruction
Distended right colon	Cecal volvulus
Distended left colon loop	Sigmoid volvulus
Stool-filled colon	Obstipation
Urinary tract density	Ureteral calculus
Large pelvic densities	Urinary retention Ovarian tumor Enlarged uterus
Calcifications or sentinel loop in upper abdomen	Pancreatitis
RLQ density with bowel loops Air in biliary tree	Gallstone ileus
Air in portal vein	Gangrene of bowel
Fusiform calcified outline	Aortic aneurysm
LUQ round calcified outline	Splenic artery aneurysm

Data from Young JO: Acute abdominal pain. *In* Hoffer EP (ed): Emergency Problems in the Elderly. Oradell, NJ: Medical Economics Books, 1985, pp 63–74.

ACUTE ABDOMEN

According to Long (1992), the acute abdomen is a physical manifestation of a number of conditions affecting the abdominopelvic cavity. Patients present with abdominal pain of varying intensity, location, and frequency. Systemic changes include nausea, vomiting, and changes in bowel function.

Radiography demonstrates well the conditions associated with the acute abdomen such as pneumoperitoneum, bowel obstruction, and adynamic ileus (Table 12.1). Acute appendicitis, acute cholecystitis, acute pancreatitis, renal colic, intra-abdominal abscesses, ischemic bowel disease, and ruptured abdominal aortic aneurysm are also evidenced with some incidence on radiographs, although other modalities best evaluate these conditions.

Two basic routines for the acute abdomen are: (1) the three-way abdomen routine, consisting of an AP supine abdomen, an AP erect abdomen, and a PA chest; and (2) the two-way abdomen routine, consisting of an AP abdomen recumbent and an AP erect abdomen to include the diaphragm. The value of the PA chest in the three-way routine lies in the fact that free air under the diaphragm may be missed on the upright abdomen. Another advantage is the value of the projection in searching for referred disease from the trunk.

In the three-way abdomen, a left side down decubitus may replace the upright abdomen if the patient is unable to tolerate a weight-bearing radiograph. The diaphragm must be included on the upright chest or upright abdomen in order to evaluate free air under the diaphragm.

Bibliography

Long BW: Radiography of the Acute Abdomen. Albuquerque, NM: American Society of Radiologic Technologists, 1992.

CHAPTER 13

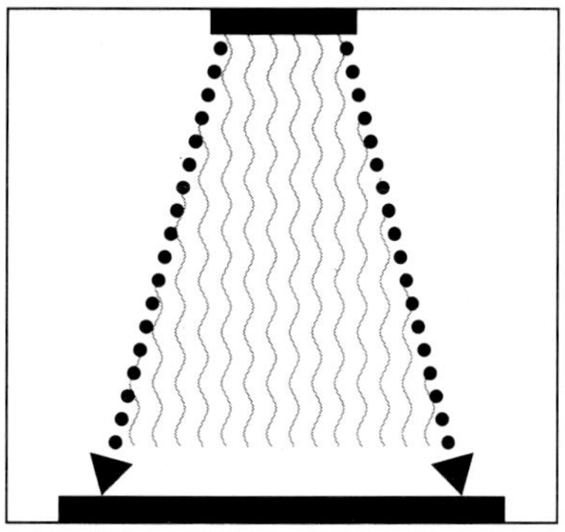

Spine

Steven B. Dowd, Ed.D., R.T.(R.)

Donna F. Burr, M.Ed., R.T.(R.)

Bettye G. Wilson, M.A.Ed., R.T.(R.), R.D.M.S.

Radiographic Anatomy

Radiographic Positioning

This chapter details the positioning of the spine and its associated anatomy. Radiography of the spine is performed in trauma and nontrauma settings to evaluate structure and function. Proper spinal radiography requires an understanding of anatomy, including embryologic development of the spine, since so many chronic conditions result from spinal development, and an understanding of technical factors, especially geometric factors.

The beam-part-film relationship is often critical in spinal radiography to visualize anatomic structures in proper perspective. For example, proper demonstration of the intervertebral foramina of the cervical region requires a longitudinal angulation of the central ray and a medial rotation of the patient (or a medial angulation of the central ray) owing to their position within the body. Proper demonstration of the intervertebral foramina of the thoracic spine, on the other hand, requires a true lateral position of the patient. Demonstration of the thoracic apophyseal joints requires a 15- to 20-degree angulation; an anterior angulation to show joints nearest the film and a posterior angulation to show the joints farthest from the film. Finally, research indicates that the PA projection for the lumbar spine places the intervertebral disk spaces at an angle more closely paralleling the divergence of the x-ray beam.

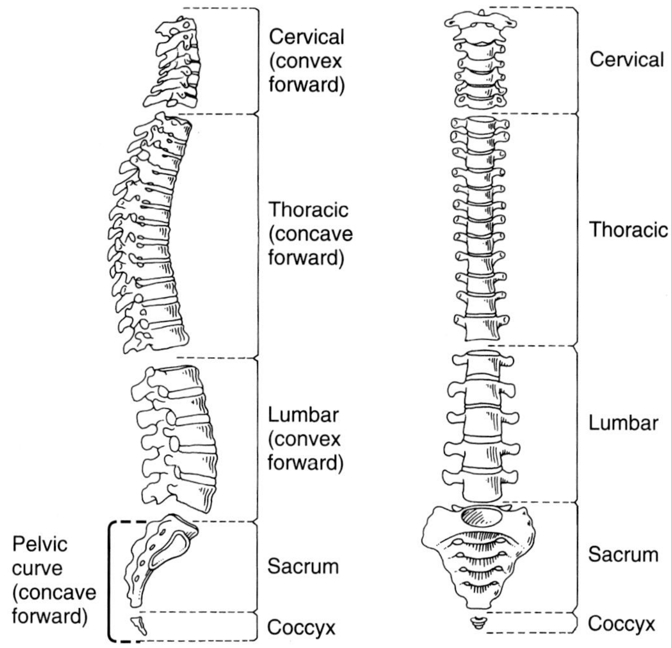

Figure 13.1. A and B, Segmental curvature of entire spine.

ANATOMY

Vertebral Column

The vertebral column consists of 24 true vertebrae and 9 other segments, divided into five sections:

- Cervical vertebrae—7, the first of which is called the atlas and the second the axis.
- Thoracic vertebrae—12.
- Lumbar vertebrae—5.
- Sacrum—5 fused segments.
- Coccyx—3 to 5 segments, with an average of 4.

The number of vertebrae may be increased by 1 in a region or decreased by 1 in another.

A lateral projection of the vertebral column shows four distinct curves: the cervical, anteriorly convex (or convex forward); the thoracic, anteriorly concave (or concave forward); the lumbar, anteriorly convex (or convex forward); and the sacrum and coccyx, anteriorly concave (or concave forward) (Fig. 13.1). Frontally, the upper thoracic vertebrae may demonstrate a slight lateral curvature, convex to the right in a right-handed person and convex to the left in a left-handed person. An abnormal lateral curvature is called scoliosis.

Common Aspects of All Vertebrae

Two distinct portions are found in each vertebra: the body anteriorly and the neural, or vertebral, arch posteriorly. These parts enclose the spinal foramen. The spinal foramen is also called the vertebral foramen. The neural arch comprises two pedicles and two laminae. Seven processes extend from the neural arch: four articular, two transverse, and one spinous.

One of the most important functions of the vertebrae is the formation of a column that supports the entire body. Each vertebra articulates closely with the one immediately above and the one immediately below it. The spinal foramina join together to form the spinal canal, which protects the spinal cord (medulla spinalis)—another important function of the spine. The spinal nerves and branches, along with the nutrient vessels, pass through the intervertebral foramina.

- Body. The body is round and is the most anterior and largest single part of a vertebra. The superior and inferior surfaces are flat and rough, and their margins form a distinct rim.
- Pedicles. There are two short and thick pedicles located bilaterally and posteriorly on each body projecting from the junction of the posterior and the lateral surfaces. The vertebral notches are the depressions located superior and inferior to the pedicles. The intervertebral foramen is formed by the inferior vertebral notch of the body of the vertebra above joining the superior vertebral notch of the body of the vertebra below. The intervertebral foramina transmit spinal nerves and blood vessels.
- Laminae. The laminae extend posteriorly and medially from the pedicles. The spinal foramen is closed posteriorly by their midline fusion.
- Processes. There are seven processes common to the vertebral bodies.

Spinous Process. The single spinous process, which can be palpated, projects posteriorly and inferiorly from the fusion of the laminae of each typical vertebrae. The spinous process of C7 can be palpated at the base of the neck (posteriorly) and may be used as a localization point.

Articular Processes. The pedicles join the laminae bilaterally to form parts of the neural arch. From these junctions extend the two superior and two inferior articular processes. The superior articular surfaces extend anteriorly. The superior facet of the body of the vertebra below articulates with the inferior facet of the body of the vertebra above. The common term for this articulation is zygapophyseal or apophyseal joint.

Transverse Processes. The juncture of the laminae with the pedicles is below the base of the superior articular process and above the base of the inferior articular process. From this site extend the transverse processes, which project laterally and minimally posterior.

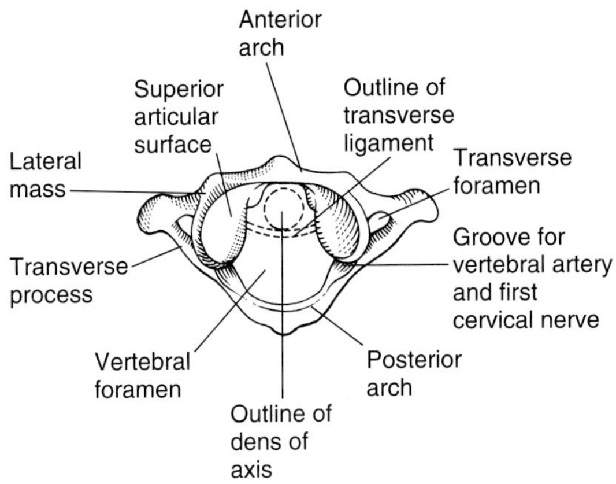

Figure 13.2. Anatomy of 1st cervical vertebra (C1) (atlas).

Cervical Vertebrae

The cervical vertebrae are small and, in relation to the thoracic and lumbar vertebrae, are the only vertebrae that contain a foramen in each transverse process. These transverse foramina transmit the vertebral arteries and veins.

C2 through C7 have two superior and two inferior articular facets (processes), one spinous process, and two transverse processes. The cervical transverse processes are small, arising from both the pedicle and the body instead of from the junction between the pedicle and the lamina. The articular pillars are situated behind the transverse processes. Each pillar has two articulating processes: a superior and an inferior articular process.

The structures of three cervical vertebrae, C1, C2, and C7, are unique from that of the others.

First Cervical Vertebra (Atlas). The head articulates in a forward and backward "rocking" motion on the ring-shaped atlas. The atlas has no body. This vertebra is usually referred to as "ring-like" in appearance. The center of the ring provides for articulation of the dens or odontoid process from C2 (axis) below. The articulation above, between the occipital bone and the atlas, is known as the atlanto-occipital junction. During embryonic development, the would-be body of the atlas (C1) fuses with that of C2 to form the dens or odontoid process of the axis. C1 has no definable body or spinous process but, instead, has a slight posterior projection from the posterior arch. Two lateral masses separate its anterior and posterior arches. Both lateral masses exhibit superior and inferior articular facets. The superior facets are deeper in concavity than those located inferiorly. The shape and depth of the superior articular facets correspond to the shape of the occipital condyles of the cranium with which they unite. The inferior articular facets of the atlas articulate with the superior articular facets of C2 (axis).

Projecting laterally from the lateral masses and posteriorly to the anterior arch are the spinous processes. The spinous processes of the axis are longer than those of the other six cervical vertebra. Within the transverse processes are located transverse foramina for the passage of blood vessels and nerves (Fig. 13.2).

Second Cervical Vertebra (Axis). The axis contains the odontoid process or dens. The dens of the axis is continuous with its body. The union of the atlas and the axis is a pivot that allows for side-to-side rotation of the head (Fig. 13.3). This union is maintained through transverse ligaments. The articular surfaces of C1 and the upper articular surface of C2 are more anteriorly situated than other cervical articulations. The spinous process of C2 exhibits the characteristic bifid tip common to C2 through C6.

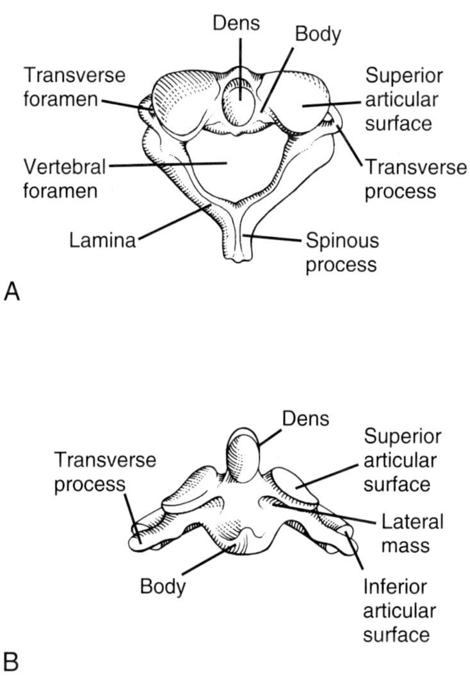

Figure 13.3. A and B, Anatomy of 2nd cervical vertebra (C2) (axis).

Seventh Cervical Vertebra. The most prominent spinous process of the cervical vertebra is located on C7. For this reason, this vertebra is called the vertebra prominens. The spinous process of C7 takes on the characteristics of the thoracic vertebra in that it extends inferiorly and loses the bifid tip common to most cervical vertebrae. The transverse processes are larger in C7 than in the others (Fig. 13.4).

Thoracic Vertebrae

The thoracic vertebrae are larger than the cervical vertebrae. They become progressively larger from T1 through T12.

The transverse processes of the vertebrae project obliquely, laterally, and posteriorly. The long spinous processes from T5 to T9 project interiorly to overlap the vertebral body below.

The costal (rib) facets are found only on these vertebrae. Each vertebrae has either a full facet or two partial facets called demifacets on each side of the body. These form the costovertebral joints in articulation with the heads of ribs. From T1 through T10, additional facets articulate with the rib tubercles.

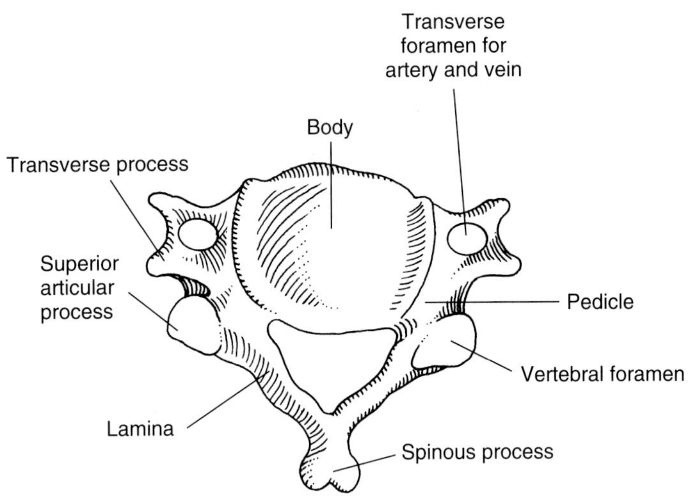

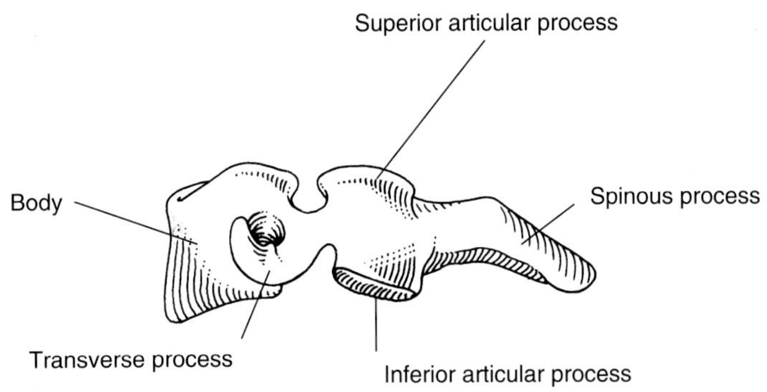

Figure 13.4. Anatomy of 7th cervical vertebra (C7) (vertebral prominence).

The differences of articulation in the thoracic vertebral bodies are:

1. The first pair of ribs articulates with the costotransverse facet and the costovertebral facet of T1. The second pair of ribs articulates with the costotransverse facet and upper costal facet of T2 and the lower costal facet of T1.
2. The third pair of ribs articulates with the costotransverse facet and upper costal facet of T3 and the lower costal facet of T2.
3. T1 through T8 have two rib articulations on each side.
4. T9 and T10 are slightly different in that the 9th pair of ribs articulates with a costotransverse facet and a costovertebral facet of T9. The 10th pair of ribs articulates with a costotransverse facet and a costovertebral facet of T10. T11 and T12 have no costotransverse facets, only costovertebral facets on each side. T12's transverse processes are replaced by three tubercles. Its inferior apophyseal joint faces in a more lateral direction than the joint above it.

Throughout the vertebral column, the superior articular facets of a body articulate with the inferior articular facets of the body above. This type of articulation is a true apophyseal articulation (apophyseal joint); an apophysis is an outgrowth (process) that has never been entirely separated from a bone. All of the apophyseal articulations (except for the inferior process of T12) angle forward 15 to 20 degrees. Each vertebral body (centrum) articulates with the intervertebral disks, the spongelike fibrocartilages located between each pair of vertebral bodies (Fig. 13.5).

Lumbar Vertebrae

The lumbar vertebrae are much larger than the thoracic vertebrae, and increase in size moving downward. The transverse processes are more prominent radiographically, although they are longer and more slender (smaller) than those of the thoracic region. The transverse processes of the first three lumbar vertebrae are truly horizontal, whereas those of the last two are inclined somewhat superiorly. The articulations of the lumbar vertebrae are identical in form to those of the thoracic vertebrae except that there are no rib articulations (Fig. 13.6). In the lumbar spine, the apophyseal joints incline posteriorly from the coronal plane. This forms an angle of 30 to 50 degrees open posteriorly from the midsagittal plane.

The thickness of L5 (anteriorly) accounts for the prominence of the lumbosacral articulation. Its spinous process is smaller, with the transverse processes thicker. Its interspace is also typically narrower. The inferior articular facets are spaced farther apart. The body of L5 may present a condition termed spina bifida occult. This condition is the result of a cleft in the vertebral arch.

The lumbosacral joint is the articulation of the last (5th) lumbar vertebra with the sacrum. When L5 is incorporated, in whole or part, in the sacrum, this is known as sacralization. When the first sacral segment is segmented and incorporated into the spine, this is known as lumbarization.

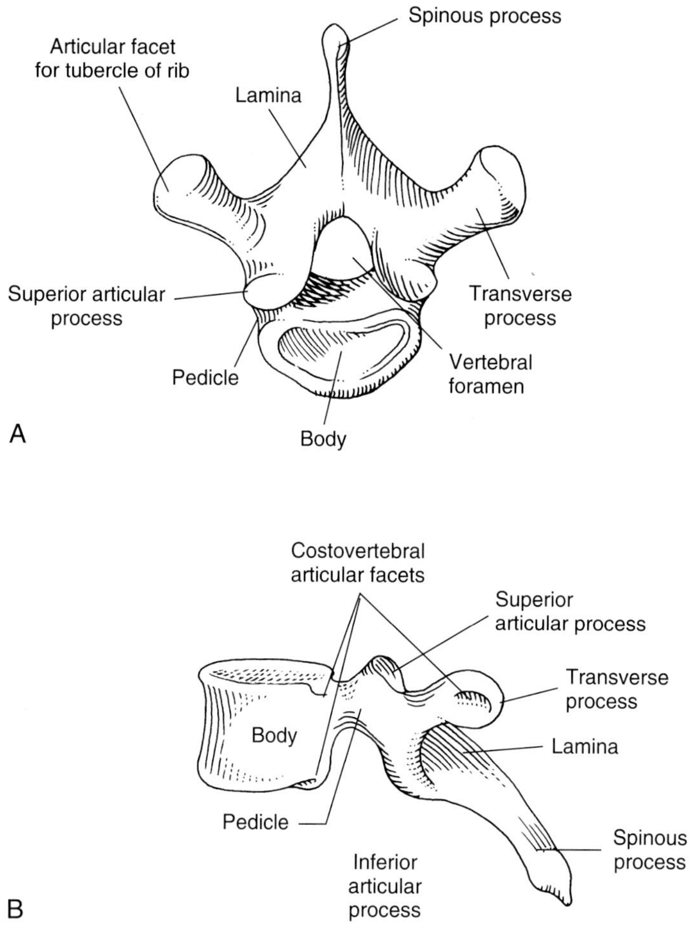

Figure 13.5. A and B, Articular facets of thoracic vertebrae.

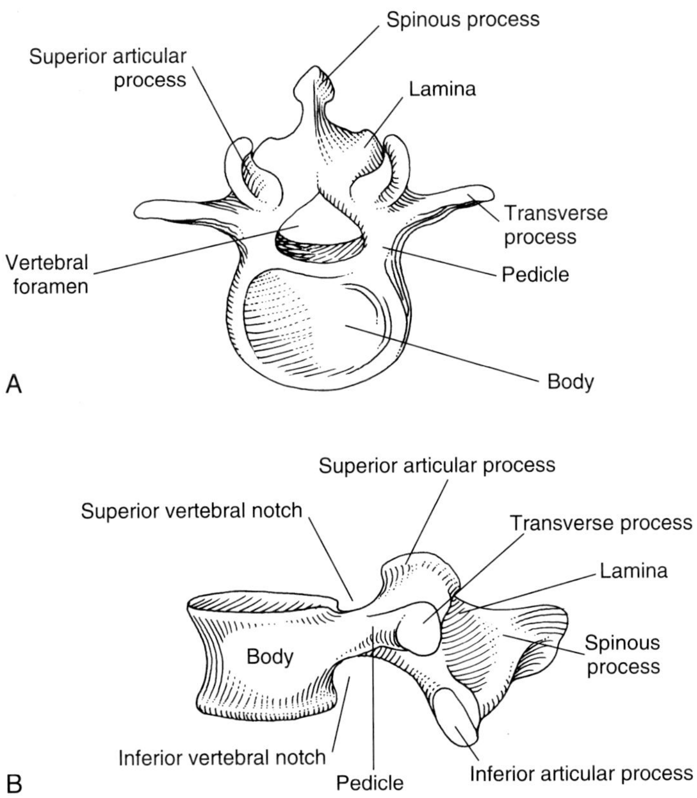

Figure 13.6. A and B, Anatomy of lumbar vertebrae.

Sacrum and Coccyx

In very young children, the sacrum and the coccyx (nine rudimentory vertebrae or segments) are distinct and separate. The proximal five segments are typically fused (ankylosed) and constitute the sacrum. The distal four segments, which articulate with the sacrum above, constitute the coccyx. At times, the coccyx may consist of three or five segments.

Sacrum. The sacrum is large and resembles a triangle with a proximal base and a distal apex. Situated between the ilia, it is inferior to L5. It forms the superior and posterior parts of the pelvic cavity. Superiorly, it articulates with the inferior surface of the last (usually 5th) lumbar vertebra, forming the lumbosacral joint. Inferiorly, it articulates with the coccyx, forming the sacrococcygeal joint.

Bilaterally, its articulations form the right and the left sacroiliac joints. The sacroiliac joints slant obliquely, posteriorly, and medially at an angle of 25 to 30 degrees, opening anteriorly to the midsagittal plane. In radiographic examinations, the sacrum and coccyx are often considered as parts of the pelvis rather than as true vertebrae. Anatomically, the sacrum and coccyx are considered as parts of the vertebral column. S1 has articular facets that articulate with the inferior articular facets of the last lumbar vertebra. The concave pelvic surface of the sacrum presents four transverse ridges that are in line with the early articulations of the five segments. The anterior sacral foramina are bilateral at the ends of these ridges. The spinal canal extends through most of the sacrum and, although it does not contain the spinal cord itself, it does contain the sacral nerves. The walls of the sacrum contain the anterior and posterior sacral foramina (Fig. 13.7).

Coccyx. None of the coccygeal segments has pedicles, laminae, or spinous processes. The proximal segment is usually separate and is the largest of these segments. The remaining segments become progressively smaller in size and are frequently fused. The apex of the coccyx is rounded, sometimes bifid, and frequently displaced to either side (Fig. 13.8).

Spinal Cord

The spinal cord is about 18 inches (45 cm) long in the adult, with termination of the cord occurring at various levels. This ranges from the middle of the body of T12 to the superior border of the body of L3. Most commonly, the cord terminates between the lower inferior body of L1 and the superior border of the body of L2. More information on the anatomy and radiographic visualization of the spinal cord can be found in Chapter 18, Myelography.

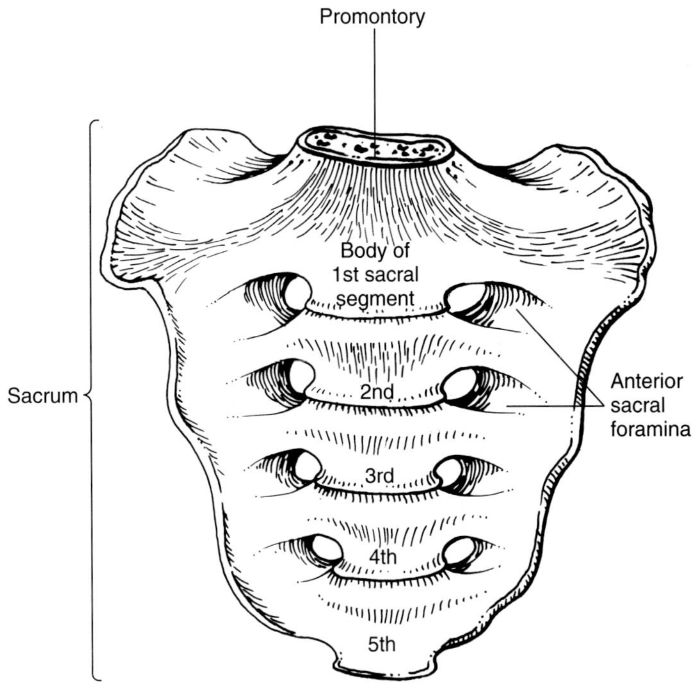

Figure 13.7. Anatomy of sacrum.

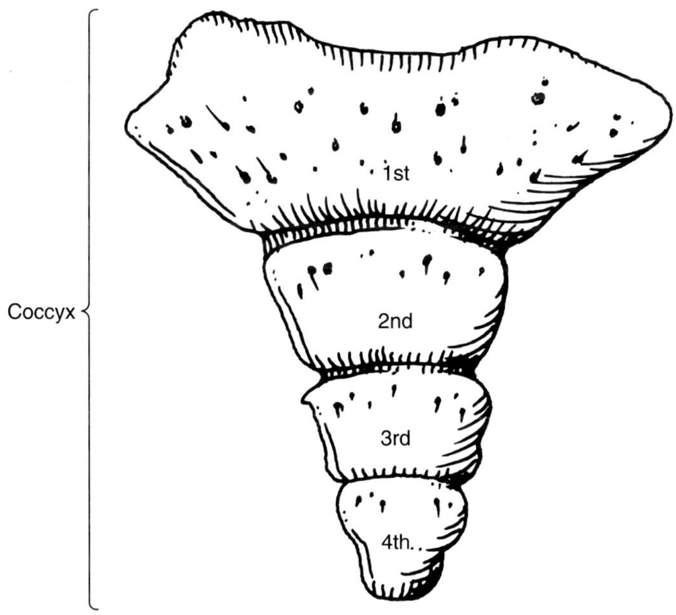

Figure 13.8. Anatomy of coccyx.

Cervical Spine

Position/Projection

AP projection

Film Size:
8 × 10 inches (20 × 24 cm)
lengthwise

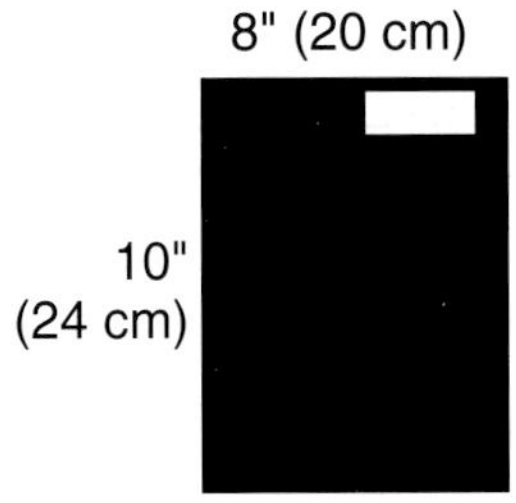

Patient Position

AP, erect or recumbent. Midsagittal plane perpendicular to plane of table. Arms alongside body; shoulders in same transverse plane (Fig. 13.9).

Part Position

Midsagittal plane centered to midline of table. Extend head to place occlusal plane and mastoid tips in same transverse plane.

Central Ray

Through 4th cervical body at an angle of 15–20° cephalad, to enter at or slightly inferior to most prominent point of thyroid cartilage.

Structures Demonstrated

Lower five cervical bodies and upper two or three thoracic bodies, interpediculate spaces, superimposed transverse and articular processes, and intervertebral disk spaces. Presence of cervical ribs may also be shown (Fig. 13.10).

Evaluation Criteria

1. Open intervertebral disk spaces.
2. Mandibular occipital shadows superimposed over C1 and C2 if central ray correctly angled; area from C3 to T2 visible.
3. Spinous processes equidistant to pedicles.
4. Mandibular angles equally distant to vertebrae.

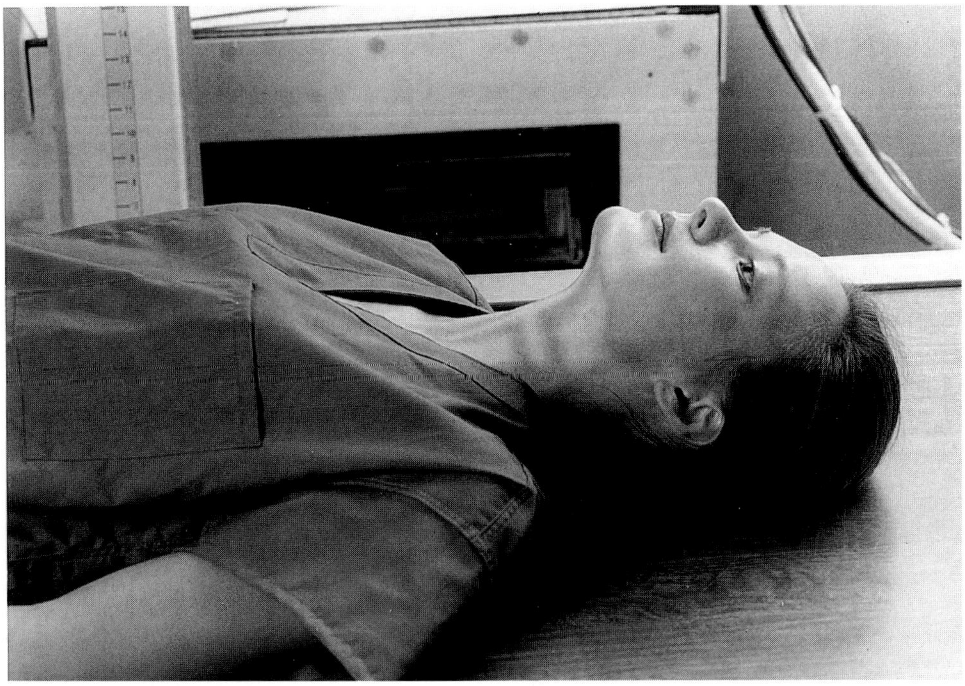

Figure 13.9. Patient in position for AP projection of cervical spine.

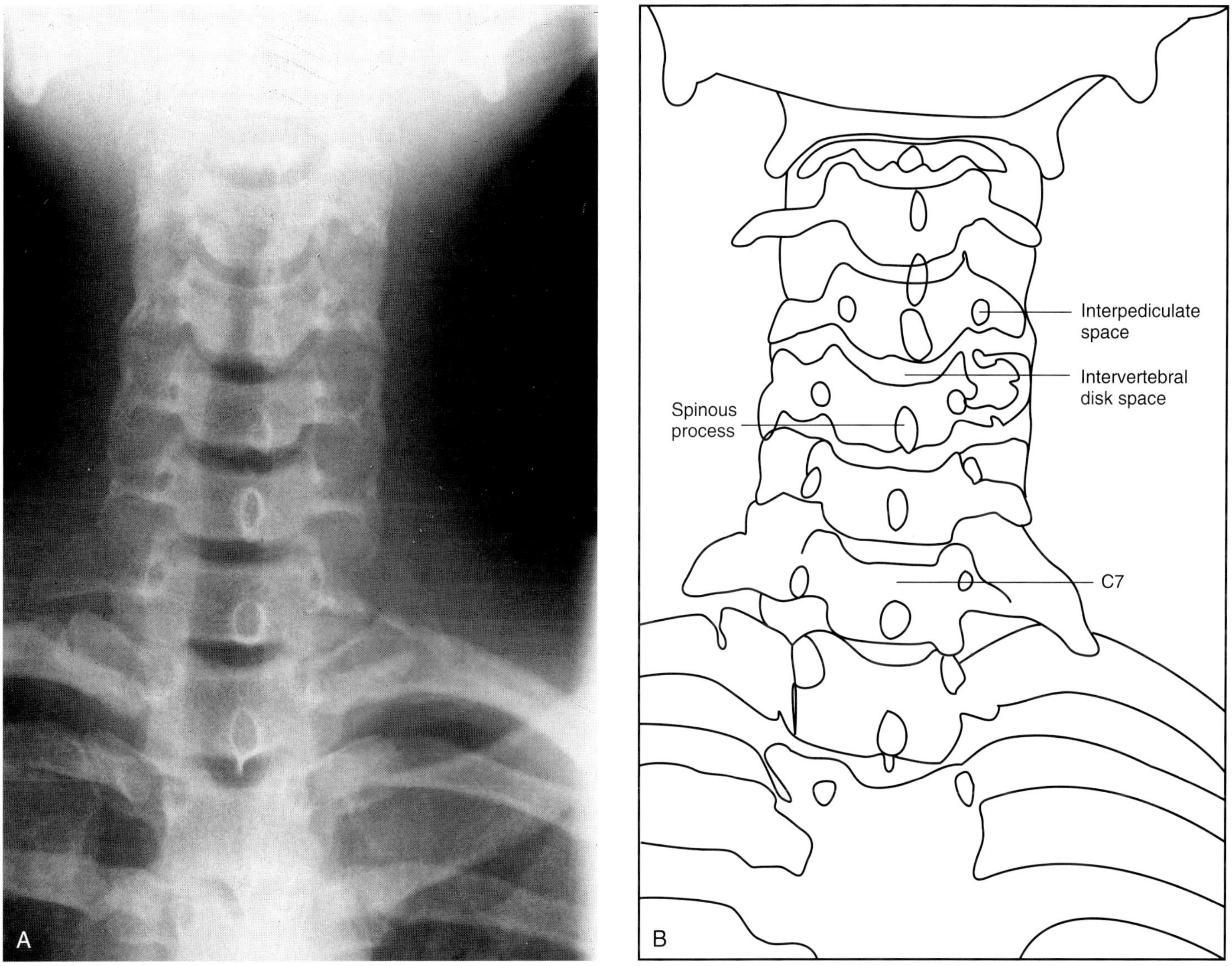

Figure 13.10. A and B, AP radiograph of cervical spine.

Cervical Spine

Position/Projection

AP; odontoid (open-mouth)

Film Size:
8 × 10 inches (20 × 24 cm) crosswise or lengthwise

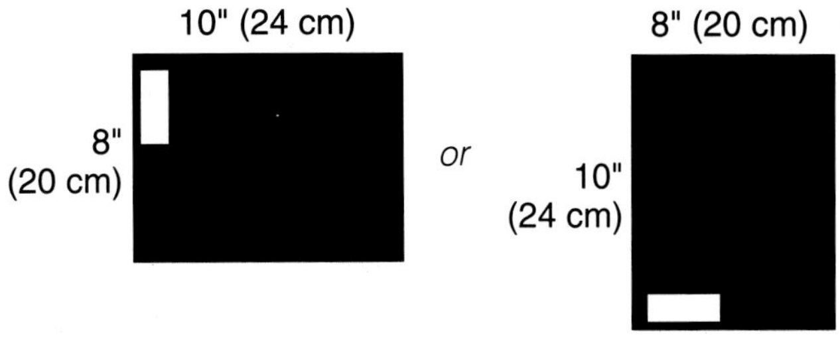

Patient Position

Supine. Midsagittal plane centered to midline of table. Arms alongside body; shoulders in same transverse plane (Fig. 13.11).

Part Position

Have patient open mouth as wide as possible. Then adjust head so that line from lower edge of upper incisors to tip of mastoid process is perpendicular to film.

Central Ray

Perpendicular to midpoint of open mouth.

Structures Demonstrated

AP projection of atlas and axis through open mouth (Fig. 13.12).

Evaluation Criteria

1. Odontoid, atlas, axis, and C1–C2 disk space are well shown.
2. Superimposition of upper teeth and base of skull with mouth wide open; tongue shadow not projected over atlas and axis.

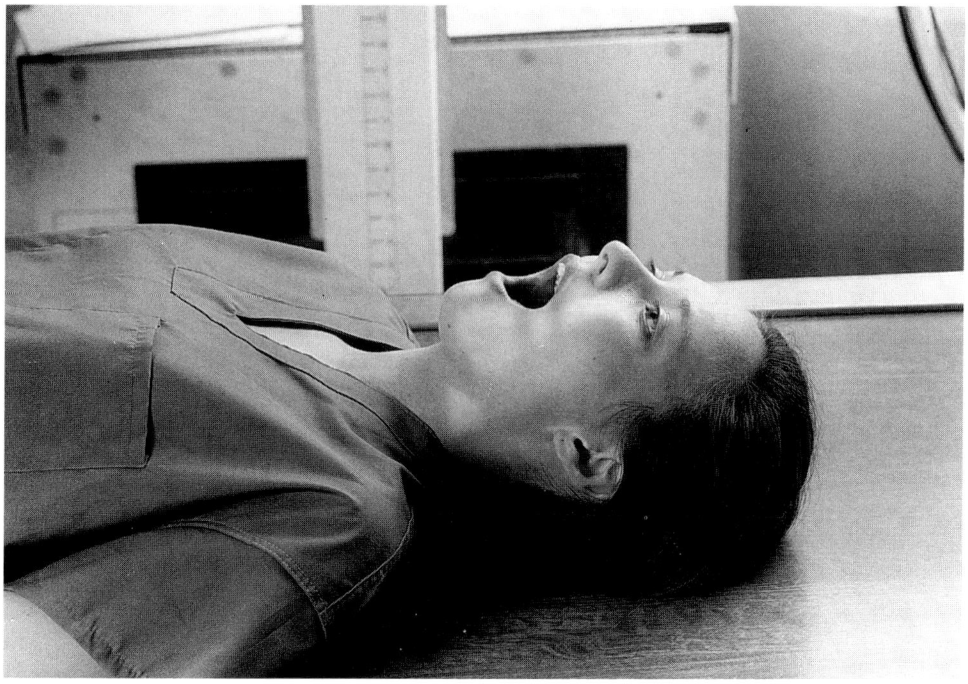

Figure 13.11. Patient in position for AP odontoid (open-mouth) view of axis.

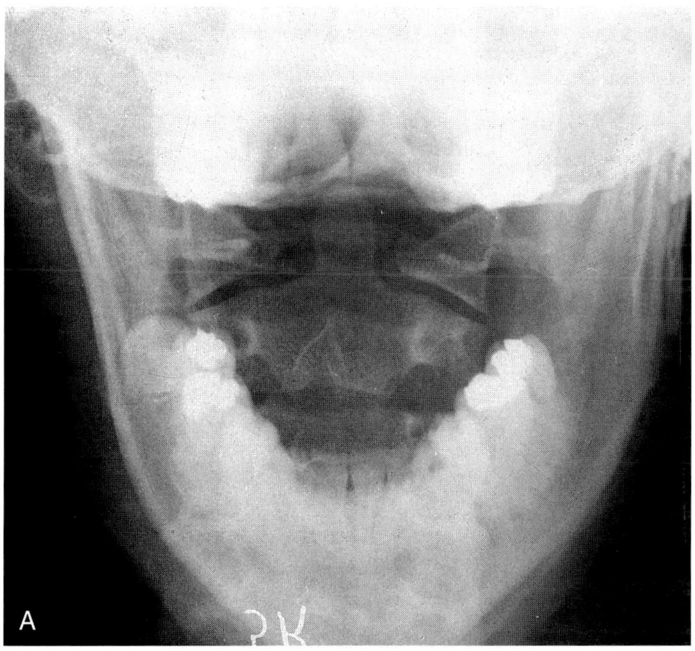

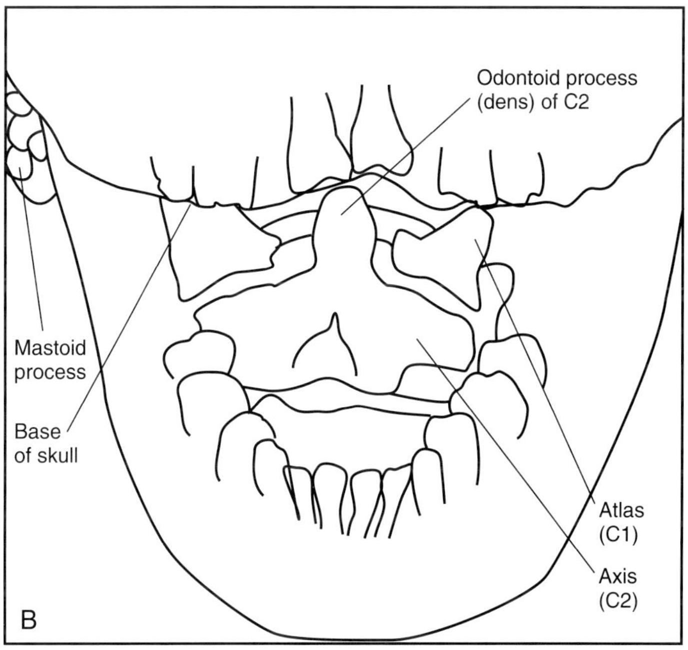

Figure 13.12. A and B, Radiograph of odontoid process of C2 (axis).

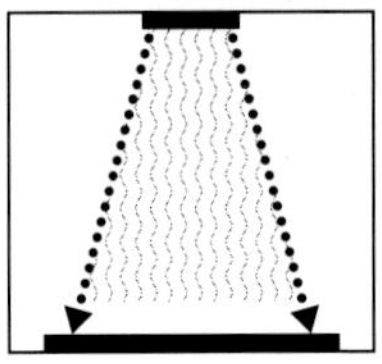

Cervical Spine

Position/Projection

AP projection, Fuchs' method for odontoid

Film Size:
8 × 10 inches (20 × 24 cm)
crosswise *or* lengthwise

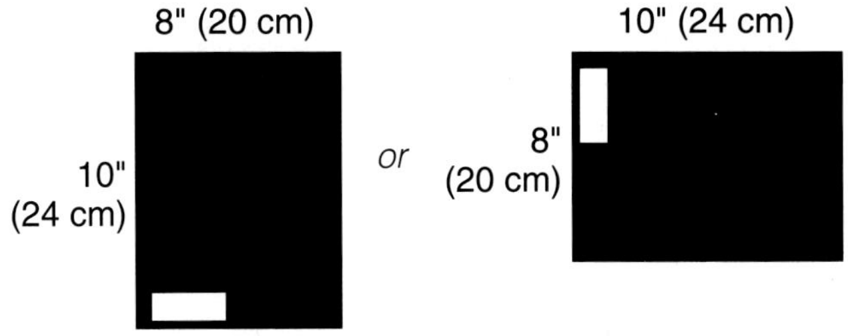

Patient Position

Supine. Midsagittal plane centered to midline of table. Arms alongside body; shoulders in same transverse plane (Fig. 13.13).

Part Position

Chin is extended until tip of chin and tip of mastoid process are vertical. Midsagittal is perpendicular to plane of table.

Central Ray

Perpendicular to midpoint of film, enters neck distal to tip of chin.

Breathing Instructions

Respiration suspended for exposure.

Structures Demonstrated

AP projection of odontoid lying in shadow of foramen magnum (Fig. 13.14).

Evaluation Criteria

1. Entire odontoid shown through foramen magnum.
2. No rotation of head or neck.

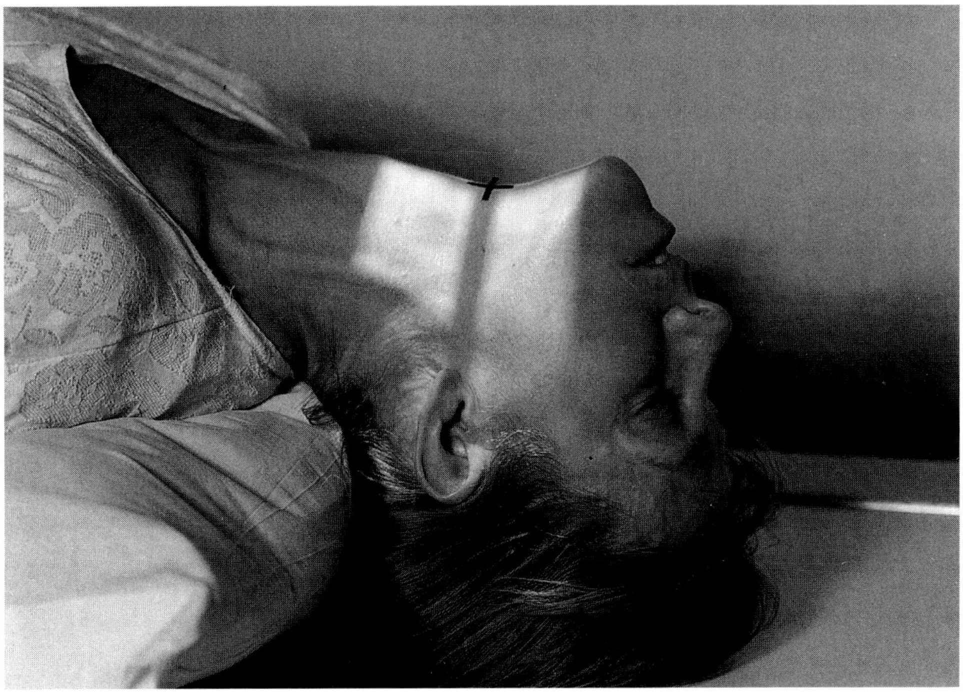

Figure 13.13. Patient in position for AP Fuchs' method for odontoid process of C2.

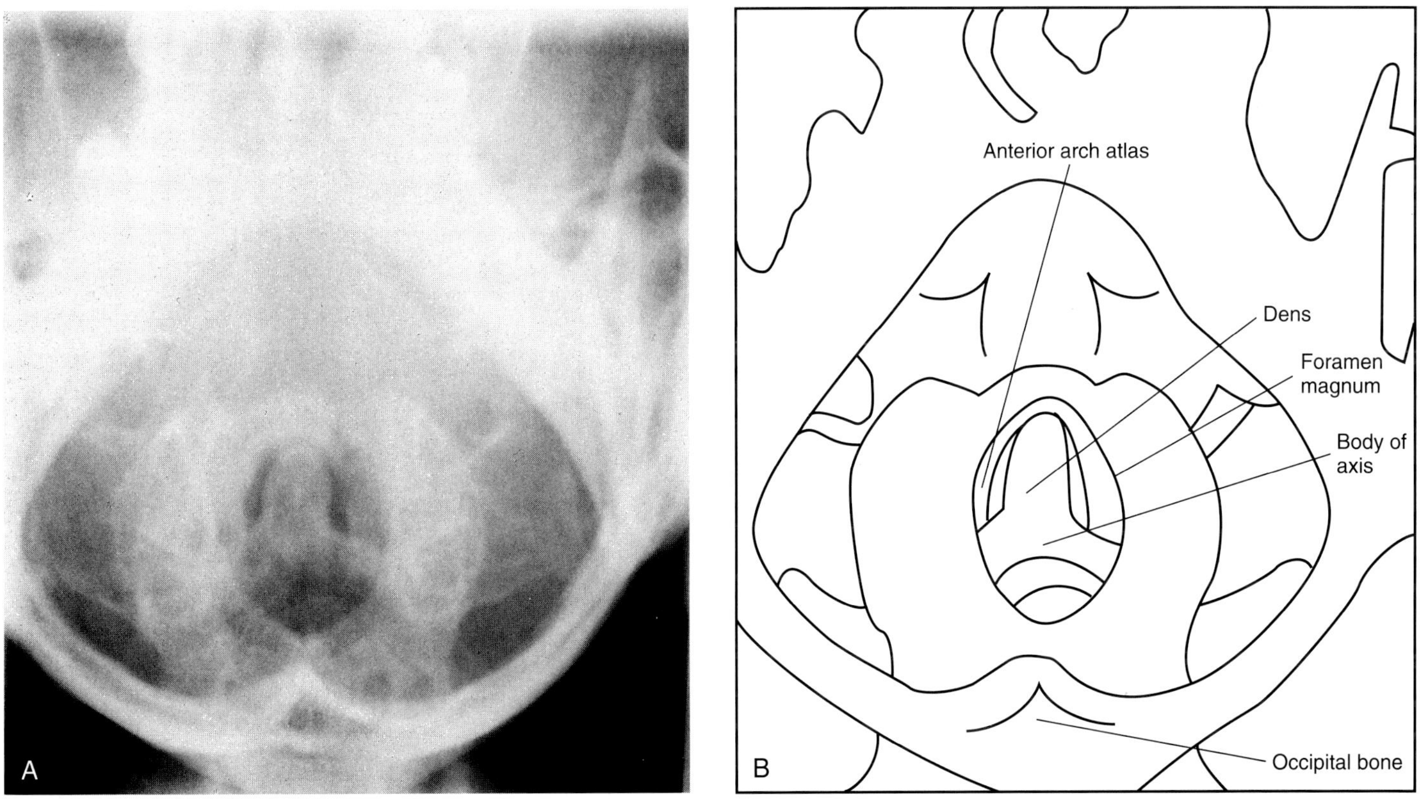

Figure 13.14. A and B, Radiograph of odontoid process in Fuchs' method.

Cervical Spine

Position/Projection

PA projection; Judd's method for atlas and odontoid

Film Size:
8 × 10 inches (20 × 24 cm)
lengthwise

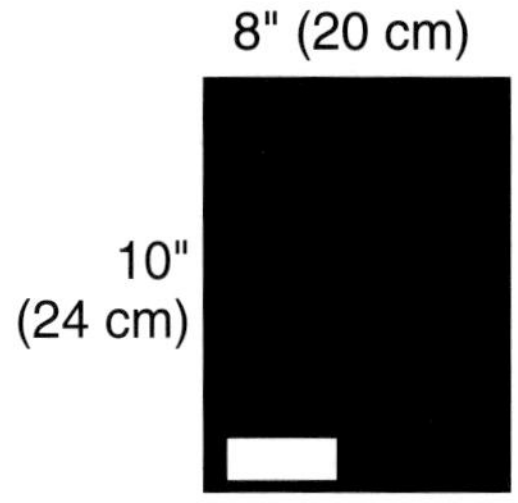

Patient Position

Prone. Midsagittal plane centered to midline of table with elbows flexed; shoulders in same transverse plane (Fig. 13.15).

Part Position

Chin extended, resting on table. Head has tip of nose 1 inch (2.5 cm) from tabletop; midsagittal plane perpendicular to table.

Central Ray

Perpendicular to midpoint of film; enters occiput posterior to mastoid tips.

Breathing Instructions

Breathing suspended for exposure.

Structures Demonstrated

PA projection of odontoid through foramen magnum (Fig. 13.16).

Evaluation Criteria

1. Entire odontoid shown through foramen magnum.
2. No rotation of head or neck.

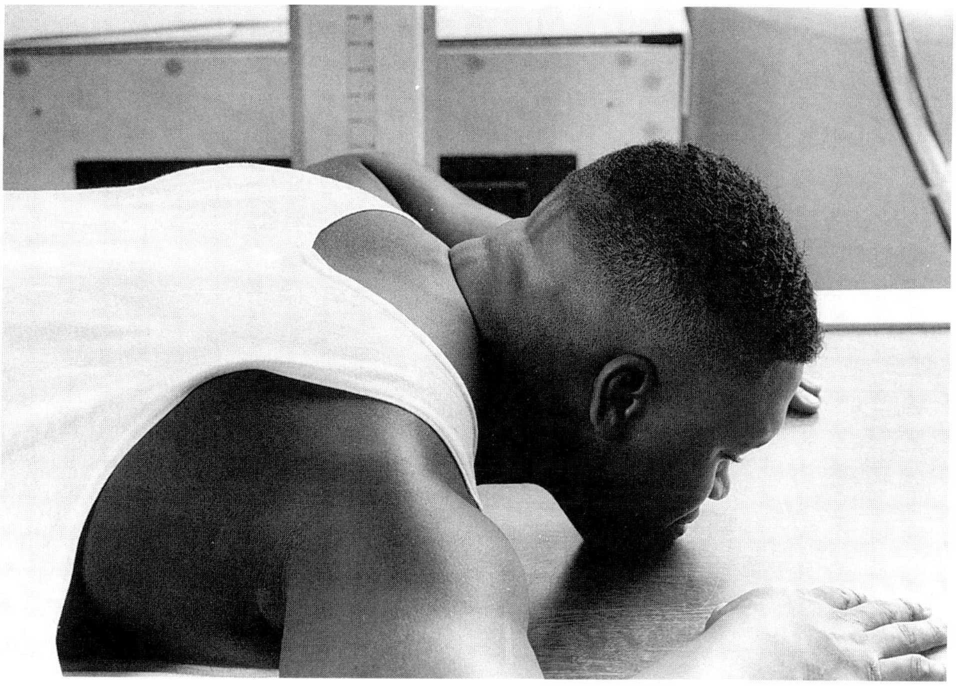

Figure 13.15. Patient in position for the Judd method for demonstration of the atlas (C1) and odontoid process of C2.

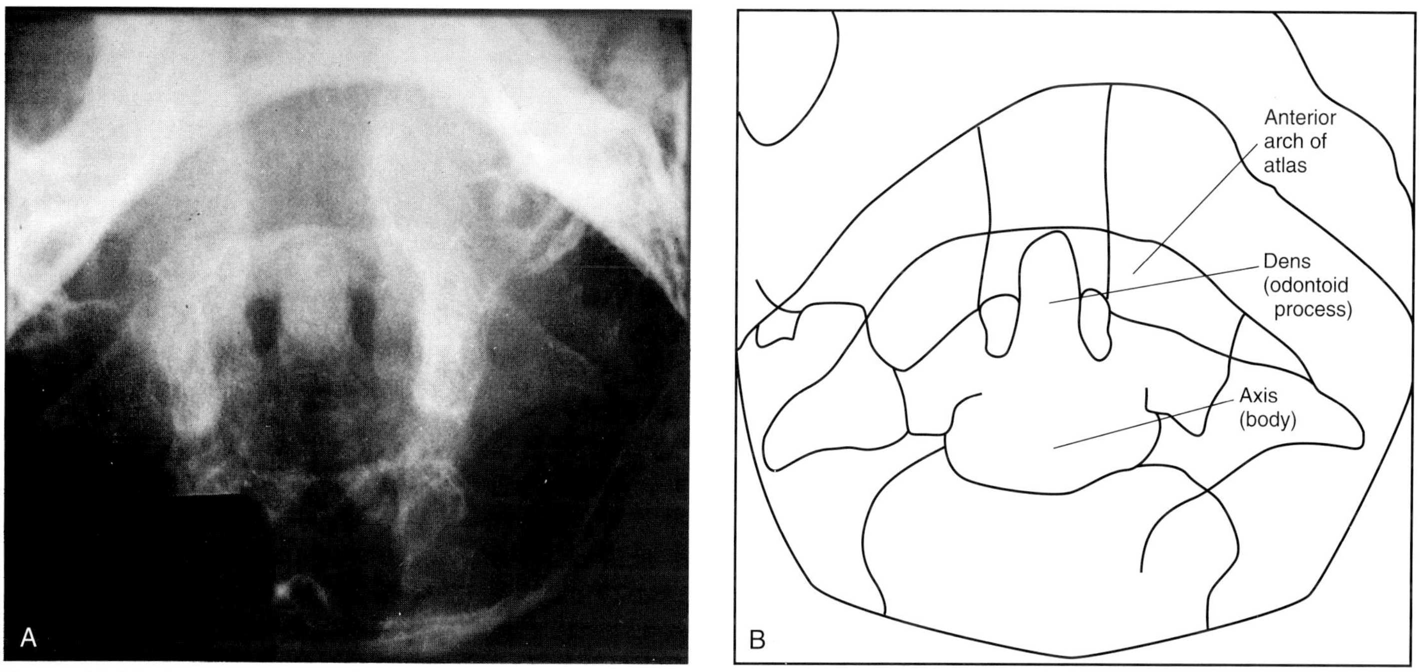

Figure 13.16. A and B, Radiograph of Judd's method of demonstrating atlas and odontoid.

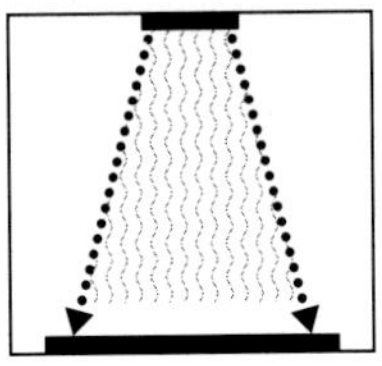

Cervical Spine

Position/Projection

AP axial oblique—Kasabach's method for odontoid

Film Size:
8 × 10 inches (20 × 24 cm)
crosswise or lengthwise

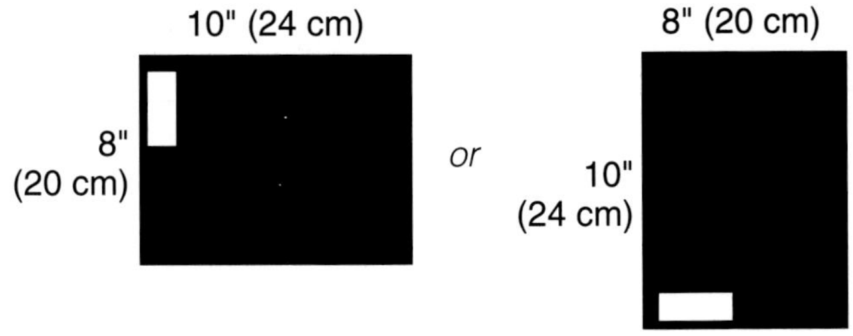

Patient Position

Supine. Midsagittal plane centered to midline of table. Arms alongside body; shoulders in same transverse plane (Fig. 13.17).

Part Position

Head rotated 40–45° away from side examined; infraorbital meatal line perpendicular.

Central Ray

10–15° caudad, centered midway between outer canthus and external auditory meatus.

Structures Demonstrated

AP view of odontoid (Fig. 13.18).

Evaluation Criteria

Odontoid process well visualized.

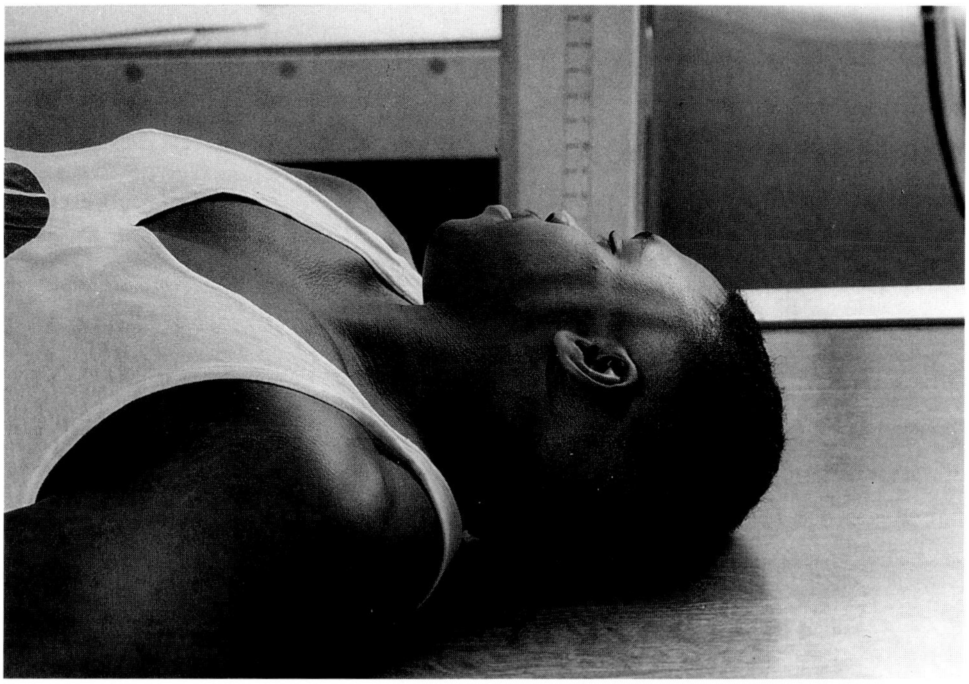

Figure 13.17. Patient in position for Kasabach's method for odontoid process.

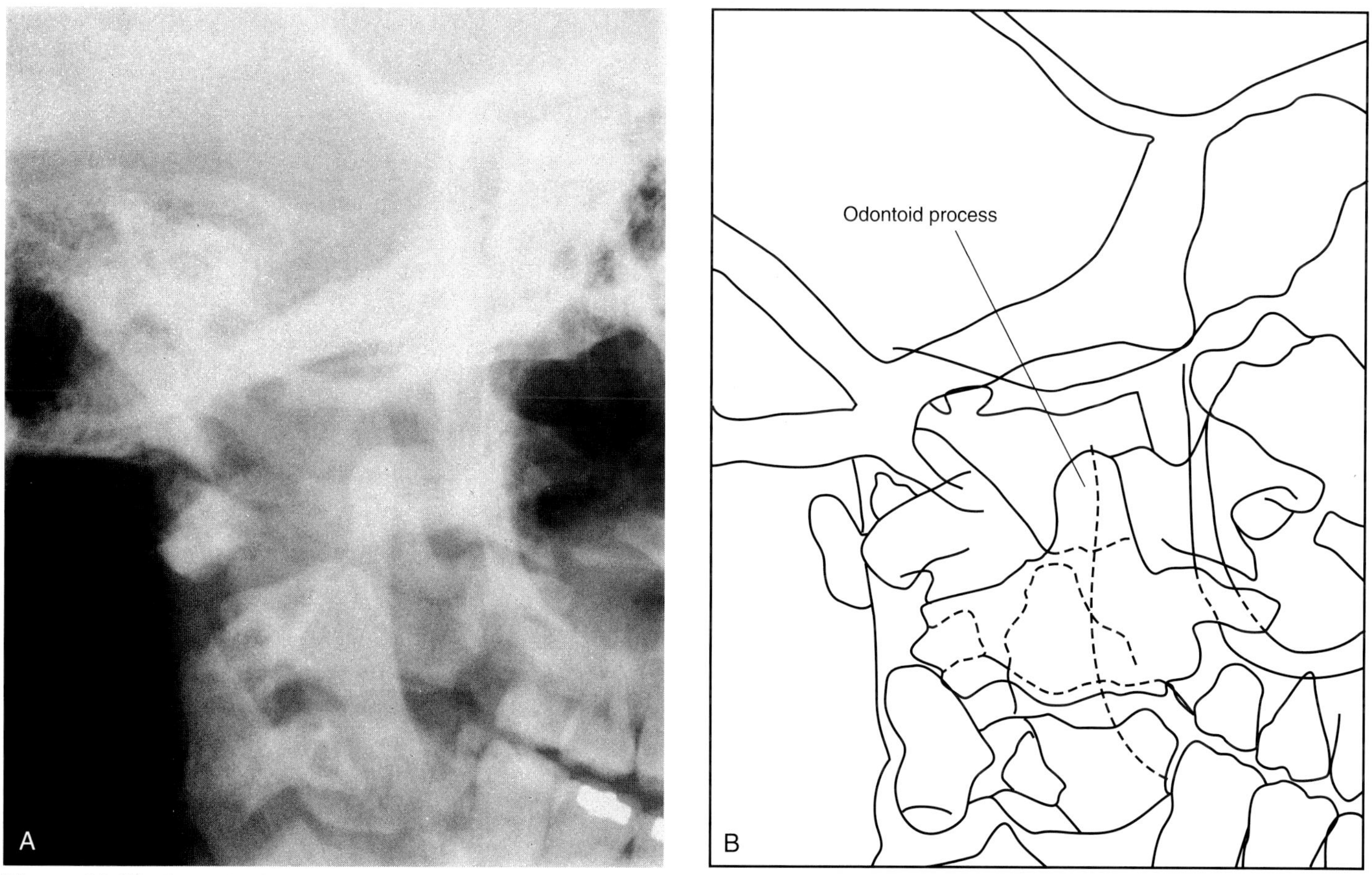

Figure 13.18. A and B, Odontoid process as visualized in the Kasabach method.

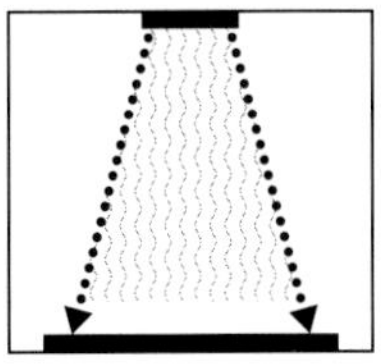

Cervical Spine

Position/Projection

PA obliques

Film Size:
8 × 10 inches (20 × 24 cm) lengthwise

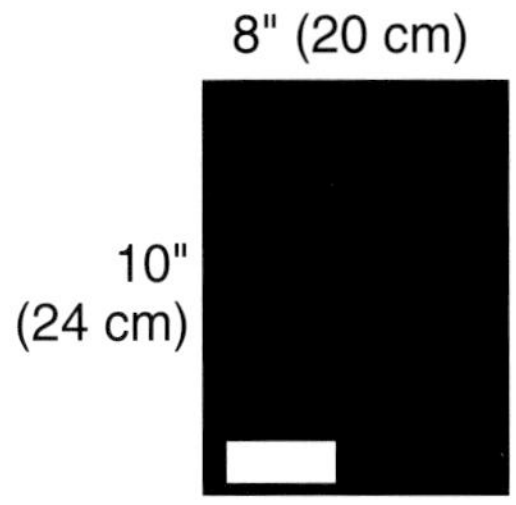

Patient Position

PA position, standing or recumbent (Fig. 13.19).

Part Position

Keeping one shoulder adjacent to film, rotate patient's entire body 45° to film. Center cassette at level of C5 segment.

Central Ray

Direct to C4 at angle of 15–20° caudad.

Structures Demonstrated

Demonstrates intervertebral foramina and pedicles closest to film and oblique projection of bodies and other parts of cervical column (Fig. 13.20).

Evaluation Criteria

1. All seven cervical vertebrae included, as well as T1.
2. Both intervertebral foramina and intervertebral disk spaces should be open and well demonstrated.
3. Occipital bone should not overlap C1.
4. Angle of mandible should not overlap C1 and C2.

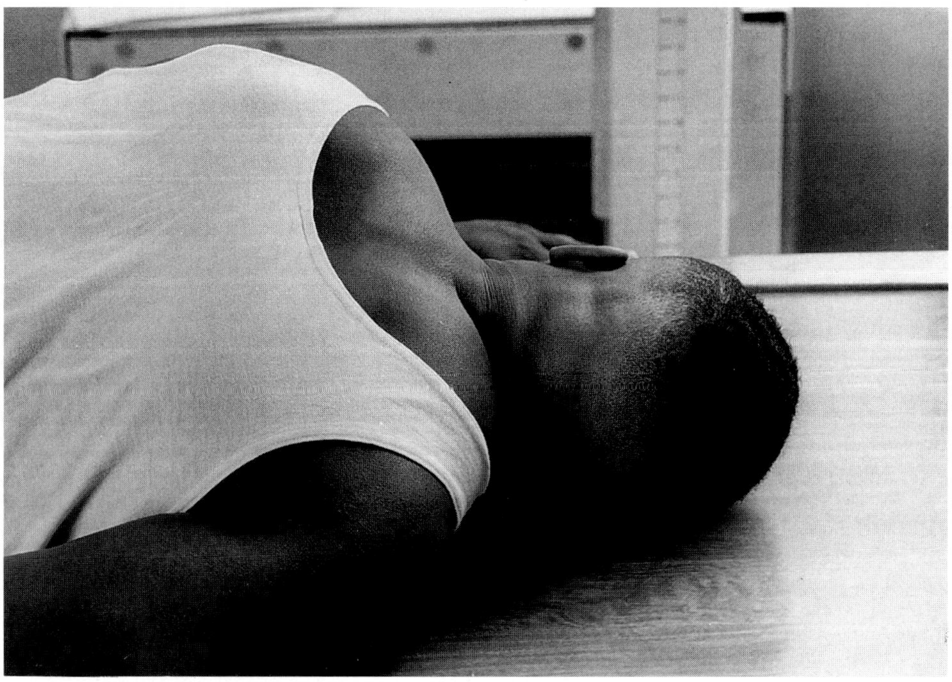

Figure 13.19. PA oblique position of cervical vertebrae.

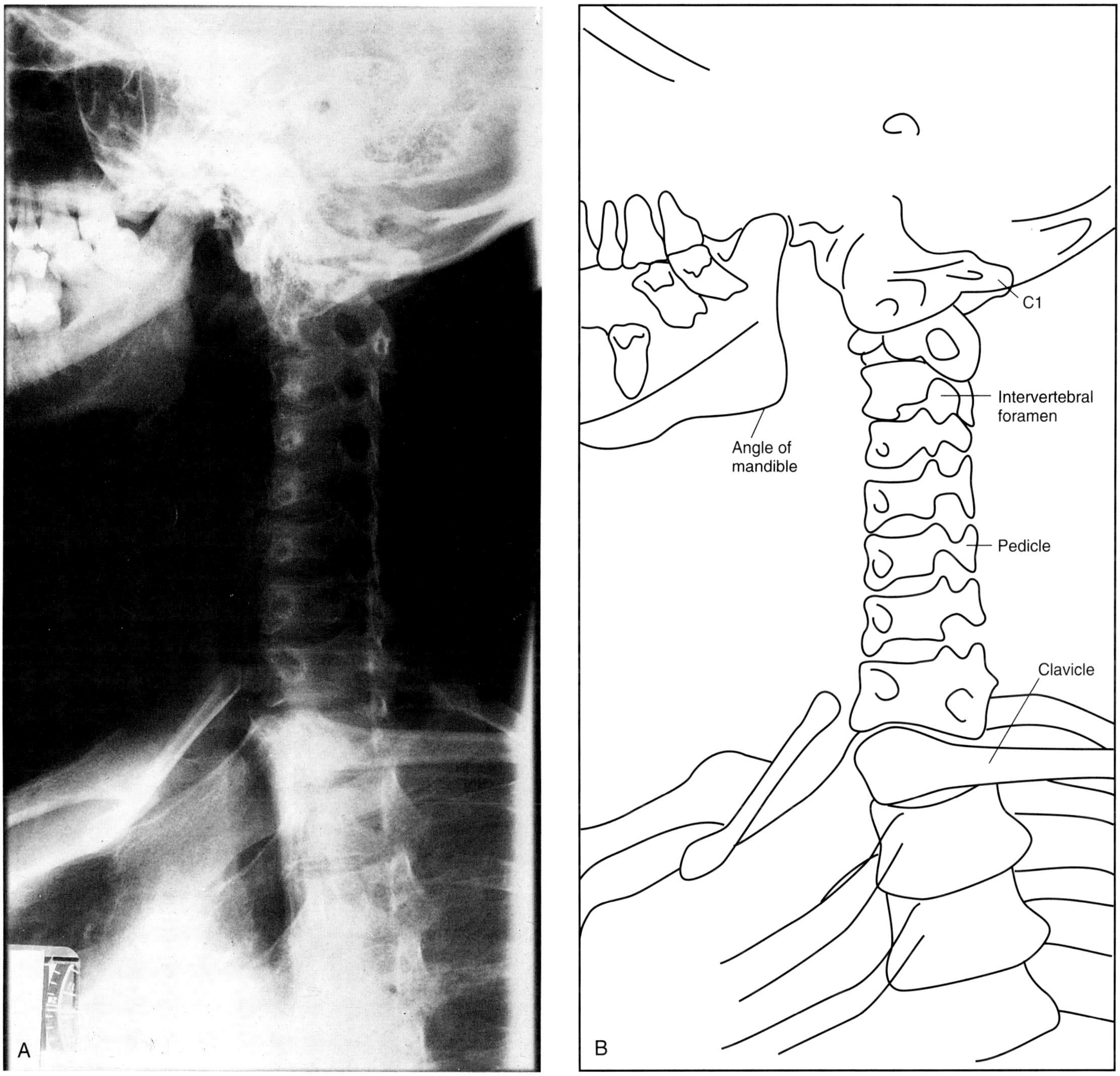

Figure 13.20. A and B, PA oblique of cervical vertebrae.

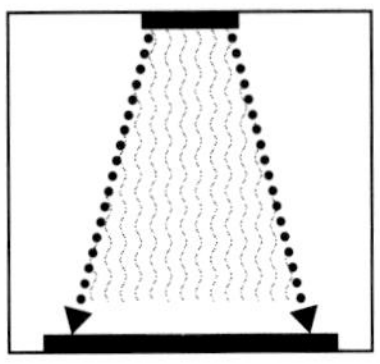

Cervical Spine

Position/Projection

AP obliques

Film Size:
8 × 10 inches (20 × 24 cm)
lengthwise

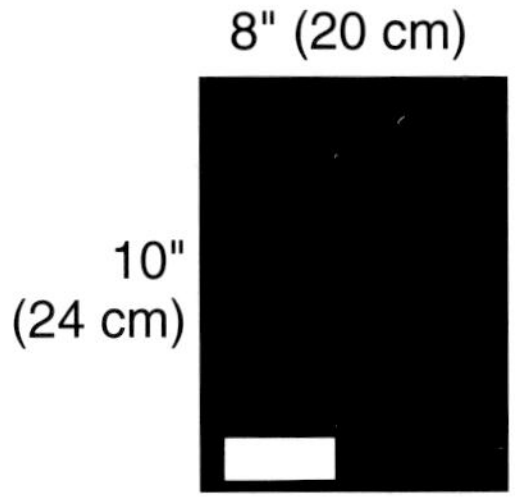

Patient Position

AP position, erect or recumbent (Fig. 13.21).

Part Position

Keeping one shoulder adjacent to film, rotate patient's entire body 45° to film. Center cassette at the level of 3rd cervical body.

Central Ray

Direct to C4 at angle of 15–20° cephalad.

Structures Demonstrated

Demonstrates intervertebral foramina and pedicles farthest from film and oblique projection of bodies and other parts of cervical column (Fig. 13.22).

Evaluation Criteria

1. All seven cervical vertebrae included, as well as T1.
2. Both intervertebral foramina and intervertebral disk spaces should be open and well demonstrated.
3. Occipital bone should not overlap C1. Angle of mandible should not overlap C1 and C2.

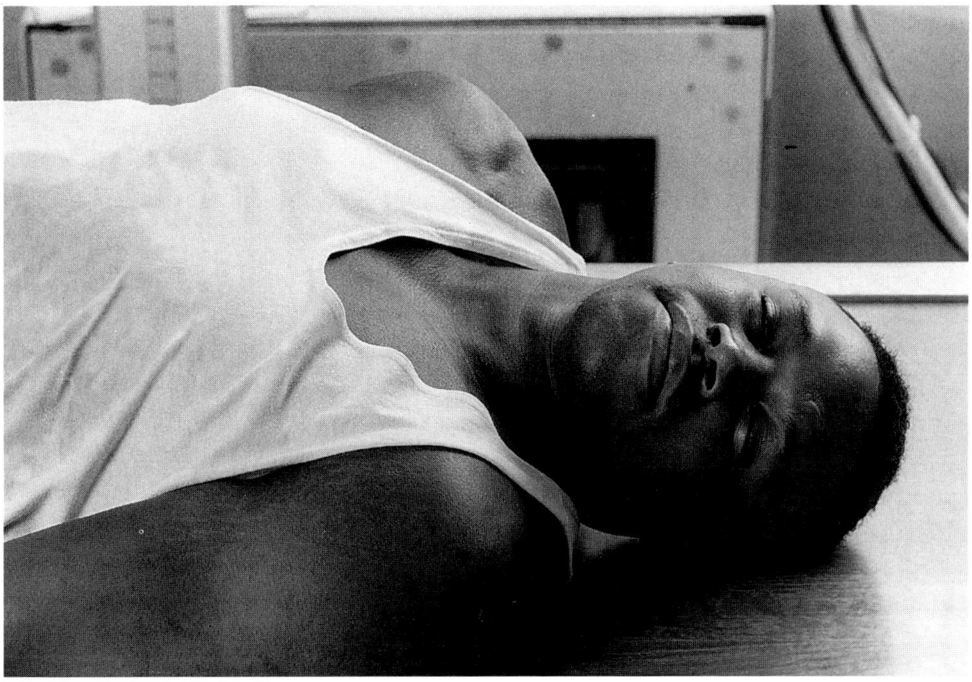

Figure 13.21. AP oblique position of cervical vertebrae.

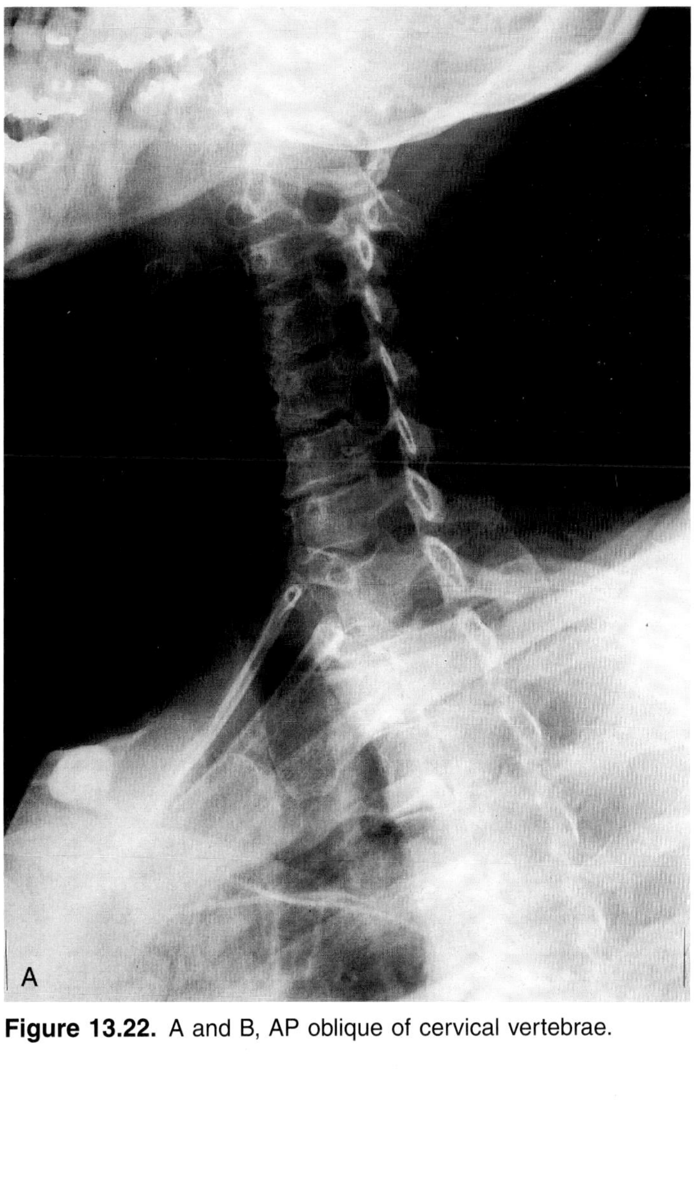

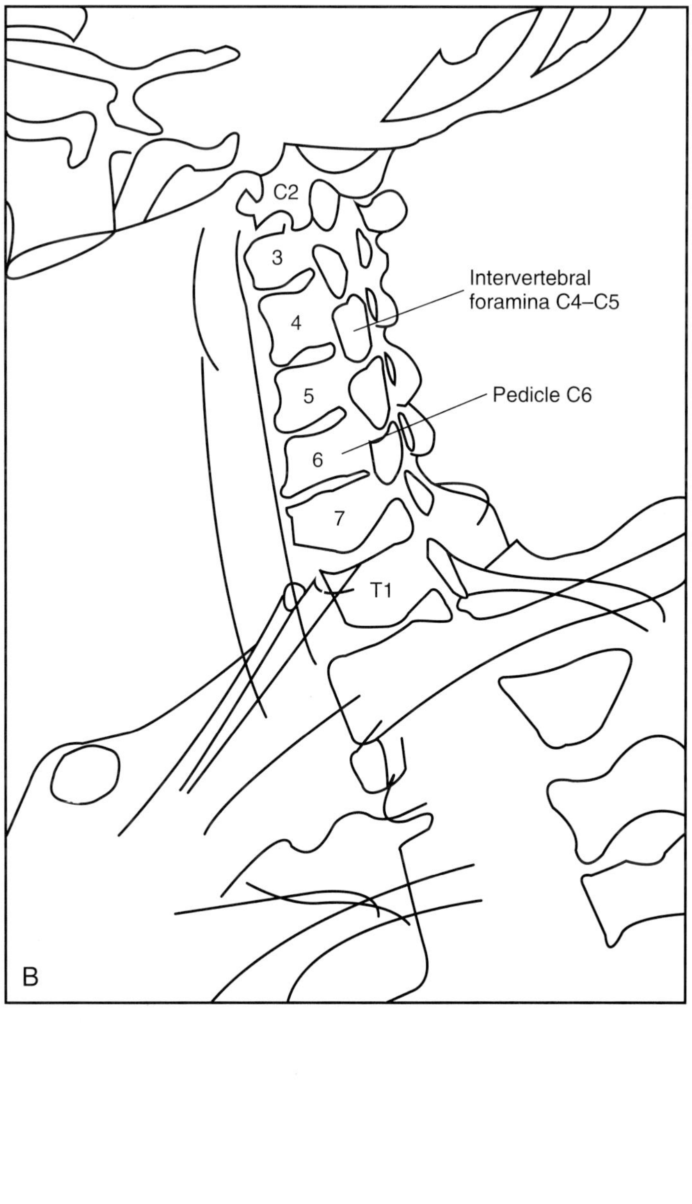

Figure 13.22. A and B, AP oblique of cervical vertebrae.

Cervical Spine

Position/Projection

Lateral

Film Size:
8 × 10 inches (20 × 24 cm)
lengthwise

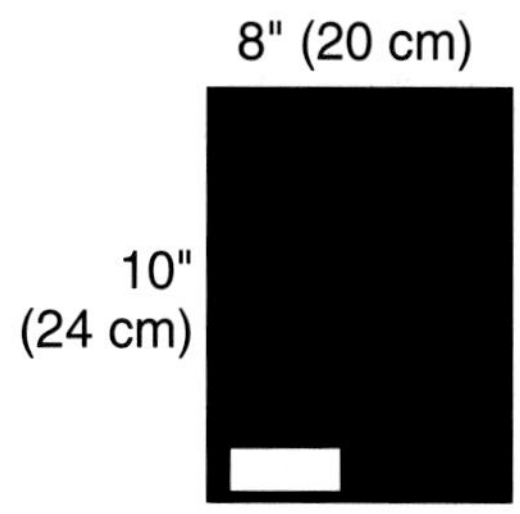

Patient Position

Lateral, seated or standing. Center cassette at level of C4 segment (Fig. 13.23).

Part Position

Center coronal plane that passes through tips of mastoid processes to midline of film. Depress shoulders as much as possible. Elevate chin slightly.

Central Ray

Horizontal to midpoint of film.

Structures Demonstrated

Lateral projection of cervical bodies and interspaces, spinous processes, lower five articular facets, and articular pillars (Fig. 13.24).

Evaluation Criteria

1. All seven cervical vertebrae. Lack of lower vertebrae requires additional view of cervicothoracic region.
2. Rami of mandible superimposed; no overlapping of C1–C2 by rami.
3. Both bony detail and soft tissue visible.

NOTE: Owing to additional part-film distance, a source-to-image receptor distance (SID) of 72 inches (183 cm) should be used to maximize definition.

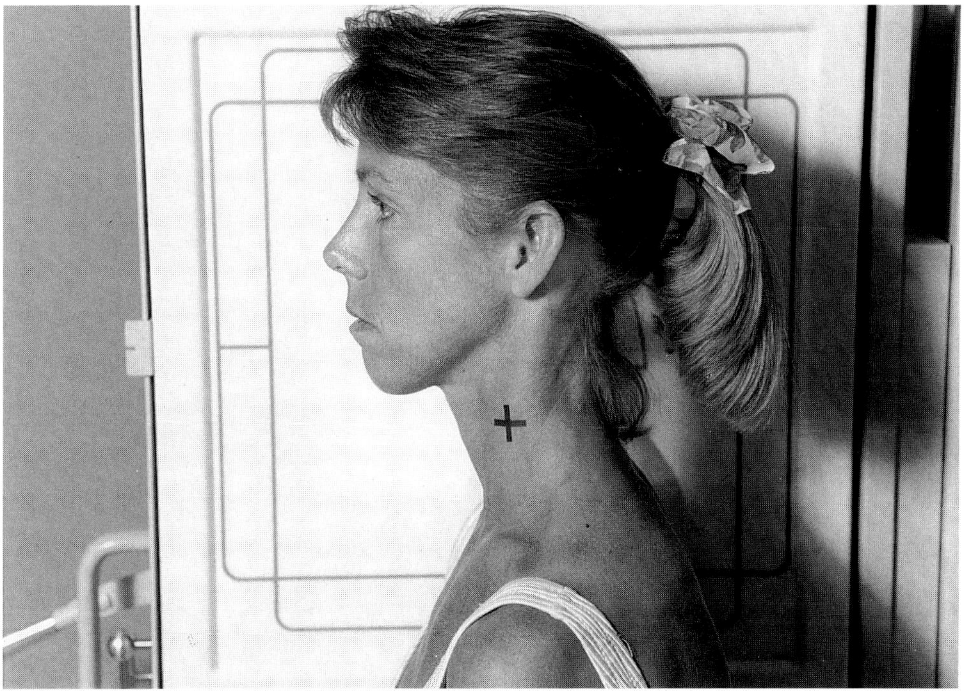

Figure 13.23. Lateral position of cervical vertebrae.

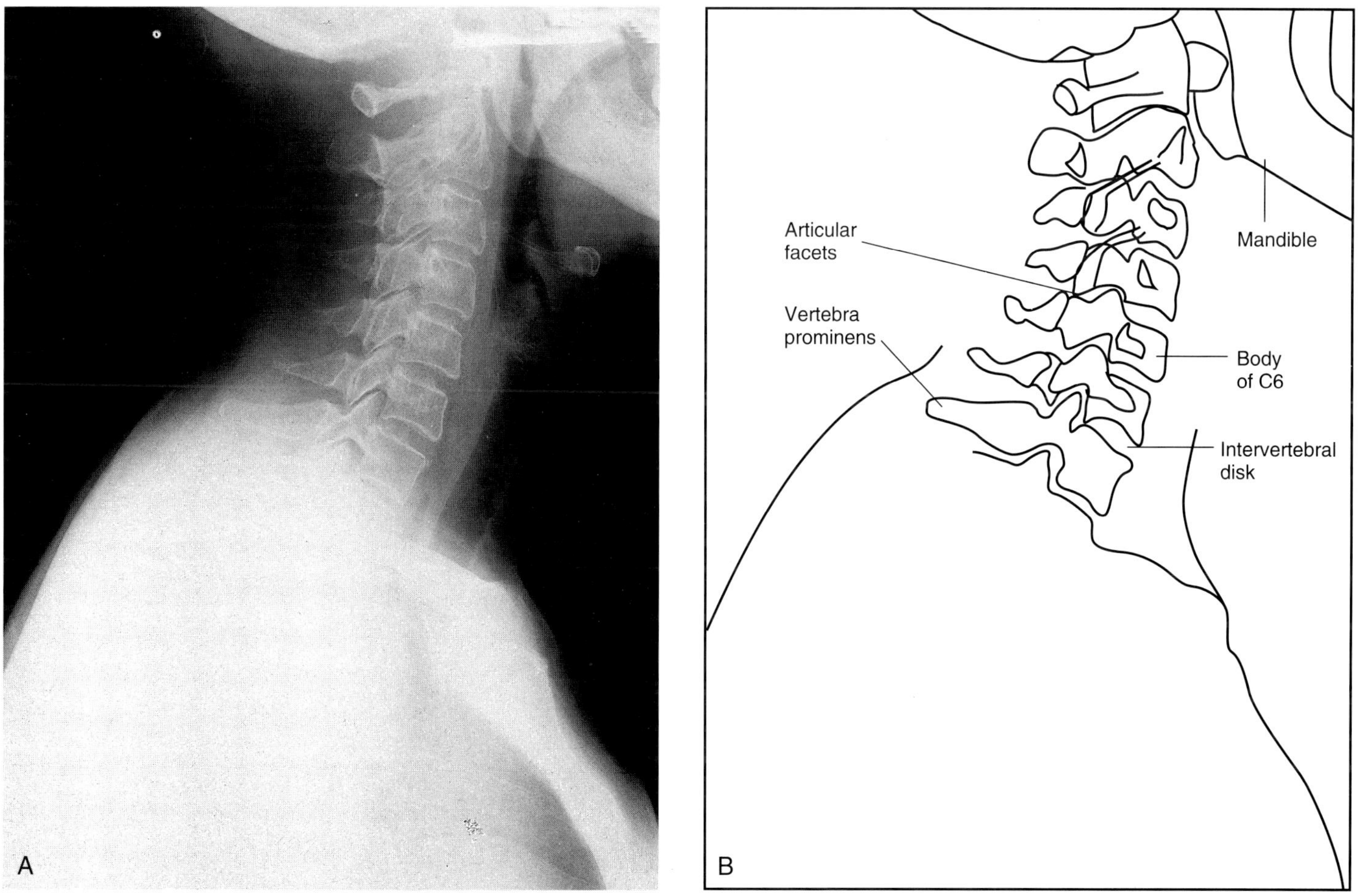

Figure 13.24. A and B, Lateral radiograph of cervical spine.

Cervical Spine

Position/Projection

Lateral—flexion and extension

Film Size:
10 × 12 inches (24 × 30 cm) lengthwise

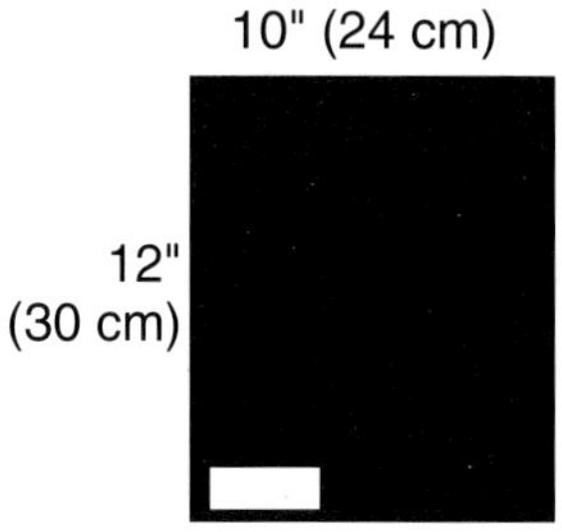

Patient Position

Lateral, seated or standing. Center cassette at level of C4 segment (Fig. 13.25).

Part Position

For Flexion Study

Keep midsagittal plane of patient's head and neck parallel with plane of film; have patient drop head forward, drawing chin as close as possible to chest.

For Extension Study

Keep midsagittal plane of patient's head and neck parallel with plane of film; have patient elevate chin as much as possible.

Central Ray

Horizontal to midpoint of film.

Structures Demonstrated

Functional demonstration of cervical vertebrae (Fig. 13.26).

Evaluation Criteria

All seven vertebrae should be seen.

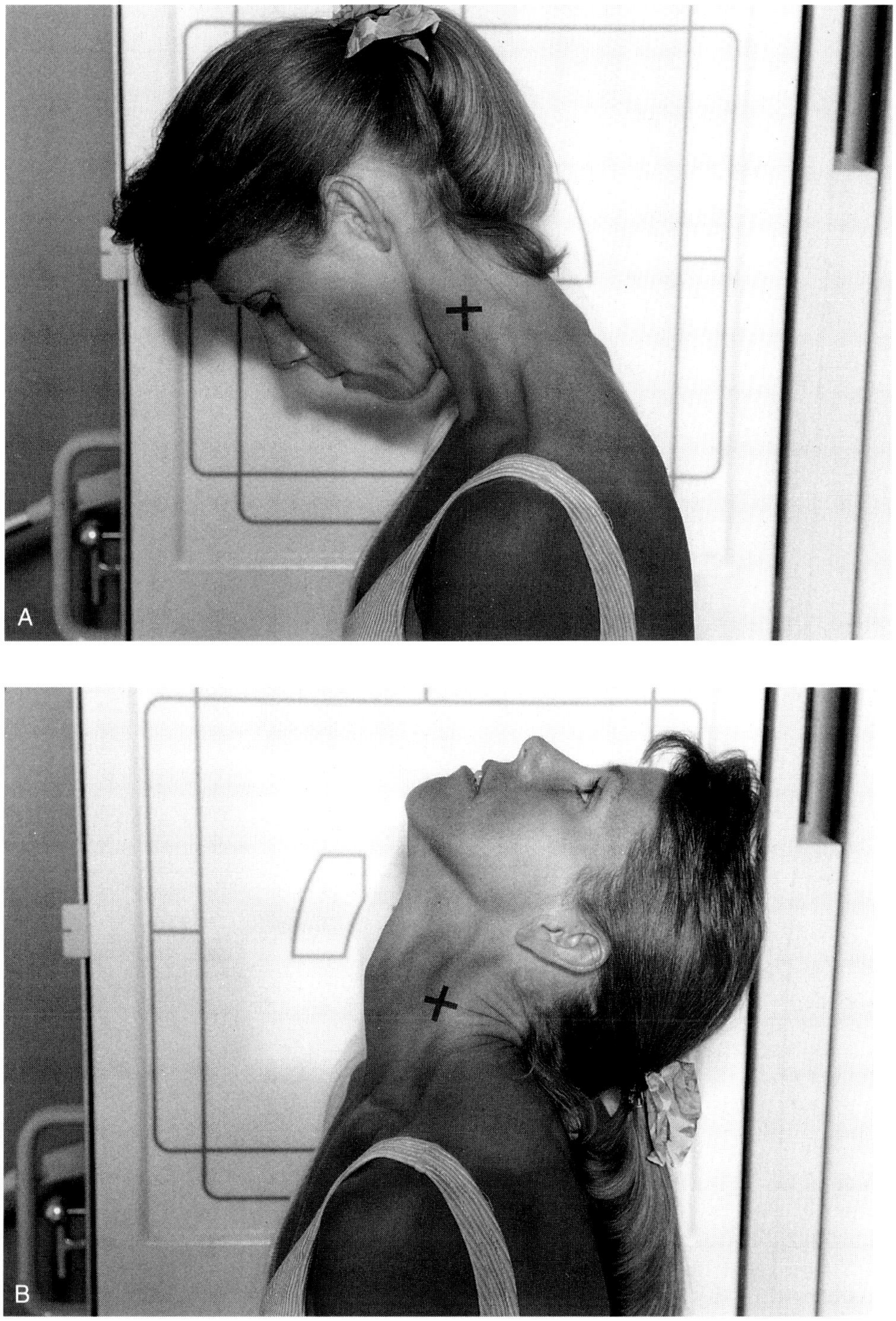

Figure 13.25. Patient in position for (A) flexion and (B) extension studies of cervical spine.

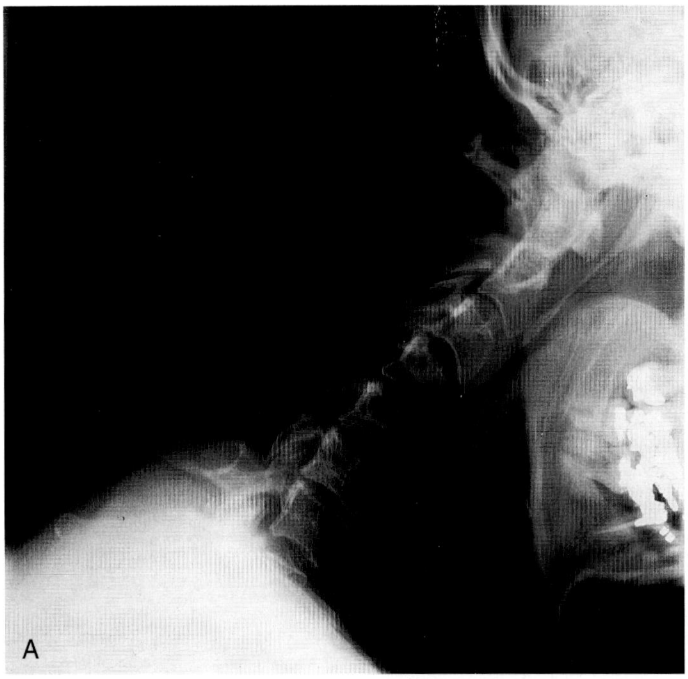

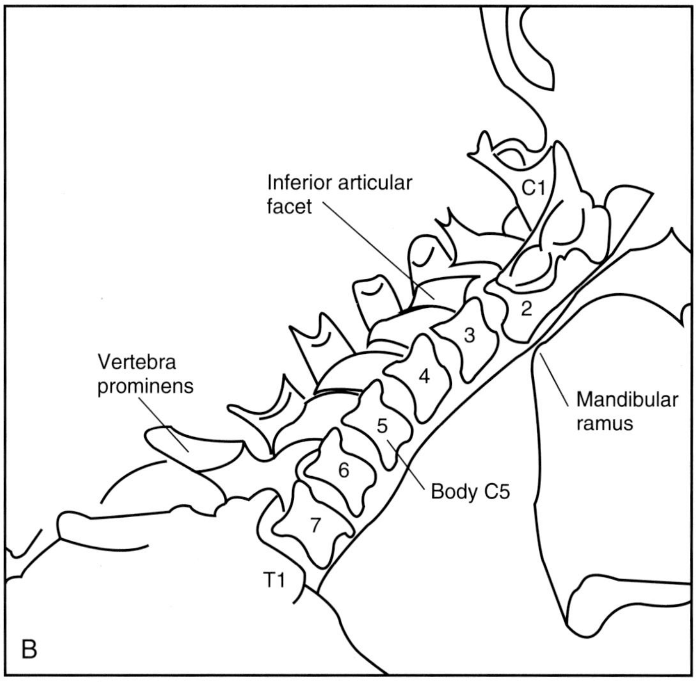

Figure 13.26. A and B, Flexion radiograph of cervical vertebrae.

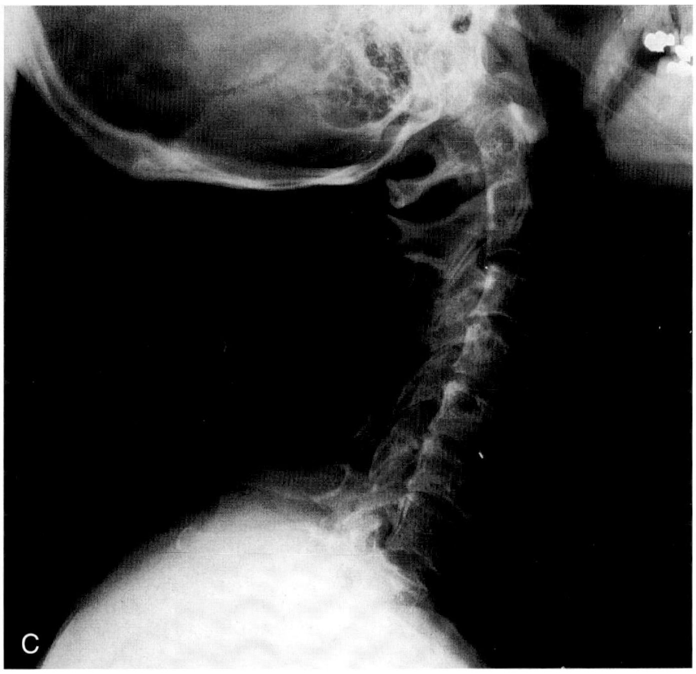

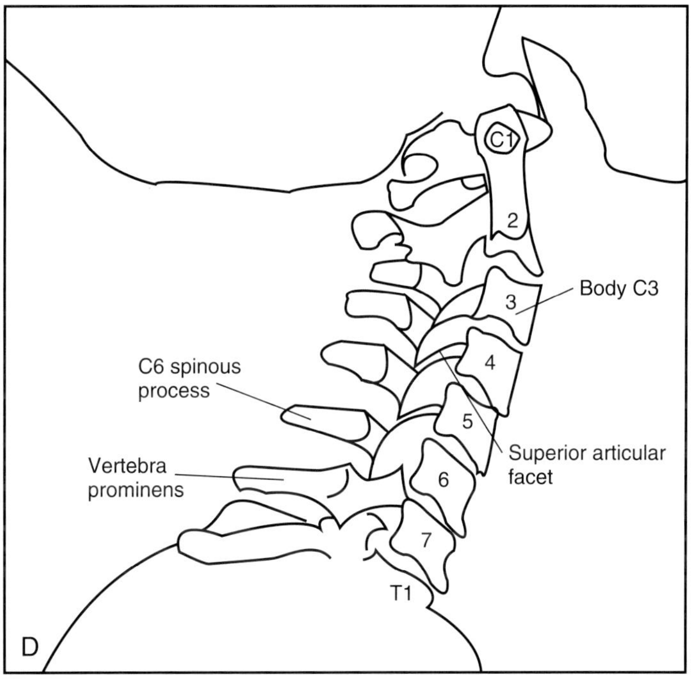

Figure 13.26 *(Continued)* C and D, Extension radiograph of cervical vertebrae.

Vertebral Arch Projections: Pillar or Lateral Mass Positions

Position/Projection

AP axial projection

Film Size:
8 × 10 inches (20 × 24 cm)
or
10 × 12 inches (24 × 30 cm) lengthwise

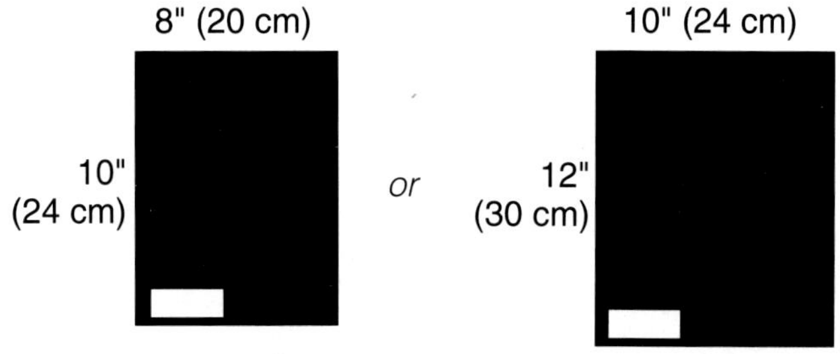

Patient Position

AP recumbent. Midsagittal plane centered to midline of table. Arms alongside body; shoulders in same transverse plane (Fig. 13.27).

Part Position

Midsagittal plane of head perpendicular to plane of table. Hyperextend neck.

Central Ray

Through C7 body at angle of 20–30° caudad. Central ray should be parallel with articular facets. Angle of central ray needs to be increased if cervical curve is accentuated. If cervical curve is diminished, angle of central ray needs to be reduced.

Structures Demonstrated

Posterior portions of cervical vertebrae and upper three or four thoracic vertebrae, articular pillar and facets, and spinous processes (Fig. 13.28).

Evaluation Criteria

1. Open zygapophyseal joints between articular facets.
2. Superior and inferior articulating processes should be demonstrated without overlapping of vertebral bodies and transverse processes.
3. Articular pillars and facets well demonstrated.

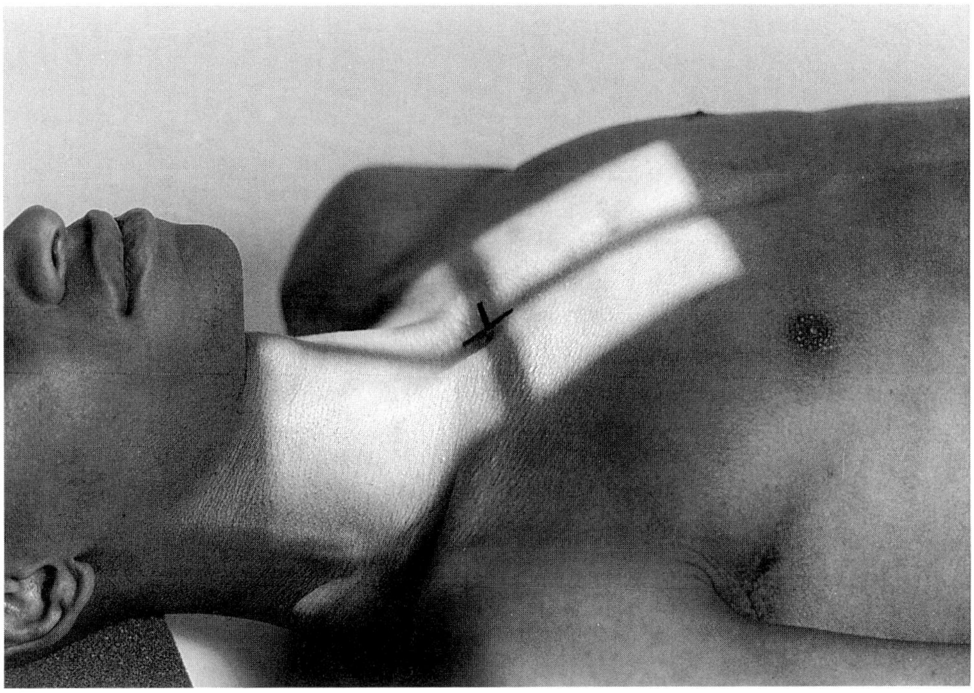

Figure 13.27. Patient in position for vertebral arch study.

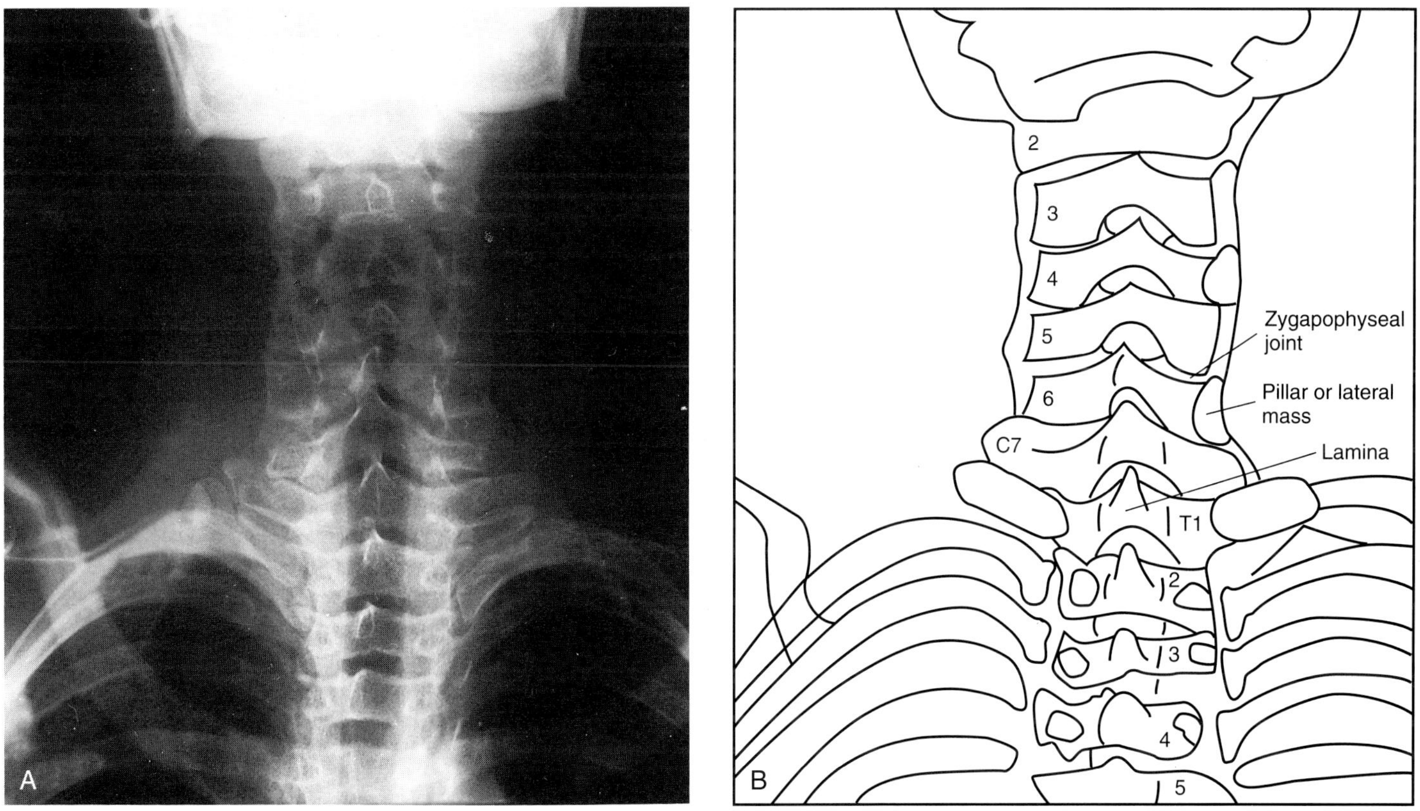

Figure 13.28. A and B, Vertebral arch radiograph.

Thoracic Spine

Position/Projection

AP

Film Size:
14 × 17 inches (35 × 43 cm) lengthwise

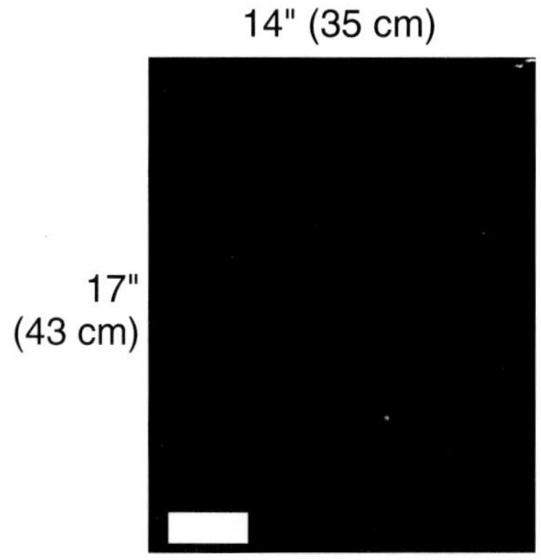

Patient Position
Recumbent or erect (Fig. 13.29).

Part Position
Midsagittal plane centered to midline of table. Center film at level of T6.

Central Ray
Perpendicular to midpoint of film.

Breathing Instructions
Respiration suspended at end of full exhalation.

Structures Demonstrated
Demonstrates AP projection of thoracic bodies, interpediculate spaces, and surrounding structures (Fig. 13.30).

Evaluation Criteria
1. All 12 thoracic vertebrae included.
2. Spinous processes at midline.
3. Vertebral column in middle of radiograph.

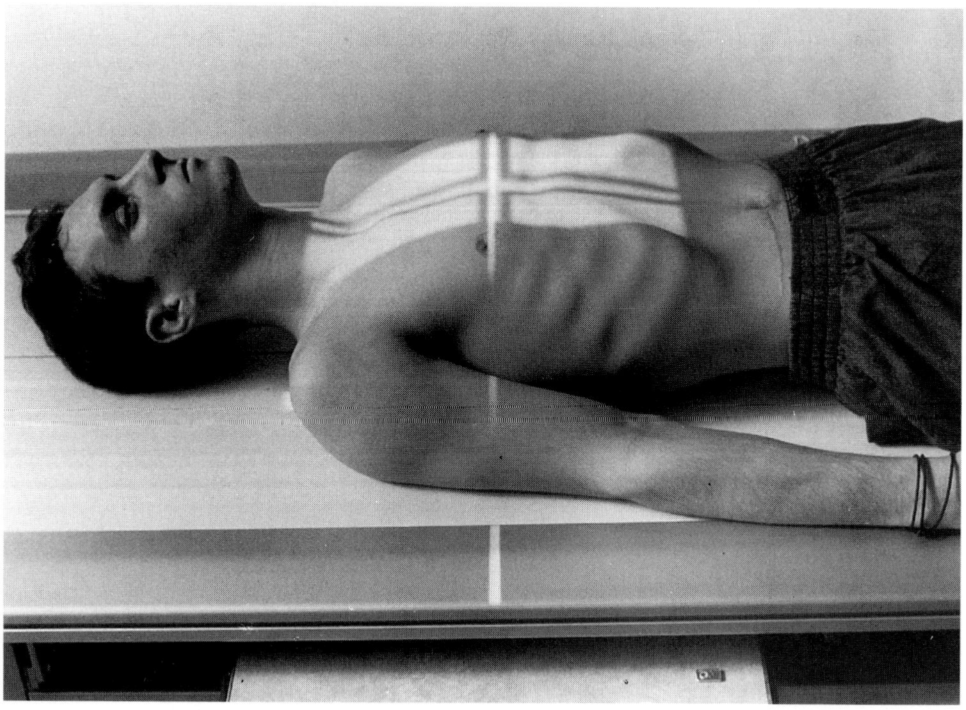

Figure 13.29. Patient in position for AP projection of thoracic vertebrae.

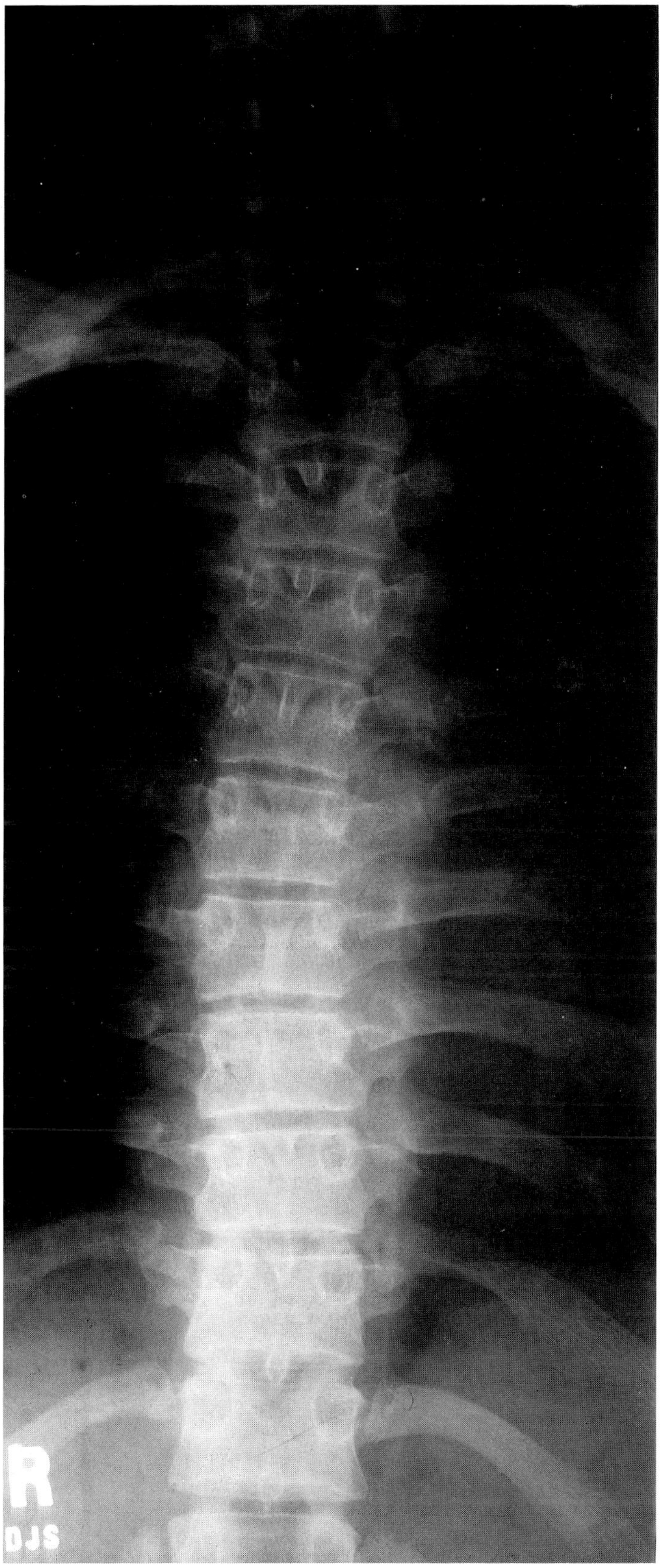

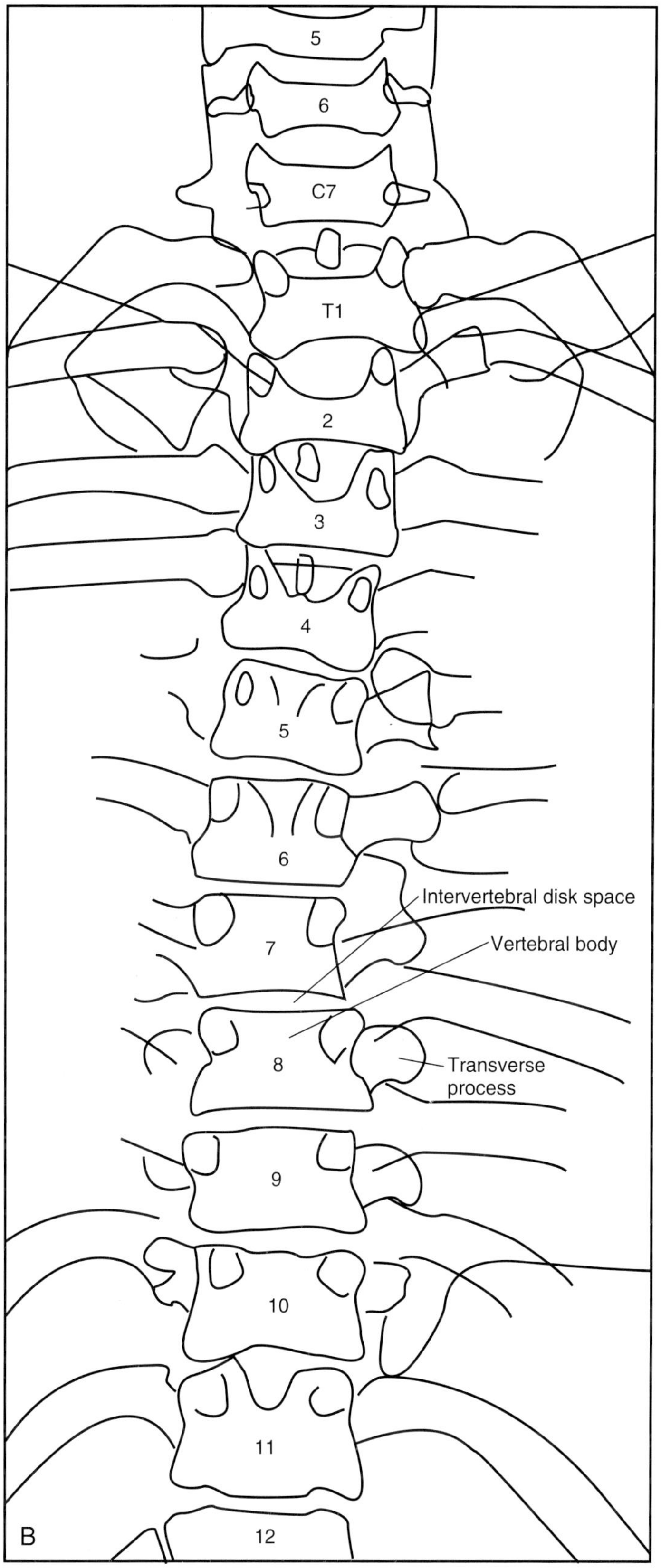

Figure 13.30. A and B, Thoracic vertebrae in AP projection.

Cervicothoracic Region

Position/Projection

Twining's method

Film Size:
10 × 12 inches (24 × 30 cm) lengthwise

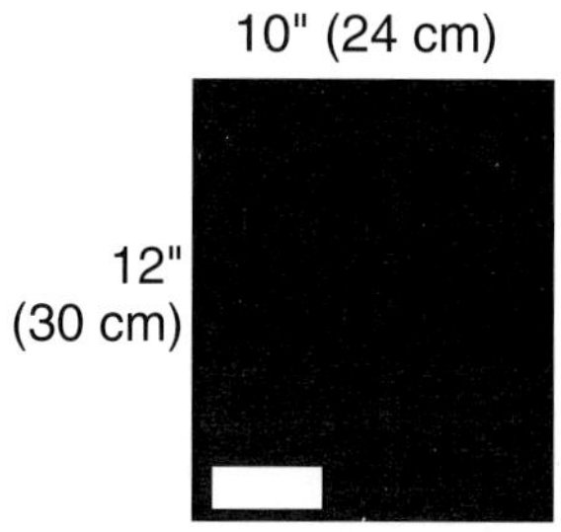

Patient Position

Lateral, erect or recumbent. Center cassette at level of T2 (Fig. 13.31).

Part Position

Center midaxillary line of body to midline of cassette. Elevate arm adjacent to film to vertical position, flex elbow, and rest forearm on patient's head. Rotate shoulder posteriorly or anteriorly. Depress shoulder farthest from film.

Central Ray

Perpendicular to midpoint of film.

Breathing Instructions

Respiration suspended at end of full exhalation or exposure can be made while patient takes shallow breaths to blur lung markings.

Structures Demonstrated

Lateral image of lower cervical and upper thoracic vertebrae (Fig. 13.32).

Evaluation Criteria

1. Vertebrae in lateral position. Area from C5 to T5 included.
2. Shoulders separated and well penetrated.

NOTE: Angle the central ray 5° caudad when the shoulder cannot be well depressed.

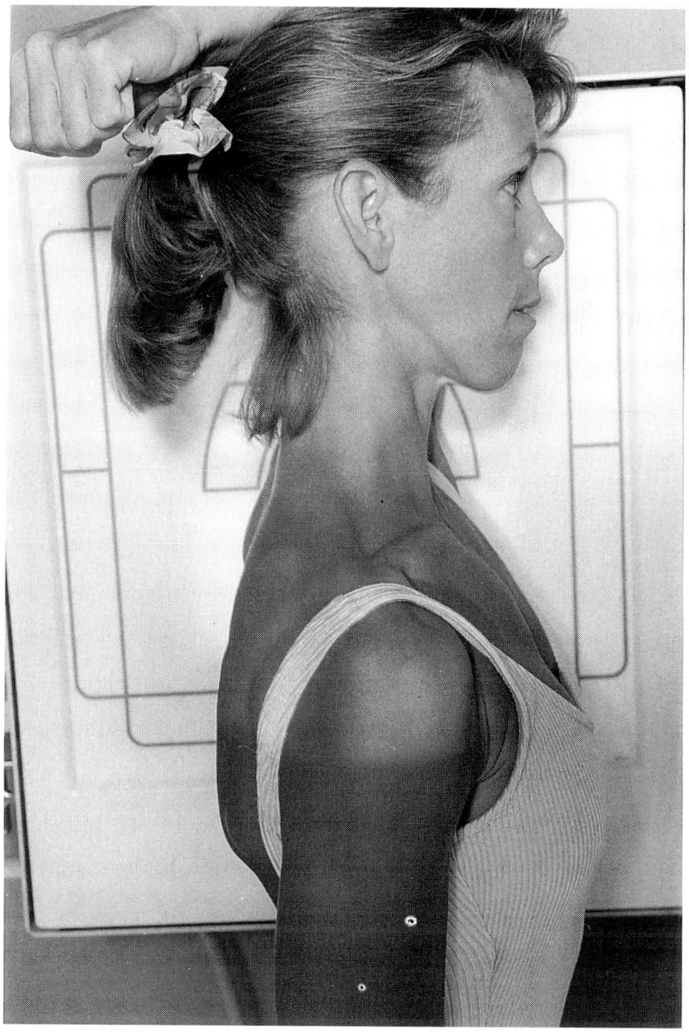

Figure 13.31. Twining's position for cervicothoracic region.

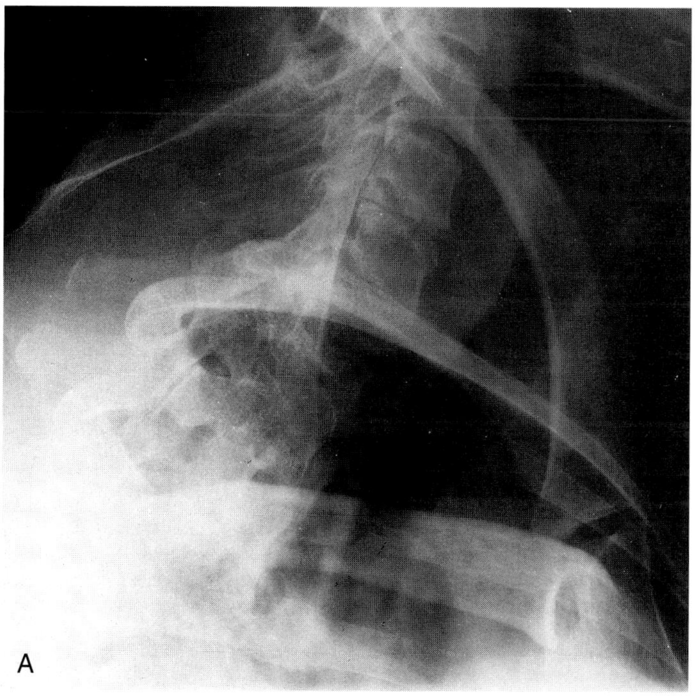

A

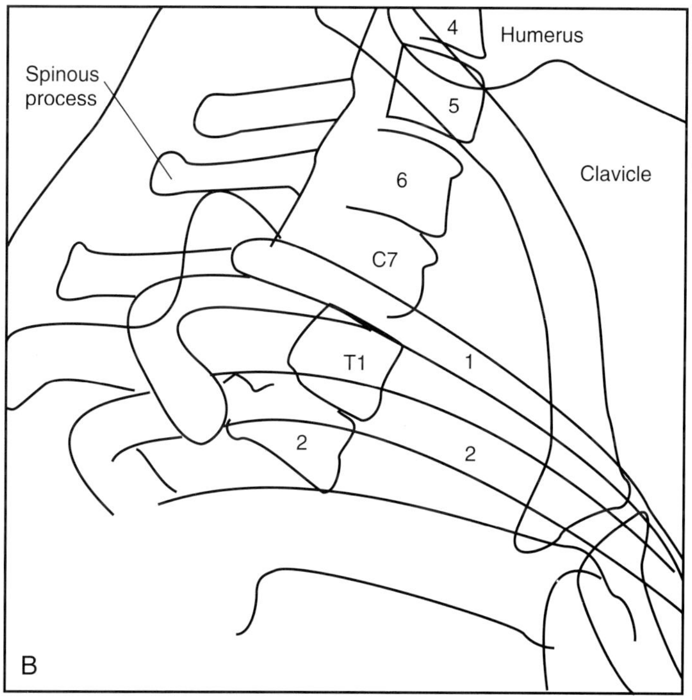

B

Figure 13.32. A and B, Cervicothoracic vertebrae as shown in Twining's projection.

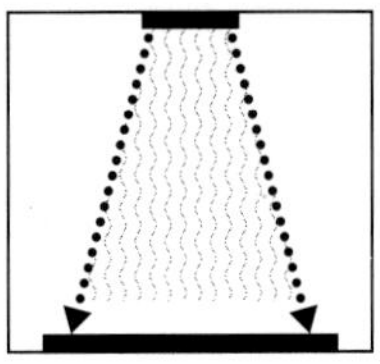

Cervicothoracic Region

Position/Projection

Lateral Projection; Pawlow's method

Film Size:
10 × 12 inches (24 × 30 cm) lengthwise

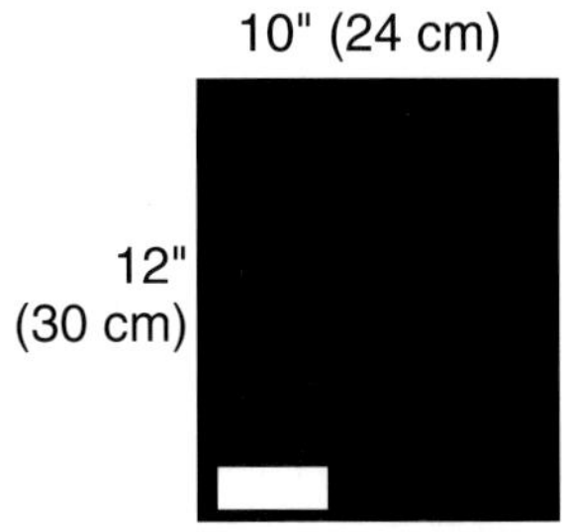

Patient Position

Lateral recumbent with head elevated (Fig. 13.33).

Part Position

Midaxillary line centered to midline of table. Dependent arm extended and adjusted to place humeral head either in front of or behind vertebrae. Uppermost arm is adjusted in opposite position. Shoulder shadows must be separated and upper shoulder immobilized. Cassette is centered at level of T2 or T3.

Central Ray

Midpoint of film; angled 3–5° caudad.

Breathing Instructions

Respiration suspended at end of full exhalation or exposure can be made while patient takes shallow breaths to blur lung markings.

Structures Demonstrated

Lateral projection of cervicothoracic vertebrae between shoulder shadows (Fig. 13.34).

Evaluation Criteria

1. Lateral without large amount of rotation.
2. Area from C5 to T5 included.
3. Shoulders separated and well penetrated.

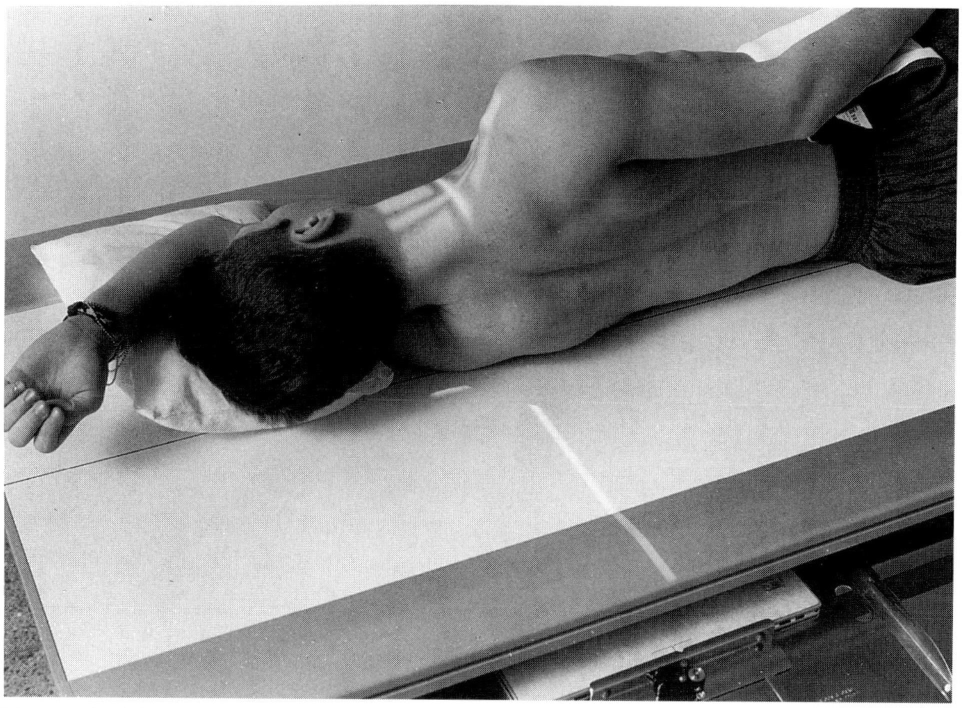

Figure 13.33. Pawlow's method for visualization of cervicothoracic vertebrae in lateral projection.

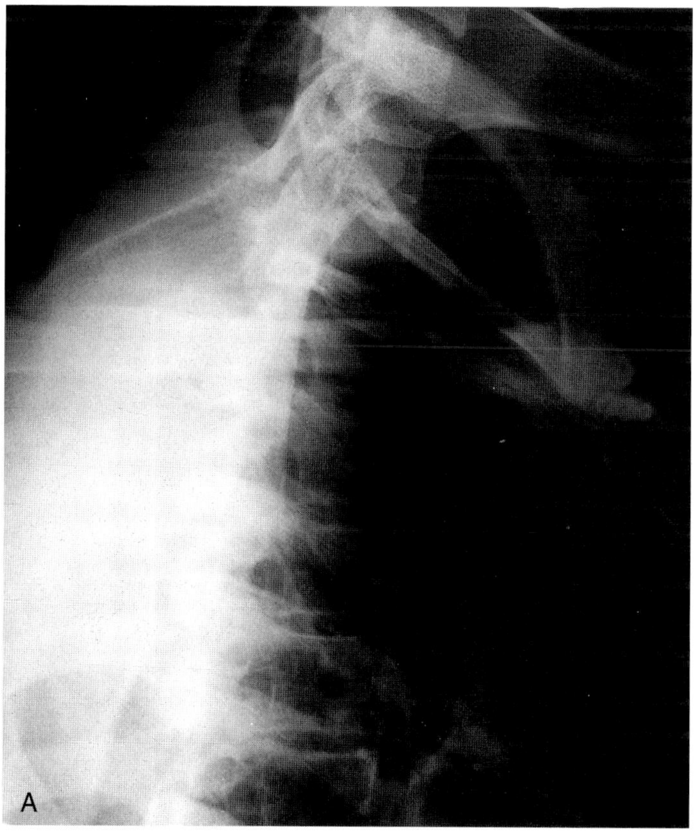

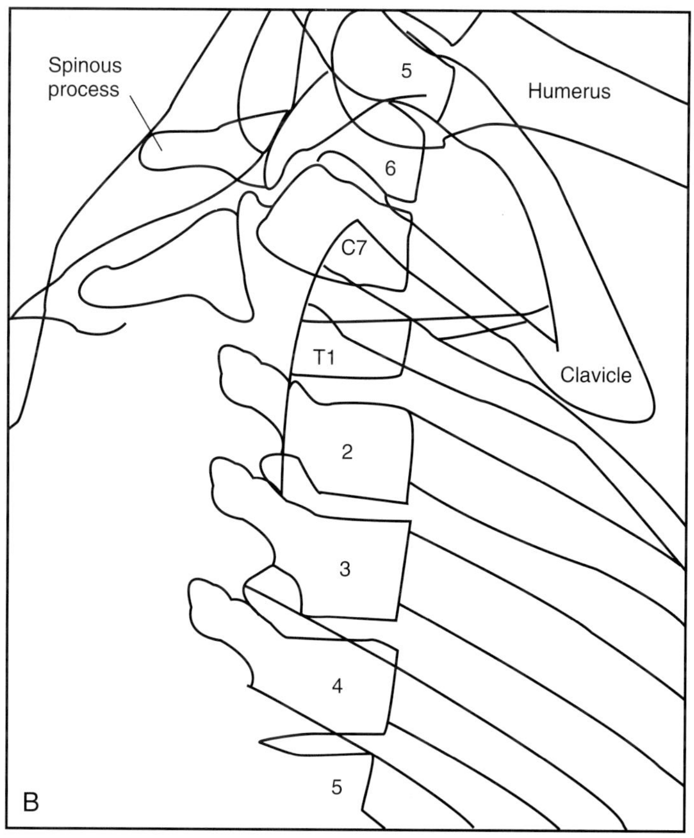

Figure 13.34. A and B, Lateral cervicothoracic vertebrae (Pawlow's method).

Cervicothoracic Region

Position/Projection

Lateral

Film Size:
14 × 17 inches (35 × 43 cm) lengthwise

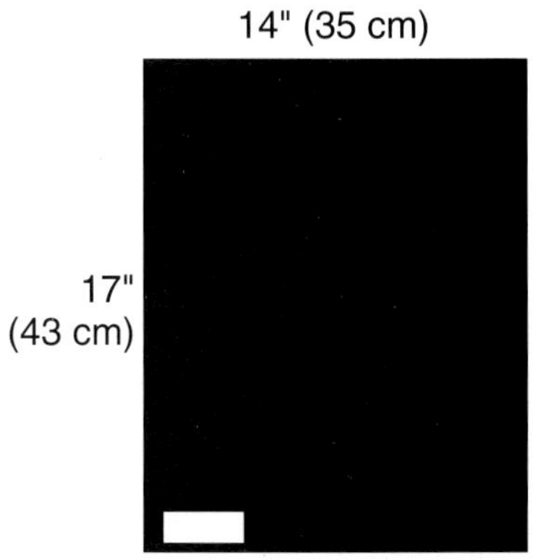

Patient Position

Lateral, recumbent or erect (Fig. 13.35).

Part Position

Flex hips and knees. Center midaxillary line of body to midline of table. Adjust arms at right angles to long axis of body. Adjust position so that long axis of vertebral column is horizontal to table.

Central Ray

Perpendicular to midpoint of film. Center at level of T6.

Breathing Instructions

Respiration suspended at end of full exhalation.

Structures Demonstrated

Lateral image of thoracic bodies is demonstrated showing interspaces, intervertebral foramina, and lower spinous processes. Because of overlapping shadows at shoulders, upper three or four segments are not demonstrated in this position (Fig. 13.36).

Evaluation Criteria

Lower thoracic vertebrae of primary interest.

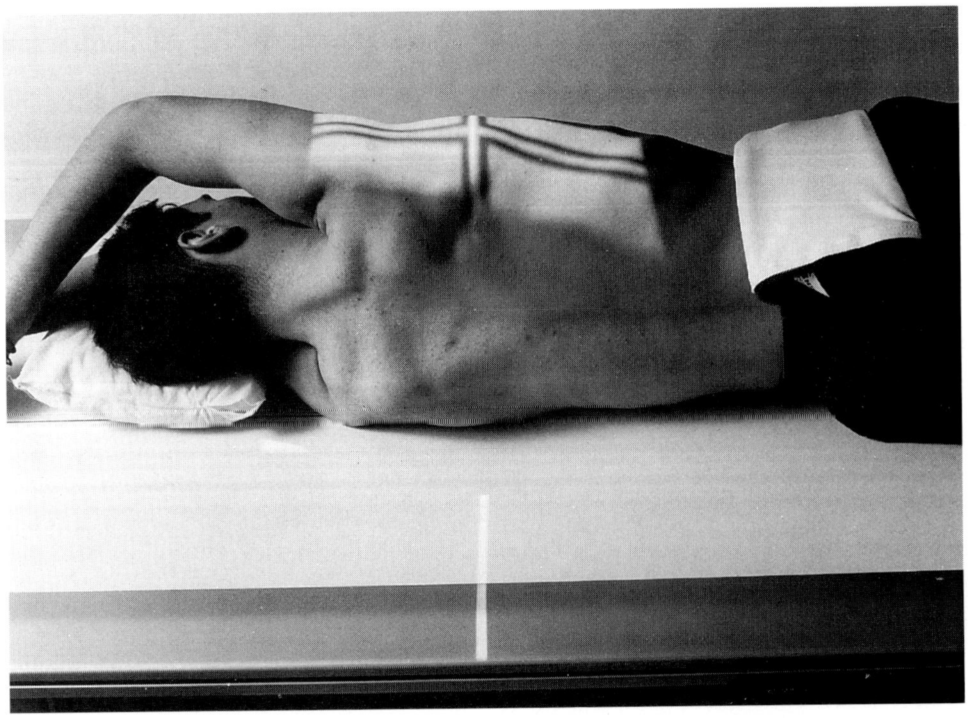

Figure 13.35. Lateral position for thoracic vertebrae.

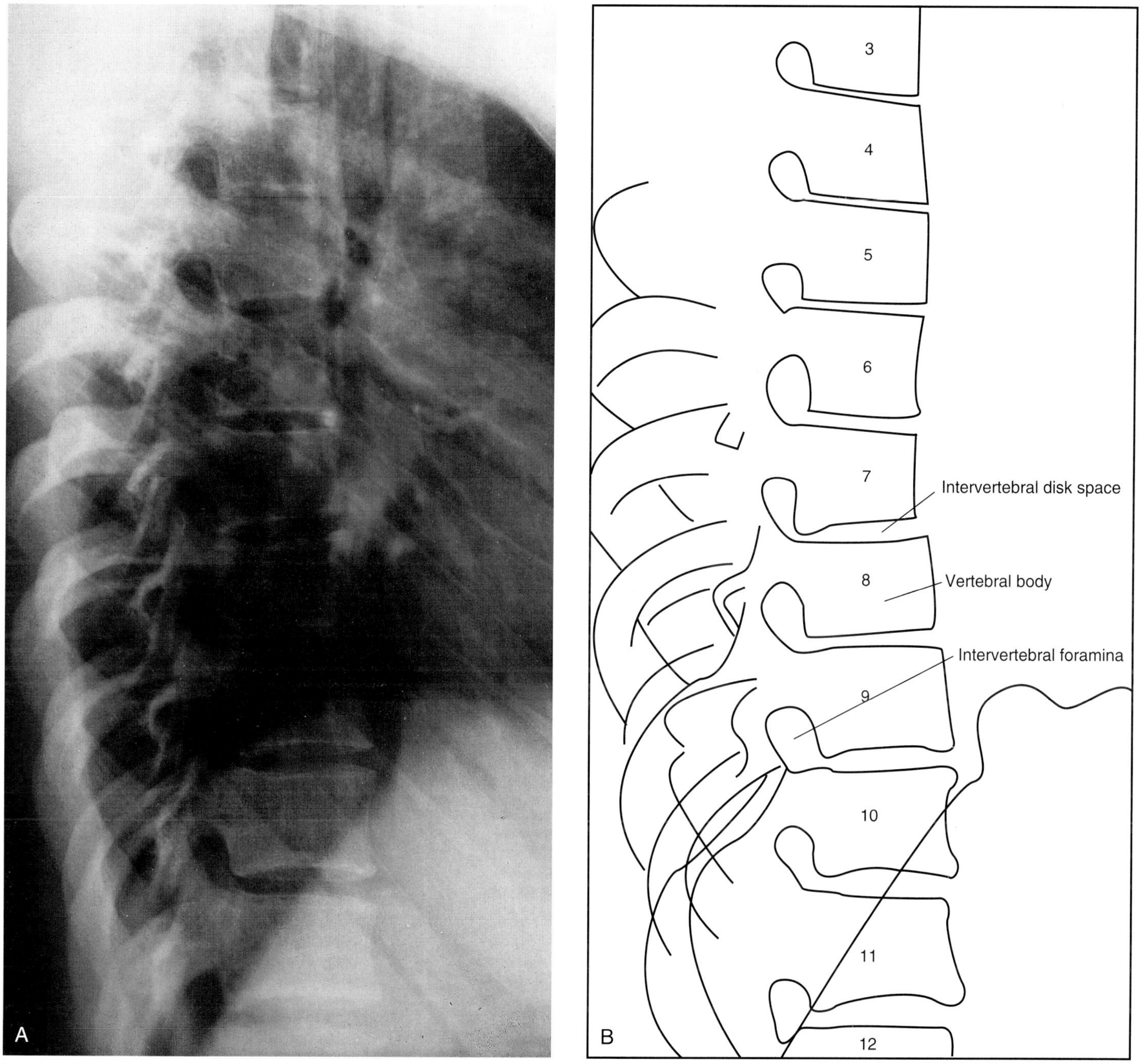

Figure 13.36. A and B, Lateral radiograph of thoracic vertebrae.

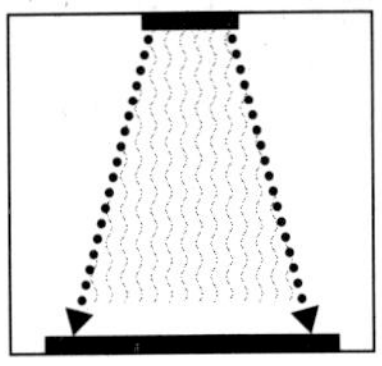

Cervicothoracic Region

Position/Projection

PA and AP obliques for apophyseal articulations

Film Size:
14 × 17 inches (35 × 43 cm) lengthwise

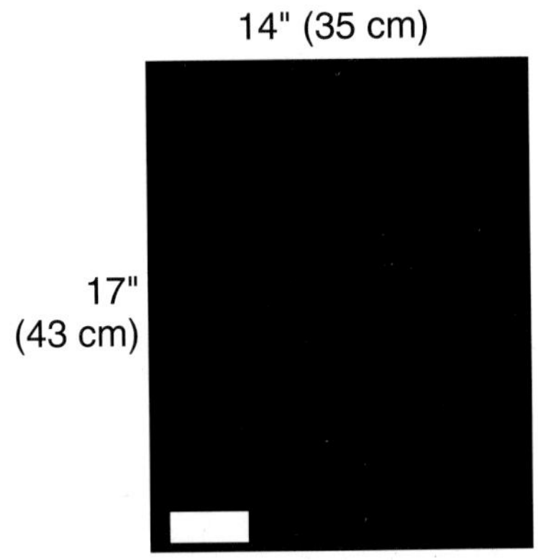

Patient Position

Erect or recumbent (Fig. 13.37).

Erect Position
Patient in lateral position in front of vertical grid. Grid should be adjusted so T6 is centered to center of cassette.

Part Position

Rotate body anteriorly or posteriorly to place coronal plane at angle of 70° from plane of cassette. Midsagittal plane forms angle of 20° to plane of cassette. Center vertebral column to midline of cassette. Place dependent shoulder against grid, flex elbow, and place hand on hip. If rotated anteriorly, patient should grasp side of grid with free hand. If rotated posteriorly, patient should place free hand on hip. Shoulders should lie in same transverse plane. Vertebral column should be parallel with cassette.

Recumbent Position
Patient in lateral recumbent position. Flex knees for comfort.

Anterior Rotation
Place dependent arm behind back.

Posterior Rotation
Position dependent arm at right angle with long axis of body and flex elbow and place hand under head. Place uppermost arm posteriorly. Rotate body anteriorly or posteriorly to place coronal plane at angle of 70° from plane of cassette. Midsagittal plane forms angle of 20° to plane of cassette; center vertebral column to midline of cassette.

Central Ray

Perpendicular to T7.

Breathing Instructions

Respiration suspended at end of full exhalation.

Structures Demonstrated

Zygapophyseal articulations of thoracic vertebrae (Fig. 13.38).

Evaluation Criteria

1. Anterior obliques demonstrate zygapophyseal articulations closest to film.
2. Posterior rotation demonstrates cervicothoracic spinous

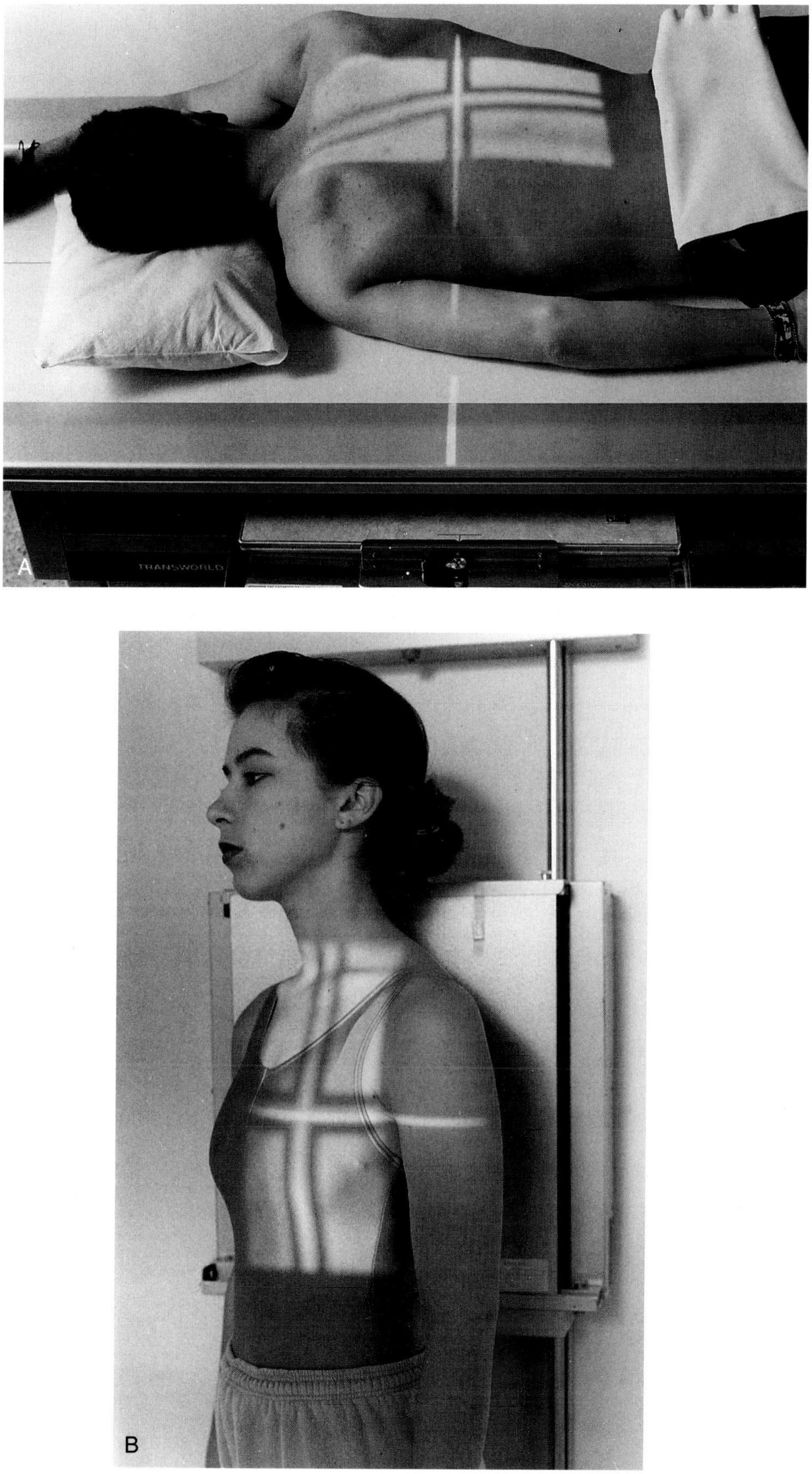

Figure 13.37. Oblique position for demonstration of apophyseal articulations A, PA. B, AP.

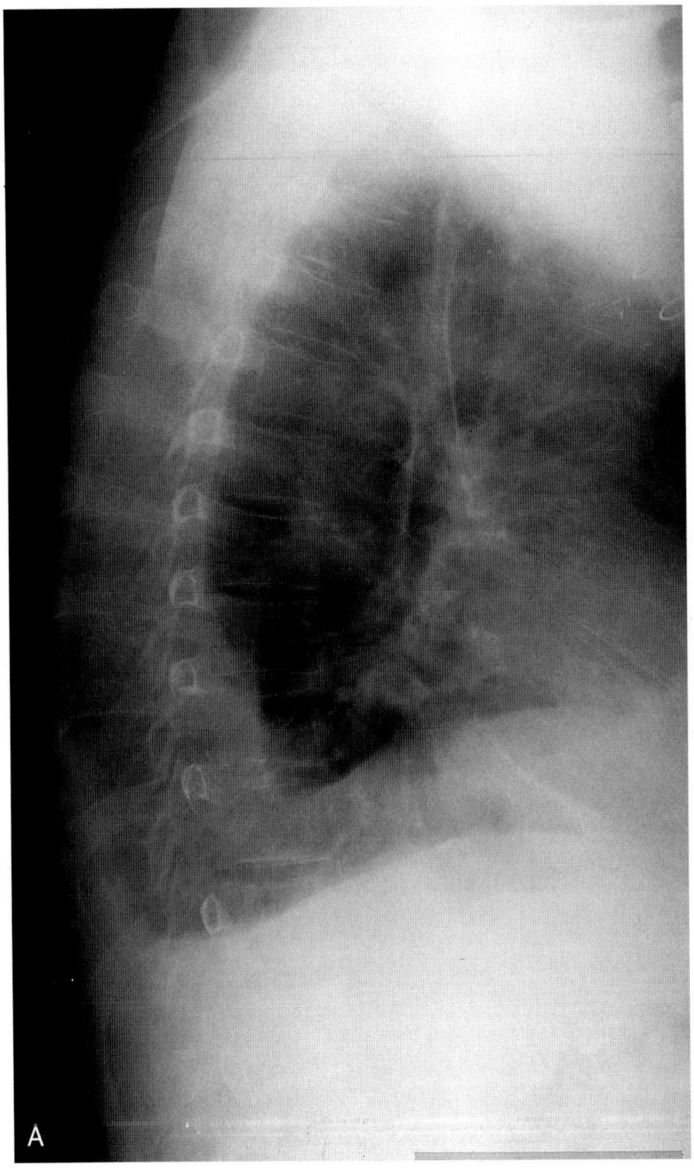

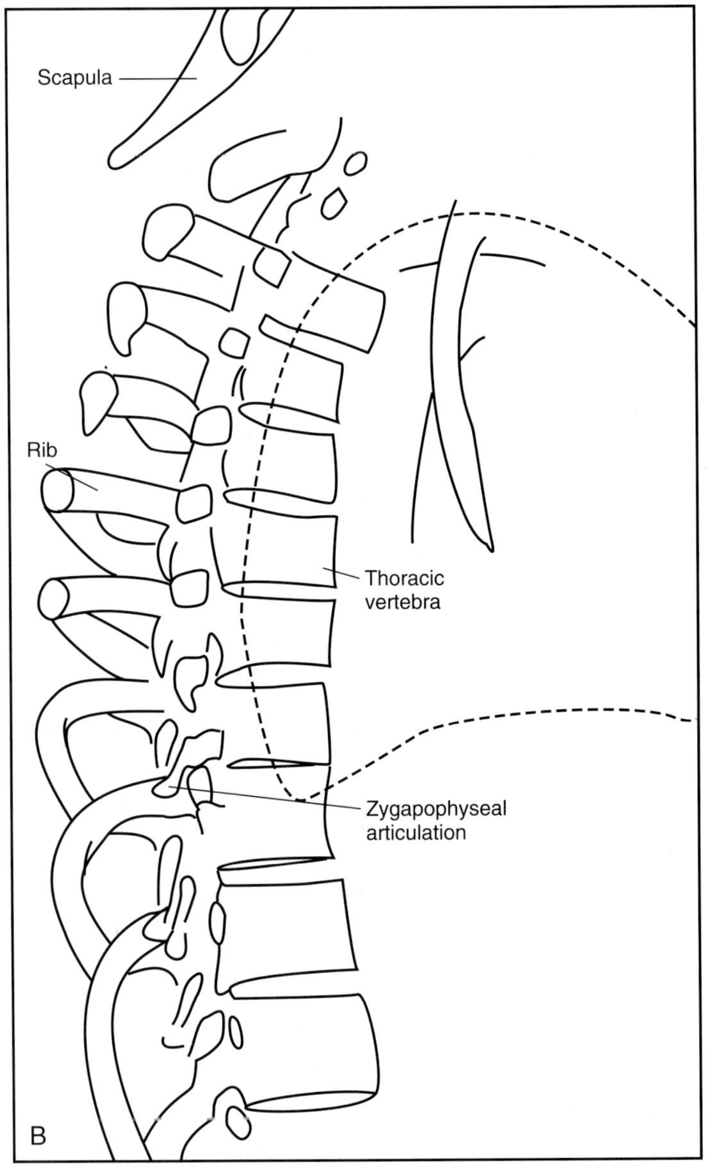

Figure 13.38. A and B, Oblique projection of apophyseal articulations.

Lumbar Spine

Position/Projection

AP

Film Size:
14 × 17 inches (35 × 43 cm)
or
11 × 14 inches (30 × 35 cm) lengthwise

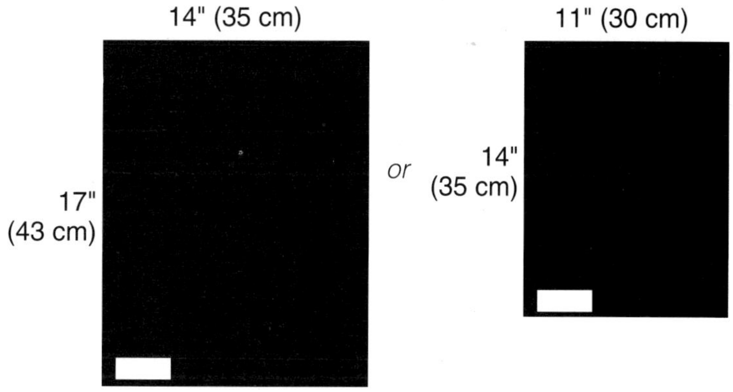

Patient Position

AP recumbent position. Midsagittal plane centered to midline of table (Fig. 13.39).

Part Position

Flex patient's elbows and place hands on upper chest. Center film at level of iliac crest.

Central Ray

Perpendicular to midpoint of cassette.

Structures Demonstrated

Lumbar bodies, intervertebral disk spaces, interpediculate spaces, laminae, and spinous and transverse processes. When larger film is used, one or two lower thoracic vertebrae, sacrum and coccyx, pelvic bones, and hip joints are included (Fig. 13.40).

Breathing Instructions

Respiration suspended at end of full exhalation.

Evaluation Criteria

1. Include area from lower thoracic vertebrae to coccyx.
2. Beam collimated to outer margin of psoas muscles.
3. Intervertebral joints open and well penetrated.
4. Sacroiliac joints equidistant from vertebral column.

NOTE: Recent evidence indicates that a PA (prone) projection may be more comfortable for the patient, places the intervertebral disk spaces at an angle more closely paralleling the divergence of the x-ray beam, and provides superior radiation protection to the patient (Ballinger, 1991; Heriard et al, 1993).

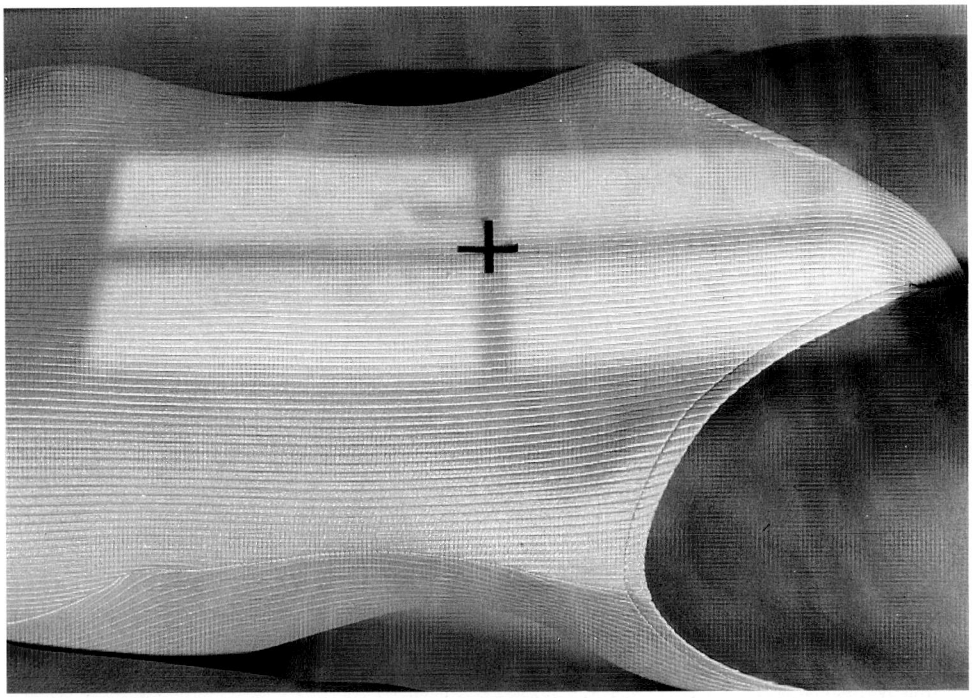

Figure 13.39. AP position for demonstration of lumbar spine.

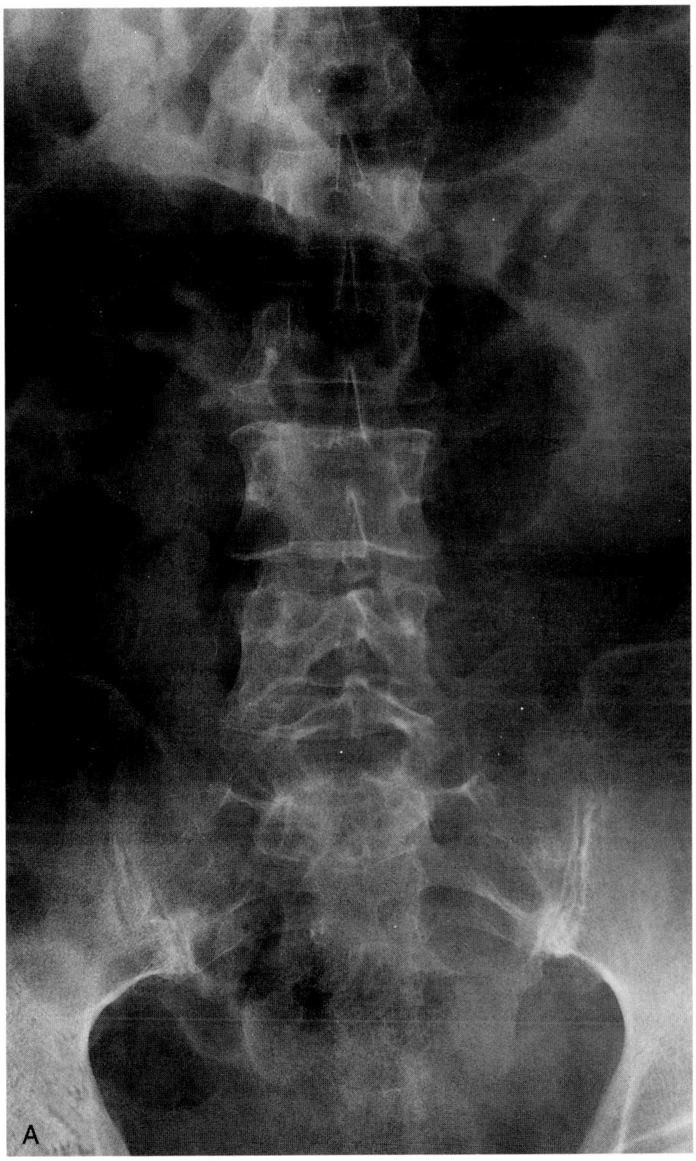

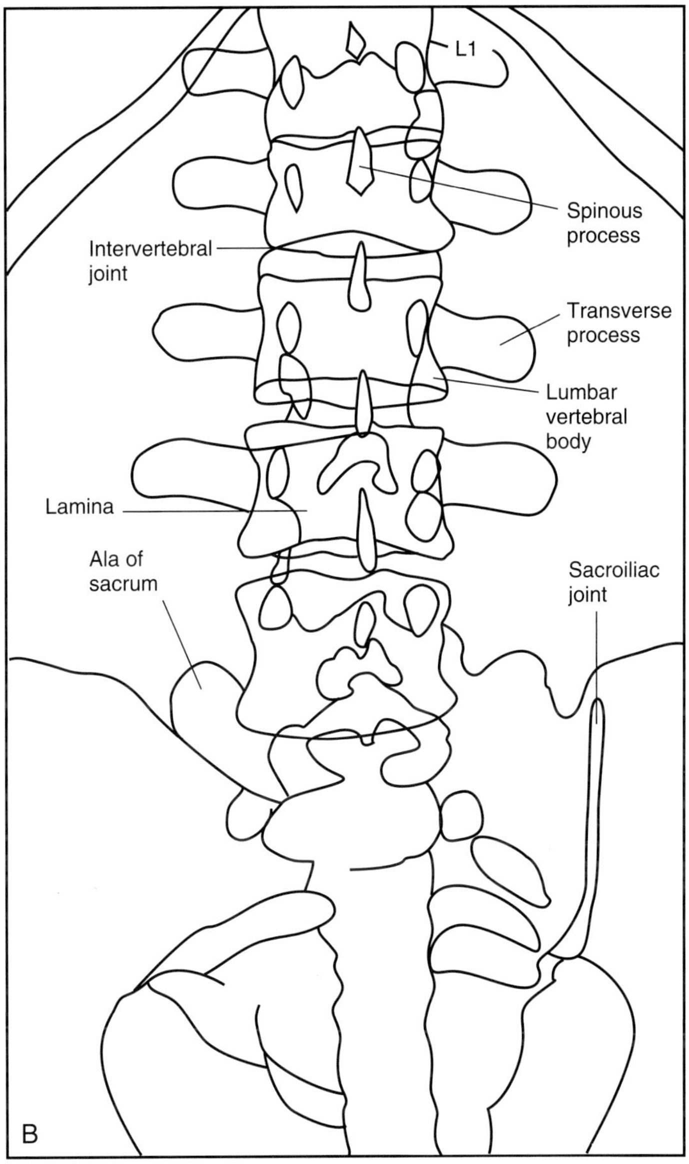

Figure 13.40. A and B, AP lumbar spine.

Lumbar Spine

Position/Projection

AP axial projection

Film Size:
8 × 10 inches (20 × 24 cm)
or
10 × 12 inches (24 × 30 cm) lengthwise

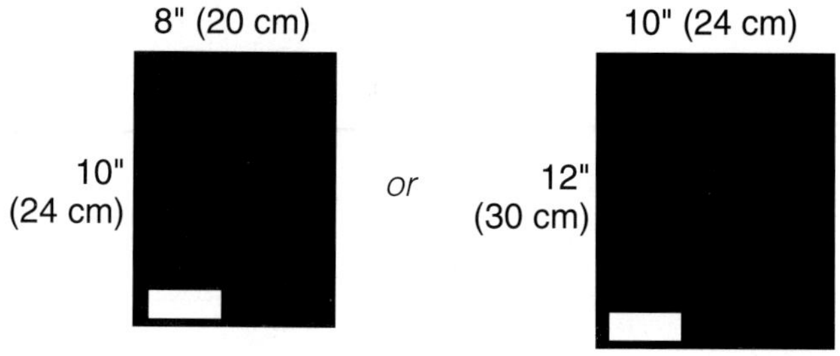

Patient Position

AP recumbent position. Midsagittal plane centered to midline of table. Lower extremities extended to remove them from path of central ray (Fig. 13.41).

Part Position

Flex elbows and place hands on upper chest. Adjust body and pelvis to place both anterior superior iliac spines (ASIS) in same transverse plane.

Central Ray

30° (for males) or 35° (for females) cephalic angle to enter midline at level of ASIS.

Breathing Instructions

Suspend respiration at end of full exhalation.

Structures Demonstrated

Lumbosacral joint should be open. Sacroiliac joints should be well demonstrated (Fig. 13.42).

Evaluation Criteria

Lumbosacral joint and sacroiliac joints should be demonstrated.

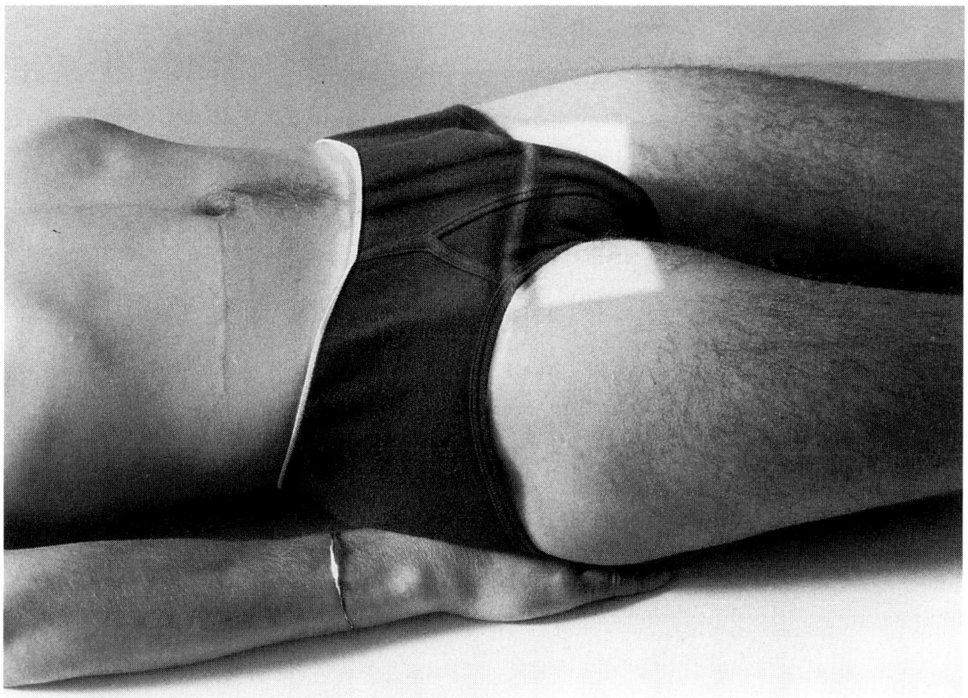

Figure 13.41. AP axial position for lumbar vertebrae.

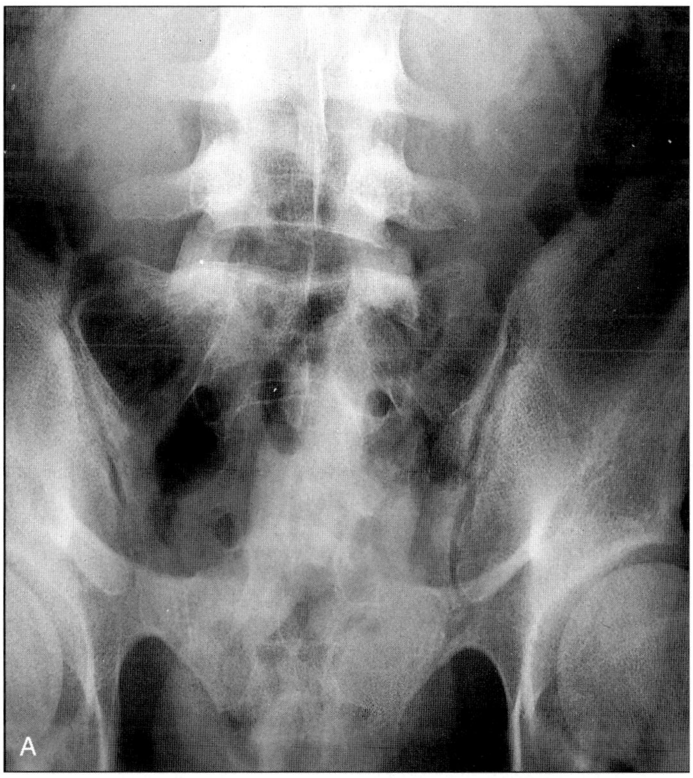

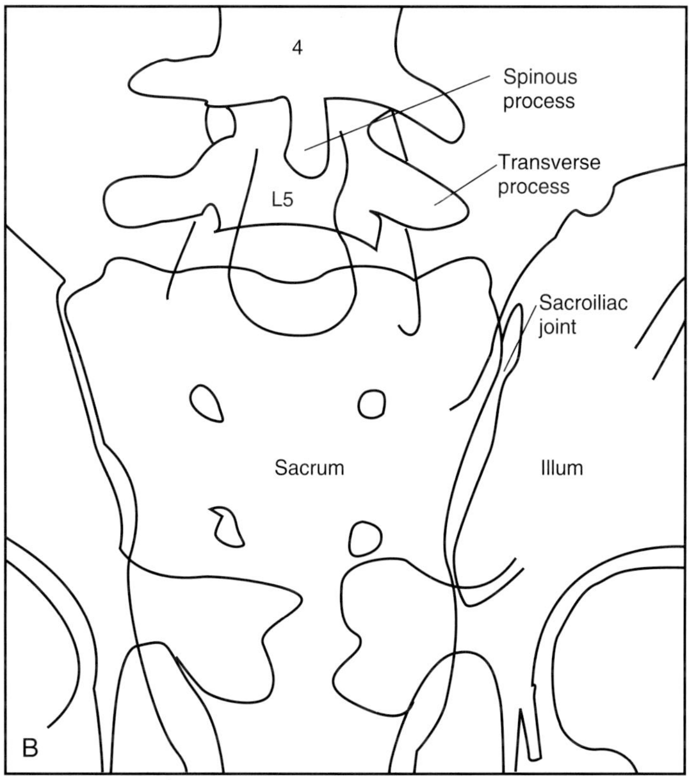

Figure 13.42. A and B, AP axial projection of lumbar spine.

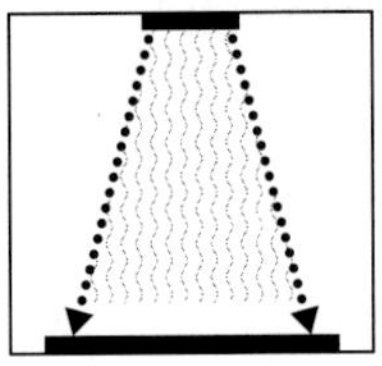

Lumbar Spine

Position/Projection

AP obliques (RPO and LPO)

Film Size:
14 × 17 inches (35 × 43 cm) lengthwise

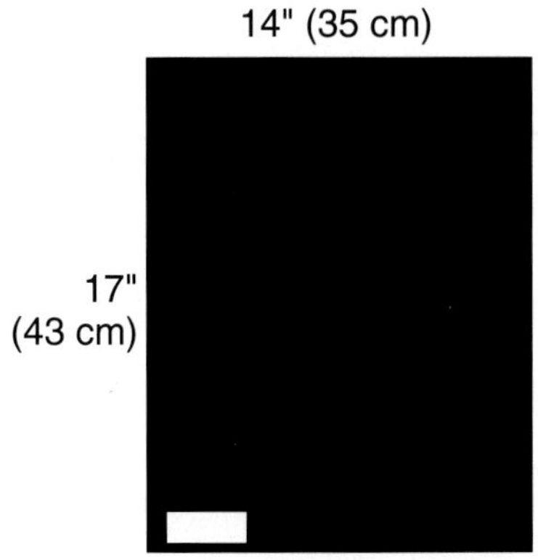

Patient Position
AP oblique recumbent position (Fig. 13.43).

Part Position
Center spine to midline of table. Adjust degree of body rotation at angle of 30°. Center cassette at the level of L3. Center midway between midsagittal plane and lateral border of abdomen.

Central Ray
Perpendicular to midpoint of film.

Breathing Instructions
Respiration suspended at end of full exhalation.

Structures Demonstrated
Oblique projection of lumbar spine. Articulating facets nearest film are demonstrated (Fig. 13.44).

Evaluation Criteria
1. Joint centered on radiograph.
2. Joint space open or with little overlap of ilia and sacrum.

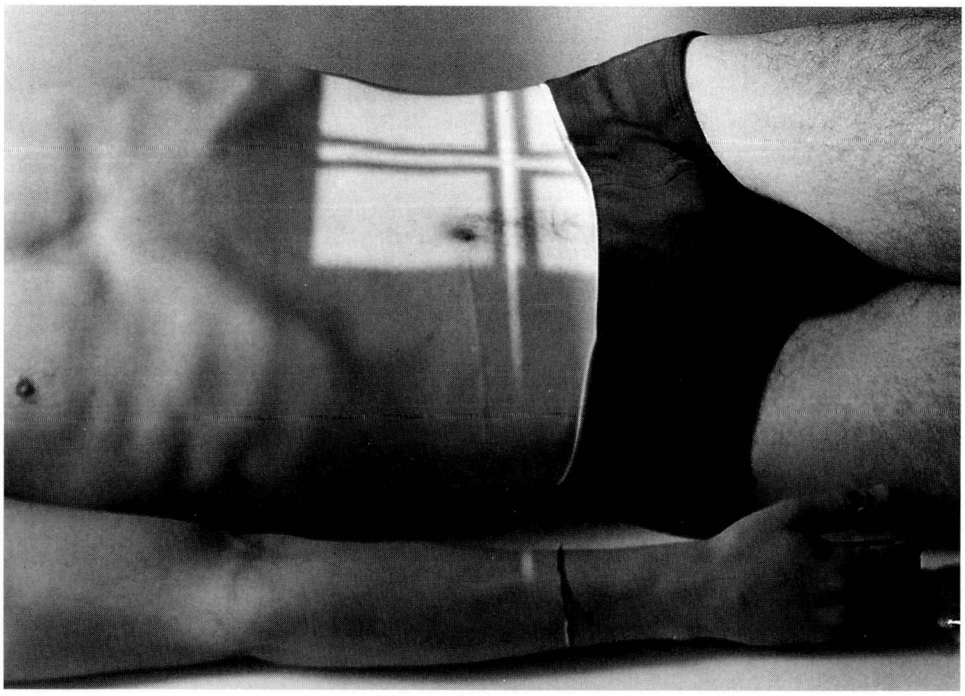

Figure 13.43. AP oblique position for lumbar vertebrae.

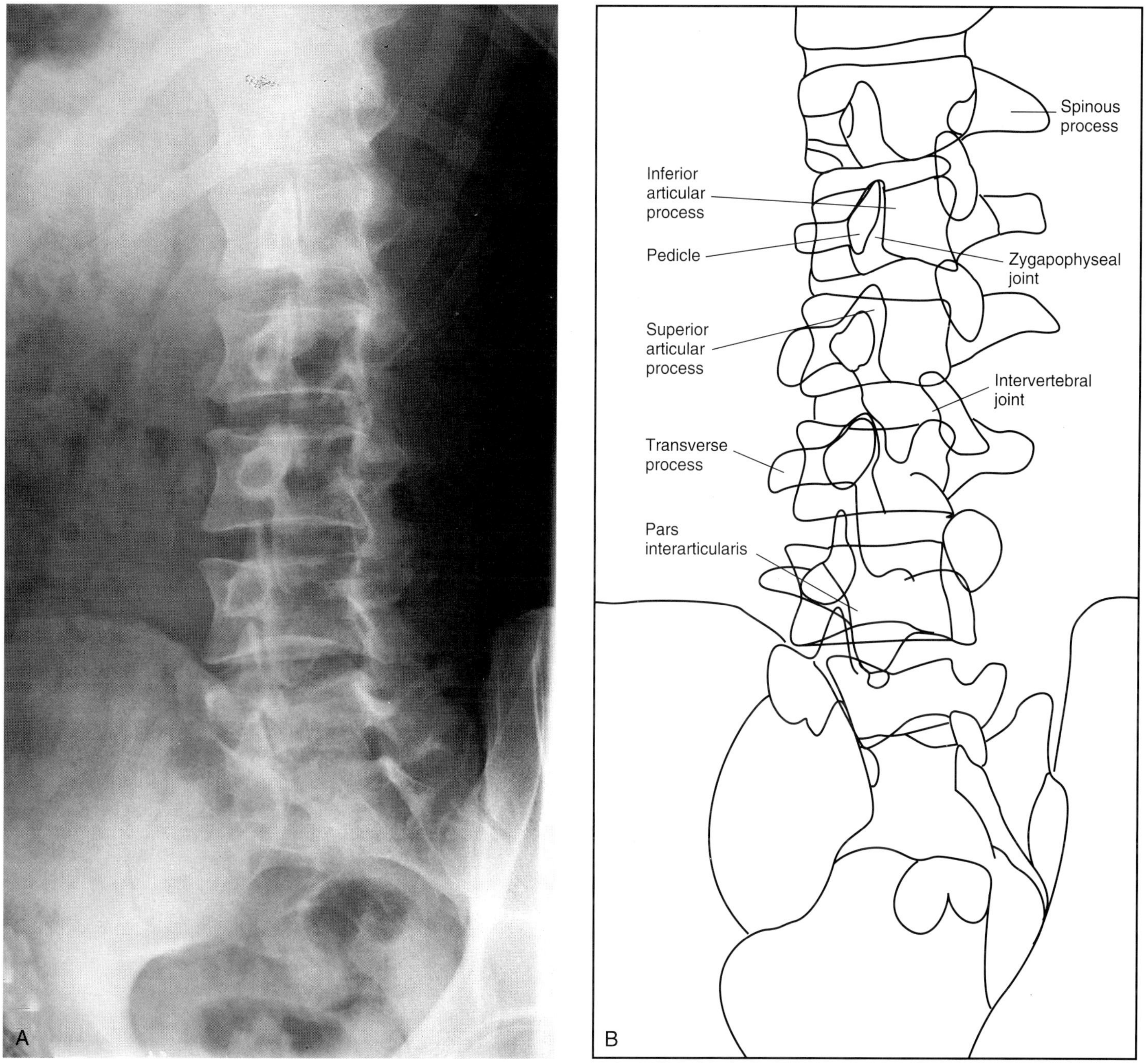

Figure 13.44. A and B, AP oblique projection of lumbar vertebrae.

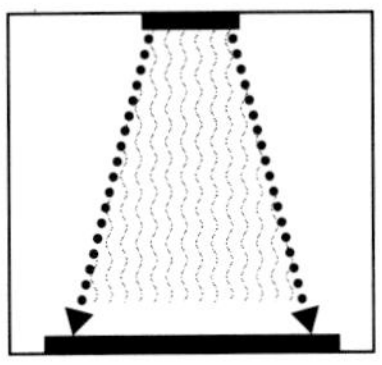

Lumbar Spine

Position/Projection

Lateral

Film Size:
14 × 17 inches (35 × 43 cm) lengthwise

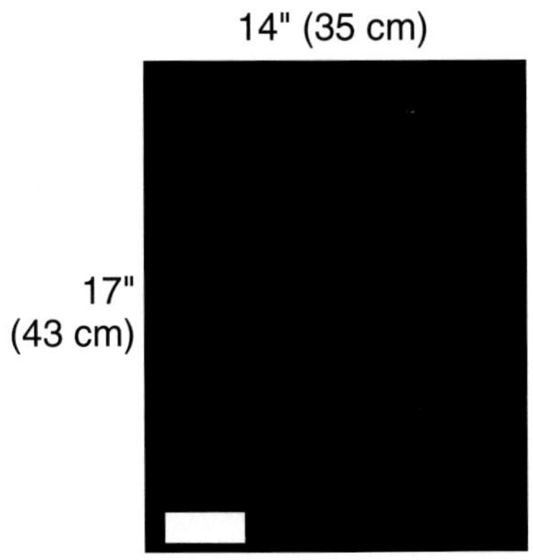

Patient Position

Lateral position. Ask patient to flex hips and knees (Fig. 13.45).

Part Position

Center midaxillary line of body to midline of table. Adjust arms at right angles to body. Adjust position so that long axis of vertebral column is horizontal to table. Center film at level of iliac crest.

Central Ray

Perpendicular to midpoint of film.

Breathing Instructions

Respiration suspended at end of full exhalation.

Structures Demonstrated

Lumbar bodies and their interspaces, spinous processes, and lumbosacral junction (Fig. 13.46).

Evaluation Criteria

1. Include from lower thoracic vertebra to coccyx.
2. Vertebra in middle of radiograph.
3. Open intervertebral disk spaces.
4. Superimposition of posterior margins of vertebral bodies.
5. Demonstration of spinous processes.

NOTE: Radiographic quality can be improved by placing a sheet of leaded rubber on the table behind the patient.

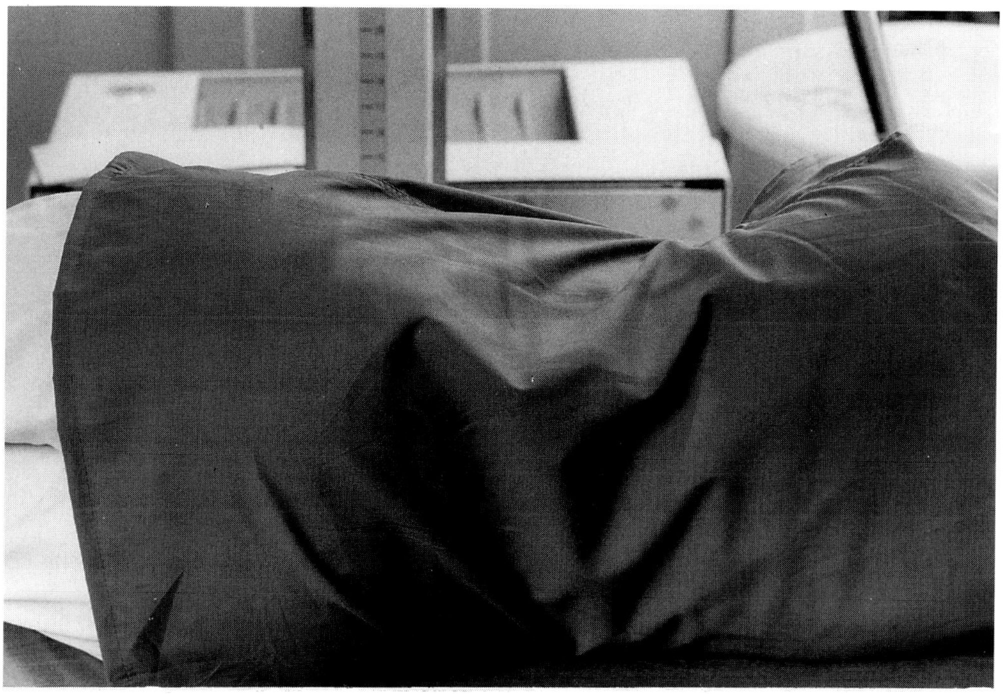

Figure 13.45. Lateral position for lumbar vertebrae.

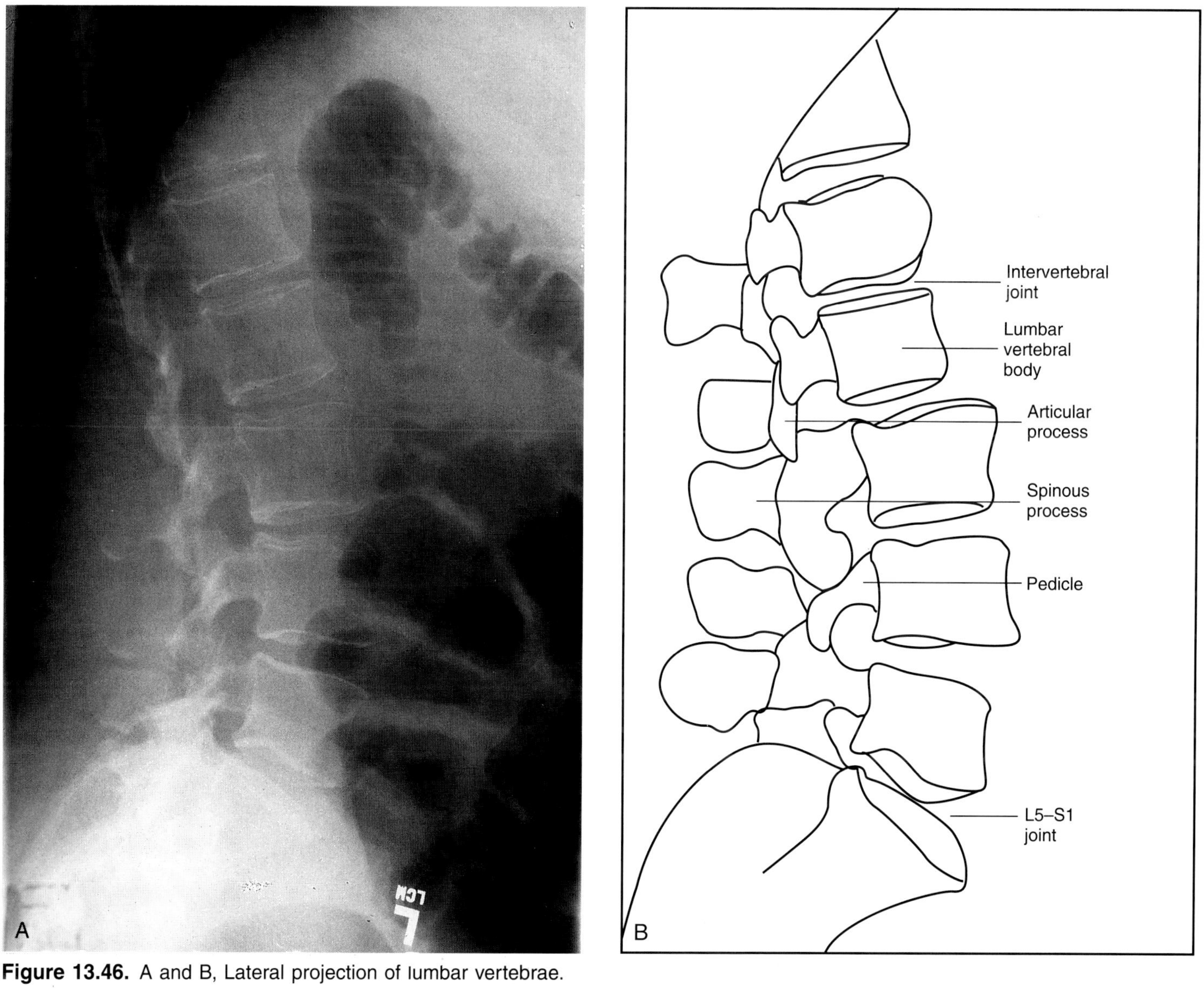

Figure 13.46. A and B, Lateral projection of lumbar vertebrae.

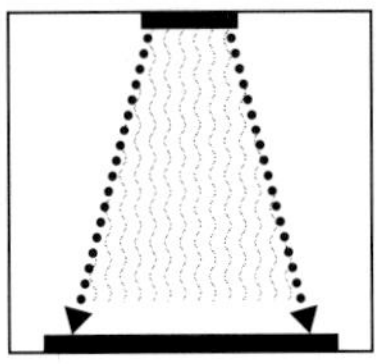

Lumbar Spine

Position/Projection

Lumbosacral spot (localized lateral projection)

Film Size:
8 × 10 inches (20 × 24 cm)
lengthwise

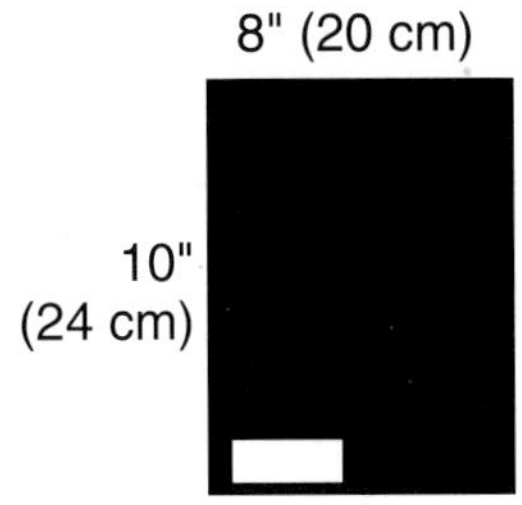

Patient Position

Lateral position. Flex hips and knees (Fig. 13.47).

Part Position

Align patient's body so that coronal plane passing 1½ inches (4 cm) posterior to midaxillary line is centered to midline of table. Adjust arms at right angles to body. Center cassette at level of transverse plane that passes midway between iliac crests and ASIS.

Central Ray

Perpendicular to midpoint of cassette. When spine is not adjusted horizontally, central ray is angled caudally 5–8°.

Breathing Instructions

Respiration suspended at end of full exhalation.

Structures Demonstrated

Lateral projection of lumbosacral joint, lower one or two lumbar vertebrae, and upper sacrum (Fig. 13.48).

Evaluation Criteria

1. Entire L5 and upper sacrum with lumbosacral joint in center of area exposed.
2. Open lumbosacral joint clearly visualized through penetration of both ilia.

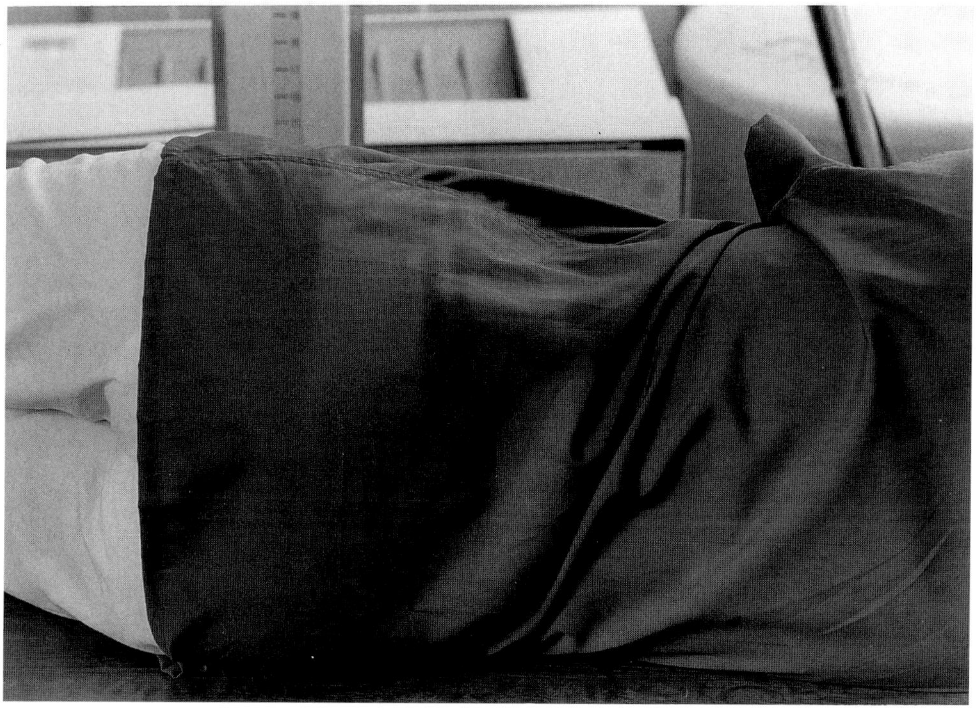

Figure 13.47. Lateral position for lumbosacral spot radiograph.

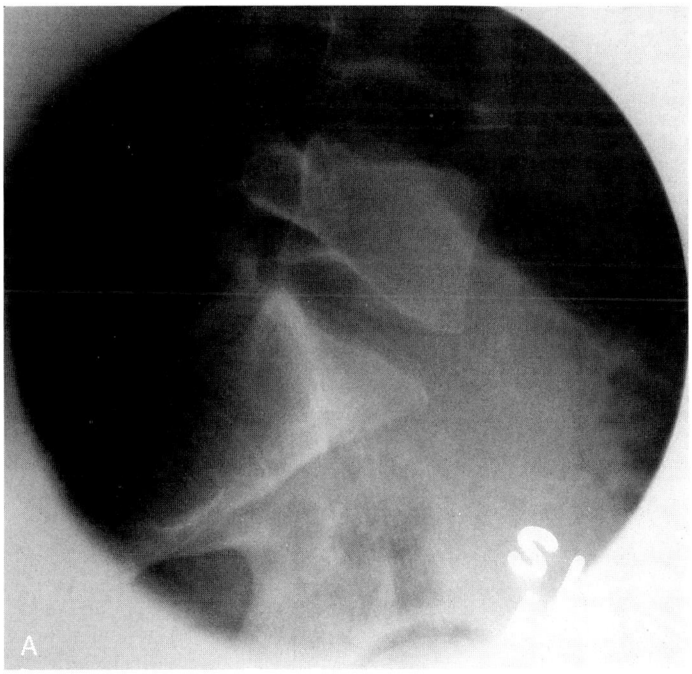

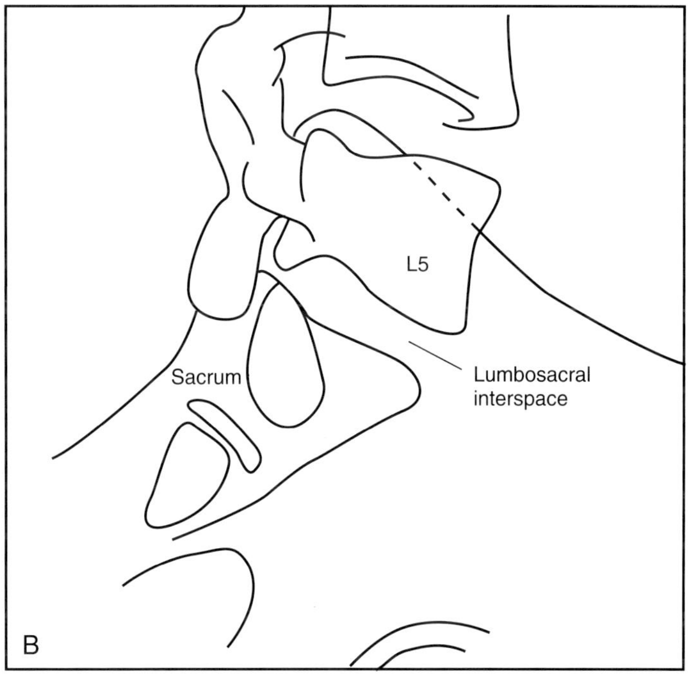

Figure 13.48. A and B, Lateral projection of lumbosacral vertebrae.

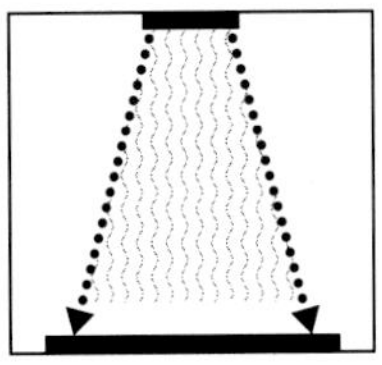

Lumbosacral Apophyseal Joints

Position/Projection

PA obliques for apophyseal articulations (RAO and LAO)

Film Size:
14 × 17 inches (35 × 43 cm)

or

11 × 14 inches (30 × 35 cm) lengthwise

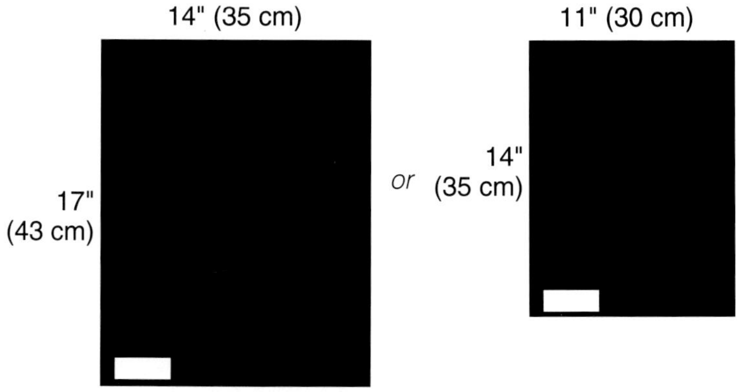

Patient Position

Prone, recumbent or erect. PA obliques demonstrate apophyseal articulations on side farthest from table (Fig. 13.49).

Part Position

Semiprone position rotated 45°. Place sagittal plane that passes 2 inches (5 cm) lateral (toward elevated side) to spinous process of L3 to midline of table.

Central Ray

Perpendicular to level of L3, enters 2 inches (5 cm) lateral (toward elevated side) to spinous process of L3.

Breathing Instructions

Suspend respiration at end of full exhalation.

Structures Demonstrated

Apophyseal articulation of side farthest from table. The "Scotty dog" will be visible if articular processes have been demonstrated. Both obliques should be done for comparison (Fig. 13.50).

Evaluation Criteria

1. Apophyseal articulations farthest from table should be demonstrated. If patient is not obliqued enough, pedicle of "Scotty dog" will appear anterior on vertebral body. If patient is obliqued too much, pedicle will appear posterior on vertebral body.
2. Vertebral column should be parallel to table with intevertebral disk spaces equal from T12 through S2.

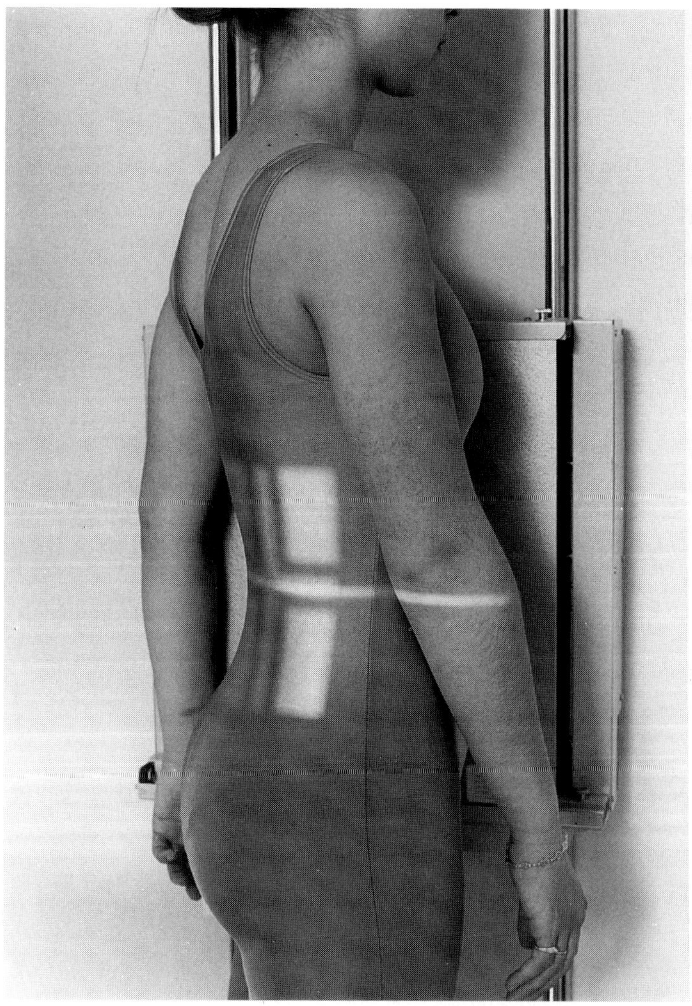

Figure 13.49. PA oblique position for demonstration of lumbar apophyseal articulations.

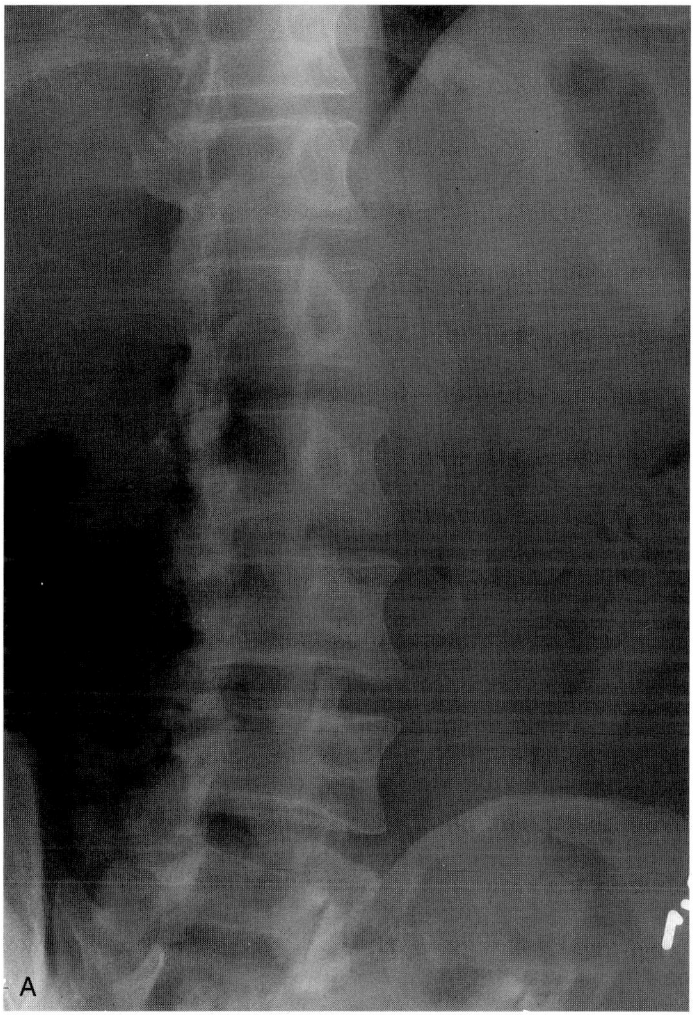

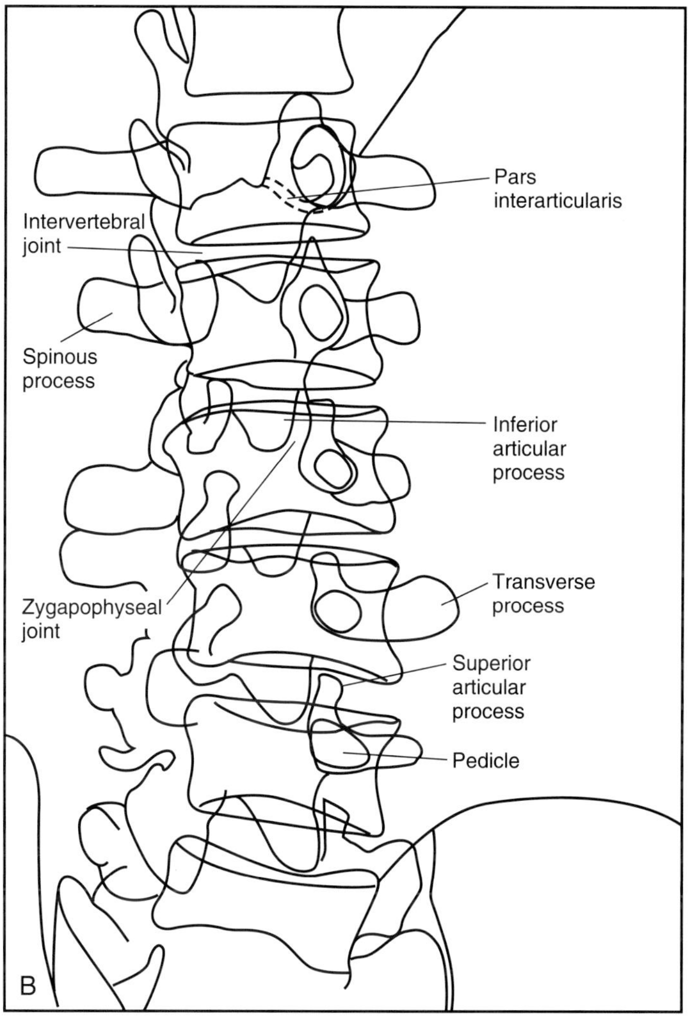

Figure 13.50. A and B, PA oblique projection of lumbar apophyseal articulations.

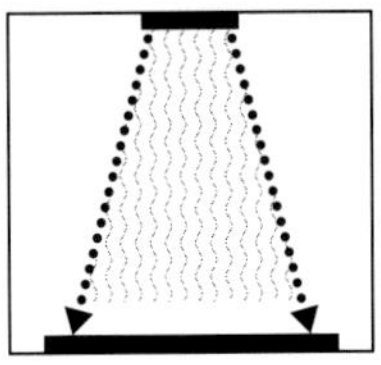

Lumbosacral Apophyseal Joints

Position/Projection

AP obliques for apophyseal articulations (RPO and LPO)

Film Size:
14 × 17 inches (35 × 43 cm)
or
11 × 14 inches (30 × 35 cm) lengthwise

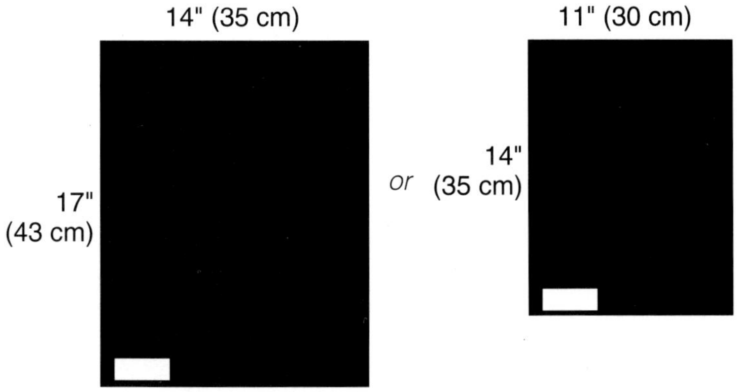

Patient Position

Recumbent or erect. AP obliques demonstrate apophyseal articulations on side closest to table (Fig. 13.51).

Part Position

Turn patient from supine position 45° toward side being examined. Place sagittal plane 2 inches (5 cm) medial from elevated ASIS to midline of table.

Central Ray

Perpendicular to midpoint of film to enter at level of L3, approximately 2 inches (5 cm) lateral to midline.

Breathing Instructions

Suspend respiration at end of full exhalation.

Structures Demonstrated

Apophyseal articulations of side closest to cassette. "Scotty dog" will be visible if articular processes have been demonstrated. Both obliques should be done for comparison (Fig. 13.52).

Evaluation Criteria

1. Apophyseal articulations closest to cassette should be demonstrated. If patient is not obliqued enough, pedicle of the "Scotty dog" will appear anterior on vertebral body. If patient is obliqued too much, pedicle of "Scotty dog" will appear posterior on vertebral body.
2. Vertebral column should be parallel to table with intervertebral disk spaces equal from T12 through S2.

NOTE: The 45° rotation demonstrates L1–L4 articular facets. To demonstrate the L5 articular facet, a 30° rotation should be used.

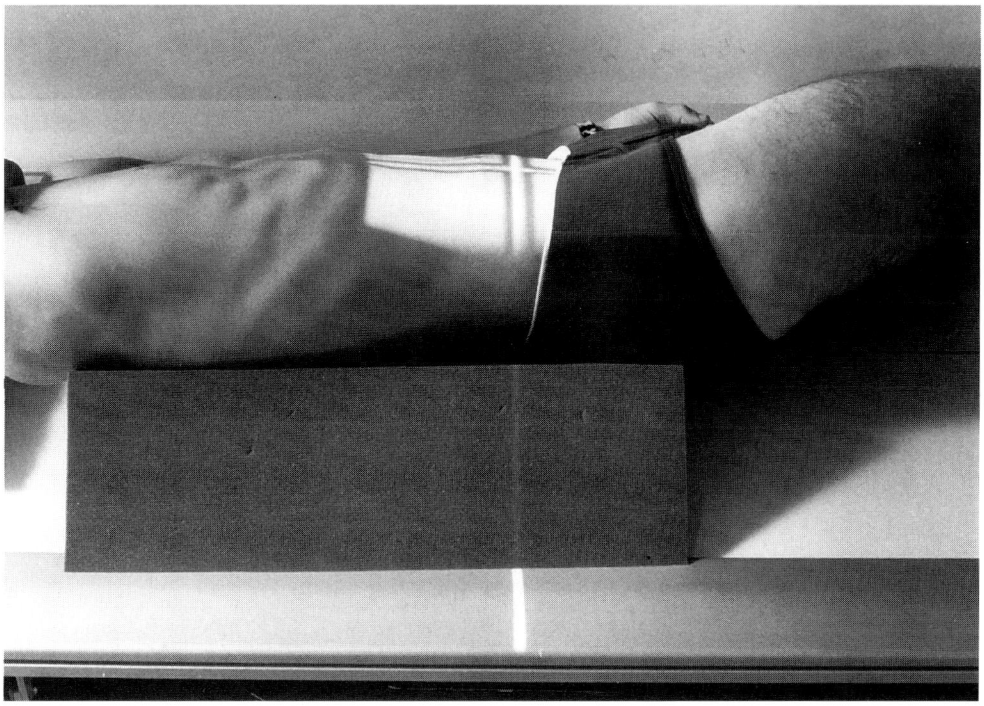

Figure 13.51. AP oblique position for demonstration of lumbar apophyseal articulations.

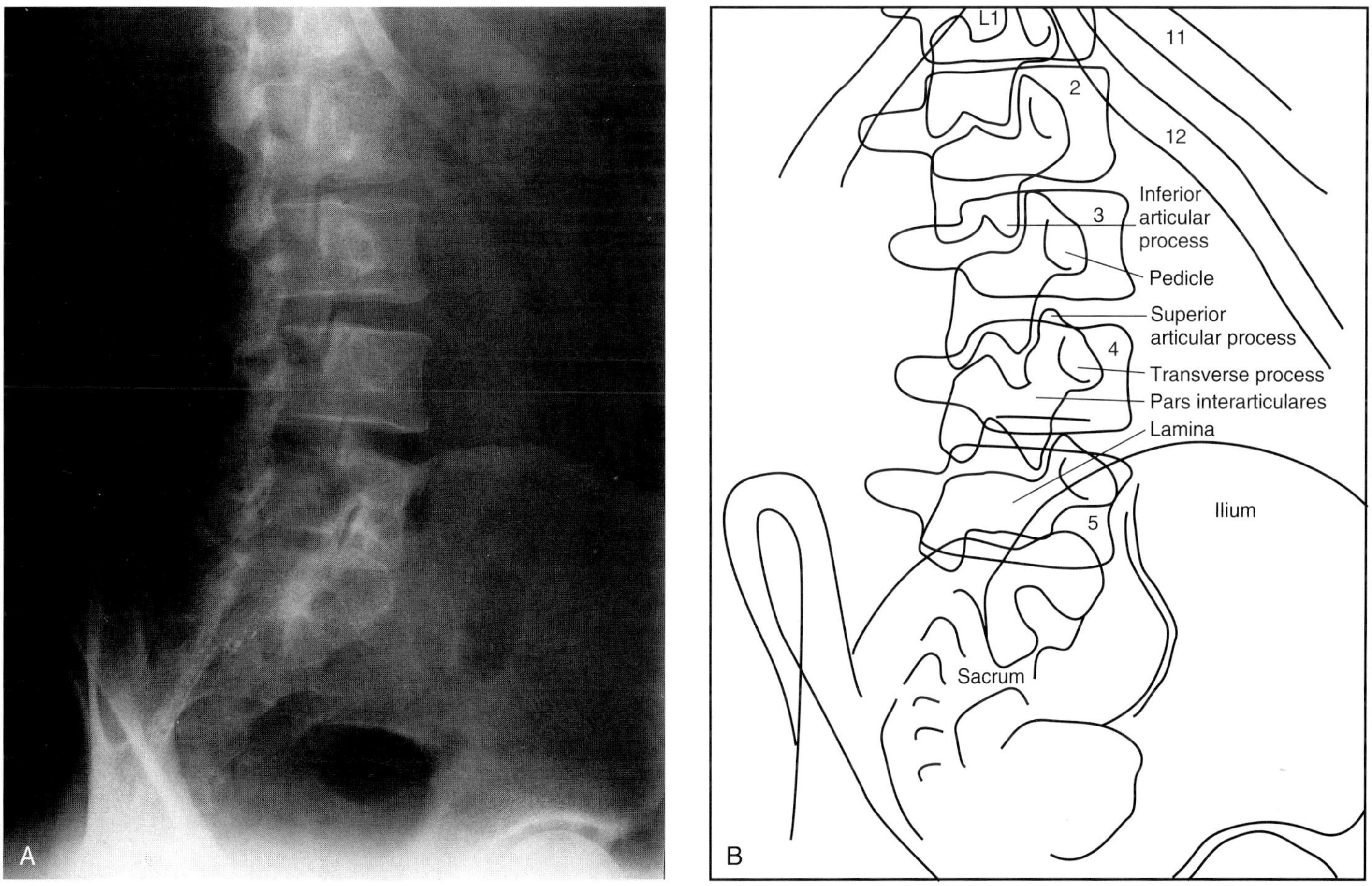

Figure 13.52. A and B, AP oblique projection of lumbar apophyseal articulations.

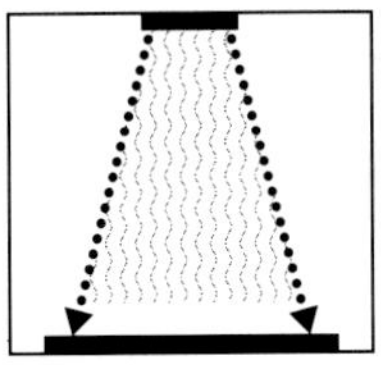

Lumbar Intervertebral Disks

Position/Projection

Weight-bearing bending studies

Film Size:
14 × 17 inches (35 × 43 cm) lengthwise

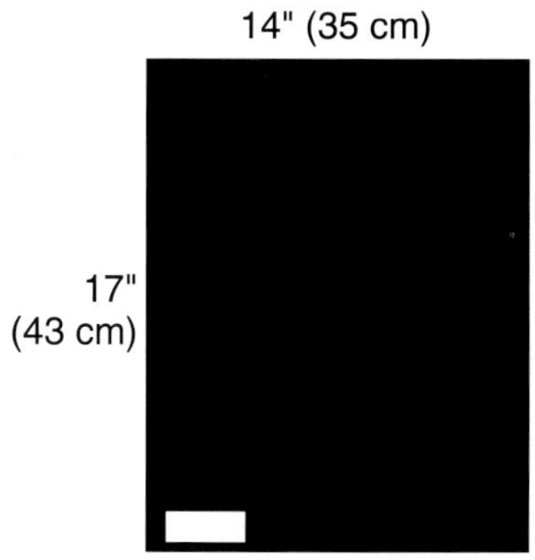

Patient Position

PA position, standing before vertical grid device (Fig. 13.53).

Part Position

Midsagittal plane to midline of vertical device. Level of L3 centered to midpoint of vertical grid device. Patient should bend laterally to left for second radiograph. Patient should lean laterally as far as possible without rotation and without lifting foot. Arms should hang by patient's side and patient should not be supported by any device.

Central Ray

Perpendicular to L3 or 15–20° caudad angle to enter at L3.

Breathing Instructions

Respiration suspended at end of full exhalation.

Structures Demonstrated

Bending projections of lower thoracic and lumbar vertebrae. Procedure is used to localize involved joint in patients with disk protrusion (Fig. 13.54).

Evaluation Criteria

1. There should be no rotation.
2. The lower thoracic vertebrae to sacrum should be demonstrated.

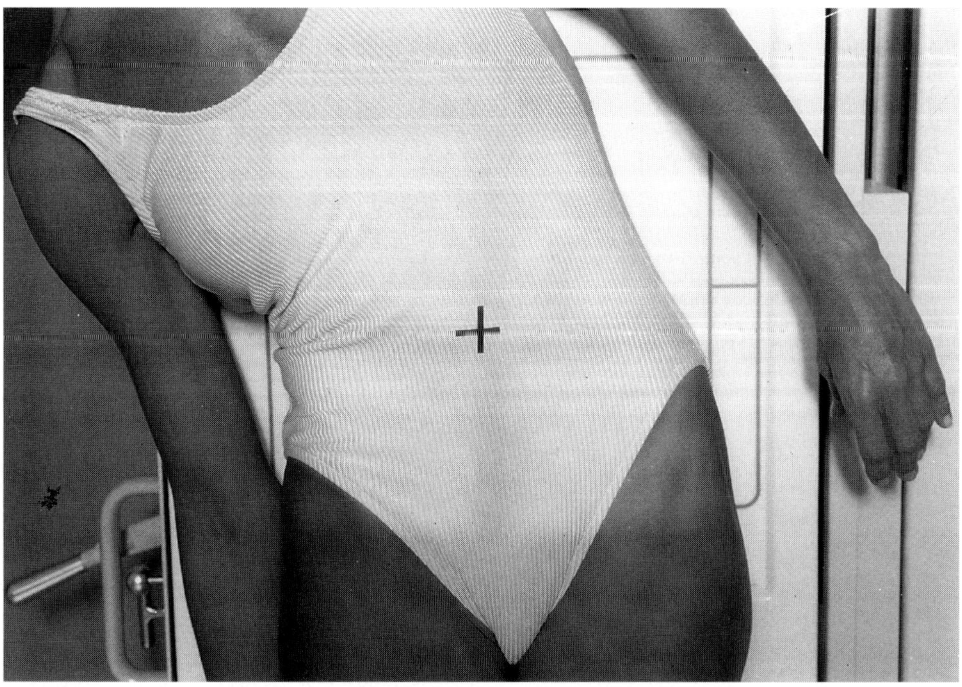

Figure 13.53. PA weight-bearing bending position for lumbar intervertebral disks.

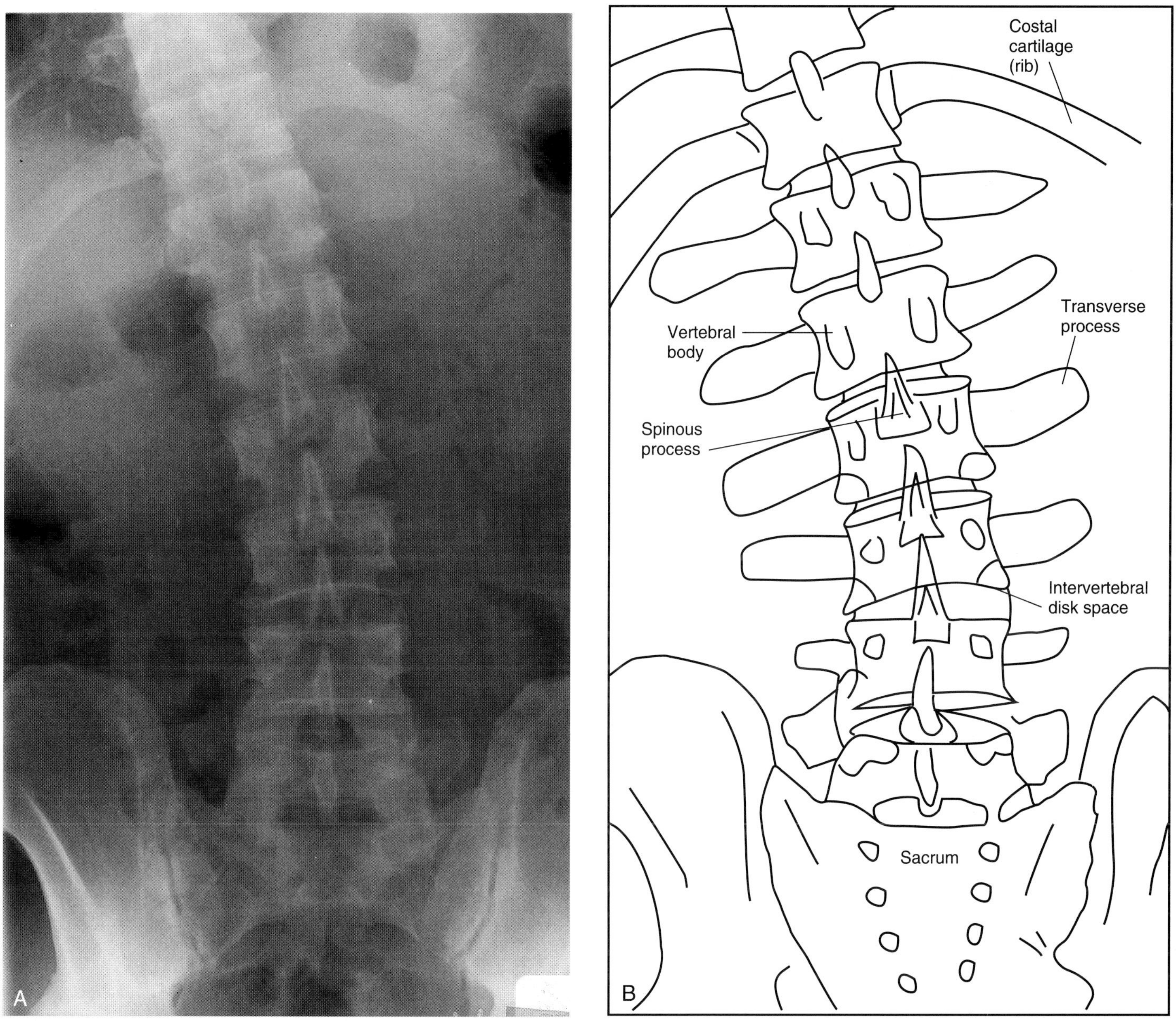

Figure 13.54. A and B, PA bending projection of lumbar spine intervertebral disks.

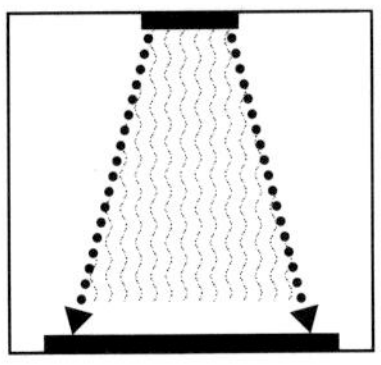

Flexion and Extension Study

Position/Projection

Lateral in flexion and extension

Film Size:
10 × 12 inches (24 × 30 cm)
or
14 × 17 inches (35 × 43 cm) lengthwise (each exposure)

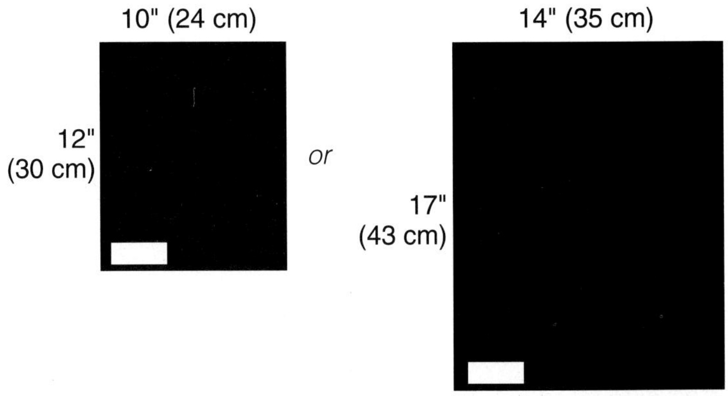

Patient Position

Lateral erect or recumbent (Fig. 13.55).

Part Position

For Hyperflexion
Patient should curve forward and pull thighs up toward chest to flex spine as much as possible.

For Hyperextension
Patient should curve backward and straighten hips and thighs as much as possible.

Central Ray

Perpendicular to level of L3, centered 2 inches (5 cm) posterior to midaxillary line.

Breathing Instructions

Suspended respiration at end of full exhalation.

Structures Demonstrated

Lateral hyperflexion and lateral hyperextension of lumbar vertebrae. Procedure is used to localize herniated disk or to demonstrate motion in area of spinal fusion (Fig. 13.56).

Evaluation Criteria

1. There should be no rotation.
2. Lumbar vertebrae should be in center of radiograph.

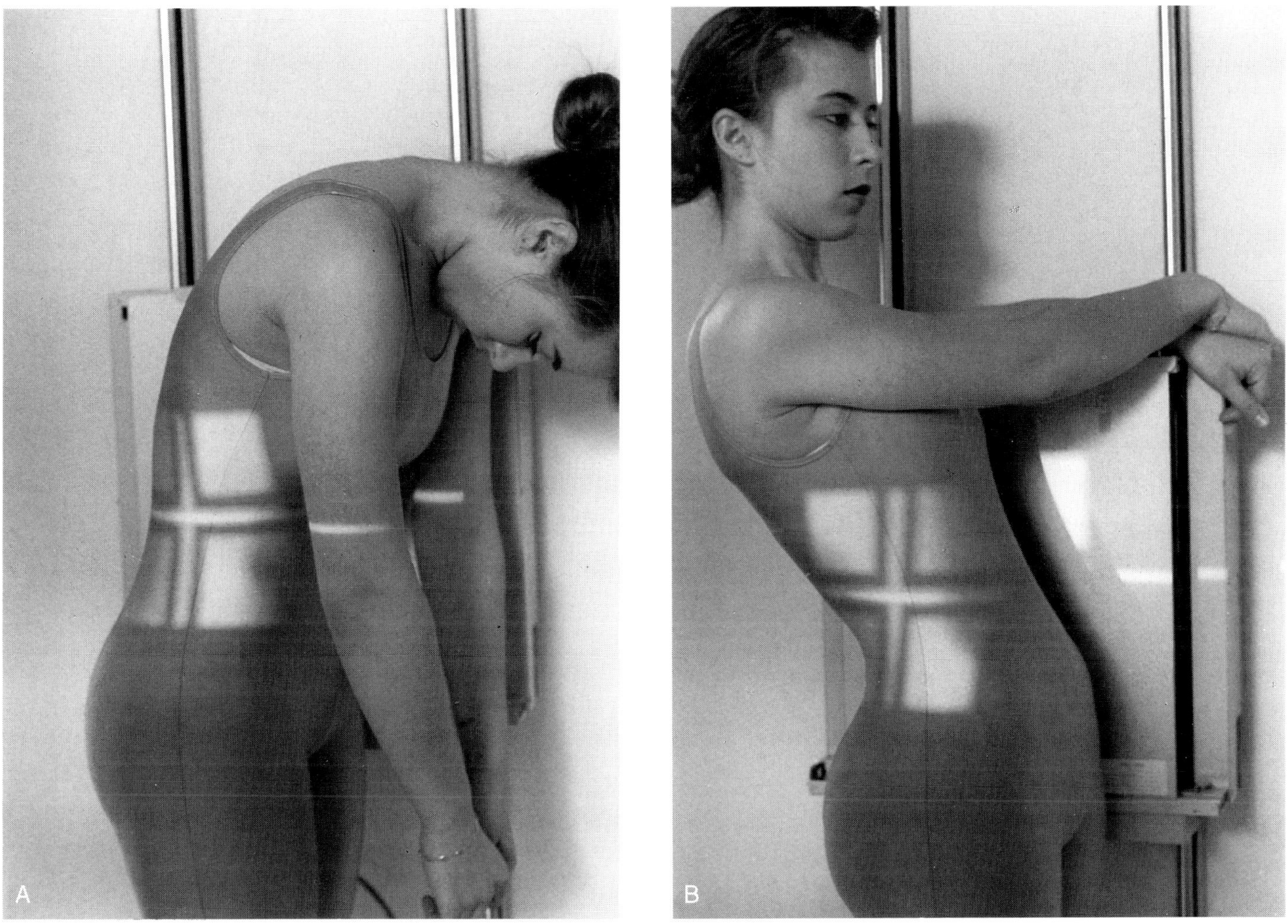

Figure 13.55. Lateral (A) flexion and (B) extension positions for lumbar vertebrae.

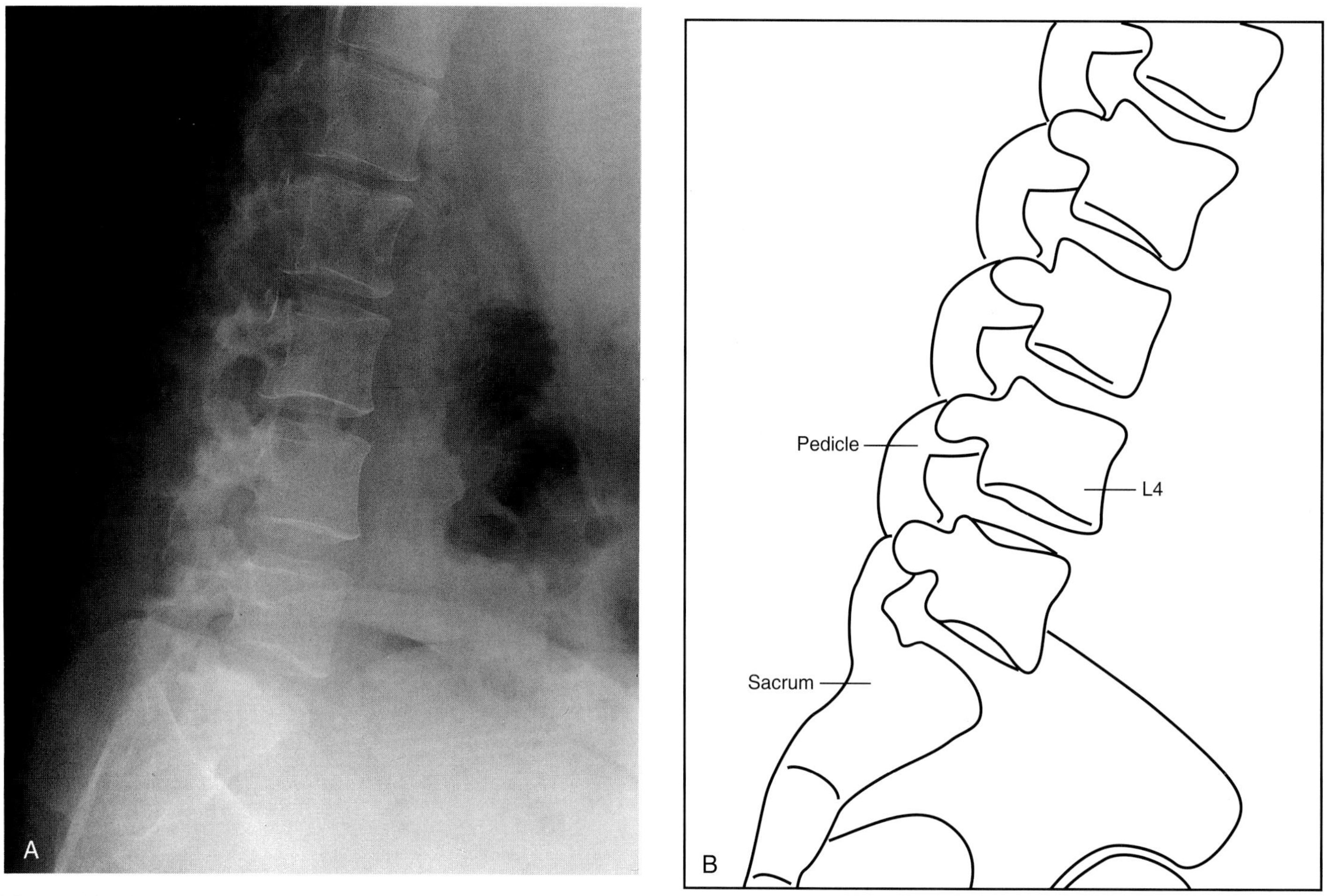

Figure 13.56. Lateral projections of (A and B) flexion and

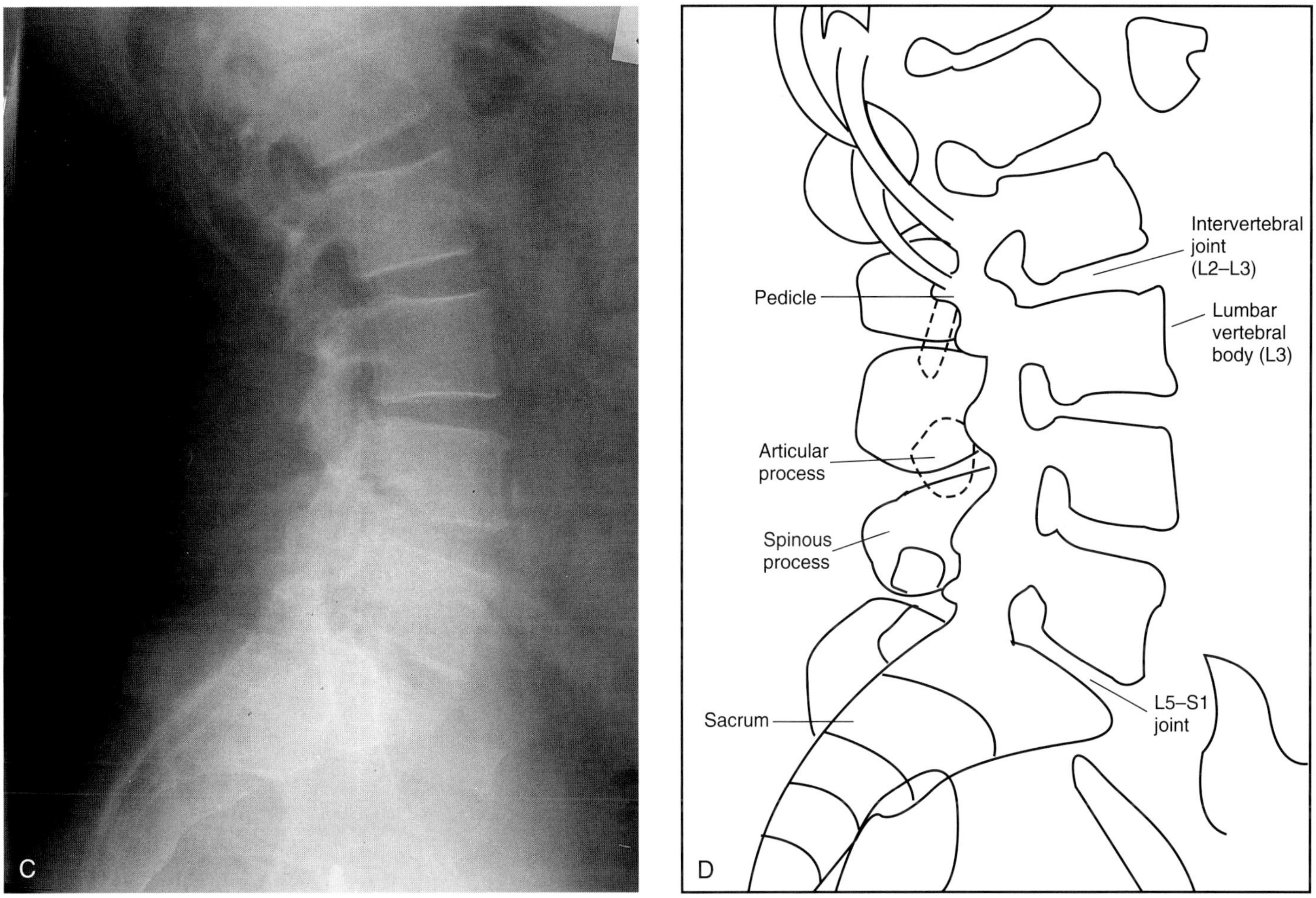

Figure 13.56 *(Continued)* (C and D) extension studies of lumbar vertebrae.

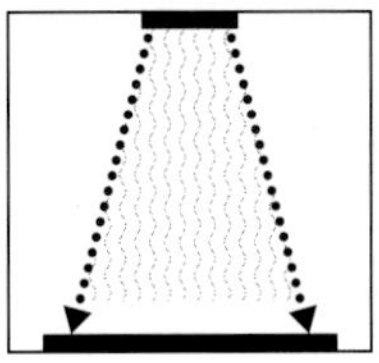

Sacrum

Position/Projection

AP and PA

Film Size:
10 × 12 inches (24 × 30 cm) lengthwise

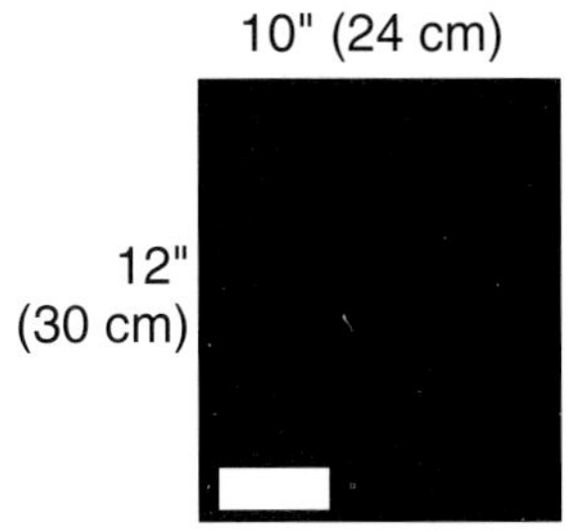

Patient Position
Prone or supine position. Midsagittal plane is centered to midline of table (Fig. 13.57).

Part Position
Midpoint of transverse plane that passes midway between pubic symphysis and ASIS.

Central Ray
15° cephalad if patient supine or 15° caudad if patient prone.

Breathing Instructions
Respiration suspended at end of full exhalation.

Structures Demonstrated
True frontal projection of sacrum (Fig. 13.58).

Evaluation Criteria
1. Straightened sacral curvature; no foreshortening.
2. Sacrum should be centered to radiograph; no rotation.
3. Lack of overlapping by pubic bones.
4. Presence of fecal material may require preparation.
5. Patient should also empty bladder before examination.

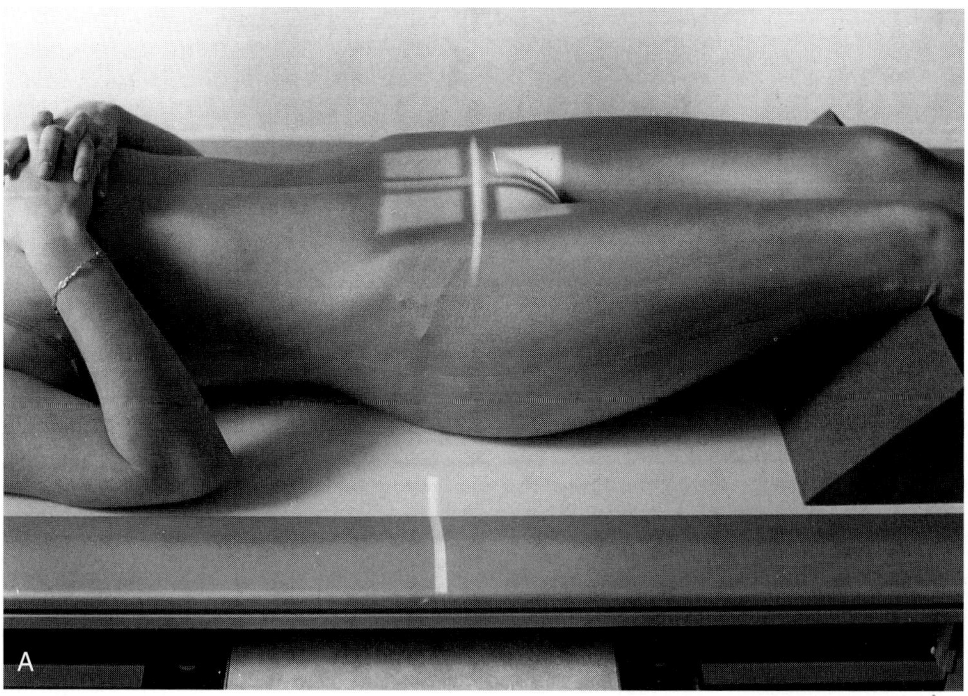

Figure 13.57. A, AP position for sacrum.

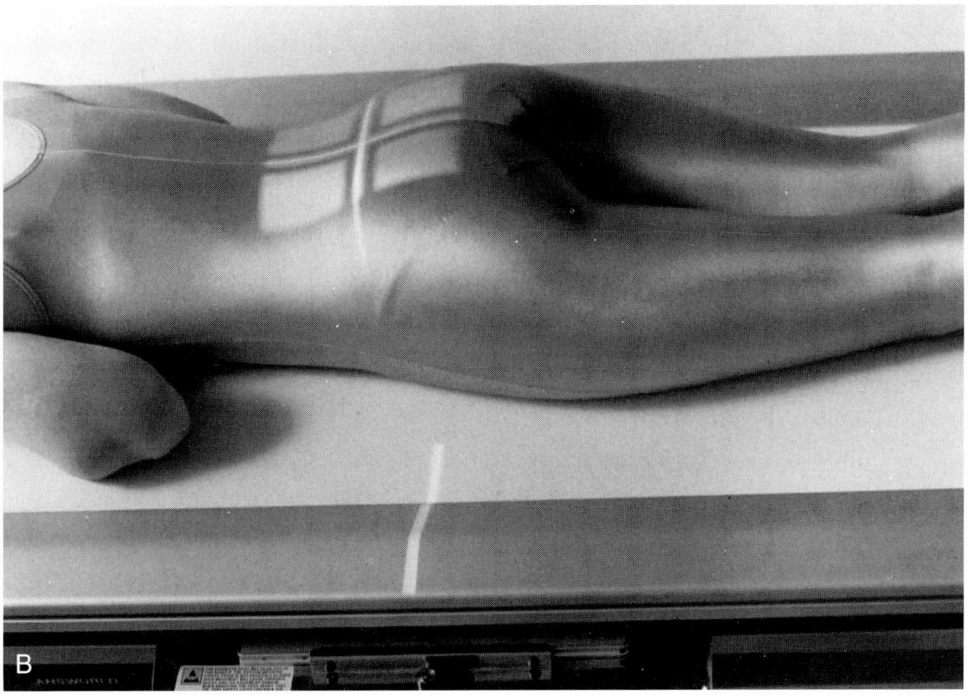

Figure 13.57. *(Continued)* B, PA position for sacrum.

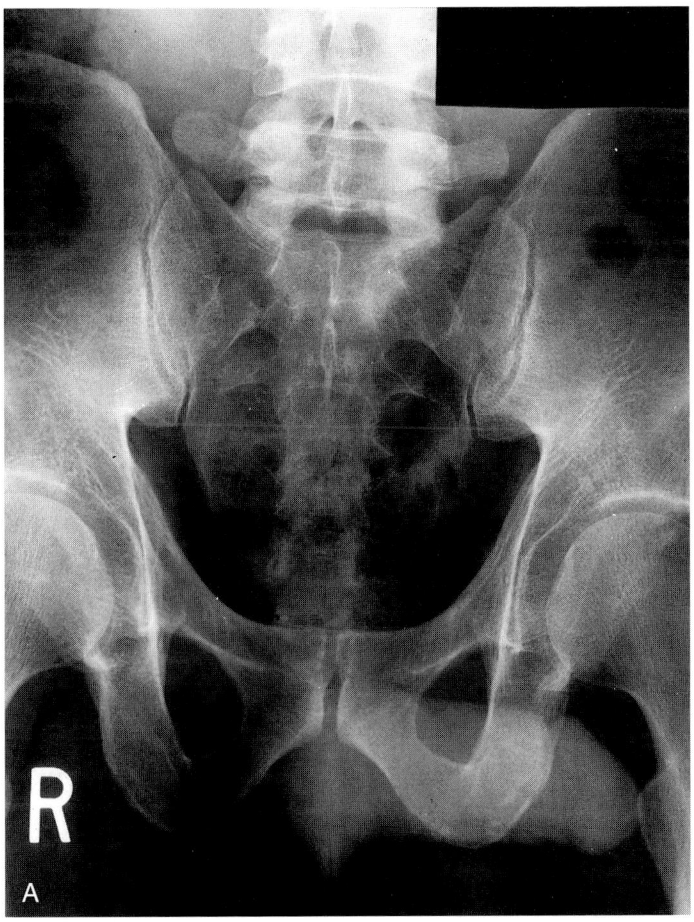

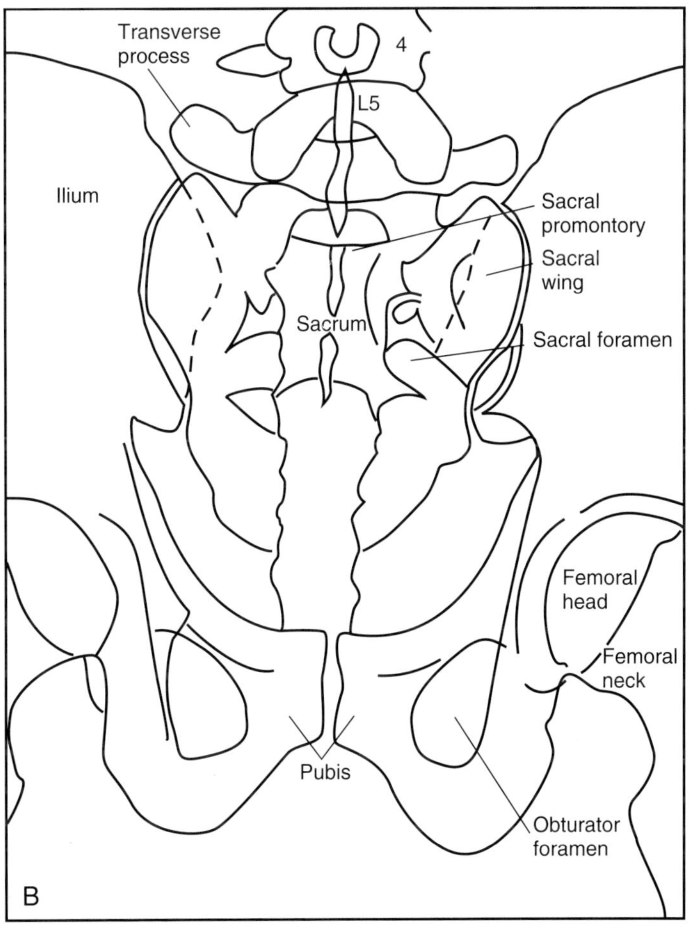

Figure 13.58. A and B, AP sacrum.

Sacroiliac Joints

Position/Projection

AP obliques (RPO and LPO)

Film Size:
8 × 10 inches (20 × 24 cm)
or
10 × 12 inches (24 × 30 cm) lengthwise

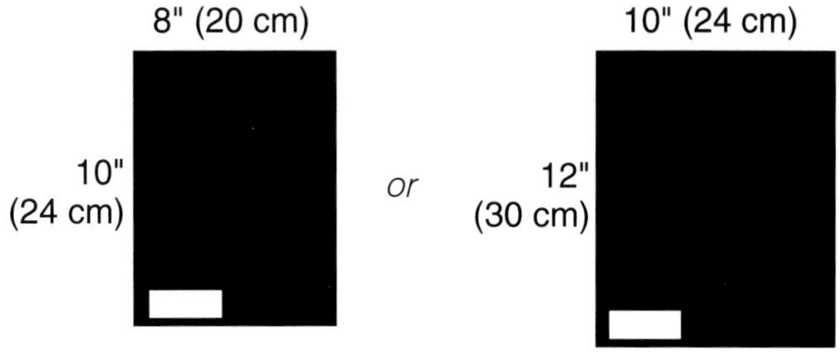

Patient Position
Supine (Fig. 13.59).

Part Position
Affected side should be elevated 25–30°. Center point 1 inch (2.5 cm) medial to ASIS of elevated side to midline of table.

Central Ray
1. Perpendicular, entering 1 inch (2.5 cm) medial to elevated ASIS.
   or
2. 20–25° cephalad angle to enter 1 inch (2.5 cm) medial and 1½ inches (4 cm) distal to elevated ASIS.

Breathing Instructions
Respiration suspended at end of full exhalation.

Structures Demonstrated
Sacroiliac joint farthest from film shown in profile. Both sides should be done for comparison (Fig. 13.60).

Evaluation Criteria
1. Joint space farthest from film should be open and in center of radiograph.
2. Both ASIS should lie in same transverse plane.

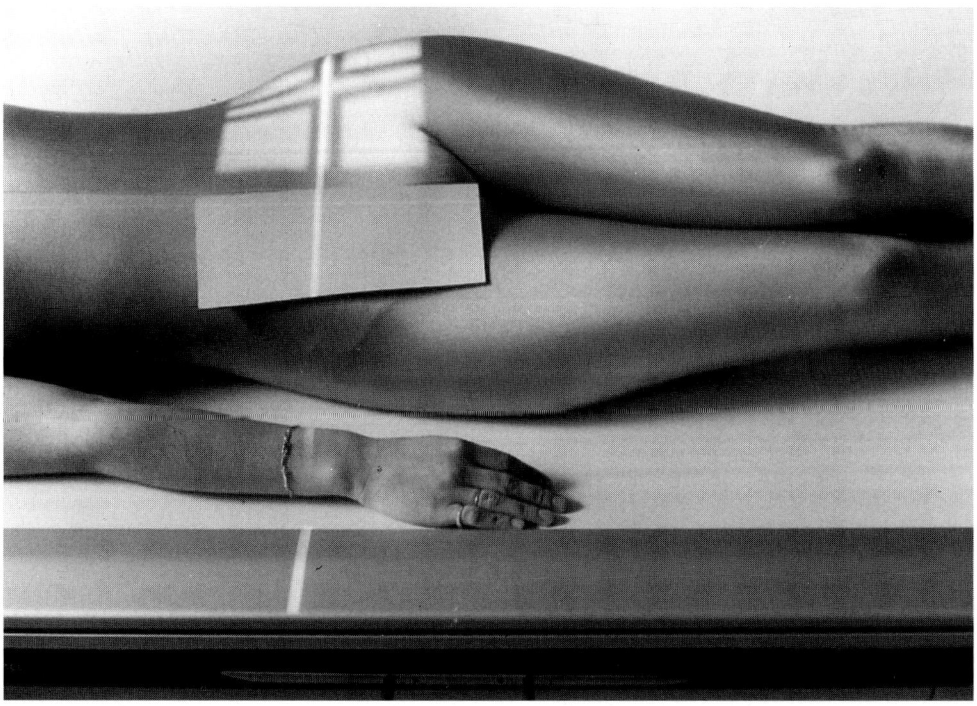

Figure 13.59. AP oblique position for sacroiliac joints.

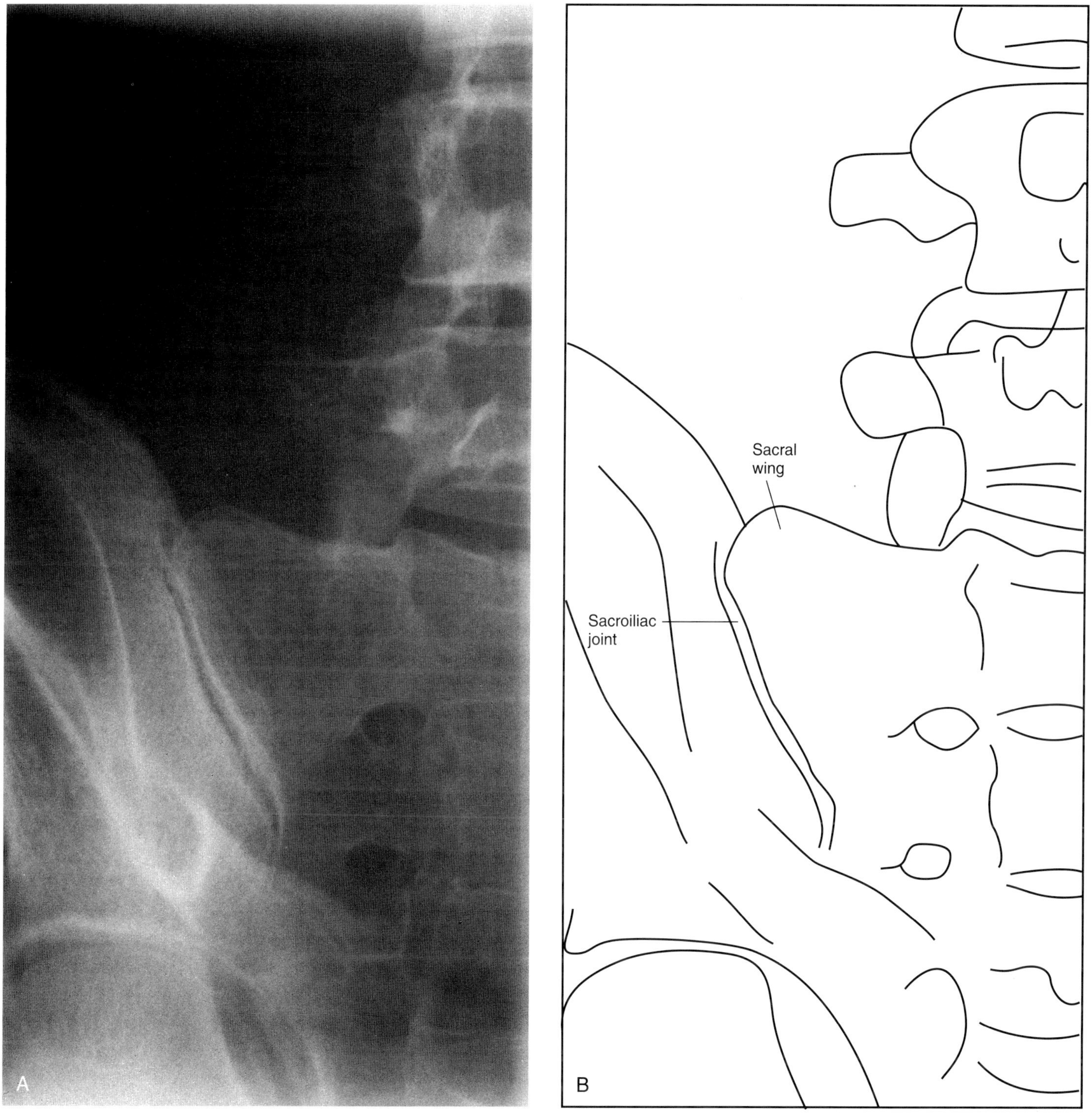

Figure 13.60. A and B, AP oblique projection of sacroiliac joints.

Sacroiliac Joints

Position/Projection

PA obliques (RAO and LAO)

Film Size:
8 × 10 inches (20 × 24 cm)
or
10 × 12 inches (24 × 30 cm) lengthwise

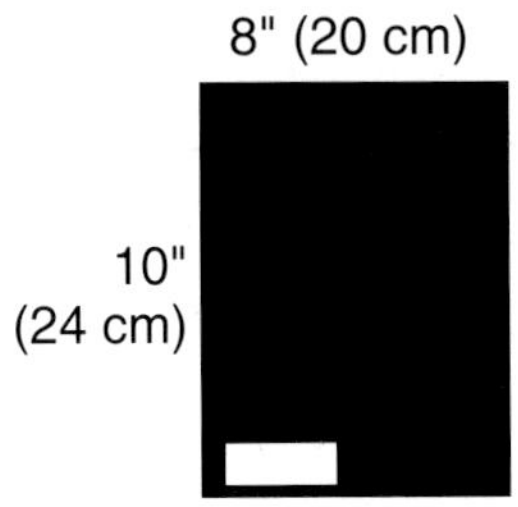

or

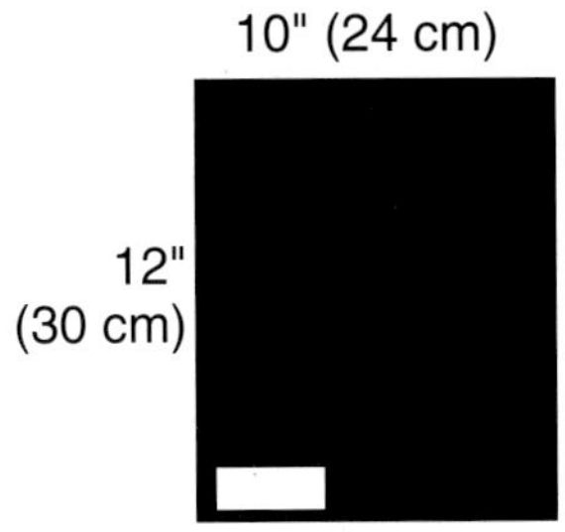

Patient Position

Semiprone. Side to be examined should be closest to table. Flex knee of elevated side (Fig. 13.61).

Part Position

Elevated side should be rotated 20–30° from plane of film. Center point 1 inch (2.5 cm) medial to dependent ASIS to midline of table.

Central Ray

1. Perpendicular, entering 1 inch (2.5 cm) medial to dependent ASIS.
   or
2. 20–25° caudad angle to enter point passing 1½ inches (4 cm) distal to L5 spinous process and exiting at level of dependent ASIS.

Breathing Instructions

Respiration suspended at end of full exhalation.

Structures Demonstrated

Sacroiliac joint closest to the film shown in profile. Both sides should be done for comparison (Fig. 13.62).

Evaluation Criteria

Joint space closest to film should be open and in center of radiograph.

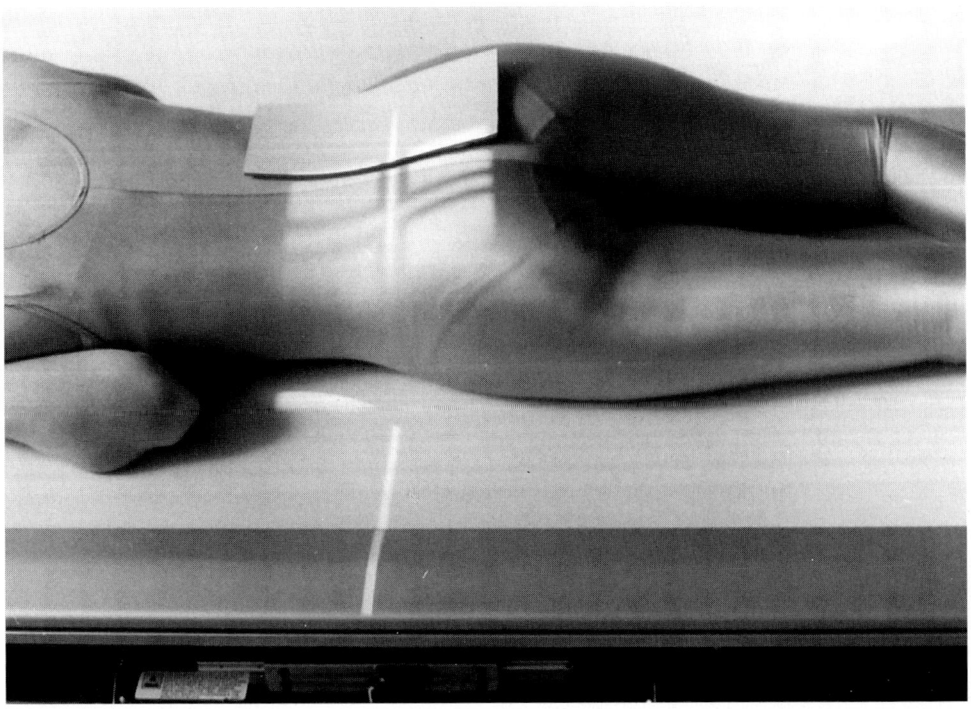

Figure 13.61. PA oblique position for sacroiliac joints.

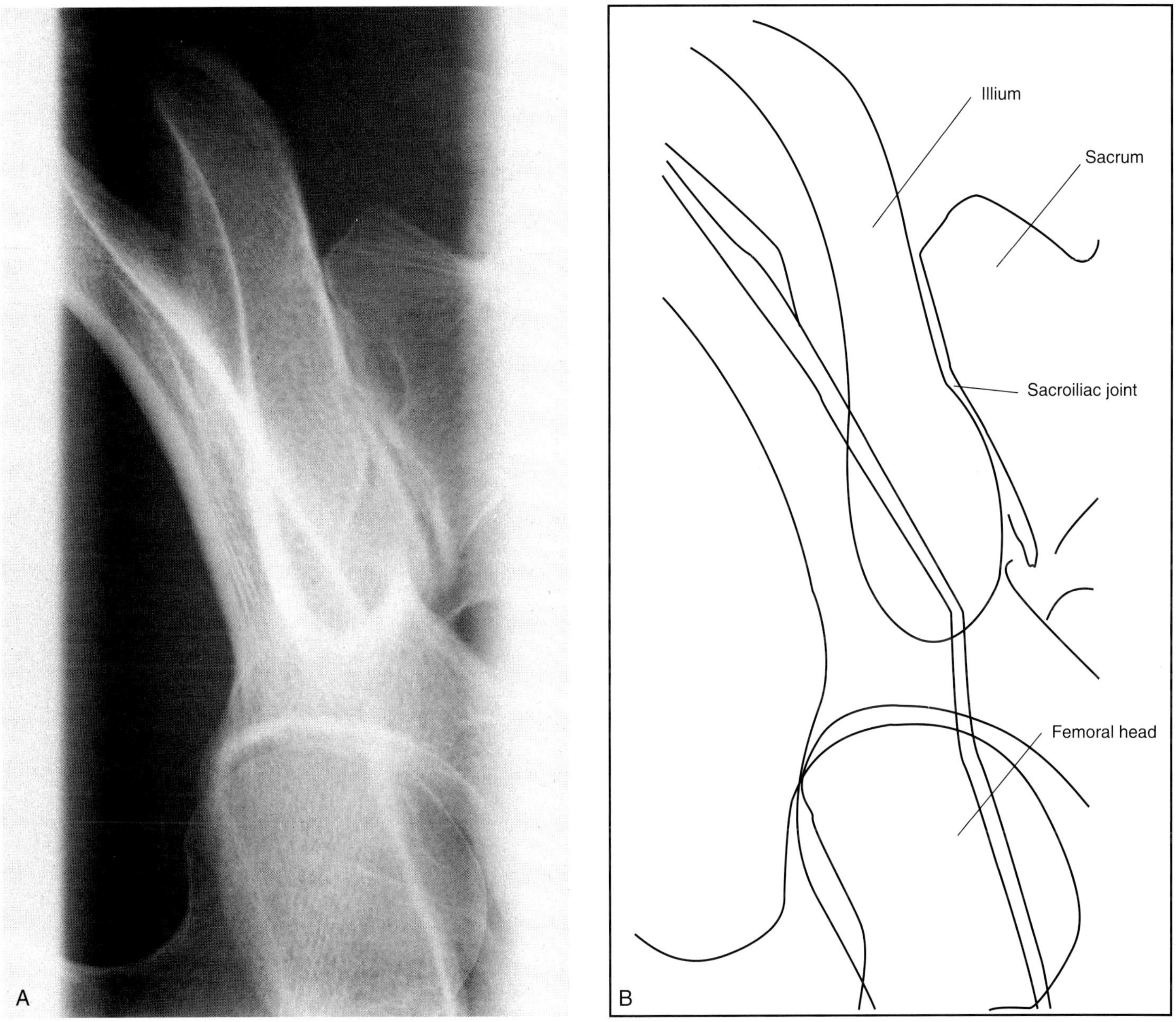

Figure 13.62. A and B, PA oblique projection of sacroiliac joints.

Sacroiliac Joints

Position/Projection

Axial projection—Nolke's method

Film Size:
8 × 10 inches (20 × 24 cm)
or
10 × 12 inches (24 × 30 cm) crosswise

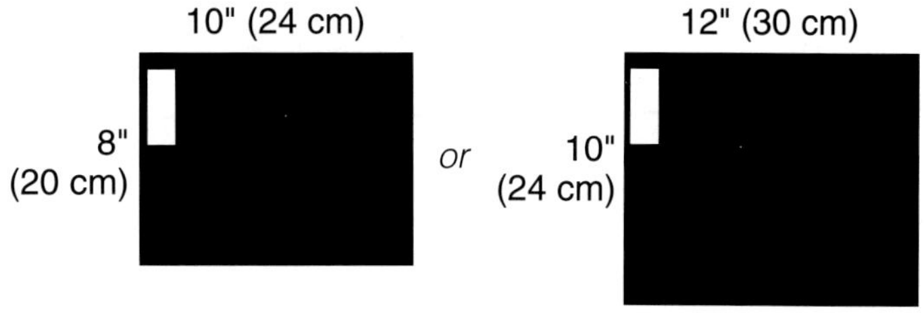

Patient Position

Seated on side table. Patient flexed varying degrees, depending on curvature of sacrum, for several regions of canal but far enough back to center midaxillary line of body to transverse axis of Bucky tray. Feet should be supported on stool or chair (Fig. 13.63).

Part Position

Midsagittal plane perpendicular to midline of table. Patient should lean forward enough to place either upper, middle, or lower segment of sacral vertebral canal vertical to table. Patient will need to hold on to legs or ankles or sides of table in order to stay in this position.

Central Ray

Perpendicular to vertical sacrum.

Breathing Instructions

Respiration suspended at end of full exhalation.

Structures Demonstrated

If patient is in acute flexion, upper sacral vertebral canal will be projected into angle that is formed by rami of ischial bones. If patient is in moderate flexion, sacroiliac joints will be demonstrated and cross-section of lower and upper sacral vertebral canal will be shown. If patient is in slight flexion, last lumbar vertebra and junction of sacrum and coccyx will be demonstrated (Fig. 13.64).

Evaluation Criteria

1. Sacral canal should be in center of radiograph.
2. There should be no lateral rotation.

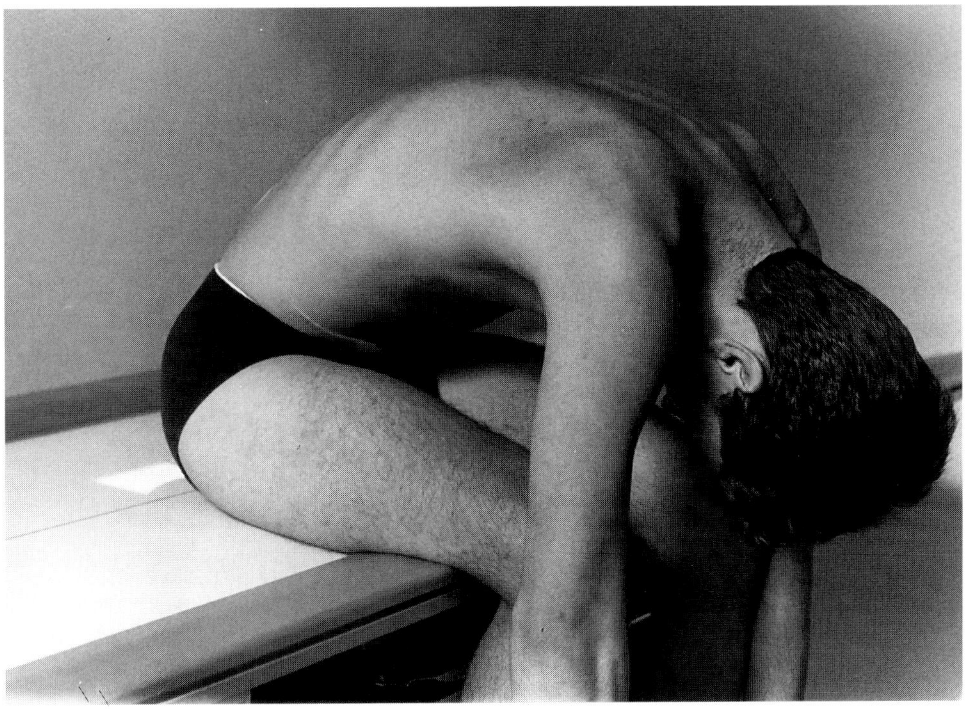

Figure 13.63. Nolke's position for axial projection of sacroiliac joints.

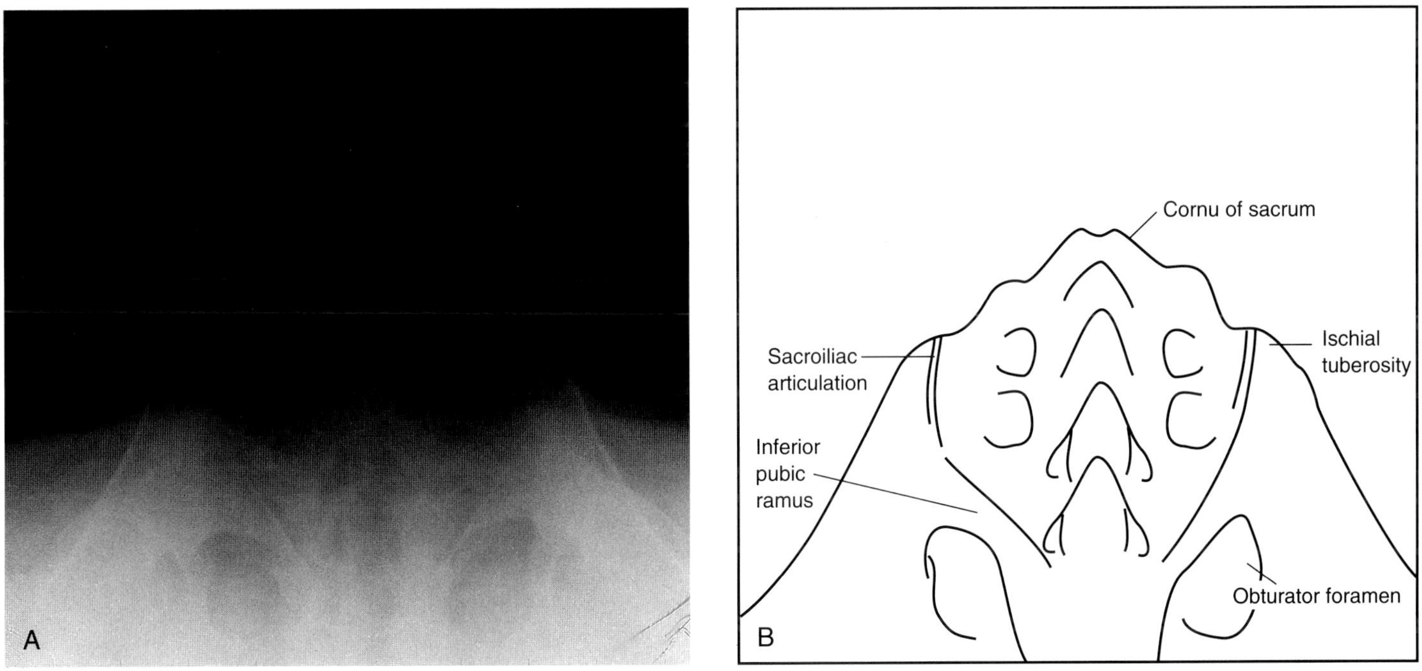

Figure 13.64. A and B, Nolke's projection of sacroiliac joints.

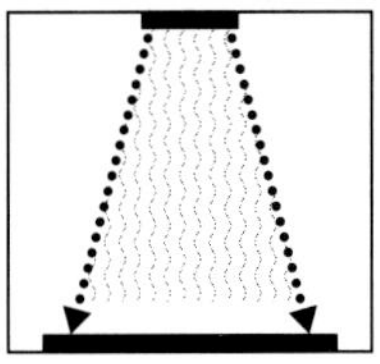

Sacrum

Position/Projection

Lateral

Film Size:
10 × 12 inches (24 × 30 cm) lengthwise

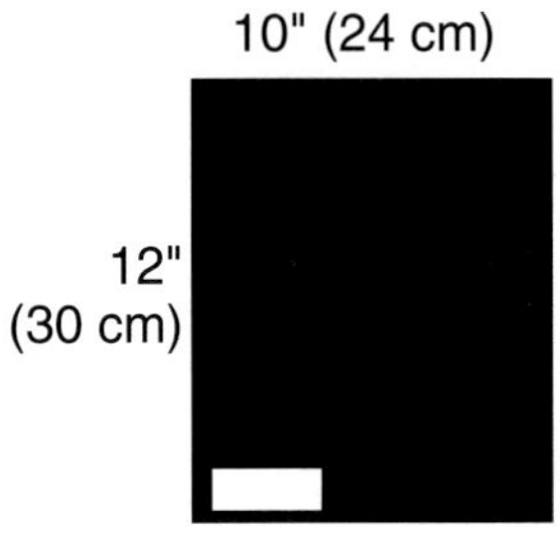

Patient Position
Lateral position. Flex hips and knees (Fig. 13.65).

Part Position
Align body so that coronal plane passing 3 inches (7.6 cm) posterior to midaxillary line is centered to midline of table. Center film at level of ASIS.

Central Ray
Perpendicular to midpoint of film.

Breathing Instructions
Respiration suspended at end of full exhalation.

Structures Demonstrated
Lateral aspect of sacrum (Fig. 13.66).

Evaluation Criteria
1. Sacrum in its entirety.
2. Short-scale of contrast is preferred.

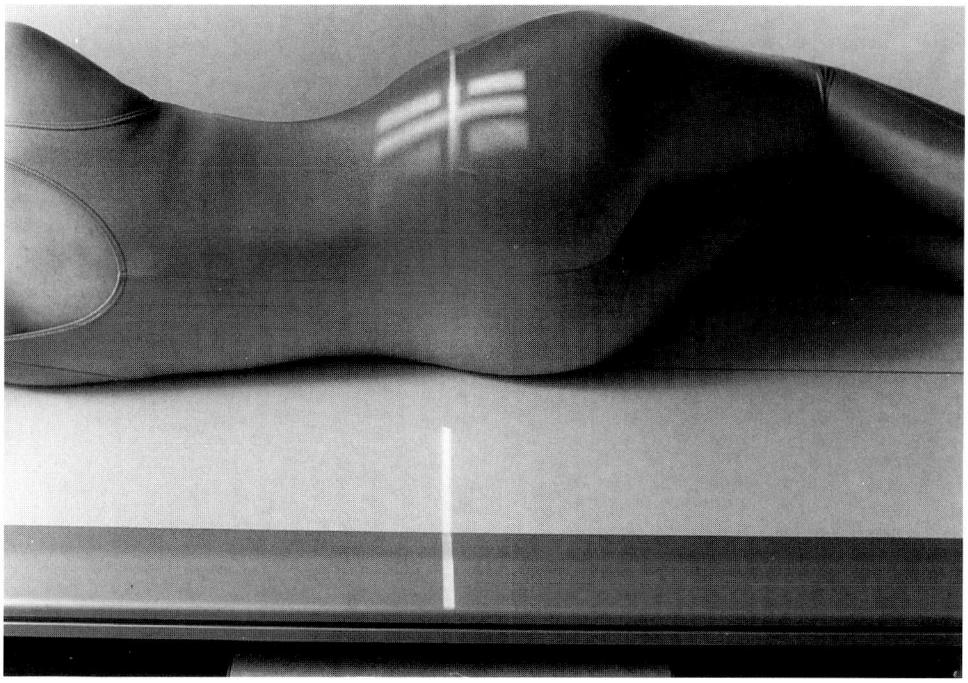

Figure 13.65. Lateral position for sacrum.

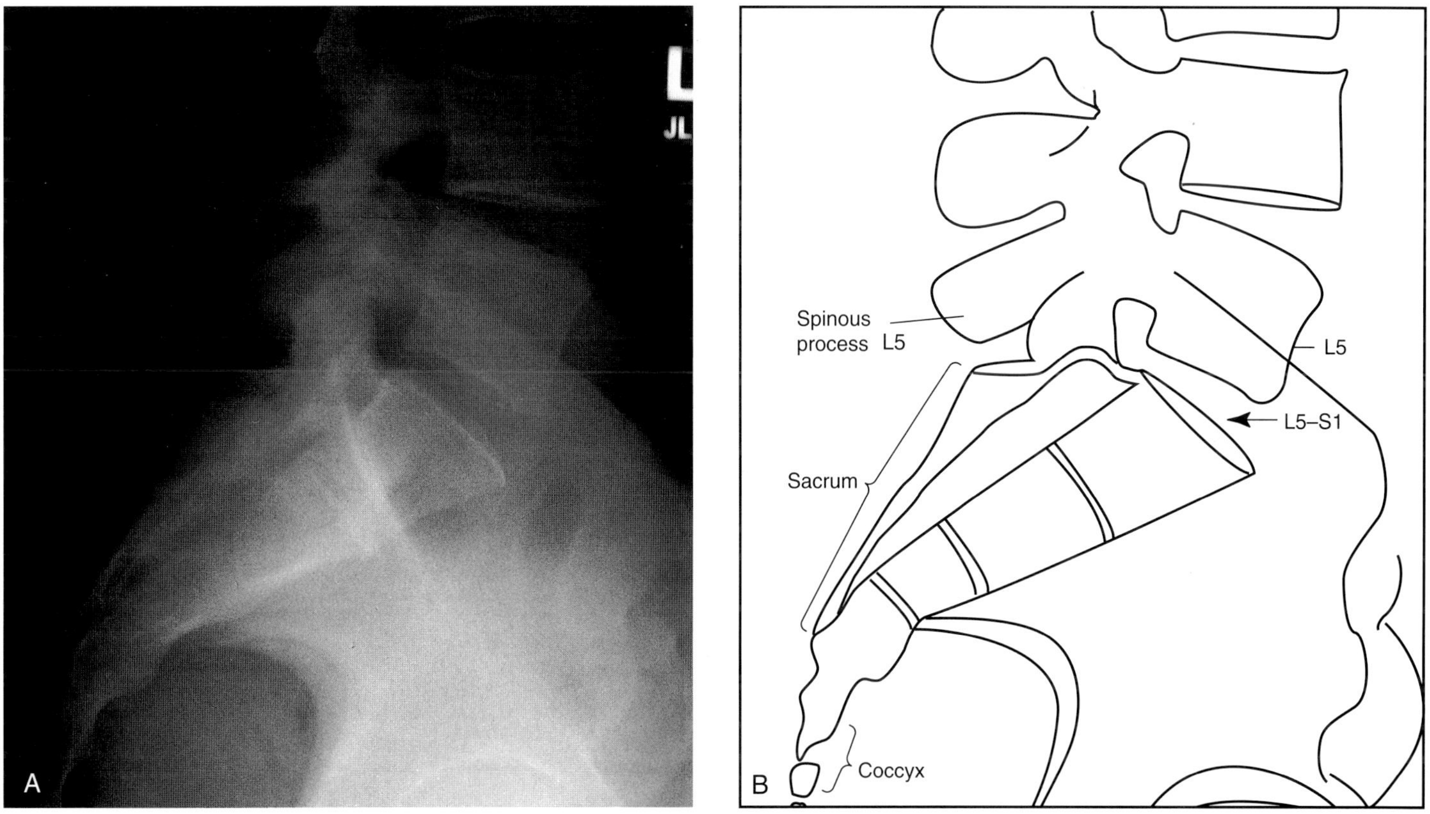

Figure 13.66. A and B, Lateral projection of sacrum.

Coccyx

Position/Projection

AP and PA

Film Size:
8 × 10 inches (20 × 24 cm)
lengthwise

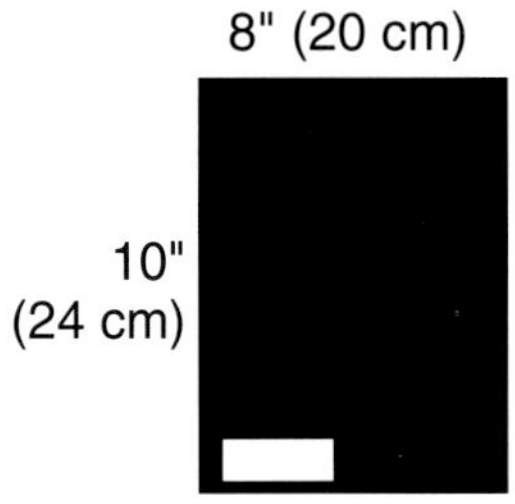

Patient Position

Prone or supine position. Midsagittal plane centered to midline of table (Fig. 13.67).

Part Position

Center central ray about 2 inches (5 cm) superior to pubic symphysis.

Central Ray

Midpoint of film at angle of 10° caudad if patient is supine, or 10° cephalad if patient is prone.

Breathing Instructions

Respiration suspended at end of full exhalation.

Structures Demonstrated

True frontal projection of coccyx (Fig. 13.68).

Evaluation Criteria

1. Coccyx centered in radiograph without rotation.
2. No superimposition of coccygeal segments.
3. Close collimation and short-scale contrast are preferred.

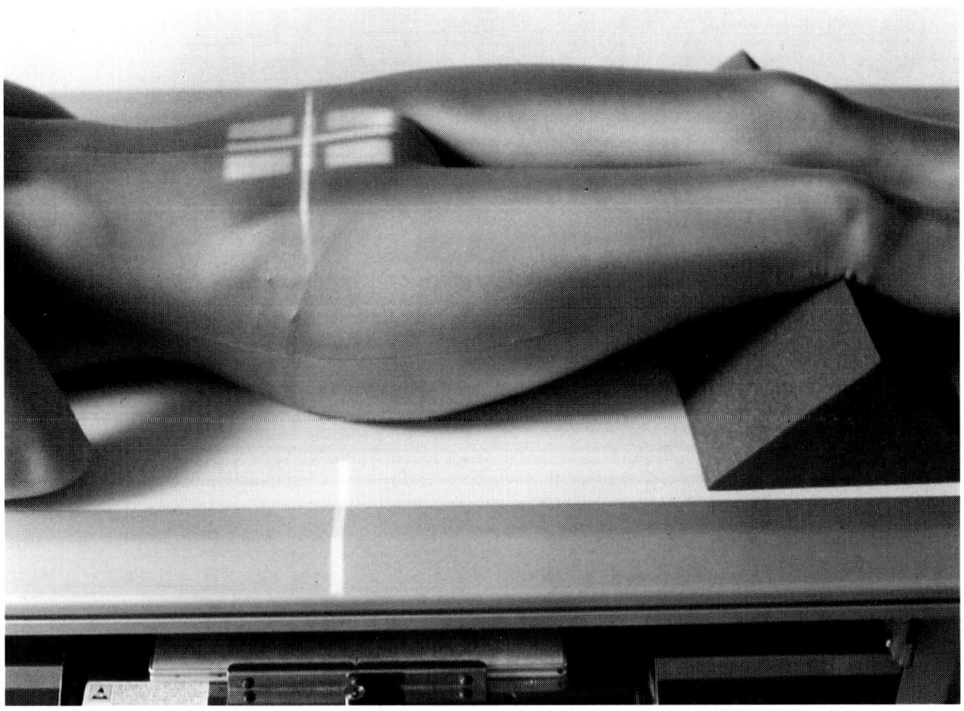

Figure 13.67. AP position for coccyx.

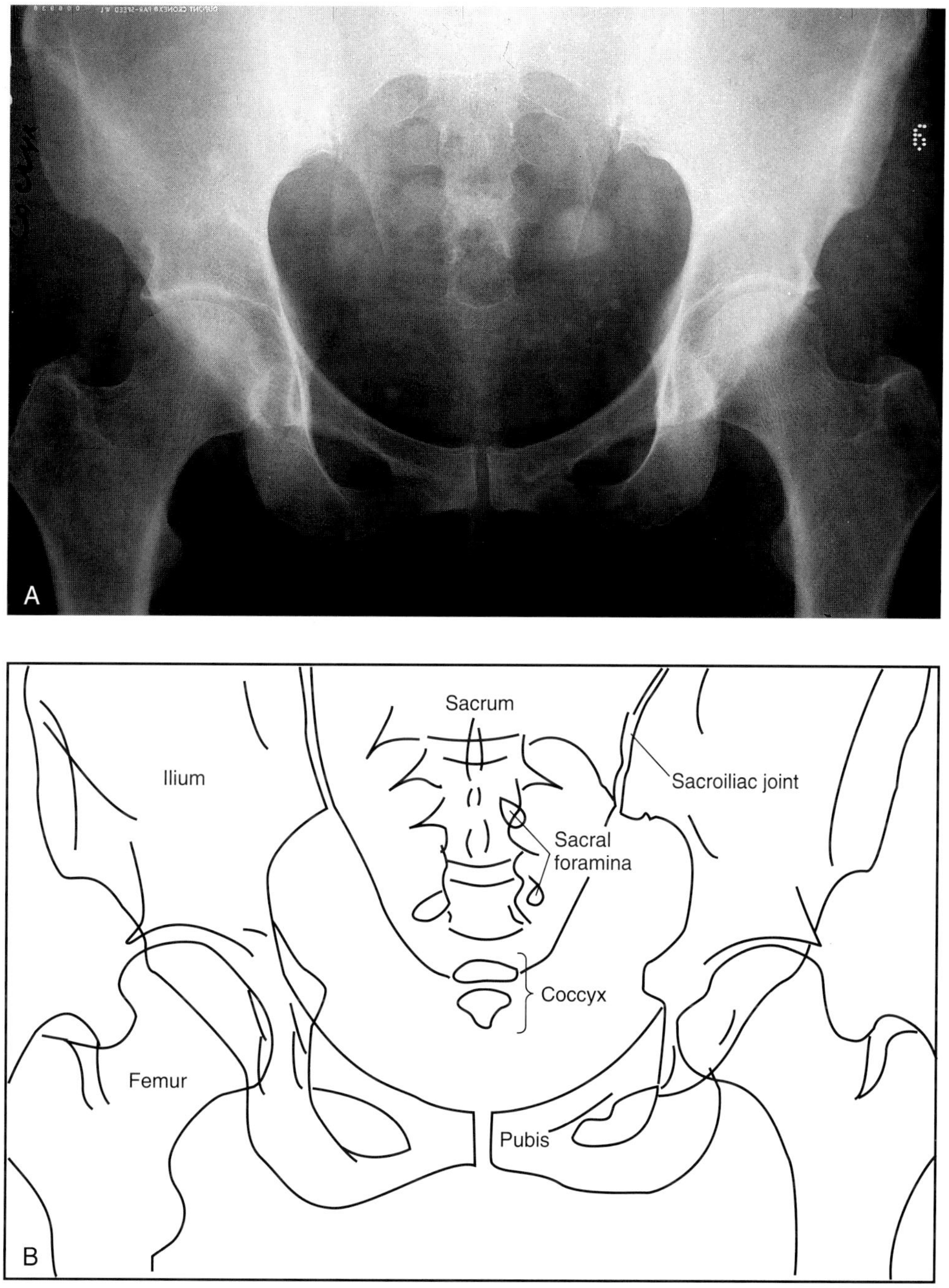

Figure 13.68. A and B, AP projection of coccyx.

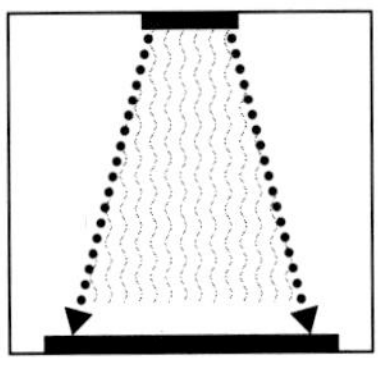

Coccyx

Position/Projection

Lateral

Film Size:
8 × 10 inches (20 × 24 cm)
lengthwise

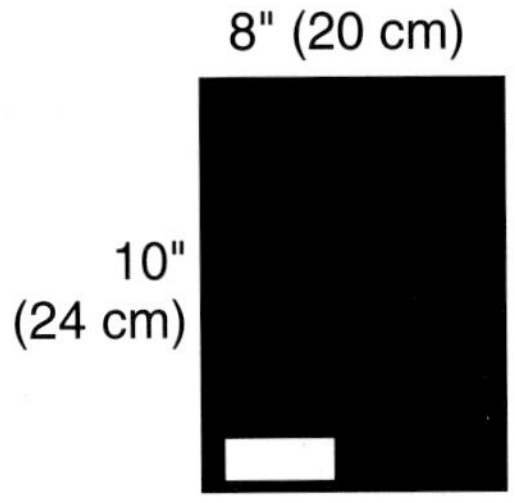

Patient Position
Lateral position. Flex hips and knees (Fig. 13.69).

Part Position
Align body so that coronal plane passing 5 inches (13 cm) posterior to midaxillary line is centered to midline of table. Center film at level of coccyx.

Central Ray
Perpendicular to midpoint of film.

Breathing Instructions
Respiration suspended at end of full exhalation.

Structures Demonstrated
Lateral aspect of coccyx (Fig. 13.70).

Evaluation Criteria
Visibility of entire coccyx with short-scale contrast.

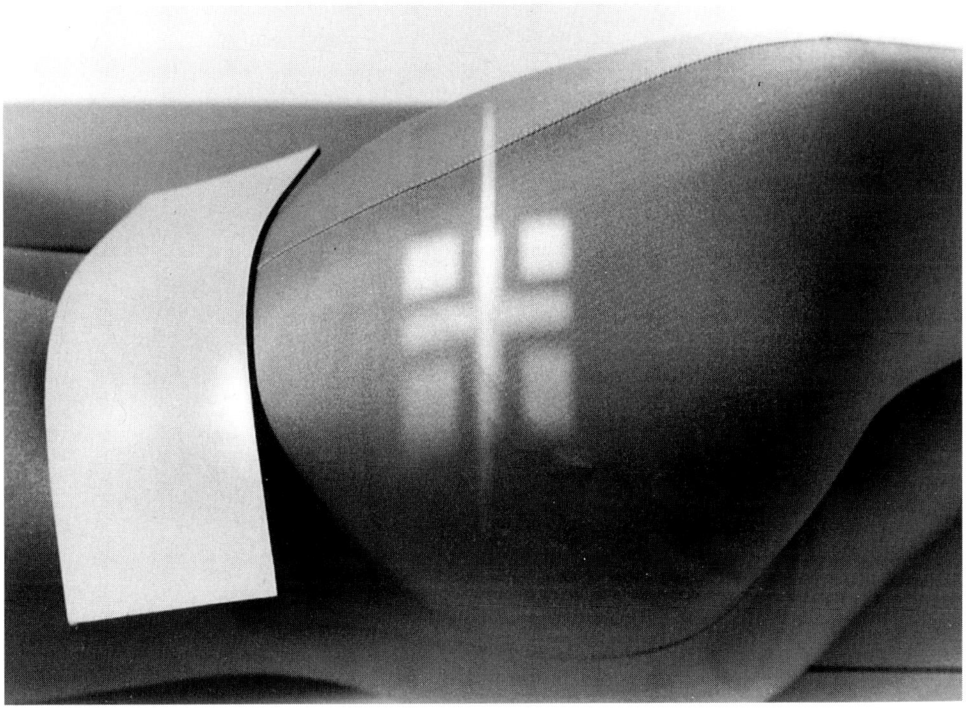

Figure 13.69. Lateral position for coccyx.

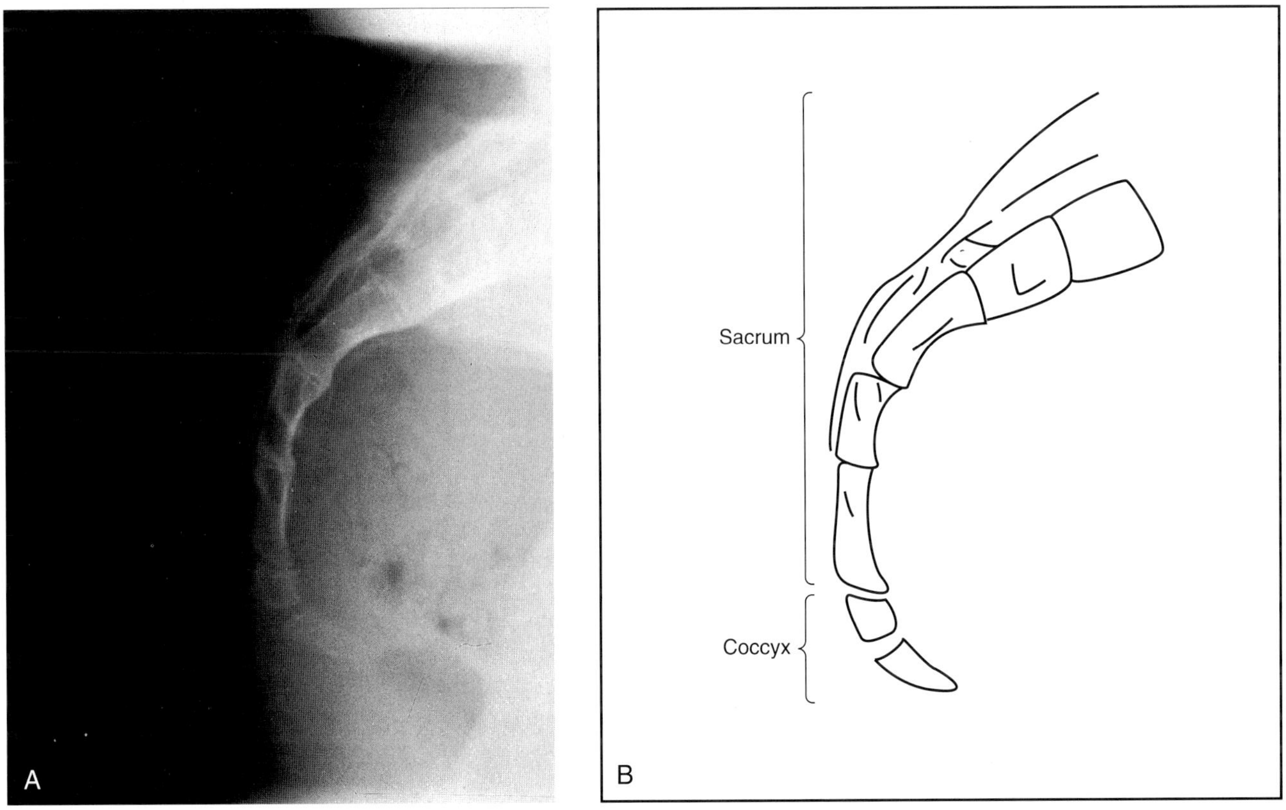

Figure 13.70. A and B, Lateral projection of coccyx.

Scoliosis Series

Position/Projection

Ferguson's method

Film Size:
14 × 17 inches (35 × 43 cm) (each exposure)

or

14 × 52 inches (35 × 132 cm) lengthwise, for entire spine, when available

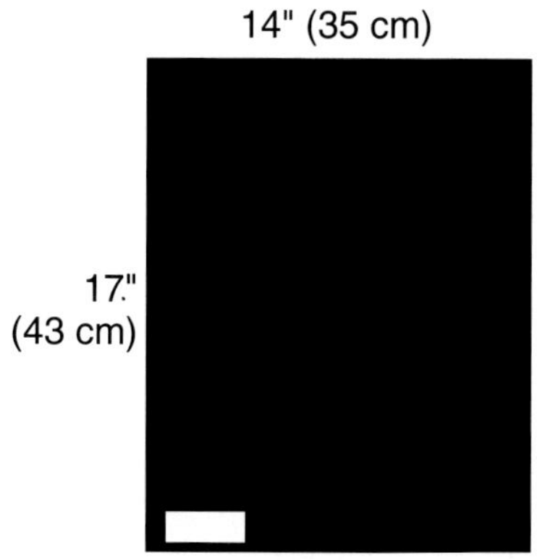

Patient Position

AP or PA, seated or standing before vertical grid device (Fig. 13.71).

Part Position

Midsagittal plane centered to midline of vertical grid for first radiograph. Second radiograph should be made by elevating hip or foot of convex side of the curve 3 to 4 inches (7.6 to 10 cm). Correct amount of elevation will cause patient to have problem maintaining position.

Central Ray

Perpendicular to midpoint of cassette. Place bottom of cassette 1 inch (2.5 cm) below iliac crest.

Breathing Instructions

Suspend respiration at end of full exhalation.

Structures Demonstrated

AP projections of thoracic and lumbar vertebrae. Procedure is used to compare deforming or primary curve with compensatory curve in scoliosis patients (Fig. 13.72).

Evaluation Criteria

1. Vertebral column should be in center of radiograph.
2. Entire thoracic and lumbar vertebrae including 1 inch (2.5 cm) of iliac crests should be demonstrated.

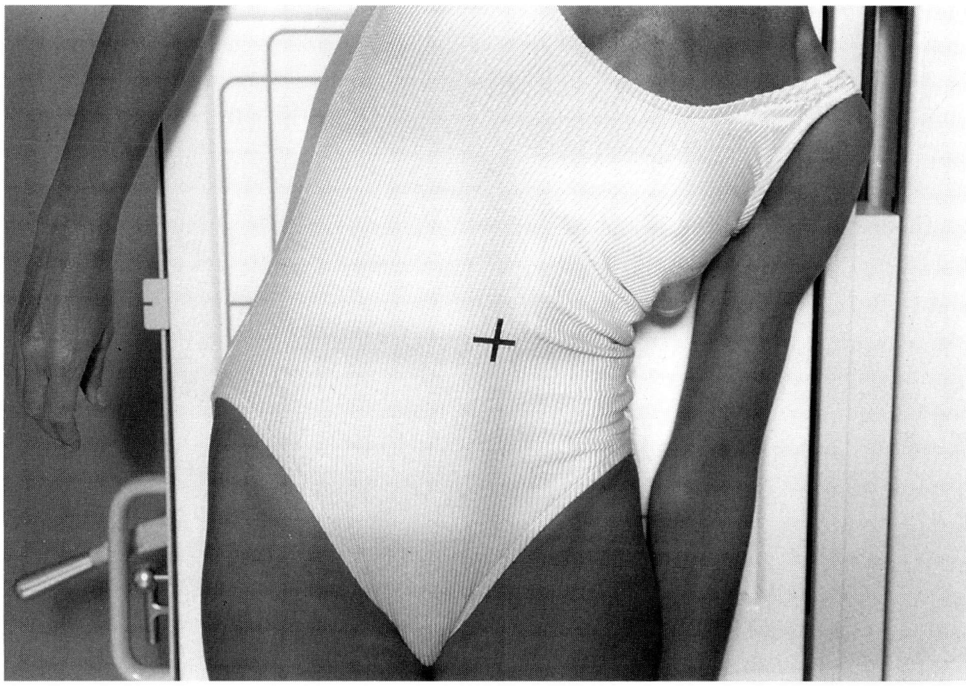

Figure 13.71. Ferguson's method for demonstration of scoliosis.

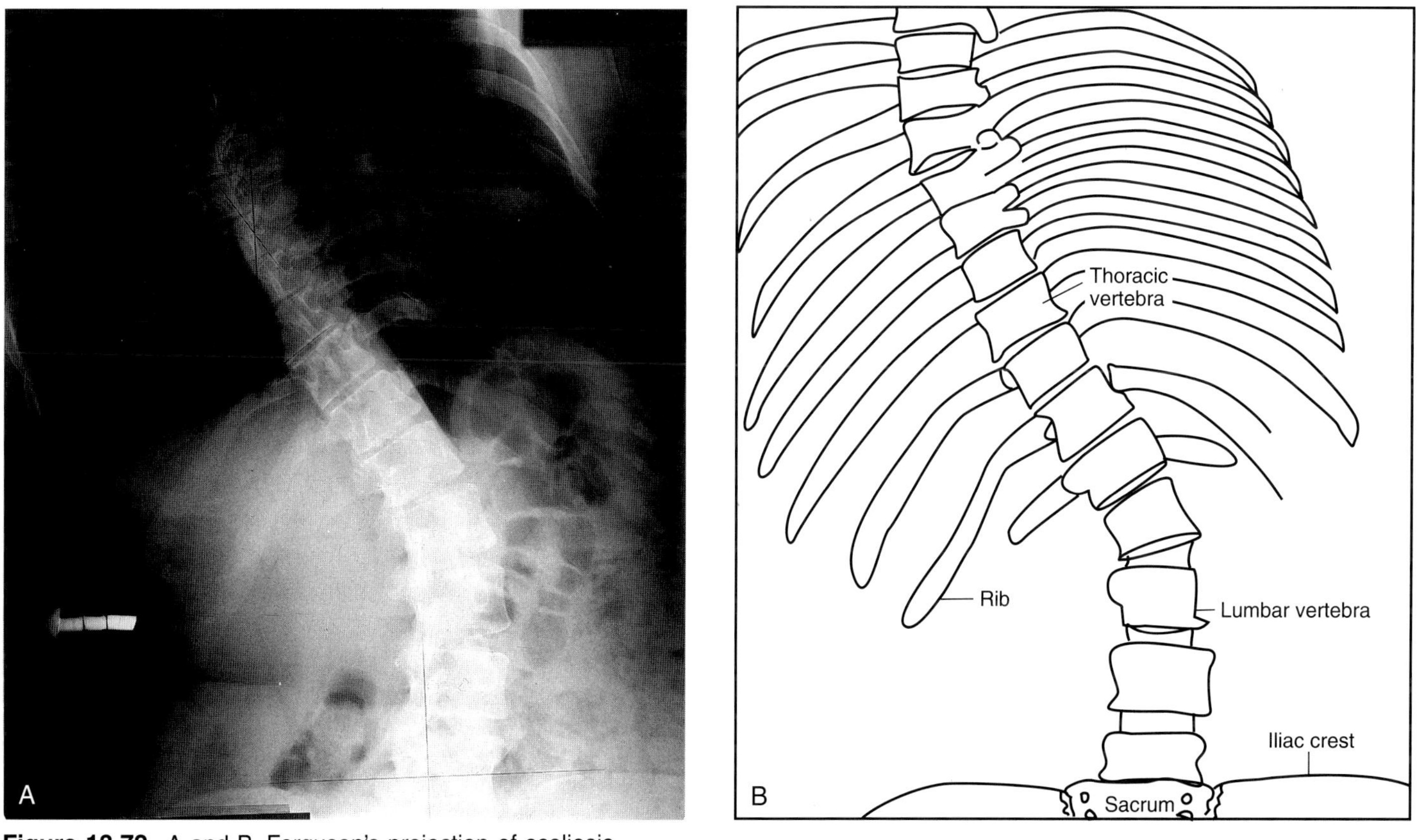

Figure 13.72. A and B, Ferguson's projection of scoliosis.

Bibliography

Ballinger PW: Merrill's Atlas of Radiographic Positions and Radiologic Procedures. 7th ed. St. Louis: CV Mosby, 1991.

Heriard JB, Terry JA, Arnold AL: Achieving dose reduction in lumbar spine radiography. Radiol Technol 1993; 65:97–103.

Meschan I: An Atlas of Anatomy Basic to Radiology. Philadelphia: WB Saunders, 1975.

GLOSSARY*

Steven B. Dowd, EdD., R.T.(R.)

A

Abduct. The opposite of adduct; to draw away from the median plane or (in the digits) from the axial line of a limb.

Abscess. A localized collection of pus.

Absorb. 1. The act of taking in or assimilating substances into or across tissues. 2. To react with radiation to cause attenuation of the beam.

Acanthion. A point located at the base of the anterior nasal spine.

Acanthomeatal line. An imaginary line extending from external auditory (acoustic) meatus to acanthion.

Accessory. Anatomically, a structure or structures that serve another main system.

Acoustic. Referring or pertaining to sound.

Acromegaly. A chronic disease caused by hypersecretion of the pituitary growth hormone and characterized by enlargement and elongation of nose, ears, jaws, fingers, and toes.

Acute. Having a sudden, sharp, short, and relatively severe onset and course. Opposite of chronic.

Addison's planes. A series of planes used as landmarks in the location of organs and viscera within the thorax and abdomen.

Adduct. The opposite of abduct; to draw toward the median plane or (in the digits) toward the axial line of a limb.

Adhesion. 1. The holding together of structures that are normally separated by new tissue that has been produced by injury or inflammation.

Adnexa. Accessory parts or appendages.

AIDS (acquired immunodeficiency syndrome). A disease caused by a virus that is the manifestation of an immunosuppresive disease that allows life-threatening infections.

Air gap. The use of increased OFD (OID) to remove scatter radiation when it arises close to the film.

Ala. A winglike structure, process, or appendage.

Alveolus. A small hollow or cavity; a small saclike dilatation.

Amphiarthrosis. A form of articulation of bony surfaces connected by elastic cartiloginous substance that permits little motion. Mobility can be exerted in all directions.

Amplitude. Largeness or fullness; extend.

Ampulla. A flasklike dilatation of a tubular structure or saclike dilatation of a duct or canal.

Anal. Pertaining to the anus or outer rectal opening.

Analgesia. 1. Relieving pain 2. Absence of normal sense of pain.

Anatomic position. The position of the human body, standing erect, with the palms of the hands turned forward.

Aneurysm. Abnormal dilatation of a blood vessel wall of an artery, a vein, or the heart.

Angiography. The visualization of blood vessels by roentgen rays following the introduction of contrast material.

Angioma. A tumor, usually benign, whose cells consist mostly of blood vessels (hemangioma) or lymph vessels (lymphangioma).

Ankylosis. Fusion and consolidation of a joint.

Anode. The positive electrode in the x-ray tube. Electrons from the filament are accelerated onto the target area of the anode to produce x-rays.

Anomaly. Marked deviation from the normal standard, usually congenital in nature.

Anterior. The opposite of posterior; pertains to in front of or in the forward part of an organ; used in reference to the ventral or belly surface of the body.

Anteroposterior (AP). From front to back of the body; in radiography, it denotes such direction of the beam.

Anthropologic baseline. An imaginary line passing from the lowest point of the inferior margin of the orbit to the center of the superior margin of external auditory meatus. Also known as Frankfurt horizontal plane, German horizontal plane, and Reid's baseline.

Antiseptic. A substance that inhibits the growth and development of infectious agents (microorganisms) without necessarily killing them.

Antrum. Any enclosed cavity or chamber; used as a general term in anatomic nomenclature, especially within a bone.

Aperture. Any opening or orifice.

Apex. A general anatomic term used to designate the top of a body, organ, or part, or the pointed extermity of a conical structure; called also tip.

Apnea. Absence or cessation of breathing.

Apophysial, apophyseal. Pertaining to or of the nature of an outgrowth or bony process that lacks a center of ossification.

Apophysis. A bony outgrowth that has never entirely separated from the bone of which it is a part, such as a process, tubercle, or tuberosity.

Apposition. The placing of things in contact with one another, especially the deposition of successive layers on those already present, as in cell walls. Called also juxtaposition.

Areola. The area surrounding the nipple of the breast.

Arteriography. Radiography of arteries after injection of radiopaque material into the bloodstream.

Artifact. Anything other than patient anatomy that was not meant to be imaged on the radiograph.

Arthrography. Radiography of the joint following instillation of contrast.

Ascites. An abnormal accumulation of serous fluid in the abdominal cavity; usually intraperitoneal in location.

Asepsis. Free from infection; the prevention or destruction of microorganisms.

Aseptic. Free from infection; sterile.

Aspiration. The process of inhaling; the removal of fluid or gases from a cavity using a suction device.

Assimilation. The transformation of food into living tissue; anabolism. It is the final stage of the nutrition process.

Asthenic. In radiography, the body habitus characterized by extremely slender build. It represents approximately 10 percent of all persons.

Atelectasis. Inadequate expansion of a lung or a portion of a lung, occurring congenitally as a primary or secondary condition or as an acquired condition. Due to resorption or expansion failure.

Atresia. Congenital absence or closure of a normal body orifice, duct, or canal; as esophageal and pulmonary atria.

Atrophy. The wasting away, or diminution in the size of a cell, tissue, organ, or part.

Auricle. That portion of the external ear not contained within the head; the pinna, or flap, of the ear.

Auricular line. An imaginary line passing through external auditory meatus; perpendicular to Frankfurt horizontal plane.

Auricular point. The center of the external auditory meatus.

Axial. The area below the shoulder joint that is bounded by the pectoralis major, the latissimus dorsi, and the humerus; the armpit.

Axis. A line about which a revolving body turns or structure would turn if it revolved.

Azygos. Singular; any unpaired part.

B

Barium. In radiography, barium sulfate (barium alone is poisonous), a nontoxic compound used as contrast.

*Some definitions taken or modified from **Dorland's Illustrated Medical Dictionary.** 28th ed. Philadelphia: WB Saunders, 1994.

Bifurcation. The site where a structure divides into branches.
Bilateral. Having two sides; pertaining to both sides.
Body mass index (BMI). A means of body habitus determination determined by dividing the body weight by the square of the stature (height).
Body-section radiography. Synonym for tomography.
Body substance precautions. Also called body fluid precautions or universal precautions (in which all patients are seen as potentially infectious); views all body substances as potentially infectious.
Bolus. A concentrated mass.
Brachial. Pertaining to the arm.
Brachiocubital. Relating to the arm and elbow or forearm.
Brachycephalic. Pertaining to having a comparatively short head with a cranial index greater than 81.
Bregma. The point on the surface of the skull at the junction of the coronal and sagittal sutures.
Bronchography. Radiography of the lung after the instillation of opaque medium in a bronchus.
Buccal. Pertaining to or directed toward the cheek.
Bucky (Bucky diaphragm, Potter-Bucky diaphragm). A grid device used in radiography that moves during the exposure to eliminate grid lines from the radiograph.
Bursa. A sac or saclike cavity filled with a viscid fluid and situated between certain tendons and the underlying bones.

C

C/kg. Coulomb per kilogram; the SI unit used to measure radiation exposure in air.
Calcification. Process whereby organic tissue becomes hardened by the deposit of calcium salts within its substance.
Calculus. Abnormal concentration, usually composed of mineral salts occurring within the animal body.
Cannula. A tube used for insertion into a duct or cavity.
Canthus. The angle of the tissue between the eyelids.
Cardioangiography. Radiography of the heart vessel.
Cassette. A light-proof container for x-ray film; contains intensifying screens.
Cathartic. To cause evacuation of the bowels.
Cathode. The negative electrode in the x-ray tube.
Cauda. A tail or tail-like appendage.
Caudad. Toward the tail.
Celiac, coeliac. Relating to the abdomen.
Centigrade. Having 100 gradations (steps or degrees); abbreviated C.
Cephalad. Toward the head.
Cephalic. Relating to the head or to the head end of the body.
Cervical. Pertaining to the neck or to the neck of any organ or structure.
Cervix. A term denoting the front portion of the collum, or neck (the part connecting the head and the trunk), or a constricted part of an organ. That portion of the uterus that protrudes into the vagina in females.
Cholangitis. Inflammation of a bile duct.
Cholangiography. Radiography of the biliary ducts after administration or injection of a contrast medium orally, intravenously, or percutaneously.
Cholecystitis. Inflammation of the gallbladder; may be acute or chronic.
Cholecystography. Radiography of the gallbladder.
Choledochogram. A radiograph of the common bile duct.
Choledochography. Radiography of the common bile duct after the administration of opaque material.
Cholegraphy. Radiographic examination of the common bile duct.
Cholelithiasis. The presence or formation of gallstones within the gallbladder.
Cholesteatoma. A cystlike mass made up of epithelial cells and cholesterol.
Chorion. In human embryology, the outermost extraembryonic membrane; composed of trophoblast lined with mesoderm, it develops villi about 2 weeks after fertilization, gives rise to the placenta, and persists until birth.
Chronic. A condition or disorder that develops slowly and persists over a long period of time.
Cleido-, cleid-. Combining form denoting relationship to the clavicle.
Clysis. The washing out of a body cavity. The infusion of fluid with therapeutic intent.
Coagulation. The process of clot formation.
Coalescence. The fusing or blending of parts.
Cohesion. The force that causes various particles to unite; the attraction between molecules that binds them.
Collateral. Secondary or accessory; indirect.
Collimation (beam restriction). Limiting the size of the beam in radiography.
Collimator. A box attached to the x-ray tube capable of limiting the beam to a specific area of the body.
Comminuted. Broken or crushed into small pieces, as a comminuted fracture of a bone.
Compensating filter. A metallic device used to adjust for variations in part thickness.
Compound fracture. An open fracture.
Concentric. Having a common center; extending out equally in all directions from a common center. Usually refers to circles or spheres.
Condyle. A rounded projection on a bone at the extremity (end) of a bone.
Congenital. Existing at and usually before birth.
Contrast. Differences in density on a radiograph.
Coracoid. Shaped like a raven's beak.
Coronal. Frontal.
Coronoid. Shaped like a crow's beak.
Crater. Circular area of a depression surrounded by an elevated margin.
Crepitation. Noise made by rubbing together the ends of a fractured bone.
Curie. The SI unit used to measure radioactivity; abbreviated Ci.
Cystography. Radiography of the bladder after injection of the organ with opaque solution.
Cystoscopy. Visual examination of the urinary tract with a cystoscope.

D

Decubitus. The position assumed when lying down. In positioning terminology, the central ray is horizontal.
Definition. Clarity and sharpness of the image.
Deglutition. Swallowing.
Dens. In radiography, another term used for odontoid process of C2.
Densitometry. Process of measuring density (the amount of blackness on a film).
Density. Blackness on a radiograph.
Development. In radiography, the conversion of a latent image into black, metallic silver.
Dextrosinistral. Extending from right to left; also applied to a person naturally left-handed but trained to use the right hand to accomplish certain tasks.
Diagnosis. The art of distinguishing one disease from another.
Diaphysis. That portion of a long bone formed from a primary center of ossification.
Diarrhea. Abnormal, frequent and liquid fecal discharges.
Diarthrosis. An articulation permitting more or less free movement; a synovial joint.
Diastole. The dilatation or period of dilatation of the heart, especially of the ventricles; period during which the cavities of the heart fill with blood. In blood pressure measurement, the second or bottom reading.
Diploe. The central layer of loose osseous tissue between the two tables of the cranial bone.
Distal. Remote; farther from any point of reference; opposite of proximal.
Distortion. In radiography, a misrepresentation of the size and shape of the object in the image.
Dolichocephalic. Long-headed; having a cephalic index of 75.9 or less.
Dorsal. Pertaining to the back or posterior surface.
Dorsal decubitus. The patient is supine; the horizontal beam enters on one side of the patient (left or right) and exits on another.

Dose equivalent limits. Used to set limits on occupational exposure.

E

Ectomorph. A body type in which tissues derived from the ectoderm predominate. A person with this body type has a propensity to linearity and fragility and has a large surface area, thin muscles and subcutaneous tissue, and slightly developed digestive viscera; the limbs predominate over the trunk.
Ectopic. Pertaining to outside the normal place; not in proper position.
Emulsion. In radiographic film, the active layer.
Endomorph. A body type in which tissues derived from the endoderm predominate. This type of person has a relative preponderance of soft roundedness, throughout the body, with large digestive viscera and accumulations of fat, large trunk and thighs, and tapering extremities. The trunk predominates over the limbs.
Endoscopy. Visual inspection of any cavity of the body by means of an instrument called an endoscope.
Endosteal. Pertaining to the endosteum; occurring or located within a bone.
Enema. A clyster or injection; a liquid injected into the rectum to evacuate the bowel.
Epicondyle. A small bony protrusion near a joint, usually above a condyle.
Epigastric region. One of three upper regions of the abdomen.
Epiphysis. The expanded articular end of a long bone.
ERCP. Endoscopic retrograph cholangiopancreatography.
Erythema. A name applied to abnormal redness of the skin that may result from a variety of causes, including radiation exposure.
Eversion. A turning inside out; a turning outward, as of the foot or eyelid.
Evert. To turn inside out; to turn outward; to overturn.
Exostosis. A benign bony growth projecting outward from the surface of a bone, characteristically capped by cartilage.
Exposure latitude. The range of exposures that may be used to obtain a radiograph demonstrating acceptable visibility of image detail.
Extension. A movement that brings the members of a limb into or toward a straight relation. The stretching out of the arm, for example.

F

Facet. A small, flat surface on a bone.
Fetography. Radiography of the fetus in utero.
Fibroma. A tumor composed mainly of fibrous or fully developed connective tissue; usually benign.
Film-screen contact. The closeness of film and screen; as contact between film and screen becomes closer, image sharpness increases.
Fissure. Any cleft or groove, normal or otherwise, especially a deep fold in the cerebral cortex that involves the entire thickness of the brain wall; sulcus.
Fistula. An abnormal passage or communication, between two internal organs or from an internal organ to the surface of the body.
Fistulography. Radiography of a fistula.
Fixation. In radiography, the process of making the visible image permanent.
Flexion. The act of bending; the condition of being bent.
Flocculent. Fluid containing downy or flaky masses.
Fluorescence. A luminescent property demonstrated by some materials when irradiated.
Fluoroscopy. Dynamic radiography; examination by means of a fluoroscope.
Focal-film distance (FFD). The distance from the anode of the x-ray tube to the film; synonymous terms are target-film distance (TFD) and source-to–image receptor distance (SID or SIRD).
Focal-object distance. The distance from the anode of the x-ray tube to the object to be radiographed.
Focal plane. The plane of tissue having maximum focus on a tomogram.
Focal spot. The area of the anode from which x-rays emanate.
Fontanel. A soft spot, such as one of the membrane-covered spaces remaining in the incompletely ossified skull of fetus or infant.
Foramen. A perforation or opening, especially into or through a bone.
Fossa. A general term for a hollow or depressed area.
Fovea. A general term for a small depression in the surface of a structure or organ.
Fowler's position. The position in which the head of a patient's bed is raised 18 to 29 inches (46 to 51 cm) above level; the knees are also elevated.
Frankfurt plane or line. See Anthropologic baseline.
Frenulum. A term for a small fold of integument or mucuous membrane that checks, curbs, or limits the movements of an organ or part. Example: linguae of the tongue.
Fulcrum. The point of support around which a lever turns; used in radiographic tomography.
Fundus. A general term for the bottom or base of an organ or the part of a hollow organ farthest from the opening or exit.
Furuncle. A painful nodule formed in the skin by circumscribed inflammation of the corium and subcutaneous tissue, enclosing a central slough or "core"; originates in a hair follicle.

G

Gall. Bile.
Gavage. Forced feeding, especially through a tube passed into the stomach.
Geometric unsharpness. Unsharpness on the radiograph due to geometric image factors (e.g., FFD, OFD, focal-spot size).
German horizontal plane. See Anthropologic baseline.
Germicide. An agent that kills pathogenic germs and microbes.
Glabella. The smooth area on the frontal bone between the supraciliary arches; above the root of the nose. The most prominent point in the midsagittal plane between the eyebrows; used as an anthropometric landmark.
Glabelloalveolar line. An imaginary line extending from glabella to upper alveolus.
Glabellomeatal line. An imaginary line extending from glabella to external auditory meatus.
Glenoid. The pit or socket of a joint.
Glossa. Tongue (lingua).
Gonads. The organs of reproduction.
Gonion. An anthropometric landmark located at the most inferior, posterior, and outward point on the external angle of the mandible.
Gray. A radiation unit (SI) used to measure absorbed dose; abbreviated Gy.
Grid. An arrangement of thin lead strips separated by a radiolucent material; used to reduce the amount of scattered radiation reaching the film.
Groin. The junctional region between the abdomen and the thigh; inguinal region.
Groove. A shallow linear depression on any surface; called also tissue and sulcus.

H

H and D curve. Hurter and Driffield curve; called also D-log E curve and characteristic curve. A plot of a series of known exposures against resulting densities; used to investigate speed, contrast, and fog exhibited on a radiograph.
Habitus. Physical characteristics of a person; in radiography, hypersthenic, hyposthenic, sthenic and asthenic.
Haustrum, haustra. A general term denoting a recess or pouch.
Hepatitis. Inflammation of the liver; hepatitis B is a contagious disease and health care workers are from 5 to 15 times more prone to contract hepatitis B owing to occupational exposure.
Herniography. The radiographic demonstration of a hernia.
Heterogeneous. Consisting of or composed of dissimilar elements or ingredients not having a uniform quality throughout; dissimilar.
Hiatus. A general term for a gap, cleft, opening, or foramen.
High (short-scale contrast). Few shades of gray (mostly blacks and whites) represented on a radiograph; gives a narrow exposure latitude; associated with low kVp.

Hilum. A general term for a depression or saclike opening at that part of an organ where vessels and nerves enter.

HIV (human immunodeficiency virus). Seen as the causative agent of AIDS.

Homogeneous. Consisting of or composed of similar elements or structure throughout.

Homologous. Corresponding in structure, position, origin, or other quality.

Hypersthenic. Relating to or characterized by hypersthenia (great strength or tonicity).

Hyperthyroid. A condition of excessive unregulated activity of the thyroid gland.

Hypertrophic. Pertaining to or marked by hypertrophy (general decrease in bulk of an organ, etc.).

Hypertrophy. The enlargement of overgrowth of an organ or part owing to increase in size of its constituent cells.

Hypogastric region. One of three lower regions of the abdomen; called also pubic region.

Hyposthenic. Pertaining to or characterized by hyposthenia (an enfeebled state; weak). In radiography, seen as a modification of the asthenic type, with about 35 percent of the population falling into this category.

Hysterosalpingography. Radiography of the uterus and uterine tubes after the injection of contrast.

I

Impacted. Driven firmly in; closely or firmly lodged in position, as an impacted tooth or fecal material in the intestine.

Incident light. The light that is transmitted through the radiographic viewbox; used in a ratio with transmitted light to determine film density.

Inferior. Situated below or directed downward; a term used in reference to the lower surface of an organ or other structure.

Infiltration. A diffusion or accumulation in tissue or cells of substance not normal to it or in amounts in excess of normal.

Infraorbitomeatal line. An imaginary line from the inferior orbital rim to the external auditory meatus.

Inguinal. Pertaining to the groin.

Inion. The most prominent point of the external occipital protuberance of the cranium.

Injection. The act of forcing a liquid into a part, as into the subcutaneous tissues, or an organ.

Instillation. Administration of a liquid drop by drop.

Insufflation. The act of blowing a vapor, gas, or air into a body cavity.

Intensifying screens. Glow with visible light when struck by x-ray; mounted in the radiographic cassette.

Interpupillary line. An imaging line between the pupils.

Interstitial. Pertaining to or situated between parts or interspaces of a tissue.

Inverse square law. States that changes in the intensity of ionizing radiation are inversely proportional to the square of the change in distance; thus, doubling distance reduces the intensity of radiation to one quarter of the original value, and halving distance increases the intensity of radiation fourfold.

Inversion. A turning inward.

Involuntary. Performed independently of the will.

Ipsilateral. Situated on, pertaining to, or affecting the same side; opposite to contralateral.

J

Joint mouse. Small, movable body made of calcium in or near a joint.

Juxtaposition. Apposition.

K

Kilovoltage. The "push" that accelerates electrons from the cathode to the anode of the x-ray tube; controls penetration of the beam; affects contrast of the radiograph.

KUB. Refers to a radiograph of the abdomen to include the kidneys, ureters, and urinary bladder.

kVp. Kilovolts peak; peak kilovoltage of x-ray beam; determines the penetrating ability of the beam.

L

Lacrimography. Radiography of the tear ducts.

Lacuna. A small pit or hollow cavity.

Lambda. A point at the site of the posterior fontanel where the lambdoid and the sagittal sutures meet.

Laminectomy. Excision of the posterior arch of a vertebra.

Laminography. Radiography of the lamina.

Laryngography. Radiography of the larynx after instillation of a radiopaque substance.

Latent image. The invisible image on a radiographic film found before processing but after exposure.

Lateral decubitus. Patient is lying on either side (right or left). When patient is lying on left side (right side is up) this is called a left lateral decubitus. When the patient is lying on right side (left side is up), this is called a right lateral decubitus. The beam enters at either front or back of patient and exits the other side.

Lavage. The irrigation or washing out of an organ.

Laxative. An agent that acts to promote evacuation of the bowel by increasing the volume of the feces.

Left anterior oblique (LAO). The patient is semiprone or standing, with the left side closest to the film.

Left hypochondriac region. One of three upper regions of the abdomen.

Left iliac region. One of three lower regions of the abdomen; called also left inguinal region.

Left inguinal region. One of three lower regions of the abdomen; called also iliac region.

Left lateral region. One of three middle regions of the abdomen; called also left lumbar region.

Left lower quadrant. A division of the abdomen.

Left lumbar region. One of three middle regions of the abdomen; called also left lateral region.

Left posterior oblique (LPO). The patient is semisupine or standing, with the left side closest to the film.

Left upper quadrant. A division of the abdomen.

Linea. A line.

Lithotomy position. The patient in dorsal recumbent position with the hips and knees flexed and the thighs abducted and externally rotated.

Localized. Not general; restricted to a limited region or to one or more spots.

Lordosis. The anterior concavity in the curvature of the lumbar and cervical spine as viewed from the side.

Low (long-scale) contrast. Many shades of gray represented on a radiograph; gives a wide exposure latitude; associated with high kVp.

Lumbar. Pertaining to the loins, the part of the back between the thorax and the pelvis.

Lymphography. Radiography of the lymph vessels.

M

Magenblase. A collection of gas in the upper portion of the stomach showing dark on a stomach radiograph.

Malignant. Tending to become progressively worse and to result in death.

Mammography. Radiography of the mammary gland.

mAs. Milliampere-seconds; the product of amperage and time applied to the x-ray tube; determines the amount of x-ray generated.

Maximum permissible dose (MPD). Occupational limits designed to quantify "safe" exposures. Now dose equivalent limits used.

Mediad. Toward a median line or plane.

Medial. Pertaining to the middle; closer to the median plane or the midline of a body or structure.

Median. Situated in the median plane or in the middle of a body or structure.

Median plane. The imaginary plane passing longitudinally through the middle of the body from front to back and dividing it into right and left halves; called also midsagittal plane.

Meniscus. Used to describe a cartilage in the knee.

Mesion. The plane that divides the body into right and left symmetric halves.

Mesocephalic. Characterized by or pertaining to a skull having an average breadth-length index, with a cephalic index of 75.0 to 79.9.
Mesomorph. A body type in which tissues derived from the mesoderm predominate. This type of person has a relative predominance of muscle, bone, and connective tissue and usually a hard, heavy physique of rectanglar outline.
Metaphysis. The wider part at the extremity of the shaft of a long bone, adjacent to the epiphyseal disk.
Method. Refers to the originator of a position or projection.
Midaxillary plane. The coronal or frontal plane that divides the body into equal front and back halves; called also midcoronal plane.
Midcoronal plane. The coronal or frontal plane that divides the body into equal front and back halves; called also midaxillary plane.
Midsagittal plane. The plane passing longitudinally through the middle of the body from front to back and dividing it into right and left halves; called also median plane.
Milliamperage. The amount of electrons generated at the cathode; with time of exposure, controls the amount of x-rays generated and film density.
Motion unsharpness. Unsharpness (lack of detail or added penumbra) owing to motion (primarily motion of the patient).
Myelography. Radiography of the spinal cord after injection of a contrast medium into the subarachnoid space.

N

Nares. The external orifices of the nose; called also the nostrils.
Nasion. A landmark located at the junction of the intranasal and nasofrontal sutures.

O

Object-to-film distance (OFD). The distance from the part of the film; called also object–image receptor distance (OID).
Object-to-image receptor distance (OID). The distance from the object being imaged to the image receptor or film; called also object–to-film distance (OFD).
Oblique. The patient is rotated between supine and prone.
Occlusal. Pertaining to the occlusion; in radiography, used to refer to the occlusal film, a small film used in dental radiography.
Occlusal line. The alignment of the occluding surfaces of the teeth in a horizontal plane.
OSHA. The Department of Labor's Occupational Safety and Health Administration; responsible for monitoring employee exposure to HIV and HBV as well as establishing and enforcing safety and health guidelines in other occupations.
Opacity. An inability to be penetrated by light.
Orbitomeatal line. The line extending from the outer canthus to the center of the tragus.
Ossicle. A small bone.

P

Palpable. Perceptable to touch.
Parenchyma. The essential elements of an organ; functional elements of an organ as opposed to the framework or stroma.
Parietal. 1. Of or pertaining to the walls of a cavity. 2. Pertaining to or located near the parietal bone.
Parotid. Situated or occurring near the ear, as the parotid gland.
Parturition. The act or process of giving birth to a child.
Pedicle. A footline, stemlike, or narrow basal part or structure.
Pelvimetry. Measurement of the dimensions and capacity of the pelvis.
Penumbra. The area of unsharpness on a radiograph (pen = around; umbra = image or area of sharpness).
Percutaneous. Performed through the skin.
Periosteum. A specialized connective tissue covering all bones of the body and possessing bone-forming potentialities.
Periphery. Outer part or edges.
Peristalsis. The movement by which the alimentary canal propels its contents.
Petrous. Resembling a rock; hard; stony.
Phlebogram. Radiography of a vein filled with contrast medium.
Phosphor-layer thickness. The thickness of crystals in the imaging receptor; affects screen unsharpness and density.
Phrenic. Pertaining to the diaphragm.
Placentography. Radiologic visualization of the placenta after the injection of a contrast medium.
Plane. A surface such that a straight line connecting any two of its points lies wholly in the surface.
Planigraphy. Body section radiography.
Position. The position of the body or part when being radiographed.
Posterior. Situated in back of or in the back part of; affecting the back part of a structure.
Posteroanterior (PA). From back to front.
Projection. Path of the x-ray beam as it passes through the body.
Pronation. The act of assuming the prone position; the state of being prone.
Prone. Lying face downward.
Proximal. Nearest; closer to any part of reference; opposed to distal.
Pubic region. One of three lower regions of the abdomen; called also hypogastric region.
Purgative. Cathartic; causing evacuation of the bowels.
Pyelo-. Combining form denoting relationship to the renal pelvis.
Pyo-, Py-. Combining form denoting relationship to pus.

Q

Quadrant. Any one of four corresponding parts or quarters, as of the abdominal surface or of the eardrum.
Quadrate. Square or squared; four-sided.
Quantum mottle. A form of noise due to the use of screens with insufficient mAs.
Quickening. The first recognizable movements of the fetus, usually appearing between the 16th and the 18th week of pregnancy.

R

Rad. The traditional unit used to measure absorbed dose of radiation.
Radio-. Combining form denoting relationship to the radius or to radiant energy such as ionizing radiation.
Radiograph. An exposed and processed x-ray film.
Radiographer. A professional certified by the American Registry of Radiological Technologists; an individual who performs radiologic procedures.
Radiologist. A physician specializing in radiology.
Radiolucent. Permit passage of rays or other forms of ionizing radiation with little attenuation; radiolucent areas dark on exposed film.
Radiopaque. Not easily penetrated by x-rays or other forms of ionizing radiation; radiopaque areas appear light or white on exposed film.
Radioparent. Radiolucent.
Rarefaction. The condition of being or becoming less dense; diminuation in density and weight, but not in volume.
Reciprocity law failure. Exposures (generally more than 6 seconds or less than 10 msec) in which all combinations of the same mAs will not ensure a similar density.
Recorded detail. Geometric representation of parts on a radiograph.
Recumbent. Lying down.
Regurgitation. To flow back.
Reid's baseline. See Anthropologic baseline.
Rem. Traditional unit for dose equivalence (occupational exposure).
Retrograde. Moving backward or against the usual direction of flow, as in retrograde pyelography.
Right anterior oblique (RAO). The patient is semiprone or standing, with the right side closest to the film.
Right hypochondriac region. One of three upper regions of the abdomen. Located to the right of the epigastrium (epigastric region), which is the middle upper region.
Right iliac region. One of the three lower regions of the abdomen; called also right inguinal region.
Right inguinal region. One of three lower regions of the abdomen; called also right iliac region.

Right lateral region. One of the three middle regions of the abdomen; called also right lumbar region.
Right lower quadrant. A division of the abdomen.
Right lumbar region. One of three middle regions of the abdomen; called also right lateral region.
Right posterior oblique (RPO). The patient is semisupine or standing, with the right side closest to the film.
Right upper quadrant. A division of the abdomen.
Roentgen. Traditional unit used for radiation exposure as measured in air; named for the discoverer of x-ray, Wilhelm Konrad Roentgen (1845–1923).

S

Sacralization. Anomalous fusion of L5 to the first segment of the sacrum, so that the sacrum consists of six segments.
Sagittal. Situated in the plane of the sagittal suture or parallel to it; said of an anteroposterior plane or section parallel to the median plane of the body.
Sagittal plane. Any vertical plane that passes through the body parallel to the median plane or sagittal suture and divides the body into right and left portions.
Salpingography. Radiography of the fallopian tubes.
Scatter. The diffusion or deviation of roentgen rays (x-rays) produced by a medium through which the rays pass; synonymous with scattered radiation.
Screen unsharpness. Unsharpness (lack of detail or added penumbra) owing to screens.
Septum. A dividing wall or partition; a general term for such a structure.
Shape distortion. Elongation and foreshortening; changes in the shape of the object on the image owing to incorrect beam-part-film alignment.
Sialography. A radiographic demonstration of the salivary ducts by means of the injection of substances radiopaque to x-radiation.
Silhouette. An outline shadow; as in cardiac silhouette.
Silicosis. A type of pneumoconiosis.
Sims' position. The patient lies on the left side with the right knee and thigh flexed and the left arm parallel along the back.
Sinistrad. To or toward the left.
Sinstro-, sinistr-. A combining form meaning left or denoting relationship to the left side.
Size distortion. The increase in the size of the object on the image; also called magnification.
Source-to–image receptor distance (SID). The distance from the source or focal spot of the x-ray tube to the film or image receptor; called also focal-film distance (FFD).
Source-to-object distance (SOD). The distance from the source of radiation to the object being radiographed.
Sthenic. Active; strong. In radiography, the term used to denote the body habitus to which 50 percent of all people fall.
Stoma. An opening established in the abdominal wall by colostomy or ileostomy; also, the opening between two portions of the intestine in anastomosis.
Stroma. The supportive framework of an organ.
Subcostal plane. A horizontal plane transecting the trunk at the level of the lower margins of the 10th costal cartilages.
Subcutaneous. Beneath the skin.
Subluxation. Dislocation.
Submentovertex. Directed from below the chin to the vertex.
Subphrenic. Situated under the diaphragm.
Sulcus. A groove, trench, or furrow.
Supination. The act of assuming the supine position; the state of being supine.
Supine. Lying with the face upward.
Syndrome. Grouping of signs or symptoms.
Systole. The contraction or period of contraction of the heart. In blood pressure measurement, the first or top number.

T

Tangent. Touching at a point.
Tangential. Directed along or arranged in a tangent.
Tomography. The recording of internal body images at a predetermined plane.
Topical. Pertaining to a particular surface area.
Tragus. The cartilaginous projection anterior to the external opening of the ear.
Transmitted light. The amount of light that passes through a film on a viewbox; used with incident light in a ratio to determine film density.
Transpyloric plane. A horizontal plane halfway between the superior margins of the manubrium sterni and the symphysis pubis; does not usually correspond to the level of the pylorus.
Transverse. Placed crosswise; situated at a right angle to the long axis of the body or of an organ.
Transverse plane. A horizontal plane of the body dividing the body into upper and lower portions.
Trendelenburg's position. One in which the patient is supine on the table or bed, the head of which is tilted downward 30 to 40 degrees, and the table or bed angulated beneath the knees.
Trimester. A 3-month period, used in reference to pregnancy.
Tubercle. A nodule or small eminence, such as a rough, rounded eminence of bone.
Tuberosity. An elevation or protuberance.
Tumor. New tissue growth; cell multiplication is uncontrolled.

U

Umbilical region. One of three middle regions of the abdomen; located between the right and the left lumbar regions and around the umbilicus.
Umbra. The sharpness of details (umbra = the image).
Unilateral. Affecting but one side.
Ureterography. Radiography of the ureter after injection of a radiopaque medium into the ureter.
Urography. Radiography of a part of the urinary tract that has been rendered opaque by some contrast medium.
Urticaria. Hives.
Uterosalpingography. Hysterosalpingography.

V

Valsalva's maneuver. Forcible exhalation effort against a closed glottis; the resultant increase in intrathoracic pressure interferes with venous return to the heart.
Venography. Radiography of the veins after injection of contrast medium.
Ventral decubitus. The patient is prone; the beam enters on one side of the patient (left or right) and exits on another.
Ventriculography. Roentgenography of a ventricle after the injection of a contrast medium.
Vertex. The top or crown of the head.
Verticomental. Pertaining to the vertex and the chin.
View. How the x-ray film "saw" the body; not usually part of accepted practice because of the miscommunications between physican and radiographer that result from its use.
Virchow's plane. See Infraorbitomeatal line.
Viscosity. A physical property of fluids that determines the internal resistance to shear forces.
Visibility of detail. The amount to which fine structures appear on the radiograph.
Visible image. The image seen on a radiograph after processing.

W

Wedge filter. A type of compensating filter in which the thick part of the filter is placed over the thinnest part of the anatomy.

Z

Zonography. Tomography of a thick region or zone.

Index

Projections and Positions

Note: Page numbers in *italics* refer to illustrations.

M

S

U

Index

Subject

Note: Page numbers in *italics* refer to illustrations; page numbers followed by t refer to tables.

B

D

G

H

I

J

K

N

O

P

Q

R

T

W

X

Z

ISBN 0-7216-5745-1

90071

9 780721 657455